Anesthesia and the Patient with Co-Existing Heart Disease

Anesthesia and the Patient with Co-Existing Heart Disease

Edited by
JOSEPH I. SIMPSON, M.D.
Chief, Division of Cardiothoracic Anesthesiology,
Long Island Jewish Medical Center, New Hyde Park, New York

Little, Brown and Company
Boston/Toronto/London

Copyright © 1993 by Joseph I. Simpson

First Edition

All rights reserved. No part of this book may be reproduced in any form or by any electronic or mechanical means, including information storage and retrieval systems, without permission in writing from the publisher, except by a reviewer who may quote brief passages in a review.

Library of Congress Cataloging-in-Publication Data

Anesthesia and the patient with co-existing heart disease / edited by Joseph I. Simpson.
    p. cm.
  Includes bibliographical references and index.
  ISBN 0-316-79185-7
  1. Heart—Diseases—Complications. 2. Anesthesia—Complications. 3. Heart—Effect of drugs on. I. Simpson, Joseph I.
    [DNLM: 1. Anesthesia. 2. Heart Diseases—complications. WG 460 A5787]
RD87.3.H43A49 1993
617.9'6041—dc20
DNLM/DLC
for Library of Congress   92-48885
                                                                   CIP

Printed in the United States of America
MV-NY

Sponsoring Editor: Laurie Anello
Production Editor: Kellie Cardone
Copyeditor: Libby Dabrowski
Indexer: Betty Hallinger
Production Supervisor/Designer: Michael A. Granger
Cover Designer: Ethan Thomas

TO MY WIFE, JUDY,
FOR HER LOVE, ENCOURAGEMENT, PATIENCE, AND UNDERSTANDING

Contents

Contributing Authors ix
Preface xi

Introduction

1. Cardiac Anatomy 3
   Richard Stein
2. Hemodynamic Effects of the Inhalation Anesthetic Agents 13
   Joseph I. Simpson
3. Hemodynamic Effects of Intravenous Anesthetic Agents 27
   Florence J. Moses and David Amar

The Adult Patient

4. Monitoring Cardiac Patients for Noncardiac Surgery 57
   Ketan Shevde and Piyush M. Gupta
5. Ischemic Heart Disease 81
   Jose A. Melendez and Paola Marino
6. Aortic Valve Disease 109
   Joseph I. Simpson
7. Mitral Valve Disease 129
   Sheldon Goldstein and Michael S. Taragin
8. Pericardial Disease 173
   Kevin M. Glassman
9. Cardiomyopathies 191
   Pierre A. Casthely, Soom Yung Lee, and Claudia A. Komer
10. Arrhythmias and Conduction Abnormalities 215
    Pierre A. Casthely and Mark J. Badach
11. Thoracic Aortic Disease 241
    Gerald A. Schiff
12. Patients with Pacemakers 267
    David Amar and Jay N. Gross
13. Postcardiac Surgical Patients 287
    Joseph I. Simpson and Zvi Zisbrod
14. The Pregnant Patient with Cardiac Disease 299
    David Wlody
15. The Patient with Systemic Disease Affecting the Cardiovascular System 335
    Sheldon Goldstein and Michael S. Taragin

The Pediatric Patient

16. Pediatric Monitoring 387
    Robert H. McDowall, Jr.
17. Noncyanotic Heart Disease 421
    Gerald A. Schiff
18. Cyanotic Congenital Heart Disease 441
    Corey S. Scher

Index 473

Contributing Authors

David Amar, M.D.
Assistant Professor, Department of Anesthesiology, Cornell University Medical College; Attending Physician, Memorial Sloan-Kettering Cancer Center, New York

Mark J. Badach, M.D.
Assistant Professor, Department of Anesthesia, University of Medicine and Dentistry of New Jersey–New Jersey Medical School, Newark; Attending Physician, Department of Anesthesia, St. Joseph's Hospital and Medical Center, Paterson, New Jersey

Pierre A. Casthely, M.D.
Professor, Division of Cardiac Anesthesia, University of Medicine and Dentistry of New Jersey–New Jersey Medical School, Newark; Attending Physician, Department of Cardiac Anesthesia, St. Joseph's Hospital and Medical Center, Paterson, New Jersey

Kevin M. Glassman, M.D.
Attending Anesthesiologist, Long Island Jewish Medical Center, New Hyde Park, New York

Sheldon Goldstein, M.D.
Assistant Professor, Department of Anesthesiology, University of Medicine and Dentistry of New Jersey, Robert Wood Johnson Medical School, Piscataway; Attending Physician, Department of Anesthesiology, Robert Wood Johnson University Hospital, New Brunswick, New Jersey

Jay N. Gross, M.D.
Assistant Professor of Medicine, Albert Einstein College of Medicine of Yeshiva University; Assistant Attending Physician, Montefiore Medical Center, Bronx, New York

Piyush M. Gupta, M.D.
Attending Anesthesiologist, Maimonides Medical Center, Brooklyn, New York

Claudia A. Komer, M.D
Assistant Professor, University of Medicine and Dentistry of New Jersey–New Jersey Medical School, Newark; Attending Physician, Department of Anesthesia, St. Joseph's Hospital and Medical Center, Paterson, New Jersey

Soom Yung Lee, M.D.
Assistant Professor of Anesthesiology, Albert Einstein College of Medicine of Yeshiva University; Director of Cardiothoracic Anesthesia, Jack D. Weiler Hospital of the Albert Einstein College of Medicine, Bronx, New York

Paola Marino, M.D.
Research Fellow, Anesthesiology and Critical Care, Memorial Sloan-Kettering Cancer Center, New York

Robert H. McDowall, Jr., M.D.
Assistant Professor, Department of Anesthesiology, Cornell University Medical College; Attending Physician, Department of Anesthesiology and Critical Care Medicine and Pediatrics, Memorial Sloan-Kettering Cancer Center, New York

Jose A. Melendez, M.D.
Assistant Professor, Department of Anesthesiology, Cornell University Medical College; Attend-

ing Physician, Memorial Sloan-Kettering Cancer Center, New York

Florence J. Moses, M.D.
Instructor, Department of Anesthesiology, Cornell University Medical College; Attending Physician, Memorial Sloan-Kettering Cancer Center, New York

Corey S. Scher, M.D.
Assistant Professor, Department of Anesthesiology, Cornell University Medical College; Attending Physician, Departments of Anesthesiology and Pediatrics, Memorial Sloan-Kettering Cancer Center, New York

Gerald A. Schiff, M.D.
Attending Physician, Department of Anesthesiology, Long Island Jewish Medical Center, New Hyde Park, New York

Ketan Shevde, M.D.
Director, Department of Anesthesia, Maimonides Medical Center, Brooklyn, New York

Joseph I. Simpson, M.D.
Chief, Division of Cardiothoracic Anesthesiology, Long Island Jewish Medical Center, New Hyde Park, New York

Richard Stein, M.D.
Chief of Cardiology and Professor of Medicine, State University of New York Health Science Center at Brooklyn College of Medicine, Brooklyn, New York

Michael S. Taragin, M.D.
Staff Anesthesiologist, Methodist Hospital, Indianapolis

David Wlody, M.D.
Clinical Assistant Professor of Anesthesia and Director, Obstetric Anesthesia, State University of New York Health Science Center at Brooklyn College of Medicine, Brooklyn, New York

Zvi Zisbrod, M.D.
Assistant Professor of Surgery and Director, Cardiothoracic Surgery, State University of New York Health Science Center at Brooklyn College of Medicine, Brooklyn, New York

Preface

Over the past 10 years, the field of anesthesiology has grown and become increasingly subspecialized. There are now recognized subspecialists in cardiac, obstetric, pediatric, ambulatory, and neurosurgical anesthesia, in addition to the subspecialists of pain management and critical care anesthesia, and, of course, the "generalist."

Those of us who are cardiac anesthesiologists deal every day with patients who have significant heart disease and manage anesthetics for cardiac surgery. Those whose area of interest is not cardiac anesthesia, or who practice anesthesia in institutions where cardiac surgery is not performed, may not come in contact with this type of patient as often. It is not uncommon to be presented with a patient for noncardiac surgery who has significant coexisting heart disease. A worse situation yet is when such a patient, whose coexisting heart disease may or may not be hemodynamically stable, presents for emergency noncardiac surgery in the middle of the night.

Many textbooks deal with anesthesia for cardiac surgery. In contrast, this book was written for the noncardiac anesthesiologist, dealing with the anesthetic management of the patient with heart disease who presents for elective and emergent noncardiac surgery.

Conceptually, this book is divided into three parts. The first is introductory and deals with relevant cardiac anatomy and the cardiovascular effects of the various anesthetic agents, both inhalational and intravenous. The second part deals with the anesthetic management of the adult patient with heart disease who presents for noncardiac surgery. The first chapter in this section discusses adult monitoring for noncardiac surgery. The succeeding chapters deal with the specific cardiac disease states that frequently coexist in these patients, including ischemic heart disease, aortic valve disease, mitral valve disease, pericardial disease, cardiomyopathies, arrhythmias and conduction abnormalities, thoracic aortic disease, and patients with pacemakers. Another chapter deals with the patient who has recently undergone cardiac surgery and is now presenting for emergent noncardiac surgery. The last two chapters in the second part discuss patients who have cardiac disease in association with pregnancy or multiorgan disease states, such as diabetes, renal failure, lupus, and thyroid disease, among others. The third part deals with the anesthetic management of the pediatric patient with congenital heart disease who presents for noncardiac surgery, and includes discussions on pediatric monitoring and noncyanotic and cyanotic congenital heart disease.

Since this is not a manual, I have tried to avoid a "cookbook" approach and rather concentrate on applied pathophysiology of the specific disease process and its interaction with anesthetic agents, techniques, and surgery. Nevertheless, where appropriate, specific "do's and don'ts" are discussed. While this book is multiauthored, I have tried to maintain some consistency in style and to eliminate overlap wherever possible.

I would like to take this opportunity to thank the many contributing authors who have participated in this book. I would also like to thank Susan Pioli, Executive Editor at Little, Brown, for her advice and patience. I thank my sister-in-law, Sheri Hagler, and the many secretaries in the anesthesia departments of both the State University of New York Health Science Center at Brooklyn and the Long Island Jewish Medical Center for their help in manuscript preparation.

Finally, I would like to thank my wife, Judy, for her constant support and encouragement, as well as her tireless efforts in manuscript preparation and editing of the entire book, and my children, Shoshana, Tova, Tzvi, and Ariella, for their patience, understanding, and encouragement.

J.I.S.

Introduction

NOTICE

The indications and dosages of all drugs in this book have been recommended in the medical literature and conform to the practices of the general medical community. The medications described do not necessarily have specific approval by the Food and Drug Administration for use in the diseases and dosages for which they are recommended. The package insert for each drug should be consulted for use and dosage as approved by the FDA. Because standards for usage change, it is advisable to keep abreast of revised recommendations, particularly those concerning new drugs.

1
Cardiac Anatomy

Richard Stein

As an introduction to the understanding of the effect of coexisting heart disease in the surgical patient, this chapter reviews briefly some basic cardiac anatomy. The reader is referred to anatomy and physiology textbooks for more complete information.

EXTERNAL ANATOMY

The heart is situated near the midpoint of the mediastinum. When viewed anteriorly it is overlapped by the right and left lungs at its lateral borders, and is covered anteriorly by the sternum, costal cartilages, and third, fourth, and fifth ribs. The heart rests on the diaphragm, and is angled and rotated so that the bottom (apex of the left ventricle) is anterior to the base. Most of the heart is to the left of midline, and the right atria and ventricle lie anterior to the left atria and ventricle.

When seen externally (as they are after a midline sternotomy), the atria lie superiorly and are separated from the ventricles by a linear indentation—the *coronary sulcus* (also termed the *atrioventricular sulcus*). This circles the heart between atria and ventricles. A second groove, the interventricular sulcus, runs from the anterior coronary sulcus around the apex of the heart back up to the posterior coronary sulcus. This marks the interventricular septum. These sulci contain coronary arteries. The right coronary artery leaves the aorta and travels posteriorly in the right coronary sulcus. At the junction of the coronary and interventricular sulci on the posterior surface of the heart (termed the *crux* of the heart, and marking the external landmark of the posterior junction of the interatrial and interventricular septum and the location of the atrioventricular node), the artery turns downward toward the apex of the heart. The left circumflex coronary artery travels in the left coronary sulcus after its origin at the left main coronary artery, and also turns posteriorly to supply the posterior aspect of the heart at the posterior junction of the coronary and interventricular sulci. The artery traveling in the posterior interventricular sulcus is termed the *posterior descending coronary artery* and is most commonly a continuation of the right coronary artery, or less often of the circumflex coronary artery. At the crux where the posterior descending coronary artery originates, a small branch vessel takes off to supply the atrioventricular (AV) node. The left anterior descending artery leaves the left main coronary artery and travels toward the apex of the heart in the anterior interventricular sulcus [1] (Fig. 1-1).

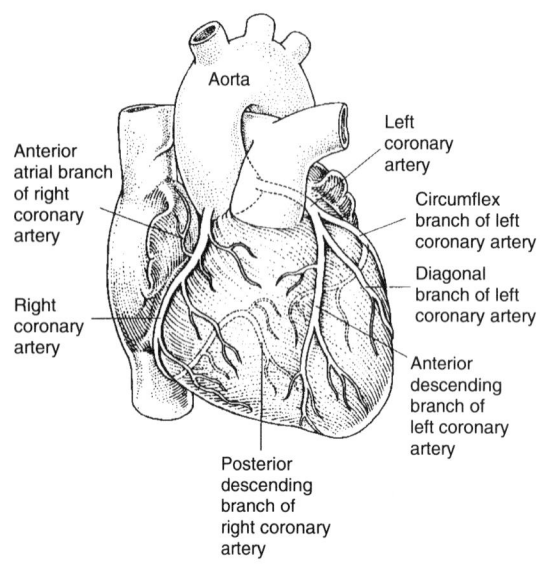

Fig. 1-1. The normal coronary circulation.

SKELETON OF THE HEART

The chambers and septa, and the valves that separate them, are anchored to a fibrous skeletal framework at the center of the heart. The major component of the framework, the *central fibrous body* (also termed the *right fibrous trigone*) is formed by the medial aspects of the mitral and tricuspid valves and the aortic root. From this central body, fibrous tissue courses to the left, anteriorly and posteriorly (this structure is called the *left fibrous trigone*) to form the annuli of the mitral and tricuspid valves. These annuli (rings) form the attachments for their respective valves as well as the atrial and ventricular muscles. Fibrous tissue extends anteriorly from the central fibrous body to form the skeletal support for the aortic root. The ligamentous extension of the aortic root skeletal support, termed the *conus ligament*, originates from the right to form the support structure of the pulmonic root. An extension of the fibrous skeletal system is the membranous interventricular septum, which extends anteriorly from the central fibrous body to the crest of the muscular interventricular septum [2]. It provides skeletal support for the right and posterior cusps of the aortic valve and is the location of major components of the conduction system of the heart, including the bundle of His and its bifurcation into left and right bundle branches.

HEART CHAMBERS

The right atrium collects the blood returning to the heart via the superior and inferior vena cava. The medial and posterior surfaces of the right atrium are smooth whereas the walls of the lateral atrium and of the atrial appendage are made up of muscle bundles, termed *pectinate muscles*. On the posterior surface is a ridge, the sulcus terminalis, which is the external representation of an internal muscle bundle, the crista terminalis, which runs from the entrance of the superior vena cava to the inferior vena cava. The sinus node usually lies near the lateral aspect of the orifice of the superior vena cava near the sulcus terminalis. The superior vena cava orifice has no valve, whereas the inferior vena cava orifice often has a rudimentary valve, the eustachian valve. The intraatrial septum is seen from the right atrium and there is a bulge, called the *torus aorticus*, caused by the right and noncoronary aortic semilunar valves. It is of note that the origin and proximal right coronary artery are near this structure. Also seen on the septum is the shallow crater of the fossa ovalis. The origin of the coronary sinus is located near the opening of the inferior vena cava and the tricuspid valve. The AV node of the conduction system is in the interatrial septum, just above the septal leaflet of the tricuspid valve (Fig. 1-2).

The right ventricle receives blood during diastole from the right atrium through the tricuspid valve. During systole right ventricular blood is ejected into the pulmonary artery. The chamber is crescent shaped with a relatively (to the left ventricle) thin wall (4–5 mm), which, on its anterior and inferior internal aspects, is lined by muscle bundles, the trabeculae carneae. These give this area of the inside of the chamber a rough surface made of crisscrossing ridges. In addition there is a muscle band, termed the *moderator band* (containing the right bundle branch of the conduction system, which travels across the right ventricular

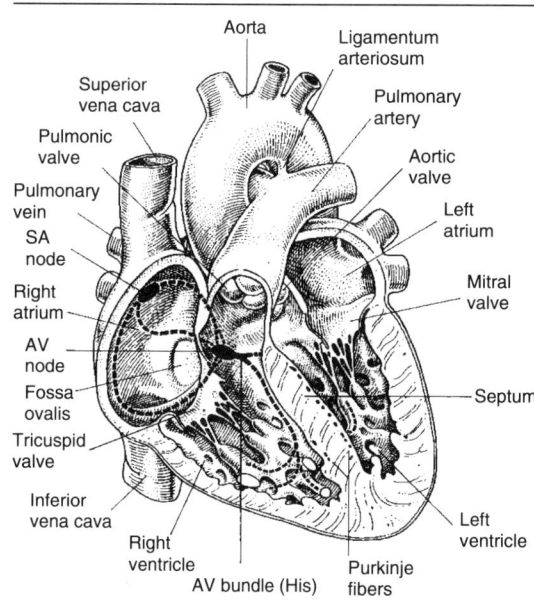

Fig. 1-2. Normal anatomy of the heart. AV = atrioventricular; SA = sinoatrial.

cavity). The right ventricle can be divided into two functional components: the inflow tract, which receives the blood from the right atrium during diastole (and consists of the tricuspid valve and the trabecular muscles of the anterior and inferior walls), and the outflow tract, which directs the blood out the pulmonary artery during systole. This latter area is also called the *infundibulum;* it is smooth walled and consists of the superior part of the right ventricle, separated from the inflow tract by a thick muscular endocardial ridge, the crista supraventricularis.

The left atrium receives blood from the pulmonary veins, collects blood during ventricular systole, and empties blood into the left ventricle during diastole. In addition, by virtue of atrial contraction at the end of diastolic filling, the ventricular volume is augmented; this is termed the *atrial kick,* as it stretches the ventricle and primes it for systole. The left atrium is a posteriorly located structure with its posterior aspect abutting the esophagus. Its wall is 3 mm thick, and receives blood from the pulmonary circulation via four pulmonary veins, which enter on the posterior atrial wall. The left atrium is smooth walled except for pectinate muscles in the appendage, and its septum has a slight indentation at the fossa ovalis [3].

The left ventricle receives blood during diastole from the left atrium via the mitral valve, and during systole ejects blood out the aorta. The left ventricle is a thick-walled (8–13 mm) ellipsoid-shaped chamber, with a septal wall (shared with the right ventricle), consisting of muscular septum and a small portion of membranous septum as its most superior aspect. The upper third of the septum is smooth, whereas the remaining interior surfaces of the ventricle are ridged by the muscle ridges, the trabeculae carneae. As is the case with the right ventricle, the left ventricle can be functionally divided into an inflow tract and an outflow tract, with the dividing structure being the anteromedial leaflet of the mitral valve. Blood entering the left ventricle is directed anteriorly and to the left by the tilt of mitral annulus and the superior aspects of the mitral leaflets and the chordae. During systole the mitral valve is closed as the intracavity pressure in the ventricle exceeds that of the atrium, and blood is expelled into the aorta.

HEART VALVES

The chambers are separated by valves that permit blood flow in only one direction. The valves that separate the ventricles from the great vessels are semilunar valves, and those that separate the atria and ventricles are two or three leaflet valves with their chordae tendineae attached to ventricular papillary muscles.

The semilunar valves are made up of three fibrous cusps, suspended from the root of the pulmonary artery (pulmonic valve) and aorta (aortic valve). Behind each cusp the root of the vessels bulges out to form the sinus Valsalva. At the center of the free edge of each cusp is a fibrous nodule called the *nodulus Arantii*. In the aortic valve apparatus, the sinus of Valsalva of the two anterior leaflets contains the ostia of the coronary arteries (right and left), and the posterior leaflet and sinus are referred to as "noncoronary." The mitral valve directs left atrial blood into the left ventricle during diastole. The fibroelastic tissue of its two leaflets (anteromedial and posterolateral) attach to the annulus fibrosus, providing a cone-shaped passage extending into the left ventricular cavity. The tricuspid orifice is larger and more superficial than the mitral orifice, and is surrounded by three leaflets. The valve leaflets of both the mitral and tricuspid valves are attached by parachute-like cords that extend from the valve leaflets (free edge of the ventricular surface) to finger-like projections of ventricular muscle, termed *papillary muscles*. The chordae allow for the even distribution of forces during systole, by permitting the valves to slightly balloon up from evenly opposed edges. Disruption of the chordae will result in failure of sustained apposition and regurgitant flow [1].

The heart is covered by two layers of thin serous tissue, termed the *pericardium*. The visceral layer surrounds the exterior surface of the heart and the parietal pericardium is a functional sac that surrounds the visceral pericardium. There is normally a small amount (10–20 ml) of clear serous fluid between the two layers. The pericardium is also innervated by cardiac vagal nerve branches, stimulation of which will decrease heart rate.

CORONARY CIRCULATION

The Coronary Arteries

The ostia of the coronary arteries are located in the upper third of their respective sinus of Valsalva of the aortic valve. The left main coronary artery is a short vessel that travels anteriorly and inferiorly to the left to emerge behind the pulmonary artery, where it bifurcates into the left anterior descending and circumflex arteries. In some instances a third vessel is generated from a trifurcation of the left main. When this occurs the middle vessel is termed an *intermediate vessel*. The left anterior descending coronary artery (LAD) is a continuation of the left main, and travels anteriorly and inferiorly in the anterior interventricular sulcus, to the inferior aspect of the apex (see Fig. 1-1). It gives off branches to the septum (septal perforators), the anterior wall of the left ventricle (diagonals), and the right ventricle (right ventricular branches). The LAD thus supplies most of the septum, and the anterior, lateral, and apical walls of the left ventricle (Fig. 1-3).

The left circumflex artery arises from the left main at an obtuse angle and turns posteriorly to travel in the left atrioventricular sulcus. About 15 percent of the time, it continues down the posterior interventricular sulcus as the posterior descending artery. In the majority of cases (85%), it terminates at the crux (junction of atrioventricular sulcus and posterior interventricular sulcus). In just less than 50 percent of cases, the sinus node artery arises from the circumflex.

The right coronary artery originates at the right sinus Valsalva and descends in the right atrioventricular groove. At the crux of the heart, it descends (in 85% of hearts) to form the posterior descending artery. In just over 50 percent of hearts, it gives origin to the sinus node artery, which travels over the anterior right atrium to encircle the superior vena cava and penetrate the sinus node. The right coronary artery supplies the sinus node (50%), the right ventricular wall, the crista superventricularis, and the right atrium. When it gives origin to the posterior descending artery, it supplies the AV node and the posterior one half of the interventricular septum [3].

Venous System

The venous system of the heart is comprised of the anterior interventricular vein, which travels in the anterior interventricular sulcus and turns behind the left atrium to become the great cardiac vein. This then becomes the coronary sinus near the crux. The posterior intraventricular vein travels with the posterior descending artery and joins the coronary sinus at its orifice or empties directly in at the right atrium. The oblique vein of Marshall travels behind the left atrium and joins the great cardiac vein as it becomes the coronary sinus. Most of the cardiac venous blood is handled by this system. A small amount of venous blood from the anterior right ventricle is handled by several small anterior cardiac veins, which receive blood from the right ventricle and right atrium, and joins the coronary sinus or drains directly into the right atrium. The thebesian veins are tiny venous tracts that drain directly into the atria and ventricle, primarily on the right side.

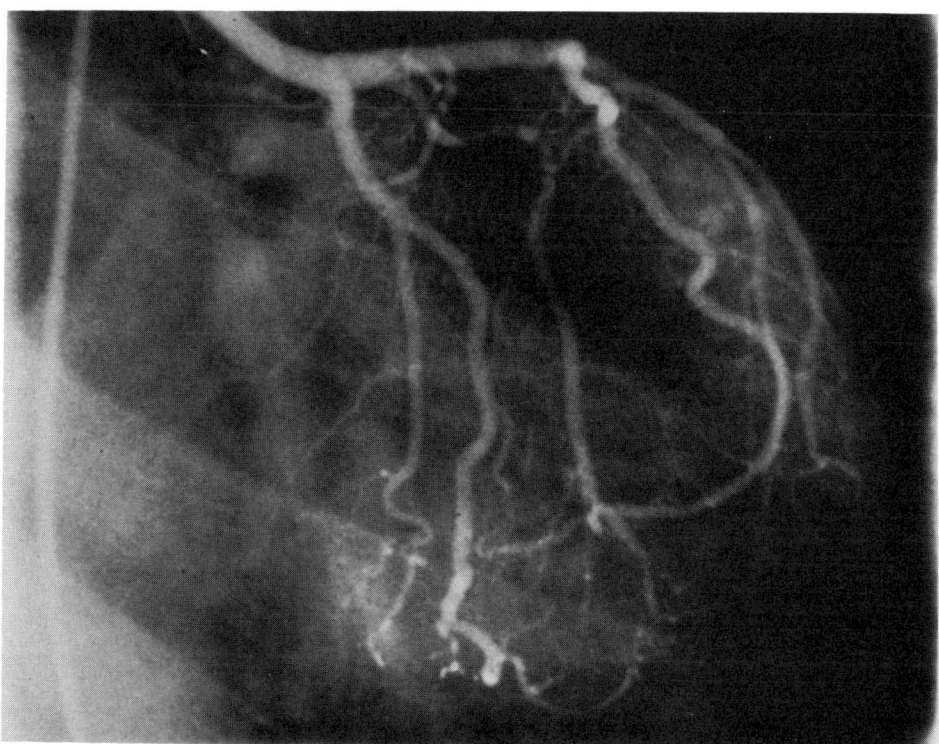

Fig. 1-3. A normal coronary angiogram of the left main, the left anterior descending, and the circumflex coronary arteries.

MYOCARDIAL BLOOD FLOW AND REGULATION

The increase in cardiac output required during exercise and other stress is, as noted previously, the result of the integration of heart rate (HR) and factors affecting left ventricular function. This increase in cardiac output is also associated with an increase in the heart oxygen requirement, the $M\dot{V}O_2$ (myocardial minute oxygen consumption). $M\dot{V}O_2$ relates to heart rate, work of contraction, and the contractile state. In clinical situations the change in the product of heart rate and systolic blood pressure (termed the *double product*) will reflect changes in $M\dot{V}O_2$. Thus, if a patient who has not had the contractile state altered by inotropic drugs, adrenergic stimulation, or other factors, has his or her double product increased by a factor of two (e.g., HR increases from 70 to 100 and systolic blood pressure increases from 100 to 140 mm Hg), then the myocardial oxygen requirement will be approximately doubled as well.

The heart is always extracting oxygen from its blood supply at a near maximal level and thus the only way it can get more oxygen to meet an increased oxygen demand is to increase coronary blood flow. Since most coronary blood flow occurs in diastole, the major mechanisms for increasing coronary blood flow are an increase in diastolic pressure and a reduction in coronary resistance effected by dilation of the coronary arteries (Fig. 1-4). Diastolic blood pressure remains unchanged or falls slightly with exercise. Thus, if the arteries are narrowed or unable to dilate, the increased oxygen demand of the heart associated with exercise or other (e.g., operative) stress will not be able to be met. The resulting imbalance between oxygen demand and supply is termed *myocardial ischemia,* and is responsible for the pathophysiology of much coronary heart disease [4].

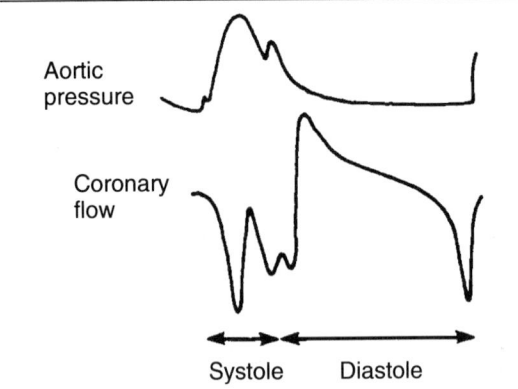

Fig. 1-4. Coronary and aortic blood flow. Note that the majority of coronary flow occurs during diastole after aortic valve closure. (Reprinted with permission from PG Barash et al. (eds), *Clinical Anesthesia*. Philadelphia: Lippincott, 1989.)

In the heart with normal coronary arteries, changing myocardial oxygen and blood flow demands are met by changes in supply through a system of regulatory actions. Coronary disease will, however, often prevent supply from meeting the increased demand associated with certain states, producing ischemia. In the normal heart, supply to heart muscle is adjusted to meet demand by autoregulation of the resistance of the coronary arteriolar beds (in distinction to the large epicardial coronary arteries). A local vasodilatory metabolite, adenosine, is postulated as the mediator of this autoregulation. Adenosine is produced by heart cell metabolism, removed by washout (blood flow), and deactivated by red blood cell enzymes. An increase in metabolism or a relative decrease in blood flow would increase interstitial adenosine and dilate arteriolar vessels to meet heart muscle demands, which would wash out or deactivate the excess adenosine, allowing a return to steady state (a classic negative-feedback loop). Other factors controlling coronary vasodilatation include arterial carbon dioxide tension ($PaCO_2$) and pH.

Coronary arterial flow is also controlled by the sympathetic and parasympathetic nervous systems. Sympathetic stimulation causes coronary vasodilatation by metabolic mechanisms while parasympathetic stimulation produces direct coronary vasodilatation by coronary artery muscarinic receptors.

The actual beating of the heart limits coronary blood flow, with a greater reduction effected in the subendocardial areas of heart muscle than in the epicardial areas. There is, thus, a blood flow gradient across the heart wall during systole that favors the epicardial area. This is due in part to greater extravascular compression caused by increased wall tension in the subendocardium. In the normal heart under normal resting conditions, distribution of blood across the heart wall is uniform during one entire cycle, indicating that the gradient in systole is matched by a reserve gradient in diastole [5].

When coronary flow is limited by coronary artery disease and muscle demand outsteps supply (Fig. 1-5), blood flow first becomes insufficient in the inner layers (subendocardial layers) of the heart. At the threshold of ischemia, autoregulation has maximally dilated arteriolar vessels and capillary beds, and thus changes in flow are determined by perfusion pressure across the coronary vascular system. This gradient can be approximated in the normal circulation by the difference in the areas under the left ventricular pressure curves and the aortic pressure curves in diastole, termed the *diastolic pressure time index*. Factors that favor a reduced value (shortening of diastole due to tachycardia, increased ventricular diastolic pressure, or a reduced perfusion pressure such as is seen in coronary occlusions) will provoke ischemia. Two additional mechanisms, coronary vasospasm and collateral blood flow, alter coronary blood flow to specific muscle fibers. In the normal heart the vasodilating effects of autoregulatory mechanisms override α-adrenergic vasoconstriction. However, autoregulation does not affect large epicardial vessels, and they can, in normal states (such as around an atherosclerotic plaque), vasoconstrict to reduce flow and cause ischemia. Coronary collateral vessels (distal connecting branches between coronary arteries) are present in variable degrees in all hearts. They are not usually of sufficient magnitude to prevent infarction following the abrupt occlusion of a coronary artery, but gradual obstruction of a coronary artery will often effect an enlargement of the collateral system that is able to supply sufficient blood to endangered myocardium [6, 7].

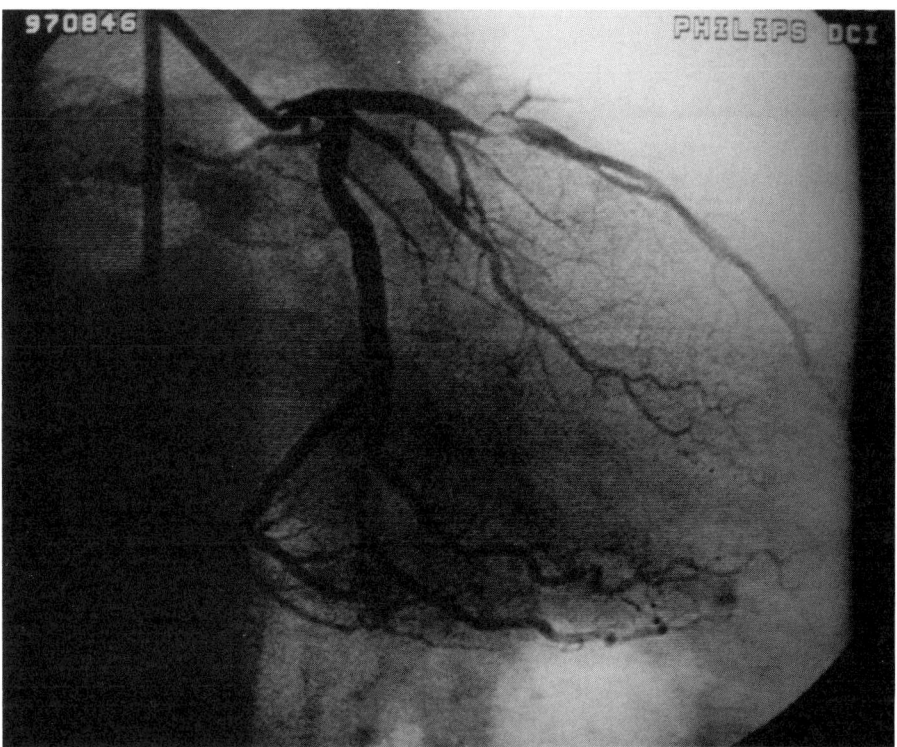

Fig. 1-5. Abnormal coronary angiogram showing proximal occlusion of the left anterior descending coronary artery.

CARDIAC CONDUCTION SYSTEM

The anatomy of the conduction system of the heart begins with the origin of the impulse, the sinoatrial node. This structure is located on the lateral aspect of the right atrium at the junction of the superior vena cava and the right atrial appendage. It is approximately 20 by 3 mm and shaped like an ellipsoid. It is perforated at its middle by the sinus node artery. Three tracts carry impulses from the sinoatrial (SA) node to the AV node. These are the anterior (termed *Bachmann's bundle*), middle, and posterior internodal tracts. The AV node is located at the base of the atrial septum. It extends anteriorly to become the bundle of His, which enters the central fibrous body at the top of the muscular septum. This structure splits into a left and right bundle. The left bundle becomes a broad band of fibers that bifurcates into anterior and posterior fascicles. The right bundle extends from the common bundle to travel to the right ventricular apex via the moderator band [8, 9]. As stated earlier, in 85 percent of people the right coronary artery supplies the AV node (AV nodal artery), bundle of His, and posterior fascicle of the left bundle. The left anterior descending coronary artery supplies the bundle of His and the anterior fascicle of the left bundle. It is easy to understand how stenosis of the right coronary artery can cause inferior wall myocardial infarction and heart block (AV nodal block and left posterior hemiblock), while stenosis of the left anterior coronary artery can cause anterior infarction with left bundle branch block or left anterior hemiblock and right bundle branch block (Fig. 1-6).

Ventricular systole begins with contraction of the chamber and rapid rise in intraventricular pressure. The mitral valve is closed almost immediately as ventricular pressure exceeds the much lower

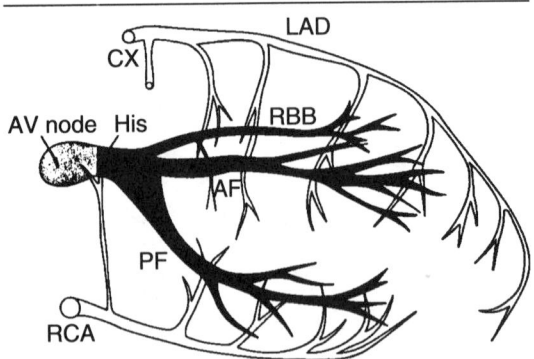

Fig. 1-6. The interventricular conduction system. Note that the right bundle branch (RBB) and the anterior fascicle (AF) of the left bundle are supplied by the left anterior descending coronary artery (LAD), while the posterior fascicle (PF) of the left bundle and the AV node are supplied primarily by the right coronary artery (RCA). (Reprinted with permission from HJJ Wellins and MB Conover (eds), *ECG in Emergency Decision-Making*. Philadelphia: Saunders, 1992.)

atrial pressure, and for a brief period as the pressure rises the ventricular volume remains constant; this is termed the *isovolumic phase* of systole. When the ventricular pressure exceeds that of the aortic root, the aortic valve is opened and blood is ejected rapidly into the aorta, the *rapid ejection phase* of systole. The rate of ejection slows (this is termed the *reduced ejection phase* of systole) and is terminated as the ejection of blood comes to an end and the aortic valve closes.

With the closure of the aortic valve, diastole begins, the ventricle starts to expand, and pressure falls (isovolumic relaxation). When the ventricular pressure falls below that of the atrium, the mitral valve opens and blood rapidly fills the ventricle from the atrium (the *rapid filling phase* of diastole). This filling slows (the *slow ventricular filling phase* of diastole) until atrial contraction and the consequent end diastolic increase in ventricular filling, which may account for 10 percent of the diastolic filling in the normal heart [10]. This sequence of ventricular contraction, relaxation and atrial contraction, and relaxation is associated with the heart sounds and the production of the arterial pulse (Fig. 1-7). The first sound (S1) is comprised of two components (MT) that occur coincident with closure of the mitral and the tricuspid valves at the onset of isovolumic contraction (the right ventricle is activated and contracts slightly later than the left). The second sound (S2), which also has two components (A_2, P_2), occurs at the onset of isovolumic relaxation and the consequent closure of the aortic and then the pulmonic valves. At times the end of rapid diastolic filling may be associated with a third heart sound (S3) and atrial contraction near the end of diastole with a fourth (S4). These sounds are considered to be generated by the acceleration and deceleration of blood and the tensing of the cardiac structures.

At the end of diastole, the left ventricle is at its greatest volume (*end diastolic volume*). With systole, a quantity of this blood is ejected into the aorta (the stroke volume), with the remaining blood in the ventricle (*end systolic volume*). This relationship can be expressed as: stroke volume = end diastolic volume − end systolic volume. The percentage of end diastolic volume ejected with systole is termed the *ejection fraction* [ejection fraction (%) = stroke volume/end diastolic volume × 100]. The ejection of the stroke volume into the aorta produces the arterial pressure pulse. The pulse rises with rapid ejection, peaking slightly after the point of maximum ventricular ejection. In the central aorta the pulse curve has a notch or shoulder that is accentuated in aortic stenosis. The end of ejection is marked by a falling of the pulse pressure wave. The closure of the aortic valve is marked by a sharp downward movement of the pressure, the incisura. As the pulse pressure is measured at distances from the aortic root in the arterial tree (e.g., brachial or femoral artery pulse waves), the rate of rise and peak systolic pressure is increased, whereas mean and diastolic pressures remain the same or fall slightly. The volume of blood that the heart pumps into the aorta each minute is termed the *cardiac output* (CO) and is the product of the heart rate and the stroke volume (CO = HR × SV). This value is measured in cardiac catheterization laboratories by utilization of the Fick equation (CO = minute oxygen consumption/arteriovenous O_2 difference) or by a thermodilution technique utilizing a thermistor catheter and injection of saline of a known temperature into the pulmonary artery [11].

The ability of the heart to supply the body's need at rest and the increased cardiac output demand

1. Cardiac Anatomy 11

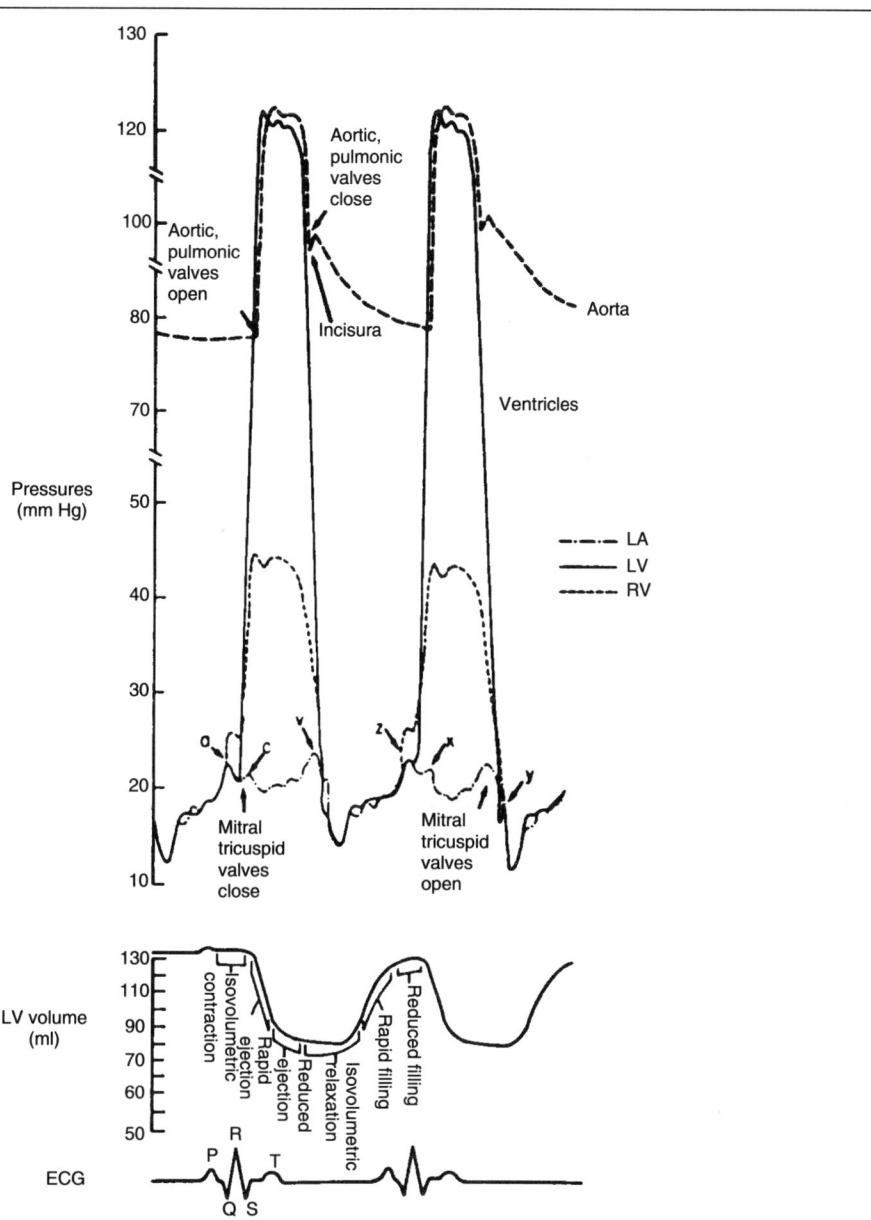

Fig. 1-7. The events of the cardiac cycle from atrial filling through ventricular emptying. (Reprinted with permission from PG Barash et al. (eds), *Clinical Anesthesia*. Philadelphia: Lippincott, 1989.)

associated with exercise or other stress are determined by the ability to increase heart rate (chronotropic reserve) and to increase stroke volume (inotropic reserve). Increasing heart rate will increase cardiac output up to a point. When the heart rate goes over 150 beats per minute, cardiac output will actually decrease, because of inadequate ventricular filling. The inotropic reserve is affected by filling volume, afterload and presystolic pressure of the left ventricle (preload). Afterload relates to peripheral vascular resistance, arterial wall stiffness, impedance to blood flow, viscosity, and the contractile state of the left ventricle.

It is common, although overly simplified, to define the health of the heart in terms of the relative contractile state of the left ventricle. In clinical situations the ejection fraction (stroke volume/end diastolic volume × 100) is often used to assess contractile state, with a normal value exceeding 45 percent. However, in addition to the contractile state, this value is dependent on the afterload (which, when elevated, will decrease ejection fraction and, when reduced, will increase ejection fraction) and on preload (which will increase ejection fraction when elevated via Starling's effect; stated simply, this describes the heart muscles' increased contractile response to enhance precontraction stretch or, in the case of the intact left ventricle, volume).

As preload increases, left ventricular contraction increases, but it is associated with an increase in end diastolic pressure. The consequence of this can be appreciated when we note that at end diastole the mitral valve is open and pressure in the left ventricle is equalized to that in the atrium and the pulmonary veins and pulmonary capillary tree. In left heart failure the increased end diastolic pressure increases the capillary pressure and when this exceeds the oncotic pressure of the blood plasma, fluid is extravasated across the capillary walls into the alveoli, resulting in pulmonary edema [4].

REFERENCES

1. Anderson, R, Becker, A. *Cardiac Anatomy*. London: Churchill Livingstone, 1980.
2. Lev, M, Bharati, S. The Fibrous Skeleton of the Heart. In JW Hurst (ed), *Update IV: The Heart*. New York: McGraw-Hill, 1982.
3. McAlpine, W. *Heart and Coronary Arteries*. New York: Springer-Verlag, 1975.
4. Cohn, P, Brown, E, Vlay, S. *Clinical Cardiovascular Physiology*. Philadelphia: Saunders, 1985.
5. Katz, A. *Physiology of the Heart*. New York: Raven Press, 1992.
6. Hurst, J. *The Heart* (6th ed). New York: McGraw-Hill, 1986.
7. Braunwald, E. *Heart Disease*. Philadelphia: Saunders, 1988.
8. Mitchell, G. *Cardiovascular Intervention*. Baltimore: Williams & Wilkens, 1956.
9. Randall, W. (ed). *Nervous Control of Cardiovascular Function*. New York: Oxford University Press, 1984.
10. Berne, R, Levy, M. *Cardiovascular Physiology*. St. Louis: Mosby Year Book, 1992.
11. Sparks, H, Rooke, T. *Essentials of Cardiovascular Physiology*. Minneapolis: University of Minnesota Press, 1987.

2
Hemodynamic Effects of the Inhalation Anesthetic Agents

Joseph I. Simpson

The modern practice of anesthesiology has advanced to the point where specific anesthetic regimens can be safely administered to patients with severe cardiovascular pathology. Advancement in the understanding of the pharmacodynamics of the various anesthetic agents and their effects on the cardiovascular system has greatly enhanced our ability to manage these patients during their perioperative period. Anesthetic agents can be divided into two broad categories: those administered intravenously and those administered by inhalation. In this chapter we discuss the cardiovascular effects of the inhalational anesthetic agents. The intravenous agents are discussed in Chapter 3.

The inhalational anesthetic agents can have varying effects on the cardiovascular system. These include effects on myocardial contractility, coronary circulation, preload, afterload, heart rate, arrhythmogenicity, antiarrhythmogenic effects, and myocardial oxygen supply and demand.

The currently available inhalational anesthetic agents include halothane, enflurane, isoflurane, and nitrous oxide. Additionally, two new inhalational agents, desflurane and sevoflurane, are in the final stages of clinical trials and may soon be introduced into clinical practice (Fig. 2-1).

NITROUS OXIDE
Myocardial Contractility

Nitrous oxide (N_2O) causes a dose-related depression of myocardial contractility. Eisele and Smith [1] found a 10 percent reduction in ballistocardiographic measurements in humans breathing 40 percent N_2O in oxygen (O_2), a dose less than that commonly used in clinical practice. Thornburn and associates [2] found that 65 percent N_2O in O_2 caused a significant reduction in cardiac output along with an increase in left ventricular end diastolic pressure (LVEDP) in dogs anesthetized with pentobarbitone. Combining nitrous oxide with any of the volatile inhalational anesthetics will worsen the myocardial depression that is normally seen with the inhalational agents alone [3–5].

When N_2O is added to an isolated heart Langendorf model, significant though mild myocardial depression ensues [6]. When N_2O is added to halothane in the presence of a critical coronary artery stenosis in a dog model, myocardial performance is worsened in both the ischemic and the nonischemic normal myocardium [7].

Nitrous oxide is a sympathomimetic and causes increased circulating levels of both epinephrine

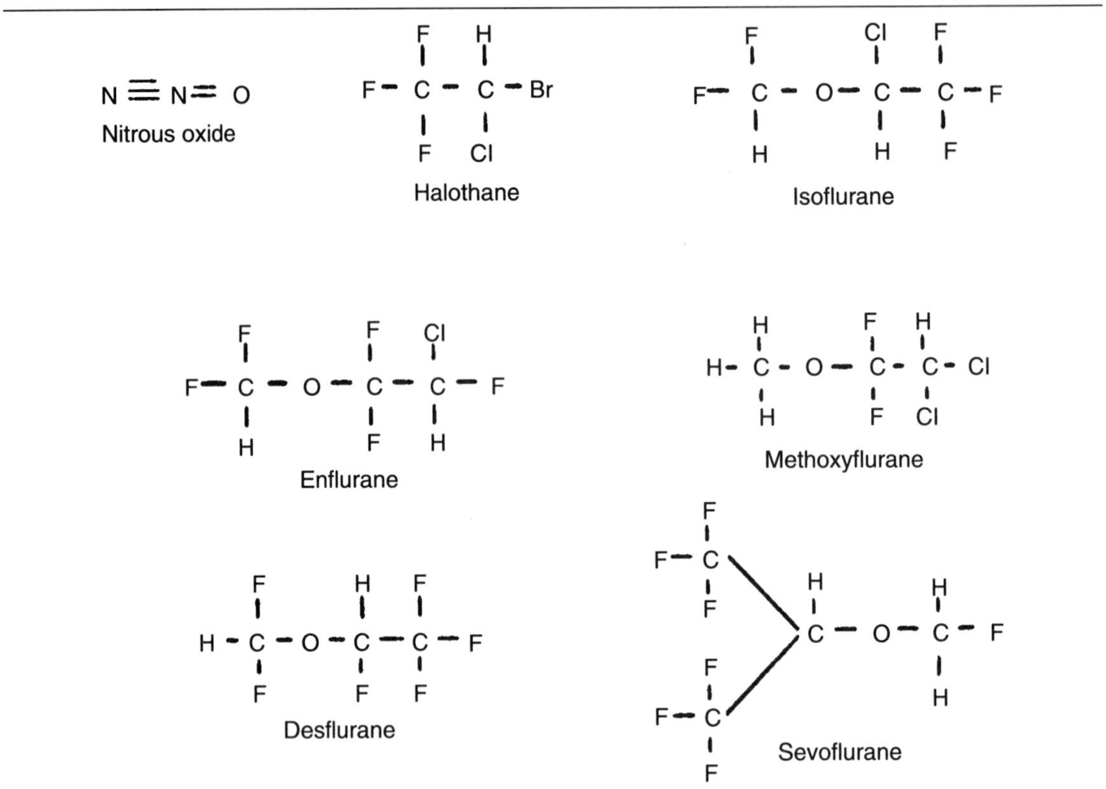

Fig. 2-1. Molecular structures of the inhalational anesthetics. (Reprinted with permission from WC Stevens and HGG Kingston, Inhalation Anesthesia. In PG Barash, BF Cullen, and RK Stoelting (eds), *Clinical Anesthesia* (2nd ed). Philadelphia: Lippincott, 1992.)

and norepinephrine [8]. This produces an increase in heart rate, blood pressure, and systemic vascular resistance (SVR). In vivo, this sympathomimetic stimulation may compensate for the myocardial depression normally caused by N_2O. The sympathetic effect of N_2O is more pronounced in the presence of the other inhalational agents than in the presence of a primarily narcotic anesthetic [8, 9]. The sympathomimetic effects of N_2O may also be blunted in states of catecholamine depletion, such as sepsis, shock, and so forth, and may not be able to adequately compensate in states of preexisting myocardial depression or β-blockade [10] (Table 2-1).

Effects on Myocardial Ischemia

The effects of N_2O on the coronary circulation and myocardial ischemia are controversial. Several studies in animals have demonstrated that N_2O may have deleterious effects on myocardial oxygen supply [11–14]. Wilkowski and associates [11] demonstrated N_2O-induced constriction of epicardial coronary arteries without effect on intramyocardial arterioles. Nathan [12] showed that when N_2O was added to isoflurane-anesthetized dogs with coronary artery stenosis, the N_2O caused a maldistribution of blood flow away from the ischemic areas and a worsening of the myocardial ischemia. In another study on dogs, N_2O worsened regional myocardial ischemia [4].

Other human studies, however, have shown minimal or no effect of N_2O on myocardial ischemia. Slavik and associates [15] demonstrated no

Table 2-1. Cardiovascular effects of 0 to 50% nitrous oxide during morphine anesthesia (means ± SD)

Cardiovascular parameter	Nitrous oxide (%)					
	0	10	20	30	40	50
Cardiac output (liters/min)[a]	5.15 ± 0.62	4.64 ± 0.38	4.29 ± 0.82	4.01 ± 0.52	3.65 ± 0.11	2.88 ± 0.80
Stroke volume (ml)[a]	57 ± 5	51 ± 6	50 ± 6	46 ± 3	42 ± 6	36 ± 4
Peripheral resistance (PRU)[b]	159 ± 24	176 ± 20	183 ± 23	204 ± 28	259 ± 11	312 ± 16
Blood pressure (mm Hg)						
Systolic[a]	124 ± 8	119 ± 6	117 ± 9	109 ± 12	104 ± 17	94 ± 9
Mean[a]	94 ± 9	90 ± 4	88 ± 8	85 ± 7	82 ± 14	73 ± 12

[a]Changes significant ($p < .01$) for all concentrations of N$_2$O, Student's test for paired data.
[b]Changes significant ($p < .05$) for all concentrations of N$_2$O, Student's test for paired data.
Source: Modified from RW McDermott and TH Stanley, The cardiovascular effect of low concentrations of nitrous oxide during morphine anesthesia. Anesthesiology 41: 89–91, 1974.

detectable change in regional wall motion abnormalities by transesophageal echocardiography in patients undergoing bypass surgery when N_2O was added to a sufentanil anesthetic. Similarly, Cahalan and colleagues [16] have demonstrated no effect on myocardial ischemia as measured by both electrocardiography and transesophageal echocardiography when N_2O was added to a fentanyl anesthetic. These results were also confirmed in patients undergoing noncardiac surgery, again with no evidence that N_2O will cause or worsen myocardial ischemia [17]. Preexisting poor ventricular function also does not seem to predispose to N_2O-induced ischemia [18]. One study by Dottori and coworkers [19] even showed an apparent increase in coronary blood flow despite a decrease in cardiac output.

Heart Rate, Arrhythmias, and the Pulmonary Circulation

Heart Rate and Arrhythmias

By its sympathomimetic effect N_2O will frequently increase heart rate when it is added to an inhalational anesthetic, as was discussed earlier. This effect is much less pronounced in the presence of a narcotic-based anesthetic. In an isolated heart model [6], N_2O had no effect on heart rate and atrioventricular (AV) conduction time. Thus, this effect on heart rate is probably not a direct result of the N_2O on the cardiac conduction system, but is rather the effect of the sympathomimetic stimulation. Nitrous oxide has also been shown to cause various dysrhythmias, especially AV junctional arrhythmias [20].

The Pulmonary Circulation

Nitrous oxide increases pulmonary vascular resistance and right heart afterload [21, 22]. This is especially true in patients with preexisting elevations of pulmonary vascular resistance, such as those with mitral stenosis, mitral regurgitation, primary pulmonary hypertension, and others. This probably occurs to a smaller degree in children, especially those with congenital heart disease.

In summary, nitrous oxide has many effects on the human cardiovascular system. It is a sympathomimetic and thus may increase heart rate, SVR, and blood pressure. It is a direct myocardial depressant that may or may not be compensated for by its sympathomimetic effects. It raises pulmonary vascular resistance and, finally, it may or may not cause or exacerbate myocardial ischemia in patients at risk.

VOLATILE AGENTS

Halothane, a halogenated alkane, is the oldest of the currently available volatile anesthetics. Enflurane and isoflurane are the other two commonly used inhalation agents. Sevoflurane and desflurane are two new agents that will be clinically available in the United States.

Myocardial Contractility

Halothane is a direct myocardial depressant [23]. Sonntag and associates [24] demonstrated a decreased left ventricular dp/dt and stroke volume with increasing preload and constant afterload when halothane was administered to human volunteers. Similarly, enflurane, isoflurane, desflurane, and sevoflurane are all negative inotropes [25, 31], though their relative effects on myocardial contractility are less well defined (see below).

The mechanism for volatile anesthetic–induced myocardial depression is probably multifactorial. Although much of the work has been done with halothane, some has been done with isoflurane/enflurane, and the mechanism is probably similar for all of them. Volatile anesthetic agents reduce calcium (Ca^{++}) availability by causing a net loss of Ca^{++} from the sarcoplasmic reticulum. This may be by limiting Ca^{++} uptake/extrusion from the sarcoplasmic reticulum [32]. Halothane may cause a reduction in the number of voltage-dependent calcium channels, leading to a reduction in Ca^{++} entry into the myocardial cell [33, 34]. Figure 2-2 is a schematic of a working myocardial cell showing the sarcoplasmic reticulum and sarcolemma, areas where volatile anesthetics exert their greatest influence on the myocardium.

The order of potency of the various anesthetics, in terms of their effects on myocardial contractility, are somewhat controversial. However, most of the studies in animals have shown that these calcium fluxes and consequently the amount of myocardial

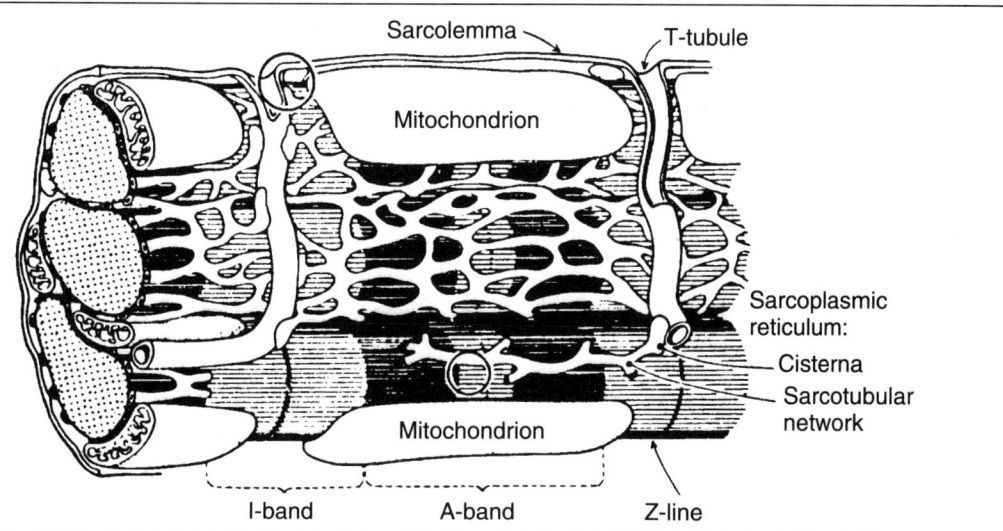

Fig. 2-2. Ultrastructure of the myocardial cell. Contractile proteins are arranged in a regular array of thick and thin filaments. The A-band represents the thick filaments into which thin filaments extend from either side. The I-band is the region of the sarcomere containing only thin filaments; these extend from the two lines that bisect each I-band. The sarcoplasmic reticulum, a membrane network that surrounds the contractile proteins, consists of the sarcotubular network at the center of the sarcomere and the cisternae, which abut on the T-tubules and the sarcolemma. (Reprinted, by permission of the *New England Journal of Medicine*. From AM Katz, Congestive heart failure: role of altered myocardial cellular control. *N Engl J Med* 293:1184, 1975.)

depression are most affected by halothane, then enflurane, and least affected by isoflurane [35–42] (Fig. 2-3). Recently, several human studies have confirmed this relationship [43–45]. One study in healthy children even showed significant depression with halothane and minimal or no depression with isoflurane [44]. Another recent study, however, suggested that the relative potency in terms of myocardial depression may be dose related, especially with regard to enflurane [46].

Desflurane, a new anesthetic, has been shown [47, 48] to cause myocardial depression similar to that produced by isoflurane [49, 50]. However, desflurane seems to sustain cardiac output better than the other inhalational anesthetics; this may be secondary to a resistance to overall hemodynamic depression because of better-maintained autonomic function [51]. Sevoflurane, another new volatile anesthetic, also appears to have myocardial depressant effects that are similar to those of isoflurane, and definitely produces less depression than halothane [52].

Effects on Peripheral Circulation

All of the volatile agents are systemic vasodilators. While halothane and enflurane do so to a much smaller extent, isoflurane, sevoflurane, and desflurane all are potent vasodilators.

Halothane will cause a mild decrease in SVR [53]. Enflurane will decrease SVR 16 to 20 percent in humans [54], while isoflurane has a profound effect on systemic vascular resistance [55]. Bernard and associates [56] and others [57] have demonstrated that sevoflurane produces a decrease in SVR similar to that of isoflurane. Similarly, Weiskopf and associates [49] and others [58] demonstrated that desflurane has a similar effect on SVR as isoflurane. The mechanism of this vasodilatation is unclear, but is probably caused by a direct effect on vascular smooth muscle by the anesthetic agent [59], and is not, as others have speculated, related to the endothelium or endothelium releasing factors [60].

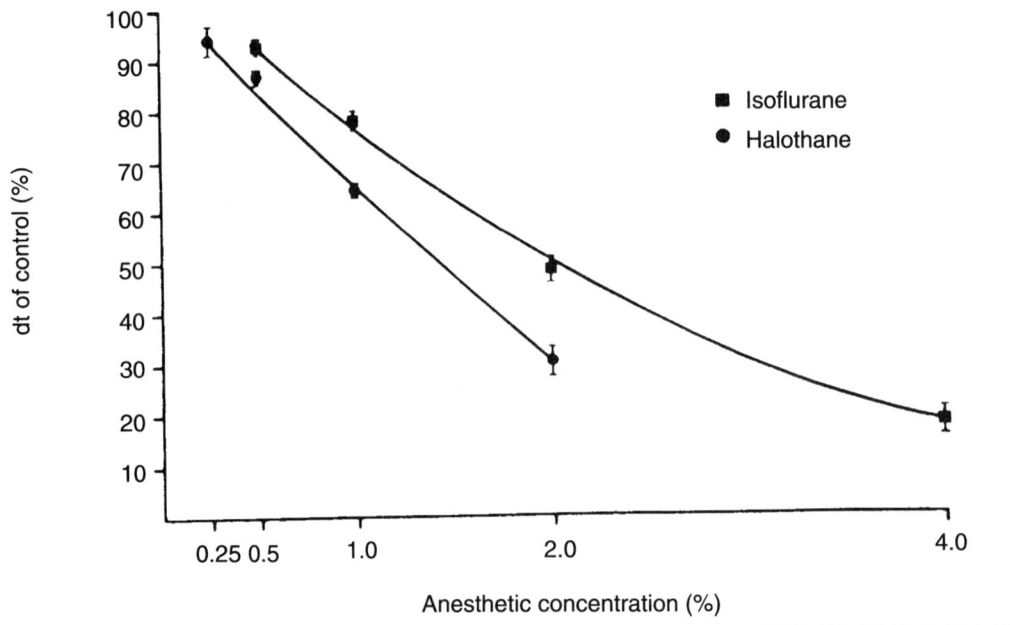

Fig. 2-3. Dose response data for alteration in dt (% of control) following halothane or isoflurane administration. (Reprinted with permission from WJ Wolf, MB Neal, BP Mathew, et al., Comparison of the in vitro myocardial depressant effects of isoflurane and halothane anesthesia. *Anesthesiology* 69:660–666, 1988.)

All of the potent inhalational anesthetic agents will inhibit hypoxic pulmonary vasoconstriction [61], although one study in dogs showed that sevoflurane may not have this effect [62]. Though they will all vasodilate the pulmonary vasculature [63], their effect on the pulmonary vasculature is less than their effect on the systemic vasculature.

Effects on Myocardial Oxygen Supply/Demand

Myocardial Oxygen Demand

All of the volatile inhalation anesthetics decrease myocardial oxygen demand (MVO$_2$). Halothane and enflurane decrease MVO$_2$ more than does isoflurane [38]. Halothane has also been shown to have protective effects in ischemic rat hearts [64], but this effect may have been related to interference with reperfusion injury. Moffitt and associates [64] demonstrated an increased coronary venous oxygen content in spite of decreased overall myocardial blood flow, implying a reduction in MVO$_2$ with halothane. However, when halothane was added to N$_2$O in a heart with a critical coronary stenosis, it caused worsening of the regional myocardial dysfunction [14].

Isoflurane also causes a decrease in MVO$_2$ even though it may cause a maldistribution of coronary blood flow and worsen ischemia [65] (see below). Isoflurane has also been shown to improve tolerance to pacing-induced myocardial ischemia in humans [66], presumably by decreasing MVO$_2$, although other recent studies have shown only halothane and enflurane to decrease MVO$_2$ while isoflurane had no effect [67, 68]. Additionally, in the dog model, halothane but not isoflurane offered protection from total myocardial ischemia. Recently, it has been shown that desflurane [57] and sevoflurane [57] both decrease MVO$_2$, in a manner similar to that of isoflurane.

Effects on Coronary Blood Flow

Isoflurane is a potent coronary vasodilator and will increase coronary blood flow out of proportion to the increase in $M\dot{V}O_2$. This is in contrast to halothane, which will increase coronary blood flow in response to an increase in $M\dot{V}O_2$ [69]. In canine hearts, intracoronary isoflurane causes a marked direct vasodilatory action [70]. It is not clear what area of the coronary circulation is most affected by isoflurane. In a study on dogs, Sill and associates [71] demonstrated no effect on the large epicardial coronary arteries, with a significant dilatation of the smaller intramyocardial coronary arterioles. In two very recent studies, Bollen and colleagues demonstrated minimal effects of isoflurane as compared to halothane, on both human [72] and porcine [73] epicardial coronary arteries.

While sevoflurane is also a coronary vasodilator and will increase coronary blood flow, some authors suggest that its effect may not be as pronounced as that of isoflurane. In a study on isolated rat hearts, sevoflurane in high concentrations decreased coronary flow reserve only 48 percent, compared with 100 percent decrease seen with isoflurane [74]. This is also confirmed in the intact rat model [57]. On the other hand, several studies have shown sevoflurane's effect on coronary blood flow to be very similar to that of isoflurane [56].

Desflurane, like isoflurane, is a coronary vasodilator. In isolated guinea pig hearts, desflurane caused an increase in coronary blood flow, though not as much as isoflurane [48]. Similarly, in a dog model [51] isoflurane caused a greater increase in coronary blood flow than did desflurane. On the other hand, Merin and associates [58] showed the increase in coronary blood flow to be similar for desflurane and isoflurane.

The mechanism for volatile anesthetic–induced coronary vasodilation is not entirely clear, though once again interference with calcium influx may play a role [75].

Coronary Steal

For development of coronary steal, one must have steal-prone coronary anatomy. Coronary steal can develop in an area of myocardium supplied by a stenosed coronary artery when this myocardium is also supplied by collaterals, which are in turn supplied by another coronary artery that also has a significant coronary lesion (Fig. 2-4). Steal is produced when flow in this second coronary artery is decreased by coronary vasodilatation, which

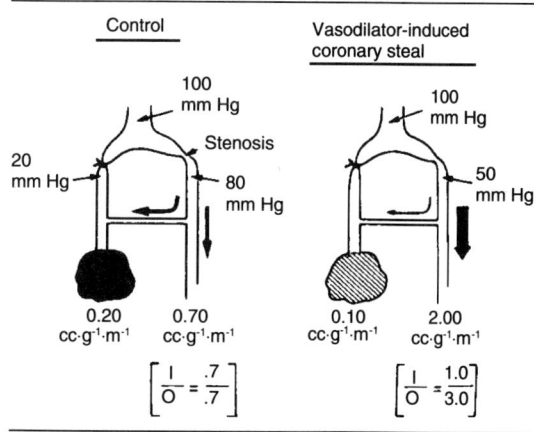

Fig. 2-4. Schematic representation of proposed mechanism of arteriolar vasodilation–induced coronary steal. During the control state (*left*), collateral flow to the underperfused area distal to the occlusion (*shaded area*) is determined by the pressure gradient between the collateral supplying artery (80 mm Hg) and the vascular bed distal to the occlusion (20 mm Hg). At rest, the proximal stenosis of the supply artery results in a clinically insignificant distal pressure drop (100 to 80 mm Hg). Following distal coronary vasodilatation (*right*), flow to the normally perfused area increases by a factor of almost 3, but becomes maldistributed between endocardium (I) and epicardium (O), as reflected by the I/O ratio of well below 1. There is a pronounced flow-related pressure drop across the stenosis (from 100 to 50 mm Hg) that will reduce the pressure gradient across the collateral bed. As a result, flow to the (already) underperfused area will decrease by another 50%. Not that proximal perfusion pressure remains unchanged throughout. (Reprinted with permission from BA Cason, ED Verrier, MJ London, et al., Effects of isoflurane and halothane on coronary vascular resistance and collateral myocardial blood flow: Their capacity to induce coronary steal. *Anesthesiology* 67:665–675, 1987.)

therefore causes a further worsening of myocardial oxygen supply in the collateral-dependent myocardium.

Whether or not isoflurane causes coronary steal has been the subject of much controversy in the anesthesia literature. Priebe [76] demonstrated that isoflurane as compared to halothane caused severe myocardial regional dysfunction in dogs with a critical coronary artery stenosis. In a study in humans with coronary artery disease, Khambatta and associates [77] demonstrated that isoflurane but not halothane caused increased lactate production.

Reiz and Ostman [78] demonstrated isoflurane to cause regional myocardial ischemia. In 21 patients with coronary artery disease anesthetized with isoflurane who were about to undergo major vascular surgery, isoflurane caused a decrease in coronary perfusion pressure and decreased coronary vascular resistance while coronary sinus blood flow remained stable. Myocardial oxygen consumption and extraction were reduced. Of the 21 patients, 10 developed ST-T depression or T-wave inversion consistent with myocardial ischemia, these changes were seen in combination with a simultaneous decrease in myocardial lactate extraction. When perfusion pressure was restored with phenylephrine and nitroglycerin, three patients had persistent signs of myocardial ischemia.

In a dog model Tatekawa and associates [65] demonstrated decreased left circumflex artery blood flow (with left circumflex stenosis) caused by isoflurane, although no ischemia was seen. In perhaps the two most convincing animal studies, Buffington and colleagues [79] and Priebe and Foex [80] demonstrated regional myocardial dysfunction produced by isoflurane (but not halothane) in collateral-dependent canine myocardium.

Coronary blood flow autoregulation is also disrupted by all the volatile anesthetic agents [81]. Sahlman and associates [82] studied a group of 21 patients undergoing coronary artery surgery. Isoflurane induced myocardial ischemia in two patients (as measured by lactate production) even in the absence of hypotension. Conzen and colleagues [83], on the other hand, demonstrated that decreased coronary blood flow caused by isoflurane in collateral-dependent regions was dependent on blood pressure, and that when pressure was normalized, blood flow to the collateral-dependent zone was also normalized.

In a study of 1,178 patients undergoing coronary artery bypass surgery anesthetized with either isoflurane or enflurane, the isoflurane patients had a higher rate of myocardial infarction and perioperative death (1.8 and 4.0%, 0.3 and 2.1%, respectively) [84].

In spite of all of the above evidence (and more), several studies have shown no effect on coronary steal by isoflurane. In a chronically instrumented single-vessel coronary disease dog model, Hartman and associates [85] demonstrated that high-dose isoflurane decreased subepicardial, subendocardial, and transmural blood flow in both normal and collateral-dependent myocardium equally. They also demonstrated that all of these blood flows returned to normal when the blood pressure was normalized. In a multivessel coronary disease model [86], adenosine but not isoflurane caused a dose-related relative decrease in collateral flow. Similarly, in other multivessel coronary artery disease models in dog [87] and swine [88] neither halothane nor isoflurane caused a decrease in coronary blood flow to the collateral-dependent zone.

When isoflurane is compared to other anesthetics in humans, the results seem to indicate that isoflurane is safe. Leung and associates [89] compared isoflurane and sufentanil anesthesia in patients undergoing coronary bypass surgery and showed no difference in the incidence of myocardial ischemia. Slogoff and colleagues [90] demonstrated no difference in ischemia in patients who had steal-prone coronary anatomy between those anesthetized with halothane, isoflurane, enflurane, and sufentanil. In another study by Slogoff [91], no difference was seen in new ST depression, postoperative myocardial infarction, and/or death between patients anesthetized with enflurane, halothane, isoflurane, or sufentanil. Similarly, Tuman and coworkers [92] found no difference between fentanyl, sufentanil, halothane, and diazepam-ketamine techniques when myocardial infarction and inhospital death were studied.

There is even some evidence that isoflurane may be protective for the ischemic heart. As discussed earlier, Tarnow and associates [66] showed that isoflurane protects against pacing-induced myocardial ischemia. Davis and Sidi [93] demonstrated that isoflurane decreased the area of myocardial necrosis following left anterior descending (LAD) artery occlusion in the dog. Similarly, isoflurane and halothane were shown to improve recovery of stunned myocardium in the dog model [94].

Recently, desflurane, a coronary vasodilator, has been shown not to redistribute blood away from collateral-dependent myocardium [95]. When desflurane was compared to sufentanil [96] for coronary artery bypass graft surgery, no difference was seen in the incidence of ischemia during maintenance of anesthesia when hemodynamics were tightly controlled. However, during induction, desflurane was associated with more hemodynamic changes and myocardial ischemia.

In summary, there is a significant amount of evidence that isoflurane may cause coronary steal in patients with steal-prone collateral-dependent myocardial anatomy. Nevertheless, isoflurane decreases $M\dot{V}O_2$ and coronary vasodilates, and may in certain circumstances protect the ischemic myocardium.

Effects on Arrhythmias

Halothane can suppress automaticity in normal pacemaker fibers. Halothane and, to a smaller extent, enflurane and isoflurane can sensitize the myocardium to epinephrine and other catecholamine-induced ventricular arrhythmias (Fig. 2-5). Atlee and Rusy [97] demonstrated reentry-type ventricular arrhythmias produced by enflurane and halothane in dogs. Takaori and Loehning [98] demonstrated ventricular tachycardia and fibrillation when aminophylline was given to halothane-anesthetized dogs. Roizen and Stevens [99] also showed ventricular tachycardia due to an interaction between halothane and aminophylline. Aminophylline is not the only potential drug interaction. Takaori and Loehning [100] demonstrated similar interactions with isoproterenol and ephedrine. Johnston and associates [101] showed an increased arrhythmogenicity of epinephrine in the presence of halothane, enflurane, or isoflurane. The lowest dose of epinephrine needed to produce ventricular arrhythmias was seen during halothane anesthesia, and the highest dose of epinephrine needed to produce ventricular arrhythmias was seen during isoflurane anesthesia. Similar results were obtained by Joas and Stevens [102].

Halothane, enflurane, and isoflurane increase the rate of automaticity in normal Purkinje fibers exposed to epinephrine by enhanced phase 4 depolarization [103]. Halothane will decrease both the heart rate and atrial conduction time [104], which is a possible explanation for the atrial arrhythmias sometimes caused by halothane. Halothane, enflurane, and isoflurane will decrease spontaneous sinoatrial (SA) node depolarization, an

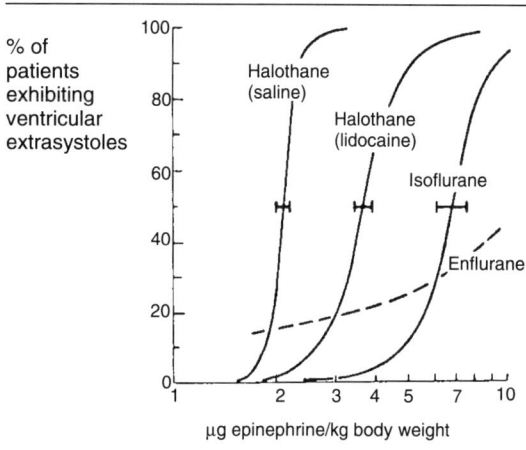

Fig. 2-5. Percent of patients exhibiting three or more ventricular extrasystoles in response to a subcutaneous injection of epinephrine. (Reprinted with permission of the International Anesthesia Research Society. From RR Johnston, EI Eger II, and C Wilson, A comparative interaction of epinephrine with enflurane, isoflurane, and halothane in man. *Anesth Analg* 55:709, 1976.)

effect that is not reversed by calcium [105]. Halothane is also known to produce junctional rhythms, especially in combination with the muscle relaxant pancuronium.

The volatile anesthetic agents can also function as antiarrhythmics, especially when these arrhythmias are caused by ischemia. In an acute ischemia/reperfusion model, halothane, enflurane, and to a lesser extent isoflurane prevented ventricular fibrillation [106]. The same is true for pacing-induced ventricular tachycardia, which was suppressed by halothane and enflurane but not by isoflurane [107] (perhaps secondary to their greater prolongation of refractory periods). In a study on Purkinje fibers from infarcted canine hearts, halothane facilitated reentrant arrhythmias while inhibiting the initiation of impulses [108]. However, based on another study by MacLeod and associates [109], it seems that halothane's antiarrhythmic effects may be species and model specific, and, therefore, extrapolation to humans may not be possible.

A review of the effects of the inhalational anesthetic agents on hemodynamics is presented in Table 2-2.

Table 2-2. Effects of the inhalational anesthetic agents on hemodynamics

Agent	Heart rate	Myocardial contractility	MVO$_2$	SVR	PVR
Nitrous oxide	+	−	+ or −	+	++
Halothane	N or −	− − −	− − −	−	−
Enflurane	N or −	− − −	− − −	−	−
Isoflurane	+	− −	− − −	− − −	−
Sevoflurane	+	− −	− −	− − −	−
Desflurane	++	− −	− −	− − −	−

PVR = pulmonary vascular resistance; − − − = strongly depressed or decreased; − − = moderately depressed or decreased; − = mildly depressed or decreased; ++ = strongly stimulated or increased; + = mildly stimulated or increased; N = no effect.

REFERENCES

1. Eisele, JH, Smith, NT. Cardiovascular effects of 40 percent nitrous oxide in man. *Anesth Analg* 51:956, 1972.
2. Thornburn, J, Smith, G, Vance, JP, et al. The effects of nitrous oxide on the cardiovascular system and coronary circulation of the dog. *Br J Anaesth* 51:937–942, 1979.
3. Smith, NT, Corbascio, AN. The cardiovascular effects of nitrous oxide during halothane anesthesia in the dog. *Anesthesiology* 27:560–566, 1966.
4. Moffitt, EA, Scovil, JE, Barker, RA, et al. The effects of nitrous oxide on myocardial metabolism and hemodynamics during fentanyl or enflurane anesthesia in patients with coronary disease. *Anesth Analg* 63:1071–1075, 1984.
5. Smith, NT, Calverley, RK, Prys-Roberts, C, et al. Impact of nitrous oxide on the circulation during enflurane anesthesia in man. *Anesthesiology* 48:345–349, 1978.
6. Stowe, DF, Monroe, SM, Marijic, J, et al. Effects of nitrous oxide on contractile function and metabolism of the isolated heart. *Anesthesiology* 73:1220–1226, 1990.
7. Ramsay, JG, Arvieux, CC, Foex, P, et al. Regional and global myocardial function in the dog when nitrous oxide is added to halothane in the presence of critical coronary artery constriction. *Anesth Analg* 65:431–436, 1986.
8. Smith, NT, Eger, EI, Stoetting, RK, et al. The cardiovascular and sympathomimetic responses to the addition of nitrous oxide to halothane in man. *Anesthesiology* 32:410–421, 1970.
9. Meretoja, OA, Takkunan, O, Heikkila, H, et al. Haemodynamic response to nitrous oxide during high dose fentanyl pancuronium anaesthesia. *Acta Anaesth Scand* 291:137–141, 1985.
10. Moffitt, EA, Sethna, DH, Gary, RJ, et al. Nitrous oxide added to halothane reduces coronary flows and myocardial oxygen consumption in patients with coronary artery disease. *Can Anaesth Soc* 30:5–9, 1983.
11. Wilkowski, DAW, Sill, JC, Bonta, W, et al. Nitrous oxide constricts epicardial coronary arteries without effect on coronary arterioles. *Anesthesiology* 66:659–665, 1987.
12. Nathan, HJ. Nitrous oxide worsens myocardial ischemia in isoflurane-anesthetized dogs. *Anesthesiology* 68:407–415, 1988.
13. Cason, BA, Demas, KA, Mazer, CD, et al. Effects of nitrous oxide on coronary pressure and regional contractile function in experimental myocardial ischemia. *Anesth Analg* 72:604–611, 1991.
14. Leone, BJ, Philbin, DM, Lehot, JJ, et al. Gradual or abrupt nitrous oxide administration in a canine model of critical coronary stenosis induces regional myocardial dysfunction that is worsened by halothane. *Anesth Analg* 67:814–822, 1988.
15. Slavik, JR, LaMantia, KR, Kopriva, CJ, et al. Does nitrous oxide cause regional wall motion abnormalities in patients with coronary artery disease? An evaluation by two-dimensional transesophageal echocardiography. *Anesth Analg* 67:695–700, 1988.
16. Cahalan, MK, Prakash, O, Rulf, ENR, et al. Addition of nitrous oxide to fentanyl anesthesia does not induce myocardial ischemia in patients with ischemic heart disease. *Anesthesiology* 67:925–929, 1987.
17. Kozmary, S, Lampe, GH, et al. Nitrous oxide does not increase myocardial ischemia during or after carotid endarterectomy. *Anesth Analg* 68:51–52, 1989.
18. Mitchell, MM, Prakash, O, Rulf, ENR, et al. Nitrous oxide does not induce myocardial ischemia in patients with ischemic heart disease and poor ventricular function. *Anesthesiology* 71:526–534, 1989.
19. Dottori, O, Haggendal, E, Linder, E, et al. The hae-

modynamic effects of nitrous oxide anaesthesia on myocardial blood flow in dogs. *Acta Anaesth Scand* 20:421–428, 1976.
20. Roizen, MF, Plummer, GO, Lichtor, JL. Nitrous oxide and dysrhythmias. *Anesthesiology* 66:427–431, 1987.
21. Lappas, DG, Buckley, MJ, Laver, MB, et al. Left ventricular performance and pulmonary circulation following addition of nitrous oxide to morphine during coronary artery surgery. *Anesthesiology* 43:61–69, 1975.
22. Schulte-Sasse, U, Hess, W, Tarnow, J. Pulmonary vascular responses to nitrous oxide in patients with normal and high pulmonary vascular resistance. *Anesthesiology* 57:9–13, 1982.
23. Deutsch, S, Linde, HW, Dripps, RD, et al. Circulatory and respiratory actions of halothane in normal man. *Anesthesiology* 23:631, 1962.
24. Sonntag, H, Donath, U, Hillebrand, W, et al. Left ventricular function in conscious man and during halothane anesthesia. *Anesthesiology* 48:320–324, 1978.
25. Priebe, HJ. Differential effects of isoflurane on regional right and left ventricular performances, and on coronary, systemic, and pulmonary hemodynamics in the dog. *Anesthesiology* 66:262–272, 1987.
26. Sato, M, Hoka, S, Arimura, H, et al. Effects of augmenting cardiac contractility, preload, and heart rate on cardiac output during enflurane anesthesia. *Anesth Analg* 73:590–596, 1991.
27. Kaplan, JA, Miller, ED, Baily, DR. A comparative study of enflurane and halothane using systolic time intervals. *Anesth Analg* 55:263–268, 1976.
28. Rao, CC, Boyer, MS, Krishna, G, et al. Increased sensitivity of the isometric contraction of the neonatal isolated rat atria to halothane, isoflurane and enflurane. *Anesthesiology* 64:13–18, 1986.
29. Mote, PS, Pruett, JK, Gramling, ZW. Effects of halothane and enflurane on right ventricular performance in hearts of dogs anesthetized with pentobarbitone sodium. *Anesthesiology* 58:53–60, 1983.
30. Brown, BB, Crout, JR. A comparative study of the effects of five general anesthetics on myocardial contractility. *Anesthesiology* 34:236–245, 1971.
31. Kemmotsu, O, Hashumoto, Y, Shimosato, S. Inotropic effects of isoflurane on mechanics of contraction in isolated cat papillary muscles from normal and failing hearts. *Anesthesiology* 39:470–477, 1973.
32. Wilde, DW, Knight, PR, Sheth, N, et al. Halothane alters control of intracellular Ca^{2+} mobilization in single rat ventricular myocytes. *Anesthesiology* 75:1075–1086, 1991.
33. Hoehner, PJ, Quigg, MC, Blanck, TJJ. Halothane depresses D600 binding to bovine heart sarcolemma. *Anesthesiology* 75:1019–1024, 1991.
34. Oshita, S, Oka, H, Hiraoka, I, et al. Halothane increases epinephrine threshold for the development of slow responses in isolated canine trabeculae. *Anesth Analg* 73:449–454, 1991.
35. Shibata, T, Blanck, TJJ, Sagawa, K, et al. The effect of halothane, enflurane, and isoflurane on the dynamic stiffness of rabbit papillar muscle. *Anesthesiology* 70:496, 1989.
36. Wolf, WJ, Neal, MB, Mathew, BP, et al. Comparison of the in vitro myocardial depressant effects of isoflurane and halothane anesthesia. *Anesthesiology* 69:660–666, 1988.
37. Stowe, DF, Monroe, SM, Marijic, J, et al. Comparison of halothane, enflurane, and isoflurane with nitrous oxide on contractility and oxygen supply and demand in isolated hearts. *Anesthesiology* 75:1062–1074, 1991.
38. Bosnjak, ZJ, Aggarwal, A, Turner, LA, et al. Differential effects of halothane, enflurane, and isoflurane on Ca^{2+} transients and papillary muscle tension in guinea pigs. *Anesthesiology* 76:123–131, 1992.
39. Conzen, PF, Hobbhahn, J, Goetz, AE, et al. Myocardial contractility, blood flow, and oxygen consumption in healthy dogs during anesthesia with isoflurane or enflurane. *J Cardiothorac Anesth* 3:70–77, 1989.
40. Housmans, PR, Murat, I. Comparative effects of halothane, enflurane, and isoflurane at equipotent anesthetic concentrations on isolated ventricular myocardium of the ferret. I. Contractility. *Anesthesiology* 69:451–463, 1988.
41. Housmans, PR, Murat, I. Comparative effects of halothane, enflurane, and isoflurane at equipotent anesthetic concentrations on isolated ventricular myocardium of the ferret. II. Relaxation. *Anesthesiology* 69:464–471, 1988.
42. Lynch, C, III, Frazer, MJ. Depressant effects of volatile anesthetics upon rat and amphibian ventricular myocardium: Insights into anesthetic mechanisms of action. *Anesthesiology* 70:511–522, 1989.
43. Lynch, C, III. Effects of halothane and isoflurane on isolated human ventricular myocardium. *Anesthesiology* 68:429–432, 1988.
44. Wolf, WJ, Neal, MB, Peterson, MD. The hemodynamic and cardiovascular effects of isoflurane and halothane anesthesia in children. *Anesthesiology* 64:328–333, 1986.
45. Murray, DJ, Forbes, RB, Mahoney, LT. Comparative hemodynamic depression of halothane versus isoflurane in neonates and infants: An echocardiographic study. *Anesth Analg* 74:329–337, 1992.
46. Seifen, E, Seifen, AB, Kennedy, RH, et al. Compari-

son of cardiac effects of enflurane, isoflurane, and halothane in the dog heart-lung operation. *J Cardiothorac Anesth* 1:543–553, 1987.
47. Pagel, PS, Kampine, JP, Schmeling, WT, et al. Influence of volatile anesthetics on myocardial contractility in vivo: Desflurane versus isoflurane. *Anesthesiology* 74:900–907, 1991.
48. Boban, M, Stowe, DF, Buljubasic, N, et al. Direct comparative effects of isoflurane and desflurane in isolated guinea pig hearts. *Anesthesiology* 76:775–780, 1992.
49. Weiskopf, RB, Cahalan, MK, Eger, EI, II, et al. Cardiovascular actions of desflurane in normocarbic volunteers. *Anesth Analg* 73:143–156, 1991.
50. Cahalan, MK, Weiskopf, RB, Eger, EI, II, et al. Hemodynamic effects of desflurane/nitrous oxide anesthesia in volunteers. *Anesth Analg* 73:157–164, 1991.
51. Pagel, PS, Kampine, JP, Schmeling, WT, et al. Comparison of the systemic and coronary hemodynamic actions of desflurane, isoflurane, halothane, and enflurane in the chronically instrumented dog. *Anesthesiology* 74:539–551, 1991.
52. Kasuda, H, Akazawa, S, Shimizu, R. The echocardiographic assessment of left ventricular performance during sevoflurane and halothane anesthesia. *J Anesth* 4:295–302, 1990.
53. Vatner, SF, Smith, NT. Effects of halothane on left ventricular function and distribution of regional blood flow in dogs and primates. *Circ Res* 34:155–167, 1974.
54. Calverley, RK, Smith, NT, Prys-Roberts, C, et al. Cardiovascular effects of enflurane anesthesia during controlled ventilation in man. *Anesth Analg* 57:619–628, 1978.
55. Brett, CM, Teitel, DR, Heymann, MA, et al. The cardiovascular effects of isoflurane in lambs. *Anesthesiology* 67:60–65, 1987.
56. Bernard, JM, Wouters, PF, Doursout, MF, et al. Effects of sevoflurane and isoflurane on cardiac and coronary dynamics in chronically instrumented dogs. *Anesthesiology* 72:659–662, 1990.
57. Conzen, PF, Vollmar, B, Habazettl, H, et al. Systemic and regional hemodynamics of isoflurane and sevoflurane in rats. *Anesth Analg* 74:79–88, 1992.
58. Merin, RG, Bernard, JM, Doursout, MF, et al. Comparison of the effects of isoflurane and desflurane on cardiovascular dynamics and regional blood flow in the chronically instrumented dog. *Anesthesiology* 74:568–574, 1991.
59. Brendel, JK, Johns, RA. Isoflurane does not vasodilate rat thoracic aortic rings by endothelium-derived relaxing factor or other cyclic GMP-mediated mechanisms. *Anesthesiology* 77:126–131, 1992.

60. Blaise, MD, Sill, JC, Nugent, M, et al. Isoflurane causes endothelium dependent inhibition of contractile responses of canine coronary arteries. *Anesthesiology* 67:513–517, 1987.
61. Marshall, C, Lindgren, L, Marshall, BE. Effects of halothane, enflurane, and isoflurane on hypoxic pulmonary vasoconstriction in rat lungs in vitro. *Anesthesiology* 60:304, 1984.
62. Okutoni, T, Ikeda, K. Sevoflurane has no inhibitory effect on hypoxic pulmonary vasoconstriction in dogs. *J Anesth* 4:123–130, 1990.
63. Coetzee, A, Brits, W, Genade, S, et al. Halothane does have protective properties in the isolated ischemic rat heart. *Anesth Analg* 73:711–719, 1991.
64. Moffitt, EA, Sethna, DH, Gary, RJ, et al. Nitrous oxide added to halothane reduces coronary flow and myocardial oxygen consumption in patients with coronary disease. *Can Anaesth Soc J* 30:5–9, 1983.
65. Tatekawa, S, Traber, KB, Hantler, CB, et al. Effects of isoflurane on myocardial blood flow, function, and oxygen consumption in the presence of critical coronary stenosis in dogs. *Anesth Analg* 66:1073–1082, 1987.
66. Tarnow, J, Markschies-Hornung, A, Schulte-Sasse, U. Isoflurane improves the tolerance to pacing-induced myocardial ischemia. *Anesthesiology* 64:147–156, 1986.
67. Stowe, DF, Marijic, J, Bosnjak, ZJ, et al. Direct comparative effects of halothane, enflurane, and isoflurane on oxygen supply and demand in isolated hearts. *Anesthesiology* 74:1087–1095, 1991.
68. Pollard, JB, Hill, RF, Lowe, JE, et al. Myocardial tolerance to total ischemia in the dog anesthetized with halothane or isoflurane. *Anesthesiology* 69:17–23, 1988.
69. Kenny, D, Proctor, LT, Schmeling, WT, et al. Isoflurane causes only minimal increases in coronary blood flow independent of oxygen demand. *Anesthesiology* 75:640–649, 1991.
70. Crystal, GJ, Kim, SJ, Czinn, EA, et al. Intracoronary isoflurane causes marked vasodilation in canine hearts. *Anesthesiology* 74:757–765, 1991.
71. Sill, JC, Bove, AA, Nugent, M, et al. Effects of isoflurane on coronary arteries and coronary arterioles in the intact dog. *Anesthesiology* 66:273–279, 1987.
72. Bollen, BA, McKlveen, RE, Stevenson, JA. Halothane relaxes previously constricted human epicardial coronary artery segments more than isoflurane. *Anesth Analg* 75:4–8, 1992.
73. Bollen, BA, McKlveen, RE, Stevenson, JA. Halothane relaxes preconstricted small and medium isolated porcine coronary artery segments more than isoflurane. *Anesth Analg* 75:9–17, 1992.
74. Larach, DR, Schuler, G. Direct vasodilation by sevo-

flurane, isoflurane, and halothane alters coronary flow reserve in the isolated rat heart. *Anesthesiology* 75:268–278, 1991.
75. Buljubasic, N, Rusch, NJ, Marijic, J, et al. Effects of halothane and isoflurane on calcium and potassium channel currents in canine coronary arterial cells. *Anesthesiology* 76:990–998, 1992.
76. Priebe, HJ. Isoflurane causes more severe regional myocardial dysfunction than halothane in dogs with a critical coronary artery stenosis. *Anesthesiology* 69:72–83, 1988.
77. Khambatta, HJ, Sonntag, H, Larsen, R, et al. Global and regional myocardial blood flow and metabolism during equipotent halothane and isoflurane anesthesia in patients with coronary artery disease. *Anesth Analg* 67:936–942, 1988.
78. Reiz, S, Ostman, M. Regional coronary hemodynamics during isoflurane–nitrous oxide anesthesia in patients with ischemic heart disease. *Anesth Analg* 64:570–576, 1985.
79. Buffington, CW, Romson, JL, Levine, A, et al. Isoflurane induces coronary steal in a canine model of chronic coronary occlusion. *Anesthesiology* 66:280–292, 1987.
80. Priebe, HJ, Foex, P. Isoflurane causes regional myocardial dysfunction in dogs with critical coronary artery stenoses. *Anesthesiology* 66:293–300, 1987.
81. Hickey, RF, Sybert, PE, Verrier, ED, et al. Effects of halothane, enflurane, and isoflurane on coronary blood flow autoregulation and coronary vascular reserve in the canine heart. *Anesthesiology* 68:21–30, 1988.
82. Sahlman, L, Milocco, I, Appelgren, L, et al. Control of intraoperative hypertension with isoflurane in patients with coronary artery disease: Effects on regional myocardial blood flow and metabolism. *Anesth Analg* 68:105–111, 1989.
83. Conzen, PF, Hobbhahn, J, Goetz, AE, et al. Regional blood flow and tissue oxygen pressures of the collateral-dependent myocardium during isoflurane anesthesia in dogs. *Anesthesiology* 70:442–452, 1989.
84. Inoue, K, Reichelt, W, El-Banayosy, A, et al. Does isoflurane lead to a higher incidence of myocardial infarction and perioperative death than enflurane in coronary artery surgery? A clinical study of 1178 patients. *Anesth Analg* 71:469–474, 1990.
85. Hartman, JC, Kampine, JP, Schmeling, WT, et al. Actions of isoflurane on myocardial perfusion in chronically instrumented dogs with poor, moderate, or well-developed coronary collaterals. *J Cardiothorac Anesth* 4:715–725, 1990.
86. Hartman, JC, Kampine, JP, Schmeling, WT, et al. Alterations in collateral blood flow produced by iso-

flurane in a chronically instrumented canine model of multivessel coronary artery disease. *Anesthesiology* 74:120–133, 1991.
87. Cason, BA, Verrier, ED, London, MJ, et al. Effects of isoflurane and halothane on coronary vascular resistance and collateral myocardial blood flow: Their capacity to induce coronary steal. *Anesthesiology* 67:665–675, 1987.
88. Cheng, DCH, Moyers, JR, Knutson, RM, et al. Dose-response relationship of isoflurane and halothane versus coronary perfusion pressures. *Anesthesiology* 76:113–122, 1992.
89. Leung, JM, Goehner, P, O'Kelly, BF, et al. Isoflurane anesthesia and myocardial ischemia: Comparative risk versus sufentanil anesthesia in patients undergoing coronary artery bypass graft surgery. *Anesthesiology* 74:838–847, 1991.
90. Slogoff, S, Keats, AS, Dear, WE, et al. Steal-prone coronary anatomy and myocardial ischemia associated with four primary anesthetic agents in humans. *Anesth Analg* 72:22–27, 1991.
91. Slogoff, S, Keats, AS. Randomized trial of primary anesthetic agents on outcome of coronary artery bypass operations. *Anesthesiology* 70:179–188, 1989.
92. Tuman, KJ, McCarthy, RJ, Spiess, BD, et al. Does choice of anesthetic agent significantly affect outcome after coronary artery surgery? *Anesthesiology* 70:189–198, 1989.
93. Davis, RF, Sidi, A. Effect of isoflurane on the extent of myocardial necrosis and on systemic hemodynamics, regional myocardial blood flow, and regional myocardial metabolism in dogs after coronary artery occlusion. *Anesth Analg* 69:575–586, 1989.
94. Warltier, DC, Al-Wathiqui, MH, Kampine, JP, et al. Recovery of contractile function of stunned myocardium in chronically instrumented dogs is enhanced by halothane or isoflurane. *Anesthesiology* 69:552–565, 1988.
95. Hartman, JC, Pagel, PS, Kampine, JP, et al. Influence of desflurane on regional distribution of coronary blood flow in a chronically instrumented canine model of multivessel coronary artery obstruction. *Anesth Analg* 72:289–299, 1991.
96. Helman, JD, Leung, JM, Bellows, WH, et al. The risk of myocardial ischemia in patients receiving desflurane versus sufentanil anesthesia for coronary artery bypass graft surgery. *Anesthesiology* 77:47–62, 1992.
97. Atlee, JL, Rusy, BF. Atrioventricular conduction times and atrioventricular nodal conductivity during enflurane anesthesia in dogs. *Anesthesiology* 47:498–503, 1977.
98. Takaori, M, Loehning, RW. Ventricular arrhyth-

mias induced by aminophylline during halothane anesthesia in dogs. *Can Anaesth Soc J* 14:79, 1967.
99. Roizen, MF, Stevens, WC. Multiform ventricular tachycardia due to the interaction of aminophylline and halothane. *Anesth Analg* 57:738, 1978.
100. Takaori, M, Loehning, RW. Ventricular arrhythmias during halothane anaesthesia: Effect of isoproterenol, aminophylline and ephedrine. *Can Anaesth Soc J* 12:275, 1965.
101. Johnston, RR, Eger, EI, II, Wilson, C. A comparative interaction of epinephrine with enflurane, isoflurane, and halothane in man. *Anesth Analg* 55:709, 1976.
102. Joas, TA, Stevens, WC. Comparison of the arrhythmic doses of epinephrine during Forane, halothane and fluroxene anesthesia in dogs. *Anesthesiology* 35:48, 1971.
103. Laszlo, A, Polic, S, Atlee, JL, III, et al. Anesthetics and automaticity in latent pacemaker fibers: I. Effects of halothane, enflurane, and isoflurane on automaticity and recovery of automaticity from overdrive suppression in Purkinje fibers derived from canine hearts. *Anesthesiology* 75:98–105, 1991.
104. Scheffer, GJ, Jonges, R, Holley, S, et al. Effects of halothane on the conduction system of the heart in humans. *Anesth Analg* 69:721–726, 1989.
105. Bosnjak, ZJ, Kampine, JP. Effects of halothane, enflurane, and isoflurane on the SA node. *Anesthesiology* 58:314–321, 1983.
106. Kroll, DA, Knight, PR. Antifibrillatory effects of volatile anesthetics in acute occlusion/reperfusion arrhythmias. *Anesthesiology* 61:657–661, 1984.
107. Deutsch, N, Hantler, CB, Tait, AR, et al. Suppression of ventricular arrhythmias by volatile anesthetics in a canine model of chronic myocardial infarction. *Anesthesiology* 72:1012–1021, 1990.
108. Turner, LA, Bosnjak, ZJ, Kampine, JP. Actions of halothane on the electrical activity of Purkinje fibers derived from normal and infarcted canine hearts. *Anesthesiology* 67:619–629, 1987.
109. MacLeod, BA, McGroarty, R, Morton, RH, et al. Effects of halothane on arrhythmias induced by myocardial ischaemia. *Can J Anaesth* 36:289–294, 1989.

3
Hemodynamic Effects of Intravenous Anesthetic Agents

Florence J. Moses
David Amar

Anesthesia for the patient with coexisting heart disease requires a thorough knowledge of the hemodynamic effects of the agents used. In this chapter we discuss the intravenous anesthetic agents, with particular focus on cardiovascular effects. Many different variables affect the hemodynamic responses of this patient population, for example, premedication, disease state, and preoperative conditions. These often differ in the literature and must be considered when the response to a particular anesthetic drug or technique is evaluated.

BARBITURATES

The barbiturates have been used for induction of anesthesia for more than 40 years because of their overall safety and lack of side effects. Today, thiamylal, thiopental, and methohexital are in common clinical use (Fig. 3-1). Derivatives of barbituric acid or of its 2-thio analogue, barbiturates are thought to act at the γ-aminobutyric acid (GABA) receptor complex. They enhance and mimic the action of GABA [1], the principal inhibitory neurotransmitter in the central nervous system (CNS).

As induction agents, barbiturates act in one arm-to-brain circulation time when used intravenously [2]. This is followed by rapid redistribution from the brain to the lean body tissue, resulting in a 5- to 8-minute duration of action. The barbiturate dose necessary to produce general anesthesia is influenced by the patient's age, premedication, and physical status.

Central Nervous System Effects

Barbiturates are hyperalgesic in subanesthetic doses, causing an exaggerated response to pain. Thiopental produces a dose-related depression on the electroencephalogram and cerebral metabolic consumption of oxygen ($CMRO_2$), with a parallel reduction in cerebral blood flow (CBF) and intracranial pressure (ICP) [3]. In contrast, epileptiform seizures have been seen after high doses of methohexital [4, 5]. Induction with either agent causes a 40 percent decrease in intraocular pressure [6].

Respiratory and Other Effects

The barbiturates all cause central respiratory depression [7]. Although safe for use in asthmatic patients despite their potential to cause histamine release, they do not produce bronchodilation, and therefore may not be the induction agents of choice. In patients with acute intermittent porphyria, barbiturates should be avoided. As a result of the induction of δ-aminolevulinic acid synthe-

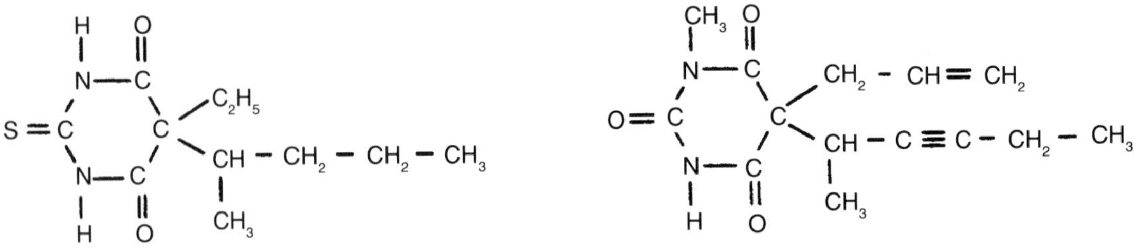

Fig. 3-1. Chemical structures of barbiturates commonly used in anesthesia.

tase and the consequent buildup of porphyrins, they can cause paralysis and death [8].

Thiopental and Thiamylal

Thiopental and thiamylal are ultra–short-acting barbiturates. After a standard induction dose of 3 to 7 mg/kg, they have a distribution half-life $(t\frac{1}{2})\alpha$ of 2.5 to 8.5 minutes and an elimination $t\frac{1}{2}\beta$ of 5 to 12 hours [9, 10]. Rapid awakening from an induction dose results from drug redistribution. Older patients require a lower induction dose than younger, healthier patients [11]. Awakening may be delayed in older patients because of either increased CNS sensitivity or alterations in metabolism [10, 12].

Thiopental and thiamylal are highly fat soluble and can accumulate in tissues, particularly when large doses are given. Clearance half-lives are likely to be prolonged in obese patients [13]. They are biotransformed in the liver to inactive metabolites that are excreted by the kidneys.

Cardiovascular Effects

The predominant cardiovascular effect of barbiturate induction is venodilation with pooling of blood in the periphery [14]. A thiopental dose of 100 to 400 mg may cause significant decreases in cardiac output (24%) and systemic blood pressure (10%). The mechanisms responsible are postulated to be a reduction in venous return secondary to an increase in venous capacitance [14, 15], a direct negative inotropic action, or transiently decreased sympathetic outflow from the CNS. Myocardial contractility is depressed, but to a lesser degree than after volatile anesthetics [16]. Contrary to initial reports [17, 18] this effect is not mediated through altered calcium uptake by cardiac sarcoplasmic reticulum [19]. The cardiac index is frequently unchanged [20–22]. Thiopental has little effect on resistance vessels, and, therefore, systemic vascular resistance (SVR) usually remains unchanged.

Induction with thiopental usually produces either an unchanged or slightly decreased mean arterial pressure (MAP) and occasionally cardiac index (CI) [21, 22]. However, a greater drop in mean blood pressure may occur in patients with valvular or congenital heart disease [23]. Normally, a 10 to 36 percent increase in heart rate is seen, probably from reflex sympathetic stimulation via the baroreceptors [20–22, 24–27]. This may be deleterious to patients with ischemic heart disease because of the associated increase in myocardial oxygen consumption [21, 25]. In one study of patients with coronary artery disease (CAD), a dose of 6 mg/kg caused parallel decreases in myocardial oxygen consumption and coronary blood flow [21]. Although thiopental is not contraindicated in patients with ischemic heart disease, if used, it should be carefully titrated with hemodynamic monitoring.

When thiopental is given in the presence of hypovolemia [28], congestive heart failure, cardiac tamponade, or a fixed cardiac output [29], a significant reduction in cardiac output and blood pressure is seen. The myocardial depressant effects of thiopental will also be unmasked when the baroreceptor reflex is blunted, in the presence of β-adrenergic blockade, insufficient myocardial reserve, high resting sympathetic tone, or myocardial ischemia. Hypotension is also greater in hypertensive patients, both treated and untreated, probably due to chronic volume contraction compared with normotensive patients [30]. The hemodynamic changes tend to be greater when thiopental is given by rapid bolus injection [24]. Tracheal intubation following induction with thiopental alone may be associated with hypertension, tachycardia, and significant cardiovascular morbidity [27, 31]. All barbiturates prolong AV junctional conduction time, by slowing initial repolarization after the action potential.

Methohexital

Methohexital is an ultra–short-acting oxybarbiturate. Its actions and uses are similar to those of thiopental, although it is approximately three times more potent. The induction dose is 1.0 to 1.5 mg/kg intravenously.

Due to increased hepatic clearance, the elimination half-life of methohexital is approximately one third that of thiopental, resulting in a more rapid return to consciousness. Despite this, there does not appear to be a significant difference in the length of time required for complete psychomotor recovery [32].

Cardiovascular Effects
Compared to thiopental, methohexital causes a mild decrease in cardiac output with a greater compensatory increase in heart rate [33]. Methohexital also dilates the capacitance vessels, and may lower total peripheral resistance [34]. In patients with cardiac disease, the same degree of cardiovascular depression is seen when methohexital or thiopental is given in equipotent doses [23, 35, 36].

BENZODIAZEPINES

The benzodiazepines act by occupying the benzodiazepine receptor [37], which modulates the inhibitory neurotransmitter, GABA [38]. The termination of action of these drugs is through redistribution. They undergo biotransformation in the liver by either hepatic microsomal oxidation or glucuronide conjugation and are excreted in the urine. Factors such as age, obesity, enzyme induction, and hepatic and renal disease influence the pharmacokinetics of the benzodiazepines. They all have hypnotic properties and produce sedation, anxiolysis, amnesia, and centrally produced muscle relaxation. They all have anticonvulsant effects. However, they lack analgesic properties. Consequently, analgesic drugs are required to block hemodynamic responses to noxious stimuli. The benzodiazepines decrease $CMRO_2$ and CBF in a dose-related manner [39].

Respiratory Effects

The benzodiazepines produce dose-related central respiratory depression. These effects are additive when combined with opioids or other respiratory depressant drugs, or in the presence of respiratory or other debilitating diseases [40]. The benzodiazepines have relatively high margins of safety. Residual or prolonged respiratory depression, sedation, and amnesia can be reversed with the specific, competitive antagonist at the benzodiazepine receptor, flumazenil [41]. Flumazenil can cause tachycardia and hypertension, although significantly less than that seen with naloxone (Narcan) [41, 42]. It can precipitate acute withdrawal symptoms in patients who are physically dependent on the benzodiazepines [43].

Diazepam

Diazepam is one of the most frequently used benzodiazepines (Fig. 3-2). It is demethylated in the liver to form the active metabolite, desmethyldiazepam, and hydroxylated to form methyloxazepam, which is then demethylated to form another active metabolite, oxazepam [44]. Diazepam has a relatively long distribution half-life (30–66 minutes) [44, 45]. The elimination half-life of diazepam is 24 to 57 hours in normal subjects, and is prolonged by liver disease [46], increased age [45], and obesity [47]. The primary active metabolite of diazepam, desmethyldiazepam, has an extremely long elimination half-life (41–139 hours) [48, 49]. The administration of diazepam in combination with cimetidine [50], an hepatic enzyme inhibitor,

30   Introduction

Diazepam

Fig. 3-2. Structural formula of diazepam.

produces a decrease in the plasma clearance of diazepam, and its hypnotic effects are extended. The administration of heparin produces similar effects as a result of a significant increase in the free (active) plasma diazepam level [51].

Cardiovascular Effects
Anesthetic induction with diazepam is usually characterized by hemodynamic stability. Neither the dose nor the speed of injection influences the hemodynamic effects of induction with diazepam [52]. In patients with CAD, when diazepam was administered in a dose of either 0.1 mg/kg [53] or 0.5 mg/kg [54], the decreases in MAP (7 and 18%, respectively) were not significantly different. Filling pressures and cardiac index were unchanged [54–57]. Likewise, there were no significant changes in heart rate (HR), left ventricular stroke work index (LVSWI), and SVR [54–56, 58, 59].

In patients with valvular heart disease, the hemodynamic changes are also mild. In a study of 60 patients with valvular heart disease, a threefold difference in dose caused similar changes in mean blood pressure and heart rate [60]. Heart rate has been reported to decrease 9 percent [58], increase 10 percent, or remain unchanged [56, 60] after diazepam (0.3–0.4 mg/kg). Mean arterial pressure was either unchanged [56, 61] or decreased (15–19%) [58, 60]. There was no change in the cardiac index [56, 58].

Diazepam has been described as having a nitroglycerin-like effect. Côté and associates [53] reported that, in patients with ischemic heart dis-

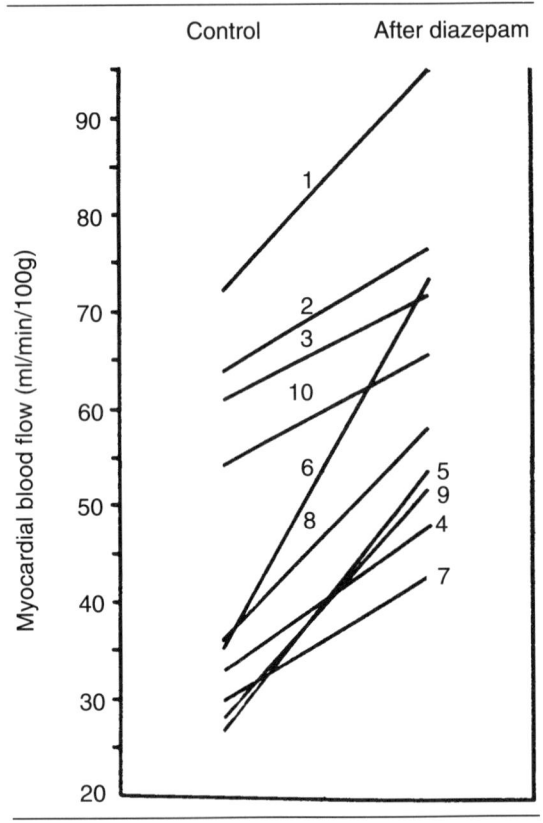

Fig. 3-3. Myocardial blood flow before and after diazepam. (Reprinted with permission from H Ikram, AP Rubin, and RF Jewkes. Effect of diazepam on myocardial blood flow of patients with and without coronary artery disease. *Br Heart J* 35:626–630, 1973.)

ease, 0.1 mg/kg diazepam produced a significant reduction in left ventricular end diastolic pressure (LVEDP) without change in coronary blood flow and cardiac index despite a decrease in systemic perfusion pressure. Diazepam, like nitroglycerin, appears to have peripheral arterial and venous effects [62]. A 73 percent increase in coronary blood flow has been reported in patients with ischemic heart disease who were given diazepam, 0.1 mg/kg [63] (Fig. 3-3). Administration of diazepam can produce a significant reduction in total myocardial oxygen consumption [53].

Diazepam has negligible effects on myocardial contractility [64] and can be used in the presence of poor ventricular function. However, it

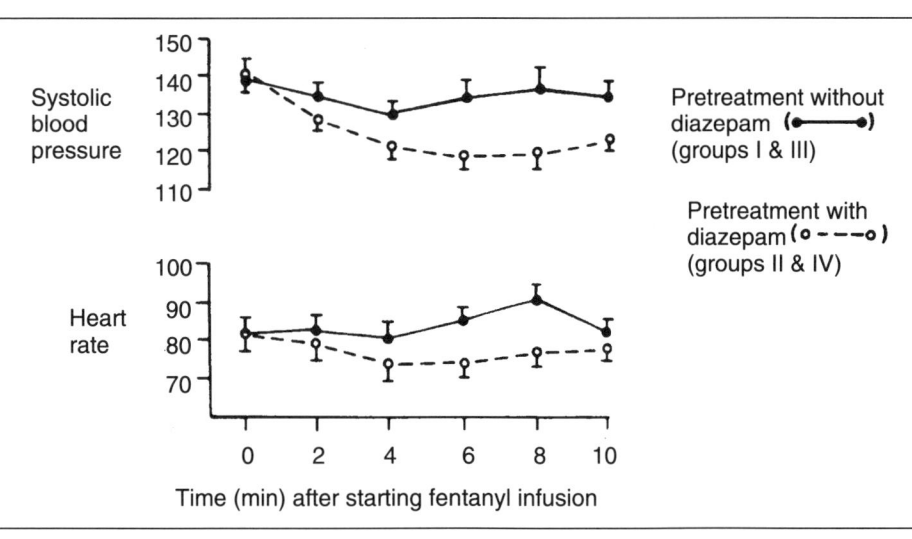

Fig. 3-4. Diazepam pretreatment (groups II and IV) before fentanyl (30 μg/kg) over 5 minutes caused significantly lower systolic blood pressures ($p = .04$) and heart rates ($p = .05$) when compared to groups I and III without diazepam pretreatment. (Reprinted with permission from the International Anesthesia Research Society. From PL Bailey, J Wilbrink, TH Stanley, et al., Anesthetic induction with fentanyl. *Anesth Analg* 64:48–53, 1985.)

has been shown to have more cardiovascular depressant effects in patients with elevated LVEDP (>15 mm Hg) and in patients with decreased ejection fractions (<38%) [65].

In a large series of American Society of Anesthesiologists (ASA) physical status III and IV patients undergoing noncardiac surgery, cardiac output and blood pressure were maintained after diazepam induction (0.2 mg/kg), in contrast to thiopental (2.0 mg/kg) [66, 67]. Of patients receiving thiopental, 85 percent sustained a 15 percent or greater fall in cardiac output, whereas fewer than 1 percent of patients in the diazepam group had a similar decrease [67]. In patients with constrictive pericarditis, hypovolemia, or cardiac tamponade, diazepam may cause significant hypotension and reductions in cardiac output [68], presumably secondary to vasodilation and reduced cardiac filling.

Although diazepam can be used safely with many anesthetic agents, the potential for hemodynamic depression exists when it is combined with opioids (Fig. 3-4). In one study diazepam, 0.25 to 0.35 mg/kg, was administered to patients with ischemic heart disease anesthetized with morphine, 3 mg/kg. Heart rate, pulmonary artery pressure (PAP), pulmonary capillary wedge pressure (PCWP), pulmonary vascular resistance (PVR), and SVR remained unchanged; however, MAP decreased from 84 to 73 mm Hg and cardiac index decreased from 2.91 to 2.36 liters/min/m^2 [69]. A greater depressant effect was seen when diazepam was combined with fentanyl. When patients with mitral valve disease who were anesthetized with fentanyl (50 μg/kg) were given diazepam (10 mg), decreases were seen in cardiac output (21%), mean blood pressure (10%), and stroke volume (17%), without change in heart rate [70, 71]. Diazepam also produces vasodilation and hypotension when combined with sufentanil or alfentanil [72]. A possible mechanism is a reduction in sympathetic tone when the drugs are used together. The addition of diazepam to nitrous oxide (N$_2$O) 50 percent in oxygen produces a greater decrease in MAP and LVSWI than is seen with N$_2$O in oxygen alone [54, 59] (Fig. 3-5).

Midazolam

Midazolam is a water-soluble benzodiazepine with a rapid onset and short duration of action (Fig. 3-6). It is biotransformed in the liver to four inactive me-

Fig. 3-5. Hemodynamic response (mean ± SDM) of 10 patients anesthetized with diazepam and oxygen and 10 patients anesthetized with diazepam and N_2O/O_2 (50:50). C = control; A = anesthesia induction; I = intubation; I + 5 = intubation plus 5 minutes; PAO = pulmonary artery occluded pressure; LVSW = left ventricular stroke work; CI = cardiac index. (Reprinted with permission from JG Reves, P Flezzani, and I Kissin. In JA Kaplan (ed), *Cardiac Anesthesia* (2nd ed), Vol. 1. Philadelphia: Saunders, 1987, P. 125.)

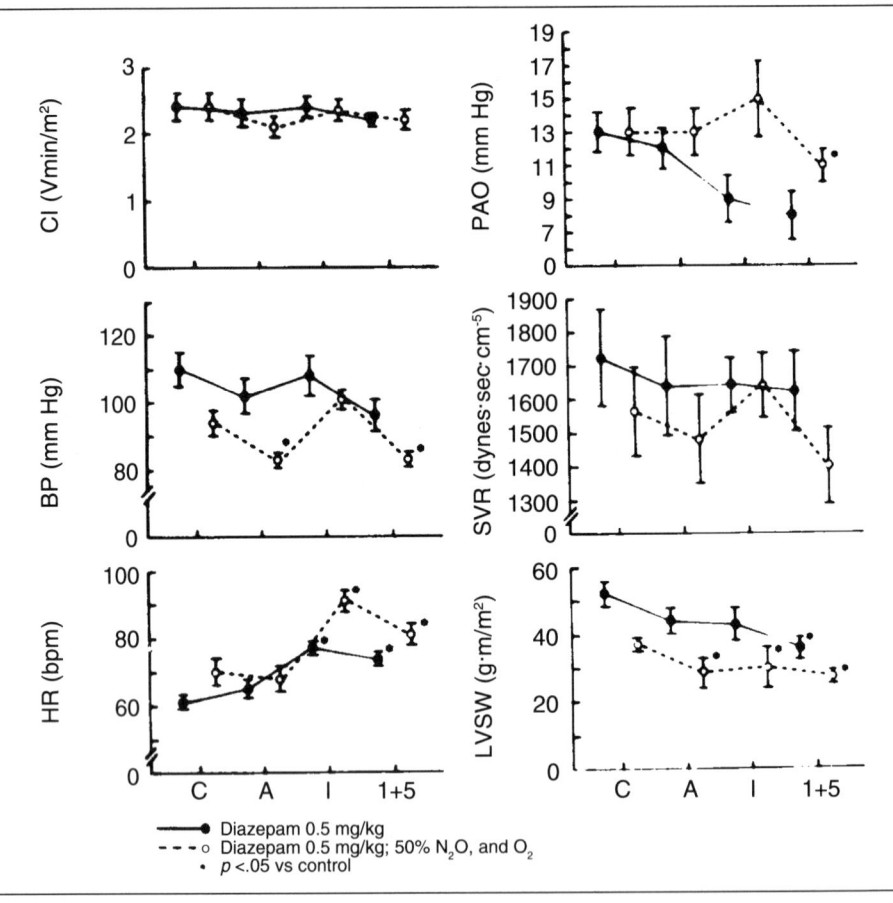

Fig. 3-6. Structural formula of midazolam.

tabolites [73]. The plasma clearance is significantly faster than for diazepam. The $t^{1/2}\alpha$ is 6 to 15 minutes [74, 75]. The $t^{1/2}\beta$ is approximately 2 hours [74–76], although this is prolonged in older patients [77, 78].

Cardiovascular Effects

The standard induction dose of midazolam (0.2 mg/kg) generally causes only minor hemodynamic

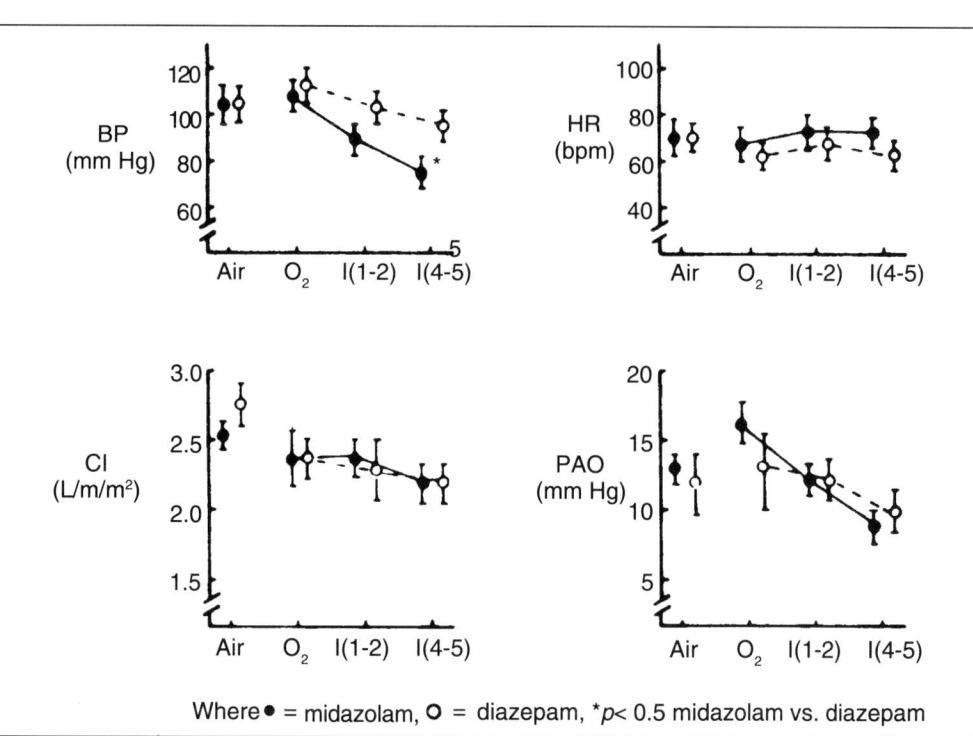

Fig. 3-7. Hemodynamic variables in patients with ischemic heart disease anesthetized with midazolam (0.2 mg/kg IV) and diazepam (0.5 mg/kg IV). HR = heart rate; BP = mean blood pressure; CI = cardiac index; PAO = pulmonary artery occluded pressure. Determinations were made breathing room air (air), breathing 100% oxygen (O_2), 1 to 2 minutes after induction [I(1−2)], and 4 to 5 minutes after induction [I(4−5)]. (Reprinted with permission from JG Reves, P Flezzani, and I Kissin. In JA Kaplan (ed), *Cardiac Anesthesia* (2nd ed), Vol. 1. Philadelphia: Saunders, 1987. P. 125.)

changes [54, 79] (Fig. 3-7). Mean arterial pressure may decrease (20%) and heart rate may increase (15%) [79]. Cardiac index, SVR, and PVR are unchanged [54, 79]. In patients with normal ventricular function, filling pressures are either unchanged or decreased [54, 79], but may be significantly decreased in patients with an elevated PCWP of 18 mm Hg or greater [79]. In a group of patients with stable coronary artery disease and PCWP greater than 18 mm Hg, anesthetic induction with midazolam (0.2 mg/kg) caused a significant reduction of PCWP. The cardiac index and heart rate increased, and MAP, LVSWI, and SVR decreased. The decrease in SVR (40%) was approximately twice that observed in patients with PCWP of less than 17 mm Hg [79]. Decreases in LVSWI and stroke index (SI) [54, 79] may reflect either decreases in myocardial contractility or PCWP [54]. Coronary blood flow is reduced by 24 percent and myocardial oxygen consumption is reduced by 26 percent [80].

In patients with either ischemic or valvular heart disease, the induction of anesthesia with midazolam is associated with minimal changes in CI, HR, and MAP [81]. Cardiac output is maintained after midazolam, in contrast to thiopental, which causes it to decrease [82], but both agents produce an increase in heart rate and a decrease in blood pressure [81].

As with diazepam, the combination of midazolam and high-dose fentanyl may produce significant hypotension [71, 83]. There is significant venous pooling and decreases are seen both in systolic blood pressure and stroke index [83]. In contrast to diazepam, midazolam causes a decrease in cardiac index without a reduction in SVR. Coronary sinus blood flow and coronary perfusion pressure decrease without change in coronary vascular resistance [83]. In a study during cardiopulmonary bypass, diazepam, 0.3 mg/kg, but not midazolam, 0.2 mg/kg, caused a transient decrease in SVR, with greater venodilation after midazolam [84]. Hemodynamic changes are rarely seen with sedative doses of midazolam (0.05 mg/kg) [85].

KETAMINE

Ketamine is a phencyclidine derivative and the only member of its class in clinical use (Fig. 3-8). After administration of an anesthetizing dose (2 mg/kg), it undergoes rapid redistribution. The t½α is 17 to 46 minutes and the t½β is 2 to 4 hours [86]. Ketamine is metabolized by the hepatic microsomal enzyme system to four known metabolites, some of which are active [87]. The metabolites are then conjugated to glucuronide derivatives and excreted in the urine [88].

Central Nervous System Effects

Unlike most other induction agents, ketamine produces profound dose-related analgesia [89]. The anesthetized state has been described as *dissociative* [90], with many protective reflexes maintained. Ketamine increases $CMRO_2$, CBF, and ICP. Its use has been limited by the undesirable psychological reactions it produces on awakening, termed *emergence reactions* or *emergence delirium*. These can be most effectively attenuated with the concomitant use of benzodiazepines [91].

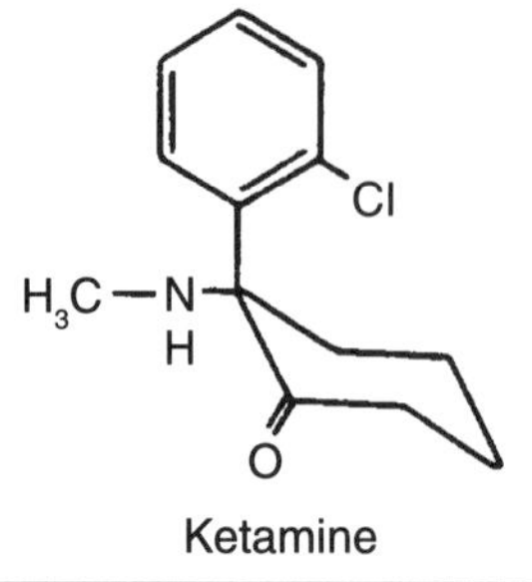

Respiratory Effects

Ketamine exerts minimal effects on the respiratory system [92]. It is a bronchial smooth-muscle relaxant [93, 94]. Increased salivation is seen.

Cardiovascular Effects

Ketamine is the only anesthetic drug that does not depress the cardiovascular system in vivo [90]. Rather, it appears to stimulate the circulatory system by a central mechanism of action [95–99]. Ketamine also causes the sympathoneuronal release of norepinephrine [100], inhibits intraneuronal uptake of catecholamines [101], and inhibits extraneuronal norepinephrine uptake [102]. In vitro, ketamine has been shown to have direct-acting negative inotropic effects that are overriden by the centrally mediated sympathetic responses [103, 104].

Ketamine's stimulatory effects are usually associated with increases in heart rate, blood pressure, and cardiac output, causing increased work and myocardial oxygen consumption. An appropriate increase in coronary blood flow has been demonstrated [105]. Ketamine increases both pulmonary and systemic vascular resistance. This effect is more pronounced on the pulmonary vascular bed in adults [106–109]. In children with congenital heart disease, this effect on PVR is minimized, while the effect on SVR is similar to that seen in adults (see Chaps. 17 and 18).

These hemodynamic changes do not appear to be dose related, and may not be seen with a second dose. On the contrary, a second dose may produce effects opposite to those of the first [110]. To block the hemodynamic effects, α- and β-adrenergic antagonists [111], vasodilators [105, 111], and the prior administration of benzodiazepines [56, 91] and volatile anesthetics [103] have been used. Ketamine is very useful in the child with cyanotic congenital heart disease, as it will frequently increase pulmonary blood flow secondary to its relative increase in SVR versus PVR.

Ketamine has been investigated as an induction agent in ASA physical status IV or V patients. Its safety has been demonstrated in hemodynamically

Fig. 3-8. Structural formula of ketamine.

unstable patients who require emergency operations [112, 113]. Most of the patients studied were hypovolemic, and despite this, blood pressure was maintained. The negative inotropic effects of ketamine may be unmasked when it is used in patients who have been severely ill for some time and who have depleted their catecholamine stores. Similarly, in the patient in whom sympathetic responses are blunted, or in the setting of deep anesthesia, ketamine can produce pronounced hemodynamic depression, particularly in the presence of halothane and enflurane [103]. A possible explanation is that the direct myocardial depressive effect is revealed when sympathetic activity normally produced by ketamine is blocked.

Because of its effects on HR, blood pressure, myocardial oxygen consumption, and myocardial work, ketamine should be used with great caution and hesitation in the patient with severe coronary disease, aortic stenosis, and mitral stenosis (see Chaps. 5–7).

ETOMIDATE

Etomidate is a carboxylated imidazole derivative (Fig. 3-9). The initial distribution half-life is 3 minutes and the elimination half-life ranges from 2.9 to 5.3 hours [114, 115]. In the liver it is hydrolyzed to an active metabolite [116].

Central Nervous System Effects

Etomidate is primarily a hypnotic agent, with a duration of action ranging from 5 to 15 minutes after an induction dose of 0.3 mg/kg [116, 117]. It has no analgesic activity. It reduces intraocular [118] and intracranial pressure, cerebral blood flow, and $CMRO_2$ without altering MAP [119]. The administration of etomidate is associated with a high incidence (10–35%) of myoclonic movements [120], unless an opioid is used before induction [121]. These movements are not associated with seizure activity on the EEG [121]. Etomidate has, however, been associated with grand mal seizures in patients with a history of epilepsy [122].

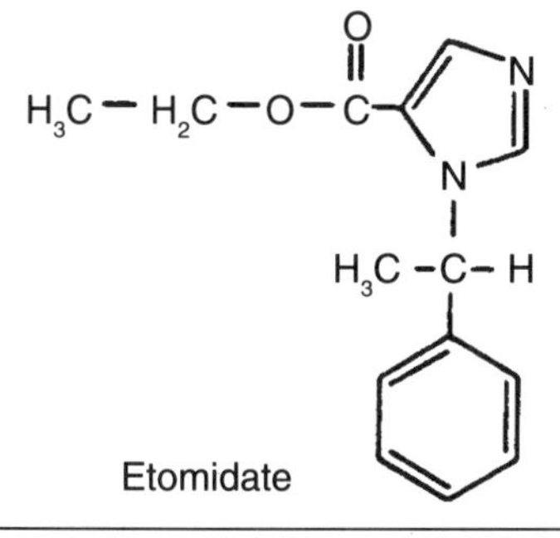

Respiratory Effects

Etomidate has minimal effect on ventilation [123].

Endocrine Effects

Etomidate infusions and single injections have been reported to suppress adrenocortical function directly. It suppresses cortisol production by blocking 11-β-hydroxylase [124–126]. Cortisol levels can be restored to normal with vitamin C supplementation [127].

Cardiovascular Effects

Compared with other anesthetic agents, induction with etomidate (0.3 mg/kg) causes the least change in hemodynamic variables [33, 128–131]. In normal patients or those with compensated ischemic heart disease, doses of 0.15 to 0.30 mg/kg do not cause significant changes in heart rate, contractility, preload, or afterload [22, 129, 131, 132]. In patients with hypovolemia, etomidate causes less hypotension than thiopental [133].

Although systemic blood pressure usually remains unchanged after induction [33, 128, 131], decreases of 10 to 19 percent may be seen in patients with valvular heart disease [128, 133, 134]. This is particularly true for patients with aortic and mitral valvular disease. They have been shown to have significant decreases in systolic and diastolic blood pressure (17–19%) [128, 133], PAP (11%) [133], PCWP (17%) [133], and SVR (17%). In these same patients, cardiac index either remained unchanged [128] or decreased 13 percent [133].

Etomidate alters the balance of myocardial oxygen supply and demand less than other intravenous anesthetics [128, 135]. The drug has been shown to

Fig. 3-9. Structural formula of etomidate.

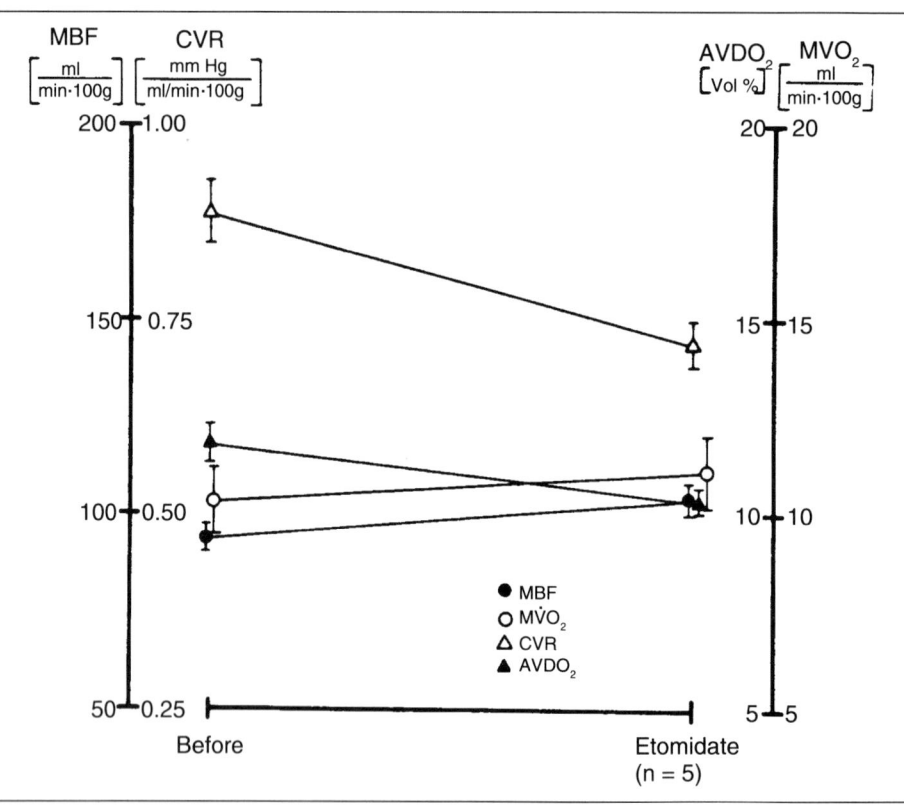

Fig. 3-10. The effect of 0.12 mg/kg/min etomidate on coronary hemodynamics and myocardial oxygen consumption in a healthy patient. MBF = myocardial blood flow; $M\dot{V}O_2$ = myocardial oxygen consumption; CVR = coronary vascular resistance; $AVDO_2$ = arteriovenous coronary oxygen difference. (Reprinted with permission from D Kettler, H Sonntag, U Donath, et al., Haemodynamics, myocardial mechanics, oxygen requirement, and oxygenation of the human heart during induction of anaesthesia with etomidate. *Anaesthesist* 23:116–121, 1974.)

decrease myocardial blood flow and oxygen consumption by 50 percent and increase coronary sinus blood oxygen saturation by 20 to 30 percent [135]. Kettler and associates [128] demonstrated a 19 percent increase in coronary blood flow with no change in myocardial oxygen consumption (Fig. 3-10). Etomidate has been described as having a mild nitroglycerin-like effect, as it decreases coronary vascular resistance by 19 percent without changing coronary perfusion pressure [128].

Administration of 66 percent nitrous oxide in oxygen does not alter the hemodynamic changes after induction with etomidate [130]. However, in cardiac patients anesthetized with a high-dose narcotic technique, etomidate has been shown to decrease CI (4–17%), HR (17–20%), SVR (14%), MAP (20%), and PAP (4–17%) [136, 137].

PROPOFOL

Propofol is an alkylphenol [138] (Fig. 3-11) with an initial distribution half-life of 2 to 8 minutes [138, 139] and an elimination half-life of 1 to 3 hours [140, 141]. In the liver it is conjugated to glucuronide and sulfate to produce inactive metabolites.

Central Nervous System Effects

Propofol is a hypnotic agent without analgesic properties. After an induction dose of 2.0 to 2.5 mg/kg, the hypnotic effect lasts for 5 to 10 minutes [142]. Propofol decreases ICP, $CMRO_2$ [143–145], and intraocular pressure (IOP) [146].

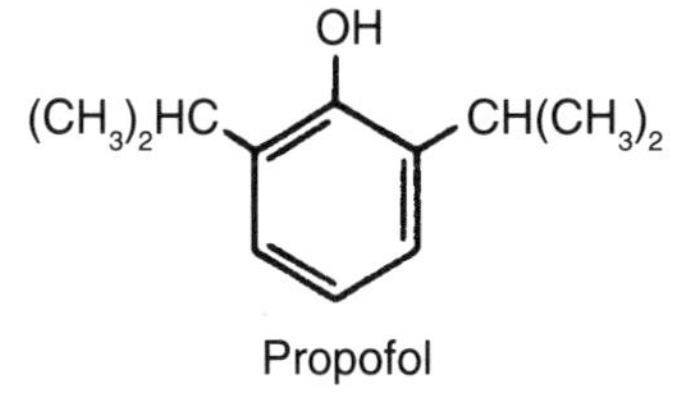

Fig. 3-11. Chemical structure of propofol.

Respiratory Effects

Apnea occurs after an induction dose of propofol, similar to that seen with the barbiturates [147–149]. The effect is greater in the presence of opioids [147].

Cardiovascular Effects

The most significant adverse cardiovascular effect produced by propofol is hypotension, which can be attenuated by slow injection. Induction with propofol combined with 67 percent nitrous oxide produces both myocardial depression [150] and vasodilatation (reducing cardiac preload) [151]. This suggests that cardiac output and arterial blood pressure can be preserved if the preload is maintained [152]. Plasma propofol concentrations have been correlated with a decrease in myocardial contractility without change in left ventricular afterload in an animal model [153]. It decreases systolic blood pressure by 20 to 35 percent, cardiac index by 11 to 29 percent, and systemic vascular resistance by 11 to 20 percent [135, 150, 151, 154–160]. Similar decreases are produced in MAP and diastolic blood pressure. LVSWI is also decreased by 30 percent [157].

Compared to the other induction agents, propofol produces a lesser degree of compensatory increase in heart rate, which may be the mechanism of hypotension [161]. Elderly patients develop more pronounced hypotension and require reduced dosages [162]. Transient falls in MAP of greater than 20 percent are also seen in the pediatric population [163].

In one series, after induction with propofol followed by continuous infusion, myocardial blood flow decreased 26 percent, myocardial oxygen consumption decreased 31 percent, and coronary vascular resistance increased 19 percent without a change in the arteriocoronary sinus oxygen content difference [164]. Myocardial lactate production, seen in a few patients, suggests the possible imbalance of regional myocardial oxygen supply-demand ratio. During propofol infusion, systolic blood pressure remains 20 to 30 percent below preinduction levels [155, 157]. SVR decreases 30 percent without change in cardiac index and stroke index [157].

In patients with impaired cardiac function, central venous pressure (CVP) decreased 16 to 29 percent and PCWP decreased 35 to 44 percent, with resultant reductions in cardiac index and MAP. SVR and PVR were unchanged in this study [159]. In patients with valvular heart disease, PAP and PCWP also decrease, suggesting a decrease in both preload and afterload [165].

OPIOIDS

The opioid class of drugs includes all agents, natural or synthetic, that have morphine-like qualities or bind at any of the several subspecies of opioid receptors with some agonist action [166]. The semisynthetic compounds are derivatives of morphine. Depending on their interactions at the various opioid receptors, opioids also can be divided into agonists, partial agonists, mixed agonist-antagonists, and antagonists (Tables 3-1 and 3-2).

Table 3-1. Effects of opioid receptors

Mu	Kappa	Sigma
Supraspinal analgesia	Spinal analgesia	Dysphoria
Respiratory depression	Respiratory depression	Hallucinations
Euphoria	Sedation	Vasomotor stimulation
Physical dependence	Miosis	Tachypnea
Bradycardia		Tachycardia
Miosis		Mydriasis
Hypothermia		
Tolerance		

Source: Modified with permission from CC Hug, Jr, *Semin Anesth* 1:14, 1982.

Table 3-2. Interactions of morphine and morphine-like drugs with opioid receptors

Drug	Receptor types		
	Mu	Kappa	Sigma
Morphine	↑	↑	0
Buprenorphine	±↑	—	0
Nalorphine	↓	±↑	↑
Pentazocine	↓	↑	↑
Butorphanol	0	↑	↑
Nalbuphine	±↑/↓	↑	↑
Naloxone	±↑/↓	↓	↓

↑ = agonist; ±↑ = partial agonist; ↓ = antagonist; 0 = no interaction.
Source: Modified with permission from CC Hug, Jr, *Semin Anesth* 1:14, 1982.

Opioids have been used during surgical anesthesia since the 1800s, but fell into disfavor following a series of postoperative deaths, probably due to respiratory depression [167]. In the 1940s, with the advent of controlled ventilation, opioids again came into use, combined with N_2O and curare.

Opioid Receptors

The opioid receptor was first described in nervous tissue in 1973 [168, 169]. All opioids are not only structurally similar, but also exhibit stereospecificity. Receptors are found in the brainstem within the periaqueductal gray matter and the solitary nuclei that receive input from the vagus and glossopharyngeal nerves. They are also found in the area postrema, which contains the chemoreceptor trigger zone; in the amygdala; and in the spinal cord in the substantia gelatinosa.

The effect produced by opioids is determined by the specific receptor to which it binds (see Tables 3-1 and 3-2). Interaction with mu receptors produces supraspinal analgesia, respiratory depression, bradycardia, miosis, hypothermia, physical dependence, and tolerance. The μ_1 receptor mediates analgesia, whereas μ_2 or delta receptors mediate respiratory depression [166, 170, 171]. The kappa receptor produces spinal analgesia, miosis, and sedation. Sigma receptors mediate dysphoric effects, hallucinations, tachypnea, tachycardia, and mydriasis. Delta and epsilon receptors have also been described [172, 173], and are thought to be specific for leucine-enkephalin and β-endorphin, respectively. A number of endogenous opioid receptor ligands have been identified, but are not discussed further in this chapter.

Central Nervous System Effects

Opioids are given primarily for analgesia, mediated by receptors in the spinal cord and brain. They are mood-altering drugs, and may produce drowsiness or sleep. Amnesia does not occur without unconsciousness [174, 175]. Most mu and kappa agonists produce miosis via excitation of the autonomic segment of the nucleus of the oculomotor nerve [166]. These drugs also have a direct suppressing effect on the cough center in the medulla [166].

At sufficiently high doses, all opioids will produce excitatory or convulsive motor activity [166, 176]. For example, very large doses of meperidine (>5 mg/kg) may induce seizures. The other opioids have been associated with myoclonic and myotonic seizure-like movements without EEG evidence of cortical seizure activity.

Opioids stimulate the chemoreceptor trigger zone producing nausea and vomiting [166]. However, at higher "anesthetic" doses, nausea is less common due to depression of the vomiting center. Opioids modestly decrease cerebral metabolic rate and intracranial pressure (10–25%). In combination with N_2O, they also cause cerebral vasoconstriction and decrease cerebral blood flow [176].

Respiratory Effects

All μ-receptor–stimulating opioids produce dose-dependent respiratory depression. They act directly on the brainstem respiratory centers and decrease the response to increases in arterial carbon dioxide tension ($PaCO_2$) [177, 178]. Both the apneic threshold and resting end-tidal $PaCO_2$ are increased by opioid administration. They also decrease hypoxic ventilatory drive [179]. At lower doses they tend to decrease respiratory rate without affecting tidal volume. When depression of the pontine and medullary centers occurs, irregular or periodic breathing may be seen [166].

Reversal of Respiratory Depression

Opioid-antagonist drugs will reverse both the respiratory depression and analgesia induced by opioid agonists. The use of naloxone has been associated with severe hypertension, tachycardia, and pulmonary edema [180, 181]. An increase of up to 60 percent in coronary blood flow and myocardial oxygen consumption has been demonstrated in animal studies [182]. Because of the short half-life of naloxone, recurrence of respiratory depression may be seen after reversal of a dense opioid state.

Hepatorenal and Gastrointestinal Effects

Opioids increase ureteral and detrusor muscle tone, which may produce urinary retention [183]. All opioid agonists may increase biliary duct pressure and sphincter of Oddi tone (choledochoduodenal sphincter) [184–186]. Morphine can also produce spasm of the sphincter of Oddi, causing a rise of pressure in the biliary tract and symptoms of biliary colic [187]. This effect can be reversed with naloxone [188] or glucagon [189], but not with atropine [189, 190]. There is no evidence, however, that opioids are directly hepatotoxic. Opioids decrease gastrointestinal tract motility [166], lower esophageal sphincter tone [191], and may delay gastric emptying for up to 12 hours, via central and peripheral mechanisms [192]. These effects can be reversed by naloxone [193].

Neuromuscular Junction and Skeletal Muscle Effects

All opioids can produce rigidity of skeletal muscles, particularly in the thorax and abdomen. This action does not appear to be mediated at the neuromuscular junctions or directly on skeletal muscle itself [194] since the rigidity can be blocked by neuromuscular blocking agents [195]. Rapid infusion of the drug [196] or the addition of nitrous oxide [197, 198] increases the incidence and severity of rigidity. It is decreased by slower administration, use of potent inhalational agents or thiopental, or pretreatment with small doses of nondepolarizing muscle relaxants [176]. Rigidity of the thoracic muscles can decrease pulmonary compliance and functional residual capacity, interfere with adequate ventilation, and cause an increase in ICP [195, 199, 200]. Opioid-induced rigidity also elevates pulmonary vascular resistance and pulmonary artery and central venous pressures [199, 201]. Succinylcholine or nondepolarizing muscle relaxants can be used to terminate the rigidity [195, 196, 202].

Pharmacokinetics and Pharmacodynamics

Morphine

Morphine (Fig. 3-12A) has an initial rapid distribution phase half-life of 1.2 to 2.5 minutes [203–205], and a second slower distribution t½ of 9.0 to 13.3 minutes. The terminal elimination half-life for morphine is 1.7 to 2.2 hours [204, 205]. Morphine is cleared from the body via hepatic metabolism to morphine-glucuronide and other metabolites that are excreted by the kidneys.

Meperidine

Meperidine (Fig. 3-12B) has a rapid distribution t½ of 4 to 17 minutes [206, 207] and an elimination half-life of 4 to 6 hours. In the liver, it is metabolized to normeperidine, meperidinic acid, and normeperidinic acid [208]. Normeperidine is an active metabolite, with twice the convulsive properties and half the analgesic effect of meperidine [208].

Fentanyl

The rapid distribution half-life for fentanyl (Fig. 3-12C) is 1.4 to 1.7 minutes, whereas the slower distribution phase is 13 to 28 minutes [209, 210]. The elimination half-life is 3.1 to 4.4 hours [209–211]. Because of its extreme lipid solubility, fat acts as a storage site for fentanyl. As the plasma concentration of fentanyl decreases following the initial rapid distribution, the fat acts as a reservoir to maintain plasma concentration, slowly releasing the fentanyl back into the plasma. This produces the relatively prolonged elimination half-life [209–211]. Fentanyl is biotransformed in the liver and the metabolites are excreted by the kidney [212].

Sufentanil

Although it is 5 to 10 times more potent than fentanyl, sufentanil (Fig. 3-12D) has pharmacokinet-

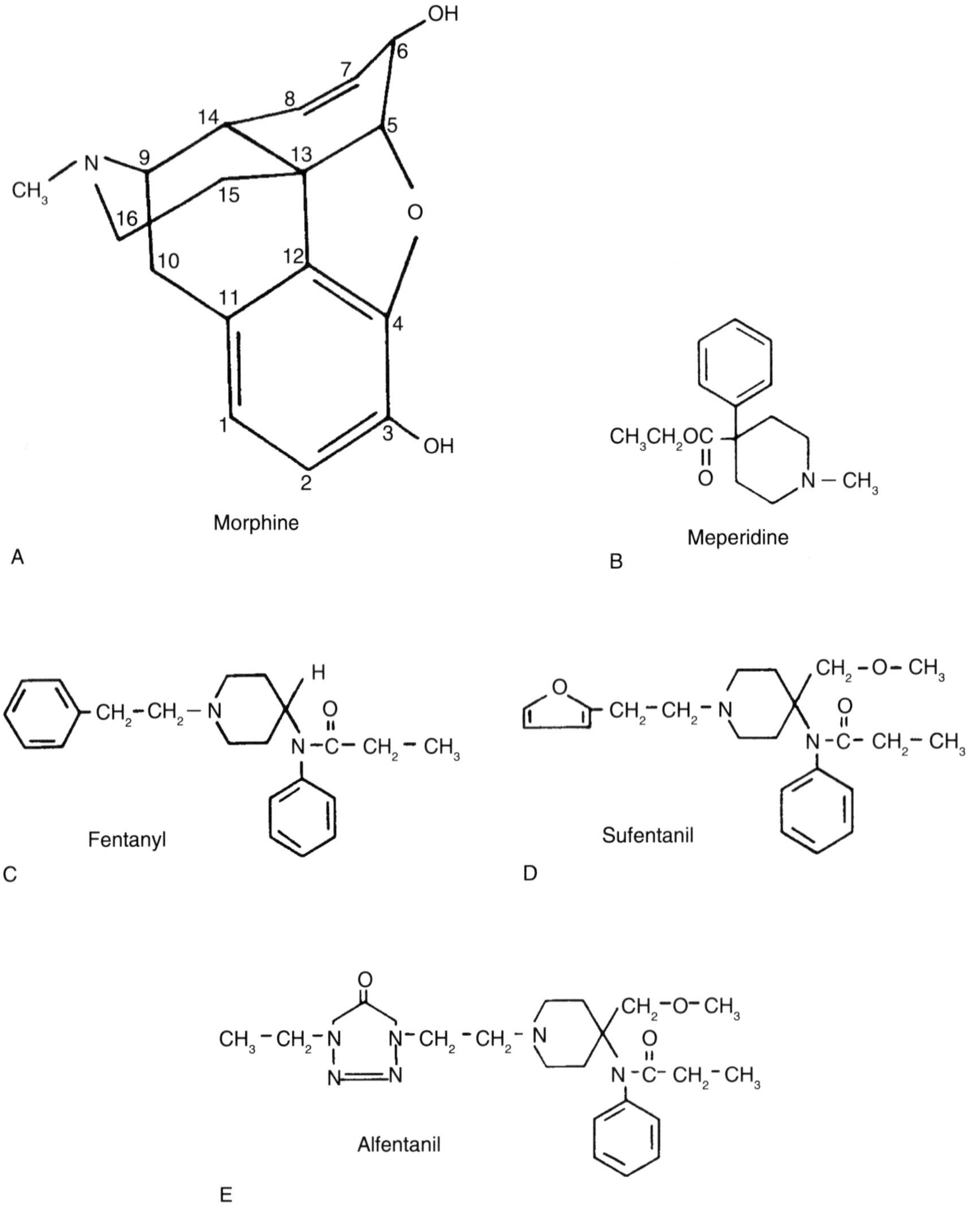

40 Introduction

Fig. 3-12. Chemical structures of opioid agonists.

ics that are similar to those of fentanyl. The rapid distribution half-life is 1.4 minutes while the slower distribution phase is 17.7 minutes. The elimination half-life is 2.7 hours [213].

Alfentanil

Alfentanil (Fig. 3-12E) is one fifth to one third as potent as fentanyl. The initial rapid distribution half-life is 1.0 to 3.5 minutes [214, 215]. The slower distribution half-life is 8.2 to 16.8 minutes [214, 215]. The terminal elimination half-life varies between 1.2 and 1.7 hours [214, 215].

Cardiovascular Effects

High-dose opioids are often chosen as the primary anesthetic technique for patients in whom myocardial depression, which may be produced by the potent inhalational agents, would not be well tolerated [216]. In large doses, opioids have been shown to suppress the hormonal and metabolic responses to surgery.

Most opioids lower sympathetic tone and enhance parasympathetic tone. Therefore, unless countered by anticholinergic or sympathetic effects (intrinsic or extrinsic), opioids can produce hypotension. Most susceptible are patients dependent on a high sympathetic tone or exogenous catecholamines for maintenance of cardiovascular function.

Although a decrease in blood pressure can occur after administration of small doses of *morphine* (5–10 mg), the decrease is much more profound after anesthetic doses (1–4 mg/kg) or rapid administration [174, 217, 218]. Morphine (1 mg/kg) was shown to increase plasma histamine, producing an increase in cardiac index and peripheral arteriolar and venous dilation, and a decrease in arterial blood pressure and SVR [219] (Table 3-3). Histamine may also cause sympathoadrenal activation and positive inotropic and chronotropic actions. These effects can be attenuated by pretreatment with both H_1- and H_2-blockers [220–222].

Morphine is also reported to have a direct action on vascular smooth muscle [219, 223, 224]. The resulting venodilation necessitates an increase in fluid administration in order to maintain adequate preload [225, 226]. Compared to patients given halothane, those anesthetized with morphine have increased fluid and blood requirements during and after surgery [226] (Table 3-4).

Morphine (2 mg/kg) in healthy volunteers has been shown to prolong the preejection period, an estimate of isovolumetric cardiac contractility [227, 228]. In clinically used doses, morphine (0.5–3.0 mg/kg) [216] or fentanyl (50–100 µg/kg) [229] had no deleterious effects on myocardial function. Higher doses of morphine (3 mg/kg) can activate the sympathoadrenal system, which may counteract some myocardial depressant effects

Table 3-3. Correlation of histamine release and hemodynamic response during administration of morphine[a]

Period	BP (mm Hg)	Diastolic BP (mm Hg)	CI (liters/min/m^2)	HR (bpm)	SVR (mm Hg/liters per min)	Venous histamine (pg/ml)
Control	88 ± 4	71 ± 3	2.4 ± 0.2	57 ± 2	15.5 ± 1	880 ± 163
Placebo	85 ± 3	67 ± 2	2.6 ± 0.1	57 ± 2	14.8 ± 1	657 ± 98
One third in	79 ± 5	61 ± 4[b]	2.8 ± 0.1[b]	58 ± 2	12.2 ± 1[b]	2,467 ± 1,208[b]
2 min after	61 ± 4[c]	45 ± 4[c]	3.0 ± 0.2[b]	59 ± 3	9.0 ± 1[c]	7,437 ± 2,684[c]
5 min after	73 ± 8	59 ± 7[c]	2.9 ± 0.3	64 ± 4	11.5 ± 1[c]	4,980 ± 1,681[c]
10 min after	74 ± 5	57 ± 5[c]	2.7 ± 0.2	59 ± 4	12.7 ± 1[c]	3,307 ± 1,090[c]

[a] Values are means ± standard error.
[b] $p < .05$ compared with control.
[c] $p < .01$ compared with control.
Source: Reprinted with permission from J Moss and CE Roscow, Histamine release by narcotics and muscle relaxants in humans. Anesthesiology 59:330–339, 1983.

Table 3-4. Blood requirements in patients anesthetized with morphine (1–4 mg/kg) plus oxygen or halothane (0.1–1.5%) plus 30% N_2O in oxygen comparison[a]

		Mean blood requirements (ml)	
Pathology	Anesthetic	Intraoperative	Postoperative
Aortic valvular disease	Morphine	2,800[b]	1,652[b]
	Halothane	1,010	757
Coronary artery disease	Morphine	2,705[b]	1,417[b]
	Halothane	1,750	722

[a]Study included 61 patients undergoing aortic valve replacement or coronary artery bypass grafting.
[b]$p < .001$, morphine group compared with halothane group.
Source: Modified with permission from TH Stanley, NH Gray, JH Isern-Amaral, and C Patton, Comparison of blood requirements during morphine and halothane anesthesia for open-heart surgery. *Anesthesiology* 41:34–38, 1974.

[230]. At unusually large concentrations (hundreds to thousands of times greater than used in clinical anesthesia), all opioids will produce direct depression of the myocardium [231–233].

Meperidine is the only opioid that has been shown to depress the myocardium directly at clinically relevant doses [231]. At doses as low as 2.0 to 2.5 mg/kg, meperidine may have a significant negative inotropic effect, producing decreases in cardiac output, arterial pressure, and peripheral resistance [176, 231, 234]. Anesthetic doses of meperidine (>10 mg/kg) markedly decrease cardiac output [234]. The tachycardia produced by meperidine may be a vagolytic effect as a result of its structural similarity to atropine, due to histamine release, or as a reflex response to hypotension. Meperidine causes histamine release more frequently than do the other opioids, the magnitude of which is correlated with the degree of hypotension [221] and a reflex increase in heart rate via its positive chronotropic effects and sympathoadrenal activation.

Fentanyl, at all dose ranges (2–100 μg/kg), seldom causes significant decreases in blood pressure, even in patients with poor ventricular function [70, 235–239]. This cardiovascular stability may be related to the lack of histamine release [219] (Fig. 3-13). Fentanyl has little or no effect on myocardial contractility [70, 219, 236, 237]. Even after anesthetic doses of fentanyl, no change is seen in arterial blood pressure, cardiac output, SVR, PVR, or PCWP [70, 219, 237–239]. If hypotension occurs it is probably secondary to the associated bradycardia and can be prevented or treated with anticholinergics, ephedrine, or pancuronium [195, 240]. Hypotension is more likely to be pronounced in patients with a high sympathetic tone. Flacke and associates [241] reported minimal hemodynamic changes after fentanyl with or without diazepam in dogs that had undergone a sympathectomy, and concluded that hypotension associated with fentanyl was indirect in nature, mediated by a decrease in CNS sympathetic outflow. Fentanyl was shown to have minimal effect on coronary vasomotor tone [242, 243].

Sufentanil, in equipotent doses, causes hypotension with similar or greater frequency than fentanyl [244]. It does not increase plasma histamine, but does cause vagally mediated bradycardia [245]. Hypotension may be due to either enhanced parasympathetic tone or direct vascular smooth-muscle relaxation [246]. Sufentanil may impair myocardial function and depress systolic blood pressure more than fentanyl, particularly in patients with poor left ventricular function or high sympathetic tone [247].

Alfentanil, in moderate doses (160 μg/kg), causes little hemodynamic change in dogs. Transient cardiac stimulation (increased left ventricular contractility, heart rate, cardiac output, PVR, and SVR) is seen at very large doses (5 mg/kg) [176]. Another study in dogs produced similar results at lower doses (200 μg/kg) [248, 249]. Others have found alfentanil to cause similar decreases in heart

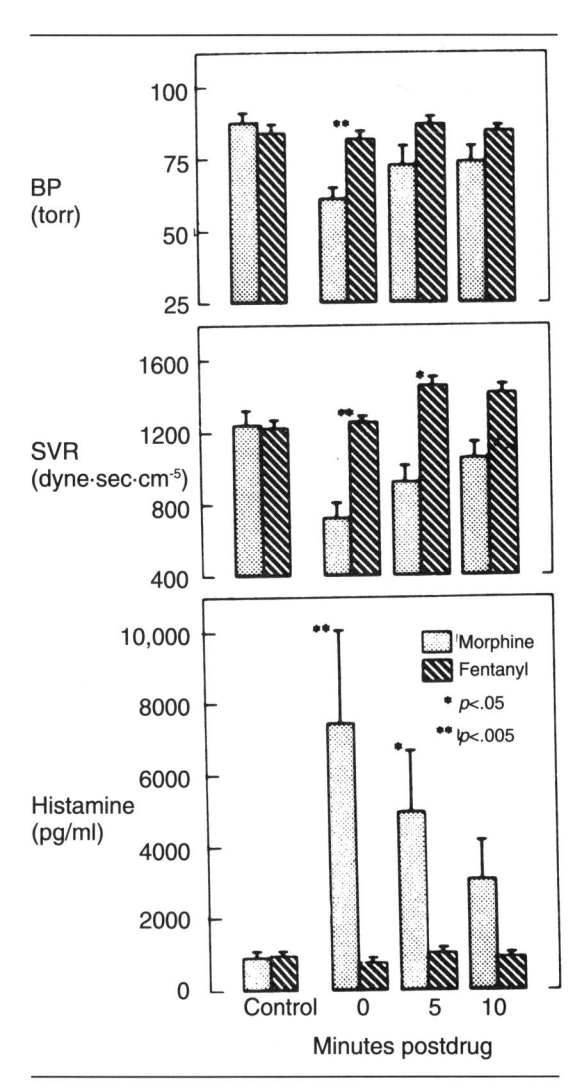

Fig. 3-13. Correlation between histamine release and decline in blood pressure and systemic vascular resistance caused by morphine, but not fentanyl. (Reprinted with permission from CE Roscow, J Moss, DM Philbin, and JJ Savarese. Histamine release during morphine and fentanyl anesthesia. *Anesthesiology* 56:93–96, 1982.)

rate, blood pressure, and cardiac index as fentanyl [250]. Alfentanil has also been shown to produce a less desirable hemodynamic profile (more hypotension and myocardial ischemia) than fentanyl or sufentanil in patients undergoing coronary artery bypass grafting [247, 251–254].

Heart Rate

Except for meperidine, all mu-receptor–stimulating opioid analgesics produce a decrease in heart rate. Subsequent doses of fentanyl cause less bradycardia than the initial dose [255] or when nitrous oxide is used [256], possibly because of the sympathomimetic effects of N_2O [257]. The degree of bradycardia may be dose dependent [258] or related to the speed of injection [255, 259]. It may be attenuated by the use of atropine, glycopyrrolate [202, 255, 259, 260], or pancuronium [261]. The mechanism of fentanyl-induced bradycardia is thought to be the stimulation of the central vagal nucleus [258, 262]. It may be prevented by bilateral vagotomy [258] or vagal block with atropine [255]. Asystole may follow opioid-induced bradycardia [263–265], often appearing during laryngoscopy and intubation. This is more common with sufentanil and alfentanil.

Drug Interactions

Increasing concentrations of opioids produce a progressive decrease in the minimum alveolar concentration (MAC) of the inhalational agents [266, 267]. Nitrous oxide can depress myocardial contractility [268], especially when combined with opioids [235, 255, 269–271]. These effects appear to be primarily caused by N_2O [272, 273] (see Chap. 2).

The addition of small doses of benzodiazepines to large doses of opioids occasionally causes a fall in blood pressure, SVR, and cardiac output [69, 70]. These effects are accompanied by decreased epinephrine and norepinephrine levels and unchanged plasma histamine levels. This may also occur when opioids are added to benzodiazepines. However, using exponentially declining infusions of lorazepam plus fentanyl in patients with CAD, a greater incidence of hypotension and bradycardia has been seen when the opioid is added to the benzodiazepine infusion, as opposed to the reverse order [274]. The hemodynamic depression may be attenuated with aggressive fluid administration [275]. When lower doses of sufentanil were combined with midazolam in patients with CAD, hemodynamic stability was maintained [276].

The combination of meperidine and monoamine oxidase inhibitors can cause agitation, labile blood pressure, hyperthermia, rigidity, convulsions, respiratory depression, hypotension, coma, and death.

REFERENCES

1. Olsen, RW. Barbiturates. *Int Anesthesiol Clin* 26: 254–261, 1988.
2. Price, HL. A dynamic concept of the distribution of thiopental in the human body. *Anesthesiology* 21: 40–45, 1960.
3. Albrecht, RF, Miletich, DJ, Rosenberg, R, et al. Cerebral blood flow and metabolic changes from induction to onset of anesthesia with halothane or pentobarbital. *Anesthesiology* 47:252–256, 1977.
4. Gumpert, J, and Paul, R. Activation of the electroencephalogram with intravenous Brietal (methohexitone): The findings in 100 cases. *J Neurol Neurosurg Psychiatry* 34:646–648, 1971.
5. Todd, MM, Drummond, JC, and U, HS. The hemodynamic consequences of high-dose methohexital anesthesia in humans. *Anesthesiology* 61:495–501, 1984.
6. Joshi, C, and Bruce, DL. Thiopental and succinylcholine action on intraocular pressure. *Anesth Analg* 54:471, 1975.
7. Hirshman, CA, McCullough, RE, Cohen, PJ, et al. Hypoxic ventilatory drive in dogs during thiopental, ketamine, or pentobarbital anesthesia. *Anesthesiology* 43:628–634, 1975.
8. Remmer, H. The role of the liver in drug metabolism. *Am J Med* 49:617–629, 1970.
9. Morgan, DJ, Blackman, GL, Paull, JD, et al. Pharmacokinetics and plasma binding of thiopental. I: Studies in surgical patients. *Anesthesiology* 54:468–473, 1981.
10. Christensen, JH, Andreasen, F, and Jansen, JA. Influence of age and sex on the pharmacokinetics of thiopentone. *Br J Anaesth* 53:1189–1195, 1981.
11. Christensen, JH, Andreasen, F, and Jansen, JA. Pharmacokinetics and pharmacodynamics of thiopentone. A comparison between young and elderly patients. *Anaesthesia* 37:398–404, 1982.
12. Sear, JW, Cooper, GM, and Kumar, V. The effect of age on recovery. A comparison of the kinetics of thiopentone and Althesin. *Anaesthesia* 38:1158–1161, 1983.
13. Jung, D, Mayersohn, M, Perrier, D, et al. Thiopental disposition in lean and obese patients undergoing surgery. *Anesthesiology* 56:269–274, 1982.
14. Eckstein, JW, Hamilton, WK, and McCammond, JM. The effect of thiopental on peripheral venous tone. *Anesthesiology* 22:525–528, 1961.
15. Flickinger, H, Fraimow, W, Cathcart, RT, et al. Effect of thiopental induction on cardiac output in man. *Anesth Analg* 40:693–700, 1961.
16. Frankl, WS, and Poole-Wilson, PA. Effects of thiopental on tension development, action potential, and exchange of calcium and potassium in rabbit ventricular myocardium. *J Cardiovasc Pharmacol* 3: 554–565, 1981.
17. Kissin, I, Motomura, S, Aultman, DF, et al. Inotropic and anesthetic potencies of etomidate and thiopental in dogs. *Anesth Analg* 62:961–965, 1983.
18. Komai, H, and Rusy, BF. Differences in myocardial depressant action of thiopental and halothane. *Anesth Analg* 63:313–318, 1984.
19. Blanck, TJJ, and Stevenson, RL. Thiopental does not alter Ca^{2+} uptake by cardiac sarcoplasmic reticulum. *Anesth Analg* 67:346–348, 1988.
20. Filner, BE, and Karliner, JS. Alteration of normal left ventricular performance by general anesthesia. *Anesthesiology* 45:610–621, 1976.
21. Reiz, S, Balfors, E, Friedman, A, et al. Effects of thiopentone on cardiac performance, coronary hemodynamics, and myocardial oxygen consumption in chronic ischemic heart disease. *Acta Anaesthesiol Scand* 25:103–110, 1981.
22. Tarabadkar, S, Kopriva, CJ, Sreenivasan, N, et al. Hemodynamic impact of induction in patients with decreased cardiac reserve. *Anesthesiology* 53:S43, 1980.
23. Lyons, SM, and Clarke, RSJ. A comparison of different drugs for anaesthesia in cardiac surgical patients. *Br J Anaesth* 44:575–582, 1972.
24. Seltzer, JL, Gerson, JI, and Allen, FB. Comparison of the cardiovascular effects of bolus v. incremental administration of thiopentone. *Br J Anaesth* 52: 527–530, 1980.
25. Sonntag, H, Hellberg, K, Schenk, HD, et al. Effects of thiopental (Trapanal) on coronary blood flow and myocardial metabolism in man. *Acta Anaesthesiol Scand* 19:69–78, 1975.
26. Tarnow, J, Hess, W, and Klein, W. Etomidate, alfathesin, and thiopentone as induction agents for coronary artery surgery. *Can Anaesth Soc J* 27:338–344, 1980.
27. Milocco, I, Lof, BA, William-Olsson, G, et al. Haemodynamic stability during anaesthesia induction and sternotomy in patients with ischaemic heart disease. *Acta Anaesthesiol Scand* 29:465–473, 1985.
28. Pedersen, T, Engbaek, J, Klausen, NO, et al. Effects of low-dose ketamine and thiopentone on cardiac

performance and myocardial oxygen balance in high risk patients. *Acta Anaesthesiol Scand* 26:235–239, 1982.
29. Graves, CL. Management of general anesthesia during hemorrhage. *Int Anesthesiol Clin* 12:1–49, 1974.
30. Prys-Roberts, C. Cardiovascular and ventilatory effects of intravenous anaesthetics. *Clin Anaesthesiol* 2:203–221, 1984.
31. Fischler, M, Dubois, C, Brodaty, D, et al. Circulatory responses to thiopentone and tracheal intubation in patients with coronary artery disease. *Br J Anaesth* 57:493–496, 1985.
32. Korttila, K, Linnoila, M, Ertama, P, et al. Recovery and simulated driving after intravenous anesthesia with thiopental, methohexital, propanidid, or alphadione. *Anesthesiology* 43:291–299, 1975.
33. Lamalle, D. Cardiovascular effects of various anesthetics in man. Four short-acting intravenous anesthetics: Althesin, etomidate, methohexital, and propanidid. *Acta Anaesthesiol Belg* 27S:208–224, 1976.
34. Bernhoff, A, Eklund, B, and Kaijser, L. Cardiovascular effects of short-term anaesthesia with methohexitone and propanidid in normal subjects. *Br J Anaesth* 44:2–6, 1972.
35. Blackburn, JP, Conway, CM, Leigh, M, et al. The effects of anaesthetic induction agents upon myocardial contractility. *Anaesthesia* 26:93A, 1971.
36. Conway, CM, and Ellis, DB. The haemodynamic effects of short-acting barbiturates. *Br J Anaesth* 41:534–542, 1969.
37. Squires, RF, and Braestrup, C. Benzodiazepine receptors in rat brain. *Nature* 266:732–734, 1977.
38. Richter, JJ. Current theories about the mechanisms of benzodiazepines and neuroleptic drugs. *Anesthesiology* 54:66–72, 1981.
39. Forster, A, Juge, O, and Morel, D. Effects of midazolam on cerebral blood flow in human volunteers. *Anesthesiology* 55:A263, 1981.
40. Sunzel, M, Paalzow, L, Berggren, L, et al. Respiratory and cardiovascular effects in relation to plasma levels of midazolam and diazepam. *Br J Clin Pharmacol* 25:561–569, 1988.
41. Haefely, W. The preclinical pharmacology of flumazenil. *Eur J Anaesthesiol* 2S:25–36, 1988.
42. File, SE, and Pellow, S. Intrinsic actions of the benzodiazepine receptor antagonist RO 15-1788. *Psychopharmacology* 88:1–11, 1986.
43. Haefely, W, Hunkeler, W. The story of flumazenil. *Eur J Anaesthesiol* 2S:3–13, 1988.
44. Mandelli, M, Tognoni, G, and Gartattini, S. Clinical pharmacokinetics of diazepam. *Clin Pharmacokinet* 3:72–91, 1978.
45. Greenblatt, DJ, Allen, MD, Harmatz, JS, et al. Diazepam disposition determinants. *Clin Pharmacol Ther* 27:301–312, 1980.
46. Klotz, U, Antonin, KH, Brügel, H, et al. Disposition of diazepam and its major metabolite desmethyldiazepam in patients with liver disease. *Clin Pharmacol Ther* 21:430–436, 1977.
47. Abernethy, DR, Greenblatt, DJ, Divoll, M, et al. Prolonged accumulation of diazepam in obesity. *J Clin Pharmacol* 23:369–376, 1983.
48. Hillestad, L, Hansen, T, and Melsom, H. Diazepam metabolism in normal man. II. Serum concentration and clinical effect after oral administration and accumulation. *Clin Pharmacol Ther* 16:485–489, 1974.
49. Smith, MT, Evans, LEJ, Eadie, MJ, et al. Pharmacokinetics of prazepam in man. *Eur J Clin Pharmacol* 16:141–147, 1979.
50. Klotz, U, Reimann, I. Delayed clearance of diazepam due to cimetidine. *N Engl J Med* 302:1012–1014, 1980.
51. Routledge, PA, Kitchell, BB, Bjornsson, TD, et al. Diazepam and n-desmethyldiazepam redistribution after heparin. *Clin Pharmacol Ther* 27:528–532, 1980.
52. Alvis, JM, Flezzani, P, Jacobs, JR, et al. Diazepam pharmacokinetics and pharmacodynamics during induction of anesthesia in CABG patients. Society of Cardiovascular Anesthesiologists Annual Meeting, Montreal, 1986.
53. Côté, P, Guéret, P, Bourassa, MG. Systemic and coronary hemodynamic effects of diazepam in patients with normal and diseased coronary arteries. *Circulation* 50:1210–1216, 1974.
54. Samuelson, PN, Reves, JG, Kouchoukos, NT, et al. Hemodynamic responses to anesthetic induction with midazolam or diazepam in patients with ischemic heart disease. *Anesth Analg* 60:802–809, 1981.
55. Rao, S, Sherbaniuk, RW, Prasad, K, et al. Cardiopulmonary effects of diazepam. *Clin Pharmacol Ther* 14:182–189, 1973.
56. Jackson, APF, Dhadphale, PR, Callaghan, ML, et al. Haemodynamic studies during induction of anaesthesia for open-heart surgery using diazepam and ketamine. *Br J Anaesth* 50:375–377, 1978.
57. McCammon, RL, Hilgenberg, JC, and Stoelting, RK. Hemodynamic effects of diazepam and diazepam–nitrous oxide in patients with coronary artery disease. *Anesth Analg* 59:438–441, 1980.
58. D'Amelio, G, Volta, SD, Stritoni, P, et al. Acute cardiovascular effects of diazepam in patients with mitral valve disease. *Eur J Clin Pharmacol* 6:61–63, 1973.

59. Samuelson, PN, Lell, WA, Kouchoukos, NT, et al. Hemodynamics during diazepam induction of anesthesia for coronary artery bypass grafting. *South Med J* 73:332–334, 1980.
60. Clarke, RS, and Lyons, SM. Diazepam and flunitrazepam as induction agents for cardiac surgical operations. *Acta Anaesthesiol Scand* 21:282–292, 1977.
61. Lyons, SM, Clarke, RSJ, and Dundee, JW. Some cardiovascular and respiratory effects of four non-barbiturate anaesthetic induction agents. *Eur J Clin Pharmacol* 7:275–279, 1974.
62. Côté, P, Noble, J, and Bourassa, MG. Systemic vasodilatation following diazepam after combined sympathetic and parasympathetic blockade in patients with coronary heart disease. *Cathet Cardiovasc Diagn* 2:369–380, 1976.
63. Ikram, H, Rubin, AP, and Jewkes, RF. Effect of diazepam on myocardial blood flow of patients with and without coronary artery disease. *Br Heart J* 35:626–630, 1973.
64. Dhadphale, PR, Behrendt, DM, Jackson, PF, et al. The effect of diazepam on contractility in the intact human heart. ASA Annual Meeting, New Orleans, LA, 1977.
65. Dauchot, PJ, Staub, F, Berzina, L, et al. Hemodynamic response to diazepam: Dependence on prior left ventricular end-diastolic pressure. *Anesthesiology* 60:499–503, 1984.
66. Knapp, RB, Dubow, HS. Diazepam as an induction agent for patients with cardiopulmonary disease. *South Med J* 63:1451–1453, 1970.
67. Knapp, RB, Dubow, H. Comparison of diazepam with thiopental as an induction agent in cardiopulmonary disease. *Anesth Analg* 49:722–726, 1970.
68. Kingston, HG, Bretherton, KW, Holloway, AM, et al. A comparison between ketamine and diazepam as induction agents for pericardiectomy. *Anaesth Intensive Care* 6:66–70, 1978.
69. Stanley, TH, Bennett, GM, Loeser, EA, et al. Cardiovascular effects of diazepam and droperidol during morphine anesthesia. *Anesthesiology* 44:255–258, 1976.
70. Stanley, TH, Webster, LR. Anesthetic requirements and cardiovascular effects of fentanyl-oxygen and fentanyl-diazepam-oxygen anesthesia in man. *Anesth Analg* 57:411–416, 1978.
71. Tomichek, RC, Roscow, CE, Schneider, RC, et al. Cardiovascular effects of diazepam-fentanyl anesthesia in patients with coronary artery disease. *Anesth Analg* 61A:217–218, 1982.
72. Silbert, BS, Roscow, CE, Keegan, CR, et al. The effect of diazepam on induction of anesthesia with alfentanil. *Anesth Analg* 65:71–77, 1986.
73. Ziegler, WH, Schalch, E, Leishman, B, et al. Comparison of the effects of intravenously administered midazolam, triazolam, and their hydroxy metabolites. *Br J Clin Pharmacol* 16:63S–69S, 1983.
74. Greenblatt, DJ, Locniskar, A, Ochs, HR, et al. Automated gas chromatography for studies of midazolam pharmacokinetics. *Anesthesiology* 55:176–179, 1981.
75. Allonen, H, Ziegler, G, and Klotz, U. Midazolam kinetics. *Clin Pharmacol Ther* 30:653–661, 1981.
76. Heizmann, P, Eckert, M, and Ziegler, WH. Pharmacokinetics and bioavailability of midazolam in man. *Br J Clin Pharmacol* 16:43S–49S, 1983.
77. Greenblatt, DJ, Abernethy, DR, Locniskar, A, et al. Effect of age, gender, and obesity on midazolam kinetics. *Anesthesiology* 61:27–35, 1984.
78. Harper, KW, Collier, PS, Dundee, JW, et al. Age and nature of operation influence the pharmacokinetics of midazolam. *Br J Anaesth* 57:866–871, 1985.
79. Reves, JG, Samuelson, PN, and Lewis, S. Midazolam maleate induction in patients with ischaemic heart disease: Haemodynamic observations. *Can Anaesth Soc J* 26S:402–409, 1979.
80. Marty, J, Nitenberg, A, Blanchet, F, et al. Effects of midazolam on the coronary circulation in patients with coronary artery disease. *Anesthesiology* 64:206–210, 1986.
81. Massaut, J, d'Hollander, A, Barvais, L, et al. Haemodynamic effects of midazolam in the anaesthetized patient with coronary artery disease. *Acta Anaesthesiol Scand* 27:299–302, 1983.
82. Lebowitz, PW, Cote, ME, Daniels, AL, et al. Cardiovascular effects of midazolam and thiopentone for induction of anaesthesia in ill surgical patients. *Can Anaesth Soc J* 30:19–23, 1983.
83. Heikkila, M, Jalonen, J, Arola, M, et al. Midazolam as adjunct to high-dose fentanyl anaesthesia for coronary artery bypass grafting operation. *Acta Anaesthesiol Scand* 28:683–689, 1984.
84. Samuelson, PN, Reves, JG, Smith, LR, et al. Midazolam versus diazepam: Different effects on systemic vascular resistance. *Arzneimittelforschung* 31:2268–2269, 1981.
85. Fragen, RJ, Meyers, SN, Barresi, V, et al. Hemodynamic effects of midazolam in cardiac patients. *Anesthesiology* 51:S103, 1979.
86. Clements, JA, Nimmo, WS, and Grant, IS. Bioavailability, pharmacokinetics, and analgesic activity of ketamine in humans. *J Pharmaceutical Sci* 71:539–542, 1982.
87. Ghoneim, MM, Korttila K. Pharmacokinetics of intravenous anaesthetics. Implications for clinical use. *Clin Pharmacokinet* 2:344–372, 1977.

88. Chang, T, Glazko, AJ. Biotransformation and disposition of ketamine. *Int Anesthesiol Clin* 12:157–177, 1974.
89. Clements, JA, Nimmo, WS. Pharmacokinetics and analgesic effect of ketamine in man. *Br J Anaesth* 53:27–30, 1981.
90. White, PF, Way, WL, Trevor, AJ. Ketamine—its pharmacology and therapeutic uses. *Anesthesiology* 56:119–136, 1982.
91. Freuchen, I, Ostergaard, J, Kuhl, JB, et al. Reduction of psychotomimetic side effects of ketamine by flunitrazepam. *Acta Anaesthesiol Scand* 20:97–103, 1976.
92. Soliman, MG, Brindle, GF, Kuster, G. Response to hypercapnia under ketamine anaesthesia. *Can Anaesth Soc J* 22:486–494, 1975.
93. Huber, FC, Jr, Reves, JG, Gutierrez, J, et al. Ketamine: Its effect on airway resistance in man. *South Med J* 65:1176–1180, 1972.
94. Corssen, G, Gutierrez, J, Reves, JG, et al. Ketamine in the anesthetic management of asthmatic patients. *Anesth Analg* 51:588, 1972.
95. Chodoff, P. Evidence for central adrenergic action of ketamine. *Anesth Analg* 51:247–250, 1972.
96. Wong, DH, Jenkins, LC. An experimental study of the mechanism of action of ketamine on the central nervous system. *Can Anaesth Soc J* 21:57–67, 1974.
97. Slogoff, S, Allen, GW. The role of baroreceptors in the cardiovascular response to ketamine. *Anesth Analg* 53:704–707, 1974.
98. Traber, DL, Wilson, RD. Involvement of the sympathetic nervous system in the pressor response to ketamine. *Anesth Analg* 48:248–252, 1969.
99. Traber, DL, Wilson, RD, Priano, LL. The effect of beta-adrenergic blockade on the cardiopulmonary response to ketamine. *Anesth Analg* 49:604–613, 1970.
100. Zsigmond, EK, Kothary, SP, Matsuki, A, et al. Diazepam for prevention of the rise in plasma catecholamines caused by ketamine. *Clin Pharmacol Ther* 15:223–224, 1974.
101. Nedergaard, OA. Cocaine-like effect of ketamine on vascular adrenergic neurones. *Eur J Pharmacol* 23:153–161, 1973.
102. Salt, PJ, Barnes, PK, Beswick, FJ. Inhibition of neuronal and extraneuronal uptake of noradrenaline by ketamine in the isolated perfused rat heart. *Br J Anaesth* 51:835–838, 1979.
103. Bidwal, AV, Stanley, TH, Graves, CL, et al. The effects of ketamine on cardiovascular dynamics during halothane and enflurane anesthesia. *Anesth Analg* 54:588–592, 1975.
104. Silvay, G. Ketamine. *Mt Sinai J Med* 50:300–304, 1983.
105. Bålfors, E, Häggmark, S, Nyhman, H, et al. Droperidol inhibits the effects of intravenous ketamine on central hemodynamics and myocardial oxygen consumption in patients with generalized atherosclerotic disease. *Anesth Analg* 62:193–197, 1983.
106. Spotoft, H, Korshin, JD, Sorensen, MB, et al. The cardiovascular effects of ketamine used for induction of anaesthesia in patients with valvular heart disease. *Can Anaesth Soc J* 26:463–467, 1979.
107. Faithfull, NS, Haider, R. Ketamine for cardiac catheterization: An evaluation of its use in children. *Anaesthesia* 26:318–323, 1971.
108. Hickey, PR, Hansen, DD, Cramolini, GM, et al. Pulmonary and systemic hemodynamic responses to ketamine in infants with normal and elevated pulmonary vascular resistance. *Anesthesiology* 62:287–293, 1985.
109. Gooding, JM, Dimick, AR, Tavakoli, M, et al. A physiologic analysis of cardiopulmonary response to ketamine anesthesia in non-cardiac patients. *Anesth Analg* 56:813–816, 1977.
110. Savege, TM, Colvin, MP, Weaver, EJM, et al. A comparison of some cardiorespiratory effects of althesin and ketamine when used for induction of anaesthesia in patients with cardiac disease. *Br J Anaesth* 48:1071–1081, 1976.
111. Nishimura, K, Kitamura, Y, Hamai, R, et al. Pharmacological studies of ketamine hydrochloride in the cardiovascular system. *Osaka City Med J* 19:17–26, 1973.
112. Lippman, M, Appel, PL, Mok, MS, et al. Sequential cardiorespiratory patterns of anesthetic induction with ketamine in critically ill patients. *Crit Care Med* 11:730–734, 1983.
113. Nettles, DC, Herrin, TJ, Mullen, JG. Ketamine induction in poor-risk patients. *Anesth Analg* 52:59–64, 1973.
114. Van Hamme, MJ, Ghoneim, MM, Ambre, JJ. Pharmacokinetics of etomidate, a new intravenous anesthetic. *Anesthesiology* 49:274–277, 1978.
115. Hebron, BS, Edbrooke, DL, Newby, DM, et al. Pharmacokinetics of etomidate associated with prolonged IV infusion. *Br J Anaesth* 55:281–287, 1983.
116. Nimmo, WS, Miller, M. Pharmacology of etomidate. *Contemp Anesth Pract* 7:83–95, 1983.
117. Doenicke, A, Löffler, B, Kugler, J, et al. Plasma concentrations and EEG after various regimens of etomidate. *Br J Anaesth* 54:393–400, 1982.
118. Thomson, MF, Brock-Utne, JG, Bean, P, et al. An-

aesthesia and intra-ocular pressure: A comparative study of total intravenous anaesthesia using etomidate with conventional inhalational anaesthesia. *Anaesthesia* 37:758–761, 1982.
119. Cold, GE, Eskesen, V, Eriksen, H, et al. CBF and CRMO$_2$ during continuous etomidate infusion supplemented with N$_2$O and fentanyl in patients with supratentorial cerebral tumor. A dose response study. *Acta Anaesthesiol Scand* 29:490–494, 1985.
120. Giese, JL, Stockham, RJ, Stanley, TH, et al. Etomidate versus thiopental for induction of anesthesia. *Anesth Analg* 64:871–876, 1985.
121. Ghoneim, MM, Yamada, T. Etomidate: A clinical and electrographic comparison with thiopental. *Anesth Analg* 56:479–485, 1977.
122. Ebrahim, ZY, DeBoer, GE, Luders, H, et al. Effect of etomidate on the electroencephalogram of patients with epilepsy. *Anesth Analg* 65:1004–1006, 1986.
123. Choi, SD, Spaulding, BC, Gross, JB, et al. Comparison of the ventilatory effects of etomidate and methohexital. *Anesthesiology* 62:442–447, 1985.
124. Wagner, RL, White, PF. Etomidate inhibits adrenocortical function in surgical patients. *Anesthesiology* 61:647–651, 1984.
125. Fragen, RJ, Shanks, CA, Molteni, A, et al. Effects of etomidate on hormonal response to surgical stress. *Anesthesiology* 61:652–656, 1984.
126. Wanscher, M, Tonnesen, E, Huttel, M, et al. Etomidate infusion and adrenocortical function: A study in elective surgery. *Acta Anaesthesiol Scand* 29:483–485, 1985.
127. Boidin, MP, Erdmann, WE, Faithfull, NS. The role of ascorbic acid in etomidate toxicity. *Eur J Anaesthesiol* 3:417–422, 1986.
128. Kettler, D, Sonntag, H, Donath, U, et al. Haemodynamics, myocardial mechanics, oxygen requirement, and oxygenation of the human heart during induction of anaesthesia with etomidate. *Anaesthesist* 23:116–121, 1974.
129. Gooding, JM, Corssen, G. Effect of etomidate on the cardiovascular system. *Anesth Analg* 56:717–719, 1977.
130. Firestone, S, Kleinman, CS, Jaffe, CC, et al. Human research and noninvasive measurement of ventricular performance: An echocardiographic evaluation of etomidate and thiopental. *Anesthesiology* 51:S22, 1979.
131. Doenicke, A, Gabanyi, D, Lemcke, H, et al. Haemodynamics and myocardial function after administration of three short-acting IV hypnotics: etomidate, propanidid, methohexital. *Anaesthesist* 23:108–115, 1974.
132. Gooding, JM, Weng, JT, et al. Cardiovascular and pulmonary responses following etomidate induction of anesthesia in patients with demonstrated cardiac disease. *Anesth Analg* 58:40–41, 1979.
133. Colvin, MP, Savege, TM, Newland, PE, et al. Cardiorespiratory changes following induction of anaesthesia with etomidate in patients with cardiac disease. *Br J Anaesth* 51:551–556, 1979.
134. Criado, A, Maseda, J, Navarro, E, et al. Induction of anaesthesia with etomidate. Haemodynamic study of 36 patients. *Br J Anaesth* 52:803–806, 1980.
135. Larsen, R, Rathgeber, J, Bagdahn, A, et al. Effects of propofol on cardiovascular dynamics and coronary blood flow in geriatric patients. A comparison with etomidate. *Anaesthesia* 43 (Suppl):25–31, 1988.
136. Lindeburg, T, Spotoft, H, Bredgaard-Sorensen, M, et al. Cardiovascular effects of etomidate used for induction and in combination with fentanyl-pancuronium for maintenance of anaesthesia in patients with valvular heart disease. *Acta Anaesthesiol Scand* 26:205, 1982.
137. Spiss, CK, Coraim, F, Haider, W, et al. Haemodynamic effects of fentanyl or alfentanil as adjuvants to etomidate for induction of anaesthesia in cardiac patients. *Acta Anaesthesiol Scand* 28:554–556, 1984.
138. James, R, Glen, JB. Synthesis, biological evaluation, and preliminary structure-activity considerations of a series of alkylphenols as intravenous anesthetic agents. *J Med Chem* 23:1350–1357, 1980.
139. Kay, NH, Sear, JW, Uppington, J, et al. Disposition of propofol in patients undergoing surgery. A comparison in men and women. *Br J Anaesth* 58:1075–1079, 1986.
140. Schüttler, J, Stoeckel, H, Schwilden, H. Pharmacokinetic and pharmacodynamic modelling of propofol ("Diprivan") in volunteers and surgical patients. *Postgrad Med J* 61 (Suppl 3):53–54, 1985.
141. Shafer, A, Doze, VA, Shafer, SL, et al. Pharmacokinetics and pharmacodynamics of propofol infusions during general anesthesia. *Anesthesiology* 69:348–356, 1988.
142. Adam, HK, Kay, B, Douglas, EJ. Blood disoprofol levels in anaesthetized patients. Correlation of concentration after single or repeated doses with hypnotic activity. *Anaesthesia* 37:536–540, 1982.
143. Stephan, H, Sonntag, H, Schenk, HD, et al. Effect of Disoprivan on the circulation and oxygen consumption of the brain and CO$_2$ reactivity of brain vessels in the human. *Anaesthesist* 36:60–65, 1987.

144. Hartung, HJ. Intracranial pressure in patients with craniocerebral trauma after administration of propofol and thiopental. *Anaesthesist* 36:285–287, 1987.
145. Vandesteene, A, Trempont, V, Engelman, E, et al. Effect of propofol on cerebral blood flow and metabolism in man. *Anaesthesia* 43:42S, 1988.
146. Mirakhur, RK, Shepherd, WFI. Intraocular pressure changes with propofol ("Diprivan"): Comparison with thiopentone. *Postgrad Med J* 61 (Suppl 3): 41–44, 1985.
147. Taylor, MB, Grounds, RM, Mulrooney, PD, et al. Ventilatory effects of propofol during induction of anaesthesia. Comparison with thiopentone. *Anaesthesia* 41:816–820, 1986.
148. Grounds, RM, Maxwell, DL, Taylor, MB, et al. Acute ventilatory changes during IV induction of anaesthesia with thiopentone or propofol in man. Studies using inductance plethysmography. *Br J Anaesth* 59:1098–1102, 1987.
149. Goodman, NW, Black, AMS, Carter, JA. Some ventilatory effects of propofol as sole anaesthetic agent. *Br J Anaesth* 59:1497–1503, 1987.
150. Brüssel, T, Theissen, JL, Vigfusson, G, et al. Hemodynamic and cardiodynamic effects of propofol and etomidate: Negative inotropic properties of propofol. *Anesth Analg* 69:35–40, 1989.
151. Profeta, JP, Guffin, A, et al. The hemodynamic effects of propofol and thiamylal sodium for induction in coronary artery surgery. *Anesth Analg* 66:S142, 1987.
152. Goodchild, CS, Serrao, JM. Cardiovascular effects of propofol in the anaesthetized dog. *Br J Anaesth* 63:87–92, 1989.
153. Coetzee, A, Fourie, P, Coetzee, J, et al. Effect of various propofol plasma concentrations on regional myocardial contractility and left ventricular afterload. *Anesth Analg* 69:473–483, 1989.
154. Grounds, RM, Twigley, AJ, Carli, F, et al. The haemodynamic effects of intravenous induction. Comparison of the effects of thiopentone and propofol. *Anaesthesia* 40:735–740, 1985.
155. Coates, DP, Monk, CR, Prys-Roberts, C, et al. Hemodynamic effects of infusions of the emulsion formulation of propofol during nitrous oxide anesthesia in humans. *Anesth Analg* 66:64–70, 1987.
156. Coates, DP, Prys-Roberts, C, Spelina, KR, et al. Propofol ("Diprivan") by intravenous infusion with nitrous oxide: Dose requirements and haemodynamic effects. *Postgrad Med J* 61 (Suppl 3):76–79, 1985.
157. Claeys, MA, Gepts, E, Camu, F. Haemodynamic changes during anaesthesia induced and maintained with propofol. *Br J Anaesth* 60:3–9, 1988.
158. Lippman, M, Paicius, R, Gingerich, S, et al. A controlled study of hemodynamic effects of propofol vs. thiopental during anesthesia induction. *Anesth Analg* 65:S89, 1986.
159. Williams, JP, McArthur, JD, Walker, WE, et al. The cardiovascular effects of propofol in patients with impaired cardiac function. *Anesth Analg* 65:S166, 1986.
160. Fairfield, JE, Dritsas, A, Beale, RJ. Haemodynamic effects of propofol: Induction with 2.5 mg/kg. *Br J Anaesth* 67:618–620, 1991.
161. Ebert, TJ, Muzi, M, Berens, R, et al. Sympathetic responses to induction of anesthesia in humans with propofol or etomidate. *Anesthesiology* 76:725–733, 1992.
162. Dundee, JW, Robinson, FP, McCollum, JSC, et al. Sensitivity to propofol in the elderly. *Anaesthesia* 41:482–485, 1986.
163. Lebovic, S, Reich, DL, Steinberg, LG, et al. Comparison of propofol versus ketamine for anesthesia in pediatric patients undergoing cardiac catheterization. *Anesth Analg* 74:490–494, 1992.
164. Stephan, H, Sonntag, H, Schenk, HD, et al. Effects of propofol on cardiovascular dynamics, myocardial blood flow, and myocardial metabolism in patients with coronary artery disease. *Br J Anaesth* 58:969–975, 1986.
165. Aun, C, Major, E. The cardiorespiratory effects of ICI 35 868 in patients with valvular heart disease. *Anaesthesia* 39:1096–1100, 1984.
166. Jaffe, JH, Martin, WR. Opioid Analgesics and Antagonists. In AG Goodman, LS Goodman, and A Gilman (eds), *The Pharmacological Basis of Therapeutics*. New York: Macmillan (7th ed), 1985. P. 491.
167. Smith, RR. Scopolamine-morphine anaesthesia, with report of two hundred and twenty-nine cases. *Surg Gynecol Obstet* 7:414–420, 1908.
168. Pert, CB, Snyder, SH. Opiate receptor: Demonstration in nervous tissue. *Science* 179:1011–1014, 1973.
169. Terenius, L. Characteristics of the "receptor" for narcotic analgesics in synaptic plasma membrane fractions from rat brain. *Acta Pharmacol Toxicol* 33:377–384, 1973.
170. Pasternak, GW. High and low affinity opioid binding sites: Relationship to mu and delta sites. *Life Sci* 31:1302–1306, 1982.
171. Ling, GSF, Spiegel, K, Nishimura, SL, et al. Dissociation of morphine's analgesic and respiratory depressant actions. *Eur J Pharmacol* 86:487–488, 1983.

172. Lord, JAH, Waterfield, AA, Hughes, J, et al. Endogenous opioid peptides: Multiple agonists and receptors. Nature 267:495–499, 1977.
173. Schulz, R, Wüster, M, Herz, A. Pharmacological characterization of the ϵ-opiate receptor. J Pharmacol Exp Ther 216:604–606, 1981.
174. Lowenstein, E. Morphine "anesthesia"—a perspective. Anesthesiology 35:563–565, 1971.
175. Mummaneni, N, Rao, TLK, Montoya, A. Awareness and recall with high-dose fentanyl-oxygen anesthesia. Anesth Analg 59:948–949, 1980.
176. de Castro, J, Van de Water, A, Wouters, L, et al. Comparative study of cardiovascular, neurological, and metabolic side-effects of eight narcotics in dogs. Acta Anaesth Belg 30:5–54, 1979.
177. Ngai, SH. Effects of morphine and meperidine on the central respiratory mechanisms in the cat; the action of levallorphan in antagonizing these effects. J Pharmacol Exp Ther 131:91–99, 1961.
178. Tabatabai, M, Kitahata, LM, Collins, JG. Disruption of the rhythmic activity of the medullary inspiratory neurons and phrenic nerve by fentanyl and reversal with nalbuphine. Anesthesiology 70:489–495, 1989.
179. Weil, JV, McCullough, RE, Kline, JS, et al. Diminished ventilatory response to hypoxia and hypercapnia after morphine in normal man. N Engl J Med 292:1103–1106, 1975.
180. Azar, I, Turndorf, H. Severe hypertension and multiple atrial premature contractions following naloxone administration. Anesth Analg 58:524–525, 1979.
181. Flacke, JW, Flacke, WE, Williams, GD. Acute pulmonary edema following naloxone reversal of high-dose morphine anesthesia. Anesthesiology 47:376–378, 1977.
182. Patschke, D, Eberlein, HJ, Hess, W, et al. Antagonism of morphine with naloxone in dogs: Cardiovascular effects with special reference to the coronary circulation. Br J Anaesth 49:525–532, 1977.
183. Kontani, H, Kawabata, Y. A study of morphine-induced urinary retention in anesthetized rats capable of micturition. Jap J Pharmacol 48:31–36, 1988.
184. Radnay, PA, Duncalf, D, Novakovic, M, et al. Common bile duct pressure changes after fentanyl, morphine, meperidine, butorphanol, and naloxone. Anesth Analg 63:441–444, 1984.
185. Hynynen, MJ, Turunen, MT, Korttila, KT. Effects of alfentanil and fentanyl on common bile duct pressure. Anesth Analg 65:370–372, 1986.
186. Vatashsky, E, Haskel, Y, Nissan, S, et al. Effect of morphine on the mechanical activity of common bile duct isolated from the guinea pig. Anesth Analg 66:245–248, 1987.
187. Radnay, PA, Brodman, E, Mankikar, D, et al. The effect of equi-analgesic doses of fentanyl, morphine, meperidine, and pentazocine on common bile duct pressure. Anaesthesist 29:26–29, 1980.
188. McCammon, RL, Viegas, OJ, Stoelting, RK, et al. Naloxone reversal of choledochoduodenal sphincter spasm associated with narcotic administration. Anesthesiology 48:437, 1978.
189. McCammon, RL, Stoelting, R, Madura, JA. Reversal of fentanyl induced spasm of the sphincter of Oddi. Surg Gynecol Obstet 156:329–334, 1983.
190. Helm, JF, Venu, RP, Geenen, JE, et al. Effects of morphine on the human sphincter of Oddi. Gut 29:1402–1407, 1988.
191. Dowlatshahi, K, Evander, A, Walther, B, et al. Influence of morphine on the distal oesophagus and the lower oesophageal sphincter—a manometric study. Gut 26:802–806, 1985.
192. Lamki, L, Sullivan, S. A study of gastrointestinal opiate receptors: The role of the mu receptor on gastric emptying: Concise communication. J Nucl Med 24:689–692, 1983.
193. Nimmo, WS, Wilson, J, Prescott, LF. Narcotic analgesics and delayed gastric emptying during labour. Lancet 1:890–893, 1975.
194. Moldenhauer, CC, Hug, CC, Jr. Use of narcotic analgesics as anaesthetics. Clin Anaesthesiol 2:107–138, 1984.
195. Hill, AB, Nahrwold, ML, de Rosayro, AM, et al. Prevention of rigidity during fentanyl-oxygen induction of anesthesia. Anesthesiology 55:452–454, 1981.
196. Jaffe, TB, Ramsey, FM. Attenuation of fentanyl-induced truncal rigidity. Anesthesiology 58:562–564, 1983.
197. Sokoll, MD, Hoyt, JL, Gergis, SD. Studies in muscle rigidity, nitrous oxide, and narcotic analgesic agents. Anesth Analg 51:16–20, 1972.
198. Freund, FG, Martin, WE, Wong, KC, et al. Abdominal-muscle rigidity induced by morphine and nitrous oxide. Anesthesiology 38:358–362, 1973.
199. Comstock, MK, Carter, JG, Moyers, JR, et al. Rigidity and hypercarbia associated with high-dose fentanyl induction of anesthesia. Anesth Analg 60:362–363, 1981.
200. Scamman, FL. Fentanyl-O_2-N_2O rigidity and pulmonary compliance. Anesth Analg 62:332–334, 1983.
201. Benthuysen, JL, Smith, NT, Sanford, TJ, et al. Physiology of alfentanil-induced rigidity. Anesthesiology 64:440–446, 1986.

202. Bailey, PL, Wilbrink, J, Stanley, TH, et al. Anesthetic induction with fentanyl. *Anesth Analg* 64: 48–53, 1985.
203. Stanski, DR, Greenblatt, DJ, Lowenstein, E. Kinetics of intravenous and intramuscular morphine. *Clin Pharmacol Ther* 24:52–59, 1978.
204. Dahlström, B, Bolme, P, Feychting, H, et al. Morphine kinetics in children. *Clin Pharmacol Ther* 26: 354–365, 1979.
205. Stanski, DR, Paalzow, L, Edlund, PO. Morphine pharmacokinetics: GLC assay versus radioimmunoassay. *J Pharm Sci* 71:314–317, 1982.
206. Mather, LE, Tucker, GT, Pflug, AE, et al. Meperidine kinetics in man. Intravenous injection in surgical patients and volunteers. *Clin Pharmacol Ther* 17:21–30, 1975.
207. Stambaugh, JE, Wainer, IW, Sanstead, JK. The clinical pharmacology of meperidine—comparison of routes of administration. *J Clin Pharmacol* 16: 245–256, 1976.
208. Szeto, HH, Inturrisi, CE, Houde, R, et al. Accumulation of normeperidine, an active metabolite of meperidine, in patients with renal failure or cancer. *Ann Intern Med* 86:738–741, 1977.
209. McClain, DA, Hug, CC, Jr. Intravenous fentanyl kinetics. *Clin Pharmacol Ther* 28:106–114, 1980.
210. Bentley, JB, Borel, JD, Nenad, RE, Jr, et al. Age and fentanyl pharmacokinetics. *Anesth Analg* 61:968–971, 1982.
211. Haberer, JP, Schoeffler, P, Couderc, E, et al. Fentanyl pharmacokinetics in anaesthetized patients with cirrhosis. *Br J Anaesth* 54:1267–1269, 1982.
212. Mather, LE. Clinical pharmacokinetics of fentanyl and its newer derivatives. *Clin Pharmacokinet* 8: 422–446, 1983.
213. Bovill, JG, Sebel, PS, Blackburn, CL, et al. The pharmacokinetics of sufentanil in surgical patients. *Anesthesiology* 61:502–506, 1984.
214. Camu, F, Gepts, E, Rucquoi, M, et al. Pharmacokinetics of alfentanil in man. *Anesth Analg* 61: 657–661, 1982.
215. Bovill, JG, Sebel, PS, Blackburn, CL, et al. The pharmacokinetics of alfentanil (R39209). A new opioid analgesic. *Anesthesiology* 57:439–443, 1982.
216. Lowenstein, E, Hallowell, P, Levine, FH, et al. Cardiovascular response to large doses of intravenous morphine in man. *N Engl J Med* 281:1389–1393, 1969.
217. Conahan, TJ, Ominsky, AJ, Wollman, H, et al. A prospective random comparison of halothane and morphine for open-heart anesthesia: One year's experience. *Anesthesiology* 38:528–535, 1973.
218. Lappas, DG, Geha, D, Fischer, JE, et al. Filling pressures of the heart and pulmonary circulation of the patient with coronary artery disease after large intravenous doses of morphine. *Anesthesiology* 42: 153–159, 1975.
219. Roscow, CE, Moss, J, Philbin, DM, et al. Histamine release during morphine and fentanyl anesthesia. *Anesthesiology* 56:93–96, 1982.
220. Fahmy, NR, Sunder, N, Soter, NA. Role of histamine in the hemodynamic and plasma catecholamine responses to morphine. *Clin Pharmacol Ther* 33:615–620, 1983.
221. Flacke, JW, Flacke, WE, Bloor, BC, et al. Histamine release by four narcotics: A double blind study in humans. *Anesth Analg* 66:723–730, 1987.
222. Moss, J, Roscow, CE. Histamine release by narcotics and muscle relaxants in humans. *Anesthesiology* 59:330–339, 1983.
223. Lowenstein, E, Whiting, RB, Bittar, DA, et al. Local and neurally mediated effects of morphine on skeletal muscle vascular resistance. *J Pharmacol Exp Ther* 180:359–367, 1972.
224. Ward, JM, McGrath, RL, Weil, JV. Effects of morphine on the peripheral vascular response to sympathetic stimulation. *Am J Cardiol* 29:659–666, 1972.
225. Stanley, TH, Gray, NJ, Stanford, W, et al. The effects of high-dose morphine on fluid and blood requirements in open-heart operations. *Anesthesiology* 38:536–541, 1973.
226. Stanley, TH, Gray, NH, Isern-Amaral, JH, et al. Comparison of blood requirements during morphine and halothane anesthesia for open-heart surgery. *Anesthesiology* 41:34–38, 1974.
227. Wong, KC, Martin, WE, Hornbein, TF, et al. The cardiovascular effects of morphine sulfate with oxygen and with nitrous oxide in man. *Anesthesiology* 38:542–549, 1973.
228. Moores, WY, Weiskopf, RB, Baysinger, M, et al. Effects of halothane and morphine sulfate on myocardial compliance following total cardiopulmonary bypass. *J Thorac Cardiovasc Surg* 81:163–170, 1981.
229. Bovill, JG, Sebel, PS, Stanley, TH. Opioid analgesics in anesthesia: With special reference to their use in cardiovascular anesthesia. *Anesthesiology* 61: 731–755, 1984.
230. Hoar, PF, Nelson, NT, Mangano, DT, et al. Adrenergic response to morphine-diazepam anesthesia for myocardial revascularization. *Anesth Analg* 60: 406–411, 1981.
231. Strauer, BE. Contractile responses to morphine, piritramide, meperidine, and fentanyl: A compara-

tive study of effects on the isolated ventricular myocardium. *Anesthesiology* 37:304–310, 1972.
232. Goldberg, AH, Padget, CH. Comparative effects of morphine and fentanyl on isolated heart muscle. *Anesth Analg* 48:978–982, 1969.
233. Sullivan, DL, Wong, KC. The effects of morphine on the isolated heart during normothermia and hypothermia. *Anesthesiology* 38:550–556, 1973.
234. Freye, E. Cardiovascular effects of high dosages of fentanyl, meperidine, and naloxone in dogs. *Anesth Analg* 53:40–47, 1974.
235. Stoelting, RK, Gibbs, PS, Creasser, CW, et al. Hemodynamic and ventilatory response to fentanyl, fentanyl-droperidol, and nitrous oxide in patients with acquired valvular heart disease. *Anesthesiology* 42:319–324, 1975.
236. Hicks, HC, Mowbray, AG, Yhap, EO. Cardiovascular effects of and catecholamine responses to high dose fentanyl-O_2 for induction of anesthesia in patients with ischemic coronary artery disease. *Anesth Analg* 60:563–568, 1981.
237. Lunn, JK, Stanley, TH, Eisele, J, et al. High dose fentanyl anesthesia for coronary artery surgery: Plasma fentanyl concentrations and influence of nitrous oxide on cardiovascular responses. *Anesth Analg* 58:390–395, 1979.
238. Waller, JL, Hug, CC, Jr, Nagle, DM, et al. Hemodynamic changes during fentanyl-oxygen anesthesia for aortocoronary bypass operations. *Anesthesiology* 55:212–217, 1981.
239. Wynands, JE, Wong, P, Whalley, DG, et al. Oxygen-fentanyl anesthesia in patients with poor left ventricular function: Hemodynamics and plasma fentanyl concentrations. *Anesth Analg* 62:476–482, 1983.
240. Liu, WS, Bidwai, AV, Stanley, TH, et al. The cardiovascular effects of diazepam and of diazepam and pancuronium during fentanyl and oxygen anaesthesia. *Can Anaesth Soc J* 23:395–403, 1976.
241. Flacke, JW, David, LJ, Flacke, WE, et al. Effects of fentanyl and diazepam in dogs deprived of autonomic tone. *Anesth Analg* 64:1053–1059, 1985.
242. Blaise, G, Sill, JC, Nugent, M, et al. Fentanyl and responsiveness of canine coronary arterial smooth muscle. *Can Anaesth Soc J* 33:S104, 1986.
243. Beland, A, Blaise, GA, Lenis, SG, et al. Effect of fentanyl on the coronary circulation in an isolated heart. *Can Anaesth Soc J* 34:S72, 1987.
244. Mathews, HML, Furness, G, Carson, IW, et al. Comparison of sufentanil-oxygen and fentanyl-oxygen anaesthesia for coronary artery bypass grafting. *Br J Anaesth* 60:530–535, 1988.
245. Roscow, CE, Philbin, DM, Keegan, CR, et al. Hemodynamics and histamine release during induction with sufentanil or fentanyl. *Anesthesiology* 60:489–491, 1984.
246. Starck, T, Hall, D, Freas, W, et al. Peripheral vascular depression with sufentanil in the dog. *Anesth Analg* 68:S277, 1989.
247. Miller, DR, Wellwood, M, Teasdale, SJ, et al. Effects of anaesthetic induction on myocardial function and metabolism: A comparison of fentanyl, sufentanil, and alfentanil. *Can J Anaesth* 35:219, 1988.
248. Schauble, JF, Chen, BB, Murray, PA. Marked hemodynamic effects of bolus administration of alfentanil in conscious dogs. *Anesthesiology* 59:A85, 1983.
249. de Bruijnn, N, Christian, C, Fagraeus, L, et al. The effects of alfentanil on global ventricular mechanics. *Anesthesiology* 59:A33, 1983.
250. Ausems, ME, Hug, CC, Jr, and de Lange, S. Variable rate infusion of alfentanil as a supplement to nitrous oxide anesthesia for general surgery. *Anesth Analg* 62:982–986, 1983.
251. Moldenhauer, CC, Griesemer, RW, Hug, CC, et al. Hemodynamic changes during rapid induction of anesthesia with alfentanil. *Anesth Analg* 62A:276, 1983.
252. Bartowski, RR, McDonnell, TE. Alfentanil as an anesthetic induction agent: A comparison with thiopental-lidocaine. *Anesth Analg* 63:330–334, 1984.
253. Lemmens, HJM, Bovill, JG, et al. Alfentanil infusion in the elderly. *Anaesthesia* 43:850–856, 1988.
254. Rucquoi, M, Camu, F. Cardiovascular responses to large doses of alfentanil and fentanyl. *Br J Anaesth* 55:223S–230S, 1983.
255. Liu, WS, Bidwal, AV, Stanley, TH, et al. Cardiovascular dynamics after large doses of fentanyl and fentanyl plus N_2O in the dog. *Anesth Analg* 55:168–172, 1976.
256. Prakash, O, Verdouw, PD, de Jong, JW, et al. Haemodynamic and biochemical variables after induction of anaesthesia with fentanyl and nitrous oxide in patients undergoing coronary artery bypass surgery. *Can Anaesth Soc J* 27:223–229, 1980.
257. Smith, NT, Eger, EI, Stoelting, RK, et al. The cardiovascular and sympathomimetic responses to the addition of nitrous oxide to halothane in man. *Anesthesiology* 32:410–421, 1970.
258. Reitan, JA, Stengert, KB, Wymore, ML, et al. Central vagal control of fentanyl-induced bradycardia during halothane anesthesia. *Anesth Analg* 57:31–36, 1978.
259. Reddy, P, Liu, WS, Port, D, et al. Comparison of

haemodynamic effects of anaesthetic doses of alphaprodine and sufentanil in the dog. *Can Anaesth Soc J* 27:345–350, 1980.
260. Stanley, TH, Philbin, DM, Coggins, CH. Fentanyl-oxygen anaesthesia for coronary artery surgery: Cardiovascular and antidiuretic hormone responses. *Can Anaesth Soc J* 26:168–172, 1979.
261. Bennett, G, Stanley, TH. Comparison of the cardiovascular effects of morphine-N_2O and fentanyl-N_2O balanced anesthesia before and after pancuronium in man. *Anesthesiology* 51:S138, 1979.
262. Laubie, M, Schmitt, H, Vincent, M. Vagal bradycardia produced by microinjections of morphine-like drugs into the nucleus ambiguus in anaesthetized dogs. *Eur J Pharmacol* 59:287–291, 1979.
263. Starr, NJ, Sethna, DH, Estafanous, FG. Bradycardia and asystole following the rapid administration of sufentanil with vecuronium. *Anesthesiology* 64:521–523, 1986.
264. Sherman, EP, Lebowitz, PW, Street, WC. Bradycardia following sufentanil-succinylcholine. *Anesthesiology* 66:106, 1987.
265. Rivard, JC, Lebowitz, PW. Bradycardia after alfentanil-succinylcholine. *Anesth Analg* 67:907, 1988.
266. Murphy, MR, Hug, CC, Jr. The anesthetic potency of fentanyl in terms of its reduction of enflurane MAC. *Anesthesiology* 57:485–488, 1982.
267. Murphy, MR, Hug, CC, Jr. Efficacy of fentanyl in reducing isoflurane MAC; antagonism by naloxone and nalbuphine. *Anesthesiology* 59:A338, 1983.
268. Eisele, JH, Smith, NT. Cardiovascular effects of 40 percent nitrous oxide in man. *Anesth Analg* 51:956–962, 1972.
269. Stoelting, RK, Gibbs, PS. Hemodynamic effects of morphine and morphine–nitrous oxide in valvular heart disease and coronary artery disease. *Anesthesiology* 38:45–52, 1973.
270. McDermott, RW, Stanley, TH. The cardiovascular effects of low concentrations of nitrous oxide during morphine anesthesia. *Anesthesiology* 41:89–91, 1974.
271. Moffitt, EA, Scovil, JE, Barker, RA, et al. Myocardial metabolism and hemodynamics of nitrous oxide in fentanyl or enflurane anesthesia in coronary patients. *Anesthesiology* 59:A31, 1983.
272. Moffitt, EA, Scovil, JE, Barker, RA, et al. The effects of nitrous oxide on myocardial metabolism and hemodynamics during fentanyl or enflurane anesthesia in patients with coronary artery disease. *Anesth Analg* 63:1071–1075, 1984.
273. Eisele, JH, Reitan, JA, Massumi, RA, et al. Myocardial performance and N_2O analgesia in coronary-artery disease. *Anesthesiology* 44:16–20, 1976.
274. Ruff, R, Reves, JG. Hemodynamic effects of a lorazepam-fentanyl anesthetic induction for coronary artery bypass surgery. *J Cardiothorac Anesth* 4:314–317, 1990.
275. Komatsu, T, Shibutani, K, Okamoto, K, et al. Comparison of sufentanil-diazepam and fentanyl-diazepam anesthesia for induction. *Anesth Analg* 65:S82, 1986.
276. Tuman, KJ, McCarthy, RJ, el Ganzouri, AR, et al. Sufentanil-midazolam anesthesia for coronary artery surgery. *J Cardiothorac Anesth* 4:308–313, 1990.

The Adult Patient

4
Monitoring Cardiac Patients for Noncardiac Surgery

KETAN SHEVDE
PIYUSH M. GUPTA

A monitor is a device that reminds or warns the clinician about a situation that can be regulated and corrected before an unfavorable outcome occurs. Anesthesia, by its very nature, necessitates the use of monitors because patients are often incapable of providing information for their wellbeing as a result of pharmacologic intervention. Although anesthetized patients have been monitored since the start of our specialty, the number and sophistication of monitoring devices have increased over the years.

To a large extent, the demand for monitoring has been prompted by our desire to provide safer anesthesia, which is warranted by the older and medically complex patient population, and, to a lesser degree, by today's legal climate, which encourages safe medical practice. A good example of the latter is the pulse oximeter, which is now mandated as a direct result of large malpractice claims made in favor of the plaintiff suffering the consequences of hypoxia during anesthetic management. In time we will be able to assess the direct result of monitoring on patient outcome and legal costs. Since the patient population and complexity of surgical procedures change with time, it is difficult to use historical data to compare previous numbers of morbidity and mortality and apply them to current conditions.

Rao and associates [1] suggested that in a group of patients with a history of previous myocardial infarction undergoing a variety of surgical procedures, invasive monitoring was in part responsible for reduced reinfarction rate and mortality. They compared their data to data on historical control subjects, who were found to have a much higher infarction rate and mortality. Although results of the study are controversial, it highlighted the fact that better monitoring provided more hemodynamic information, which facilitated patient management. In contrast, some medical centers in this country that do not routinely use pulmonary artery catheters for coronary artery bypass surgery have as good, or better, outcomes as centers that routinely use the pulmonary artery catheter for all cardiac procedures. Controversy over whether monitoring improves outcome is further complicated by the fact that information derived from monitoring is not always received and interpreted without error. For example, a transducer may be erroneously positioned, resulting in inappropriate therapy. In addition, morbidity and mortality are associated with the use of some monitoring devices; for example, a pulmonary catheter may cause rupture of the pulmonary artery, resulting in a 50 percent mortality [2]. An inadvertent carotid artery puncture during jugular venous cannulation may require an additional surgical procedure for repair of the artery. When assessing the efficacy of a monitoring mo-

58 The Adult Patient

dality, one must consider the associated complications. When used correctly, monitoring can certainly provide information vital to patient care. Since all monitoring devices have limitations, and possible complications, these should be taken into account when one chooses a monitoring device, and maximum benefit from monitoring is realized when it is used as an adjunct, not a substitute, for vigilance.

NONINVASIVE MONITORING

Blood Pressure

The first report of recorded blood pressure during anesthesia was by Cushing in 1902 [3, 4]. Though it was reluctantly accepted by skeptics in the early days, anesthesiologists have now adopted monitoring of blood pressure as a standard of care in the operating room. The Harvard Medical School Standard of Practice concerning minimal monitoring, adopted in 1985, states that, where clinically practical, every patient receiving general, regional, or monitored intravenous anesthesia should have arterial blood pressure and heart rate measured at least every 5 minutes.

Technical Aspects

The most commonly used method, known as the Riva-Rocci technique [5], makes use of audible sounds heard through a stethoscope placed on an artery. This method utilizes an inflated cuff (12–16 cm in width) placed around the arm and pneumatically inflated above the systolic pressure with the use of a sphygmomanometer. The examiner listens to the brachial artery below the cuff and slowly releases the cuff pressure until distinct sounds are heard. These are known as Korotkov sounds [6], the exact mechanisms of which are unclear, but which are postulated to be blood jetting distally through a partially open vessel during systole. The initiation of Korotkov sounds denotes systolic blood pressure. As the cuff pressure decreases and approaches diastolic pressure, sounds become muffled and low pitched, and then disappear. It is controversial as to which should be considered the true diastolic pressure, the beginning of the muffled sounds or their total cessation, and this may cause disparity in the readings taken by different clinicians (Fig. 4-1).

Other inaccuracies are associated with this method. The recommended cuff width is 20 to 30 percent of the arm circumference. If the cuff is not of adequate width in relation to the circumference of the arm, the pressure reading may be falsely

Fig. 4-1. Correlation between cuff pressure oscillations and Korotkov sounds. A = point where cuff pressure oscillations start to increase; B = amplitude corresponding to auscultatory systolic pressure; C = maximum oscillation amplitude, which signals mean pressure; D = amplitude corresponding to auscultatory diastolic pressure.

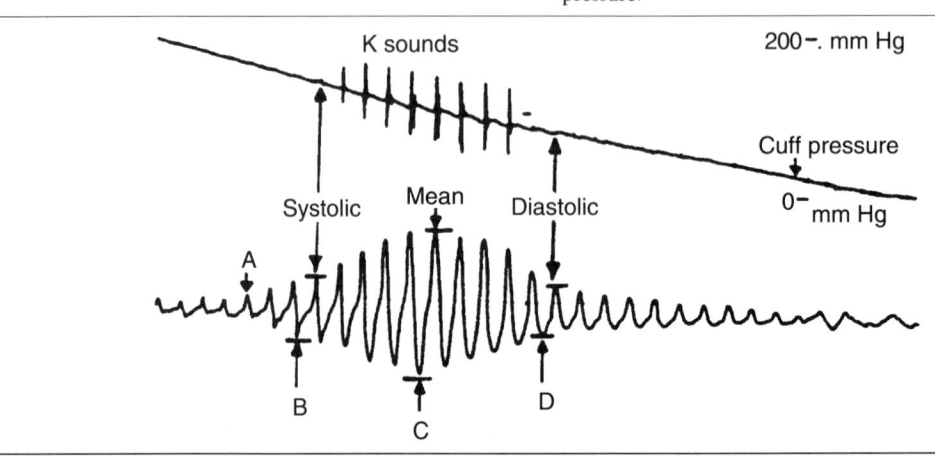

elevated. This poses an additional problem because the inflated cuff does not impart uniform pressure on the arm, falsely elevating the arterial pressure. In these patients invasive blood pressure monitoring may be indicated if the surgical procedure warrants accurate blood pressure monitoring.

The Riva-Rocci method is also inadequate in accurately measuring low blood pressures. In the critically ill, those undergoing cardiopulmonary resuscitation, and those in shock, in whom accurate measurement of low blood pressure is essential, direct intraarterial pressure monitoring is indicated. In rare instances the blood pressure cuff can be applied to the leg [7], blood pressure being palpated over the popliteal artery. Due to the extraordinary size of the thigh and difficulty in palpating the arteries of the leg, the accuracy of this method is questionable except in very lean subjects.

Intermittent Automatic Blood Pressure Monitoring

Automatic blood pressure monitoring makes use of the oscillometric principle [8] and is very commonly used in operating rooms today. Its popularity can be attributed to its reliability, accuracy, and ability to free the anesthesiologist to perform other tasks while the blood pressure is being taken. Printout capability adds to the usefulness of the monitor because it allows better record-keeping. There are several good automatic blood pressure monitors on the market. Since they also use inflatable cuffs, as in the Riva-Rocci method, they share the same cuff-related problems. The frequency of blood pressure measurements can be adjusted according to the patient's hemodynamic status. The essential component parts of the system are an inflatable cuff, which is connected to a tube used to transmit pressure changes to a transducer; a celenoid valve, which automatically allows the pressure cuff to deflate in stages; and a microprocessor, which controls the inflation/deflation sequence.

Inaccuracies in blood pressure measurements may be introduced by patient movement, which transmits pressure changes to the transducer system. Hutton and Prys-Roberts [9] have reported that the diastolic pressure may be approximately 10 mm Hg higher compared to intraarterial readings when the automatic, noninvasive blood pressure system is used. When readings seem to be inconsistent with the patient's condition, they should always be verified by another technique or monitor.

Two potential problems may be encountered: incomplete deflation of the cuff between inflations and failure of the automatic timing mechanism, which produces rapid inflation cycles that do not allow enough time for venous drainage. The result is venous stasis, swelling of the limb, and the possibility of nerve damage [10, 11].

Continuous Noninvasive Blood Pressure Monitoring

A continuous noninvasive blood pressure device, known as Finapres (Ohmeda, Englewood, CO), is available [12]. The device makes use of technology described by Penaz [13] in 1973. The monitor is a servoplethysmomanometer and utilizes a photoplethysmograph, which is built into a small cuff that can be fitted around the finger (Fig. 4-2). The diameter of the digital artery is continuously measured by transillumination. Optimum detection of change in vessel diameter is obtained by adjusting partial inflation of the cuff. Pressure changes are converted to electrical signals on the monitor screen, and the likeness of the wave form to a direct intraarterial pressure tracing is striking. The monitor does, however, require frequent calibration for accurate readings [14].

It must be cautioned that the pressure cuff may cause impairment of venous or arterial circulation to the finger, resulting in swelling and possible neurologic injury, or ischemia. Additionally, the measured pressure is that of the finger, which may be subject to local changes in arterial blood flow and may not accurately reflect blood pressure taken more proximally [15]. The device requires more extensive evaluation in clinical situations.

Electrocardiography

Electrocardiography was not routinely used in the operating room until the 1960s. Since then it has become one of the most valued noninvasive monitoring devices. In addition to being useful intraoperatively, ECG now serves as a powerful diagnostic tool in the preoperative, as well as postoperative, periods [16]. Preoperative ambulatory ECG (AECG) performed over a 24-hour period is very useful for the diagnosis of dysrhythmias and myo-

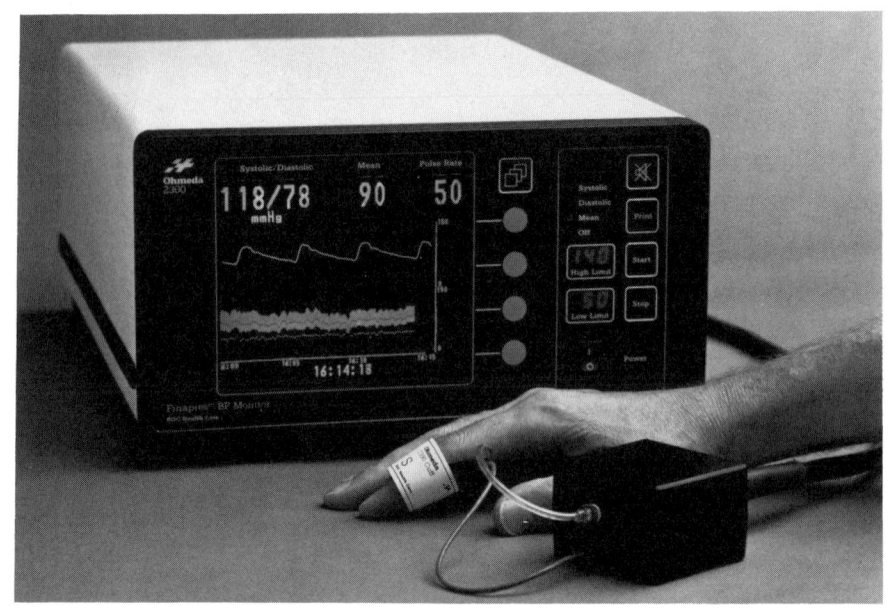

Fig. 4-2. Finapres blood pressure monitor showing the finger cuff and arterial blood pressure tracing.

cardial ischemia. Postoperatively, ECG monitoring is continued until the patient's condition is stable and he or she is ready to be discharged from the postanesthesia care unit. When ECG was introduced into the operating room, dysrhythmia detection was the main aim; however, because of the increasing age of surgical patients, the emphasis has now shifted to diagnosis of ischemia.

Diagnosis of Myocardial Ischemia
Electrocardiography is a simple, inexpensive, and noninvasive method of detecting myocardial ischemia. In the preoperative period both an exercise tolerance test and AECG are good diagnostic tests to identify patients with coronary artery disease (CAD). These tests are used for screening patients who are at high risk and identifying those with silent ischemia. They are discussed more fully in Chapter 5.

This underscores the importance of our being able to effectively diagnose intraoperative ischemia. The use of a five-lead ECG with leads II and V_5 monitoring capability enhances ischemia detection from 60 to 85 percent when compared to lead II monitoring alone. If in addition V_4 is also used, the yield is increased further to 90 percent of all detectable ischemia diagnosed by a 12-lead ECG [17, 18]. Therefore, if possible a five-lead ECG should be utilized when ischemia detection is important. If this is not available, a three-lead system can be modified to give lead II and modified V_5 readings. This is achieved by placing the right arm lead on the right shoulder, the left arm lead on the V_5 position, and the left leg lead in the usual position. Lead I is then selected to give a modified V_5 ECG [19], while lead II selection will still give a true lead II, which is the most useful lead for arrhythmia detection [17].

It has been demonstrated that intermittent visual observation of the intraoperative ECG is an unsatisfactory method of ischemia detection. This can best be overcome by a computerized system that not only picks up ischemic changes but also gives cumulative summation of all ECG changes over unit time, known as ECG ST trending [20] (Fig. 4-3). Computer technology sets the PR interval as the baseline and compares deviation of the ST segment in relation to it. A summation of all deviations can then be plotted graphically to facilitate visual appreciation of ST segment changes

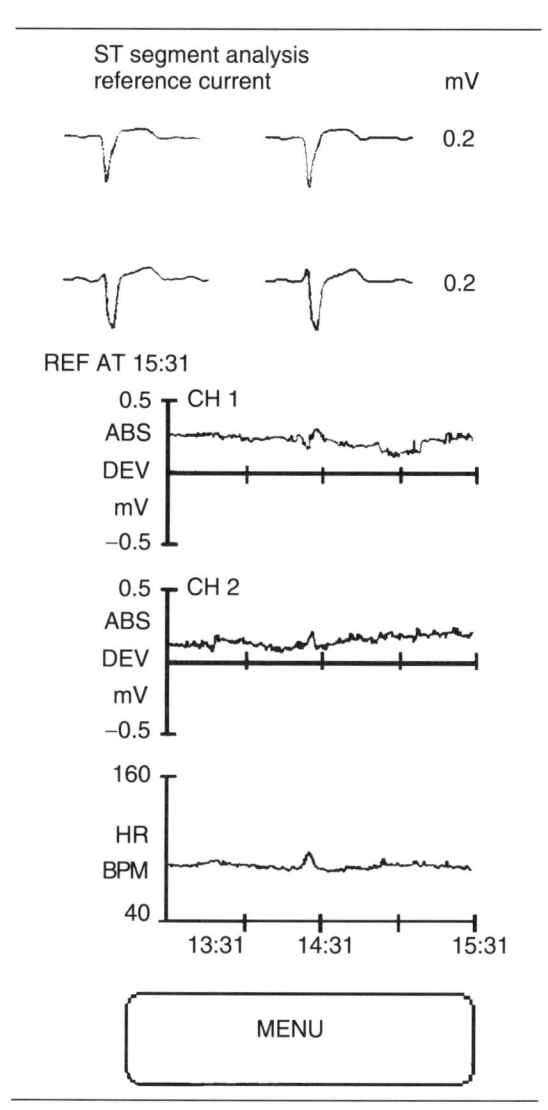

Fig. 4-3. An example of computerized ST segment analysis and trending over 2 hours. CH 1 = channel 1 = lead II; CH 2 = channel 2 = lead V_5; HR = heart rate.

in a quantitative fashion. The intraoperative ECG is also used to detect arrhythmias, which are discussed more fully in Chap. 10.

Echocardiography

Echocardiography has been used in cardiology since 1953, mainly for the diagnosis of valvular heart disease, cardiac tumors, and pericardial effusions. The transthoracic approach used by cardiologists made the use of echo difficult in the operating room. It remained exclusively a cardiology tool until Frazin inserted the echo transducer into the tip of a gastroscope for use as a transesophageal echocardiogram (TEE) [21]. This method was introduced into the operating room in 1985. This new technology made anesthesiologists the natural users of TEE in the operating room. However, TEE has brought with it a diagnostic modality that requires skill and training not readily available to all anesthesiologists. Attempts are being made at a national level to resolve this issue by setting credentialing standards so that anesthesiologists can be certified to use and interpret TEE readings [22]. Until then, it is advised that interpretation be reviewed and confirmed by a trained cardiologist and that a formal report be placed in the patient's chart as a permanent record. This becomes even more important if surgical decisions are made on the basis of echocardiographic findings interpreted by anesthesiologists.

General Information

The echocardiogram makes use of piezoelectric crystals, which, when electrically stimulated, emit sound waves greatly in excess of audible frequency (>20,000 Hz). These are known as ultrasound waves, which travel through most body tissue at a speed of 1,540 meters per second. When confronted with a tissue interface, one of three things will happen: The ultrasound can either reflect, scatter, or be absorbed by the tissue. All three result in a diminished energy with which sound can subsequently travel. The reflected waves are sensed by the transducer and converted to electrical signals as visual images. Depending on the type of transducer and equipment used, the images may either be displayed as M (motion) mode or the currently introduced two-dimensional (2D) version. The M mode is displayed as a "slice" through the heart and by sequencing many images quickly a mobile effect is generated. The 2D echo displays a triangular plane through the heart, giving a more lifelike picture, and allows better visualization of various parts of the heart. Since a good amount of echo is either scattered or absorbed, images of superior resolution are obtained close to the transducer and become

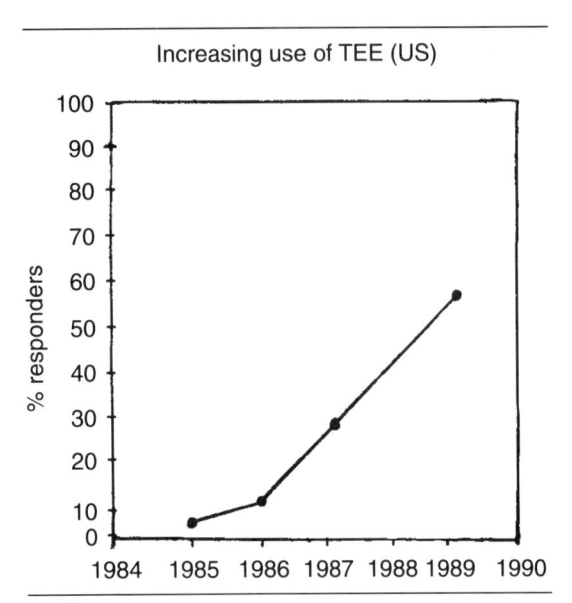

Fig. 4-4. Increase in the use of TEE in the United States.

less clear as the distance from the transducer increases. Transthoracic echo gives images of inferior clarity when compared with TEE because of interposed cartilage, ribs, and lungs, all of which interfere with the transmission of ultrasound. High-end ultrasound frequency (5–7 MHz) provides better resolution but less penetration than low-end (2.5–3.5 MHz), which gives better penetration but inferior resolution. TEE utilizes frequencies of 5 MHz or greater, whereas transthoracic echo is performed with 3.5 MHz or less.

Transesophageal echocardiography has enjoyed substantial increase in use in the past few years (Fig. 4-4), mainly because it is relatively noninvasive and is associated with a very low complication rate. Ultrasound has not been shown to be a radiation hazard and is safe to use in pregnancy. The clarity of images obtained by TEE is superior to that of transthoracic echocardiography, with excellent views of the aortic and mitral valves, the atria, the aortic outflow tract, the interventricular septum, and the left ventricular cavity. The only views that are sometimes less than satisfactory are those of the right ventricle and the tricuspid valve, because these are further away from the esophagus. Color Doppler capability allows flow visualization as an added diagnostic feature. In most instances interpretation of data is not complicated for routine clinical work [23, 24]. The system also allows for storage of images, which can be reviewed with a cardiologist.

Technical Aspects

The TEE scope is 110 cm long and has a nontraumatic tip, which, depending on the make, is approximately 14 mm long and 11 mm wide. The tip can be manipulated by a turning mechanism in a fashion similar to that used with the gastroscope. It is advisable that the scope be carefully handled and maintained, because the protective sheath that covers the tip is susceptible to damage by sharp objects (such as teeth) and this can seriously deteriorate the image quality and become an electrical hazard. The scope can be gently washed with water after use and then submerged in glutaraldehyde (Cidex) for 15 minutes before subsequent use. Before insertion it is advisable to empty the stomach and esophagus of air and other contents with a gastric tube for a clearer image. It is also recommended that a protective sheath be used around the scope when it is inserted into the patient.

When the scope reaches a depth of 30 cm, the aortic valve and the atria will come into view (Fig. 4-5). The tip of the scope can be directed in the appropriate position for best images. When the scope is inserted 2 to 3 cm further, the long-axis (four-chamber) view of the heart comes into view (Fig. 4-6). By advancing the probe further, the short-axis view of the left ventricle is seen. This view is particularly useful in the diagnosis of ventricular cavity size and segmental wall motion abnormalities (SWMA). The fluid status of the patient can be monitored easily: The circumference of the ventricular cavity is determined by mapping the perimeter with the tracer, and an estimation of ventricular contractility and ejection fraction is obtained by comparing the end diastolic and the end systolic circumferences of the ventricle. Ventricular contractility can also be assessed by using the M mode in the short-axis view and comparing the distance between the anterior and posterior walls of the ventricle in diastole and systole. In poorly contractile ventricles, the difference between systole and diastole is small, whereas in ventricles with good ejection, the systolic wall thick-

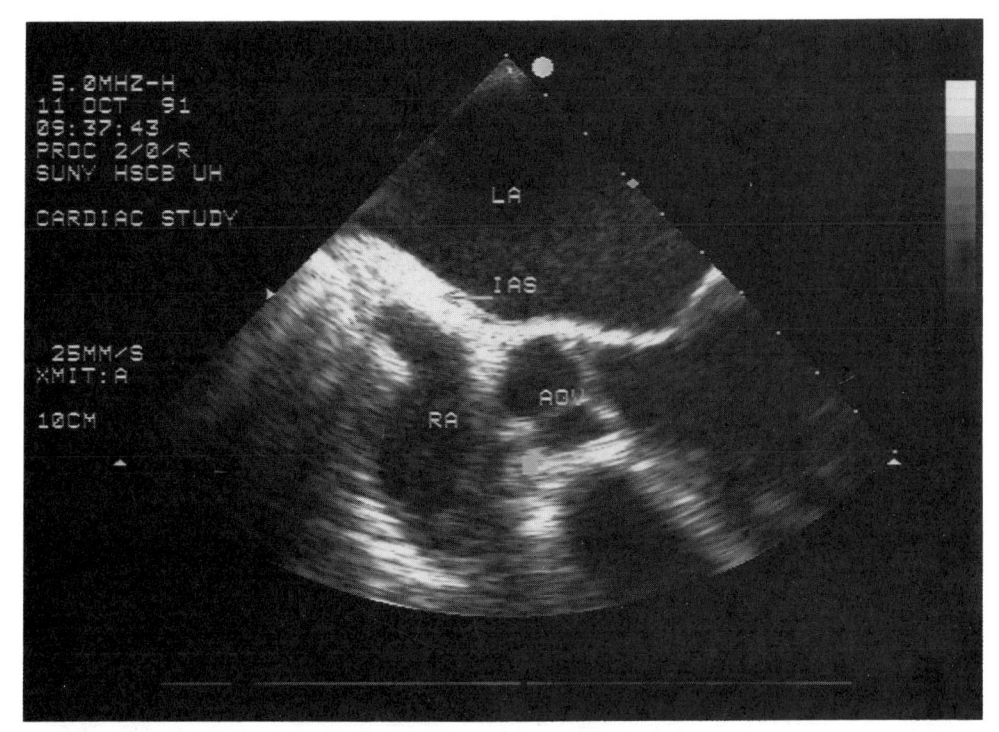

Fig. 4-5. Short-axis view of aortic valve and surrounding structures. AOV = aortic valve; RA = right atrium; LA = left atrium; IAS = intraatrial septum.

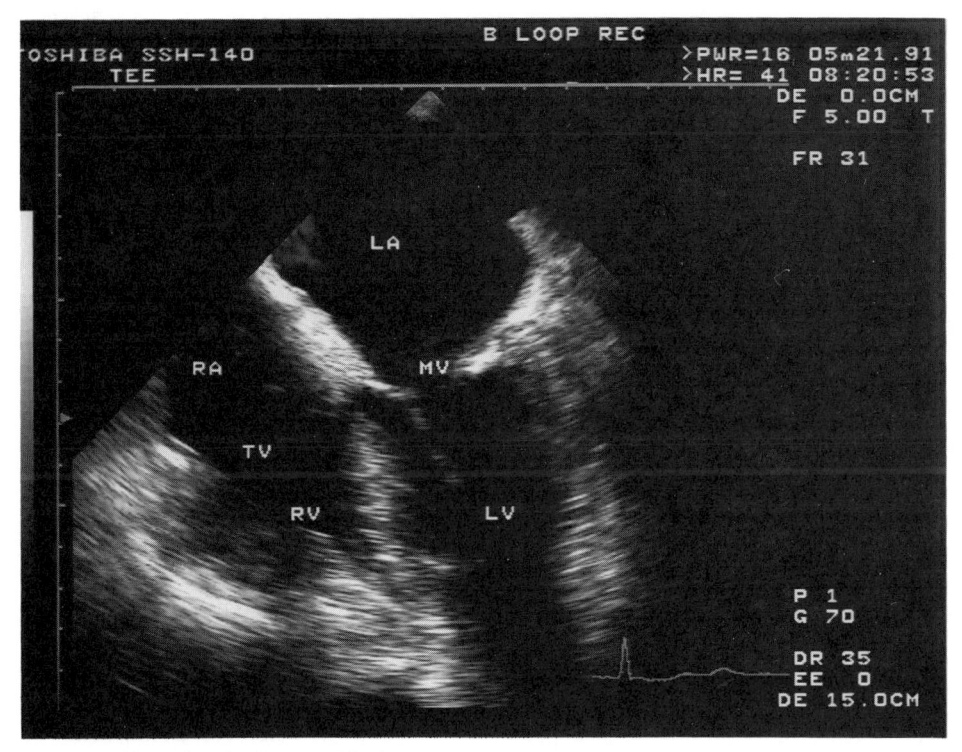

Fig. 4-6. Long-axis (four-chamber) view of the heart showing all four chambers. LA = left atrium; RV = right ventricle; TV = tricuspid valve; RA = right atrium; LV = left ventricle; MV = mitral valve.

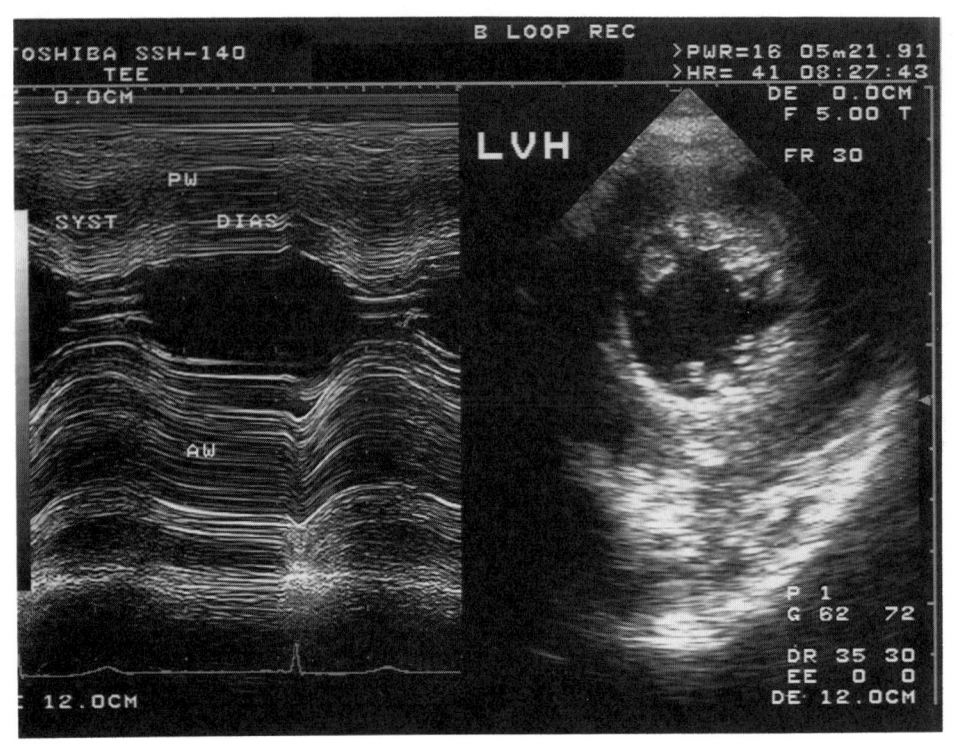

Fig. 4-7. Short-axis view of the left ventricle showing cross section through the papillary muscles. This ventricle is hypertrophied and the M mode (*left*) shows good contractility. PW = posterior wall; AW = anterior wall; syst = systole; dias = diastole.

ening is greater (Fig. 4-7), as is the difference between systole and diastole.

Ischemia Detection

The short-axis view is the most useful for detection of ischemia. Tennant and Wiggers [25] in 1935 demonstrated that dog ventricles showed signs of SWMA within seconds after occlusion of a coronary artery. This information is now being used to diagnose ischemia in humans using the echo. It is important to standardize the short-axis view in order to do this correctly. The plane should pass through both the papillary muscles. A central point in the ventricular cavity can be visually ascertained and the movement of each quadrant of the myocardium toward this point determined. Where no SWMA exists all four quadrants will move toward the center during systole with equal thickening, maintaining a uniform circular cavity, but with a decreased diameter. At this level blood is supplied to the myocardium by all three coronary arteries, that is, right coronary artery (RCA), left anterior descending (LAD), and circumflex (CIRC) coronary arteries (Fig. 4-8). When SWMA exists, one or more quadrants corresponding to one or more areas of coronary blood supply will either move less (hypokinesia), or not at all (akinesia), or move paradoxically outward (dyskinesia) [26–28]. Split-screen or quadruple-screen images can be viewed simultaneously so that prior wall motion can be compared with contemporaneous data. Such direct comparison is important in evaluating changing myocardial function so that appropriate therapeutic maneuvers can be initiated.

Since one of the main uses of TEE is to diagnose myocardial ischemia, it is important to compare its sensitivity and specificity to that of other diagnostic modalities. It has been shown that in patients undergoing coronary balloon angioplasty, SWMA were detected earlier and with greater frequency

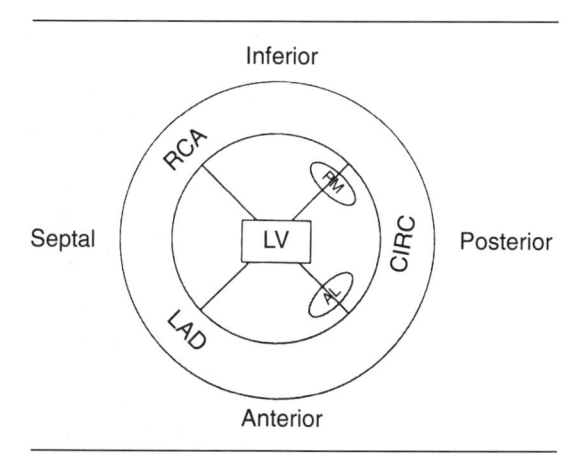

Fig. 4-8. Diagrammatic short-axis transesophageal echocardiogram at the midpapillary muscle level. LV = left ventricular cavity; AL and PM = anterior lateral and posterior medial papillary muscles. The LV is divided into four segments or walls by two perpendicular lines that bisect the papillary muscles. The walls are by convention named anterior, posterior, septal, and inferior. Coronary blood flow is supplied to these walls as indicated by the left anterior descending coronary artery (LAD), the circumflex coronary artery (CIRC), and the right coronary artery (RCA). (Reprinted with permission from MK Cahalan, Detection of Intraoperative Myocardial Ischemia. In NP de Bruijn and FM Clements (eds), *Intraoperative Use of Echocardiography*. Philadelphia: Lippincott, 1991. P. 51.)

Table 4-1. Conditions that can be detected by TEE

Intraoperative ischemia

The size of various chambers of the heart, especially the left ventricle, which is not visualized adequately by other techniques because of its posterior position even during cardiac surgery

Mitral valve pathology, i.e., mitral stenosis, regurgitation, prolapse of the mitral valve, presence of vegetations

Thrombi in the atria or ventricles

Atrial and ventricular septal defects

Aortic stenosis, incompetence, calcification, dilatation

Interventricular septal thickening at the level of the left ventricular outflow tract

Air in the heart chambers and the proximal aorta

Pericardial effusion

Tumors of the heart and extension of extracardiac tumors into the heart

Aortic dissection and aneurysm

Left main coronary artery disease

with TEE than with ECG ST changes [29]. Smith and associates [30] showed intraoperative TEE to be more sensitive in the detection of myocardial ischemia than ECG. TEE determination of ischemia is made more difficult because not all SWMA are related to ongoing ischemia, but may be due to false positives related to old infarcts or to the patient's volume status and afterload, or may be variations of normal contractility. Other common uses of the TEE include estimation of left ventricular size [31], detection of atrial thrombi [32], intracardiac air [33–35], and aortic dissection [36, 37]. A more complete list of conditions that can be detected by TEE is presented in Table 4-1.

New technology introduced by Hewlett-Packard (Andover, MA) in their latest model, HP SONOS 1500, permits continuous tracking of endocardial borders using raw acoustic data that can display cardiac chamber geometry. This technology is likely to enhance quantitative analysis of cardiac function. Biplane, 2D echo capability is also available, allowing us to view a segment of the heart in two planes, both horizontal (transverse) and vertical. Most recently, Hewlett-Packard has introduced the omniplane, TEE, 2D, color flow Doppler transducer; allowing for multiple plane analysis.

INVASIVE MONITORING

Indications for Invasive Blood Pressure Monitoring

High-risk patients, especially those with cardiac disease, are prone to hemodynamic instability in the perioperative period. Direct arterial pressure monitoring is essential in these cases, because it provides accurate, online information of the patient's hemodynamic status and at the same time frees the anesthesiologist to attend to other important tasks. Strip chart records and trending software can be installed on monitors so that a record of blood pressure readings over time can be reviewed as needed. Besides obtaining pressure readings it is possible to print out the pressure trace for further analysis of the wave form. Rise in pressure over time (dp/dt) is an important measure and gives us information about myocardial contractility. The higher the ratio of dp/dt, the stronger the myocardial contraction. A narrow pressure wave form is often indicative of constricted arterial vasculature, as in hypovolemia, or it could indicate the use of vasoconstrictor therapy. A wide pulse wave, on the other hand, is often an indication of myocardial depression due to the use of cardiac depressant drugs, such as β-blockers or inhalational anesthetic. An added use of an arterial line is for repeated arterial blood sampling. Commonly used sites of insertion of arterial cannulas include radial, femoral, axillary, and dorsalis pedis arteries.

Radial Artery Cannulation

Patency of the palmar arch before insertion of a radial artery catheter is assessed by performing Allen's test, which was first described in 1929 [38]. In this test the patient is first asked to make a tight fist. The anesthesiologist then occludes both the radial and the ulnar arteries at the patient's wrist with his or her hands. The patient is then asked to open the fist, revealing a blanched appearance of the hand. Pressure on the ulnar artery is released to allow blood flow to the hand. This maneuver should immediately change the blanched appearance to a red color starting from the ulnar to the radial side, thus ensuring adequate ulnar circulation. If this happens it is assumed that the radial artery can be safely cannulated. However, if the ulnar artery is inadequate, the radial cannulation is best avoided. Slogoff and associates [39] questioned the usefulness of Allen's test when they showed that neither a positive nor a negative test correlates with outcome. Other general guidelines could be followed. The catheter diameter should be small to allow adequate blood flow around it, yet large enough to provide a good trace and allow easy sampling [40]. A 20-gauge (G) catheter is generally optimum for radial artery cannulation.

The wrist is placed comfortably in a supine position over an arm board with a 1-in.-thick soft booster under the wrist. The arm and hand are secured in place with tape leaving the thumb free. The radial artery is then palpated just proximal to the proximal crease of the wrist and the area is appropriately prepared for a sterile technique. Lidocaine 1 percent is instilled in the subcutaneous area with a 25G needle. Several methods are used for radial artery cannulation. A 20G Arrow radial artery catheter with a spring guidewire can be used. It is inserted slowly into the anterior wall of the vessel (Fig. 4-9). Blood flashback is seen in the clear tube located distal to the catheter. The spring guidewire is then advanced into the vessel and the entire unit moved forward 2 to 3 mm before the catheter is selectively advanced into the vessel, to

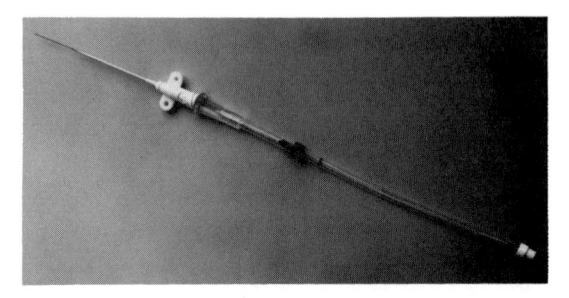

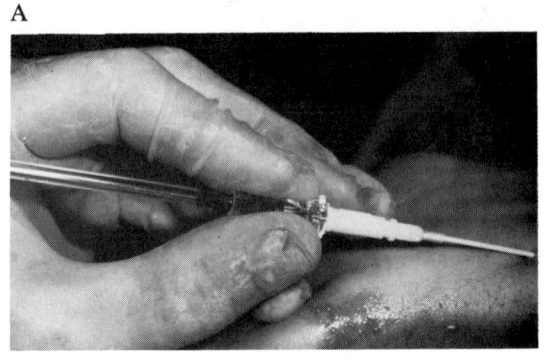

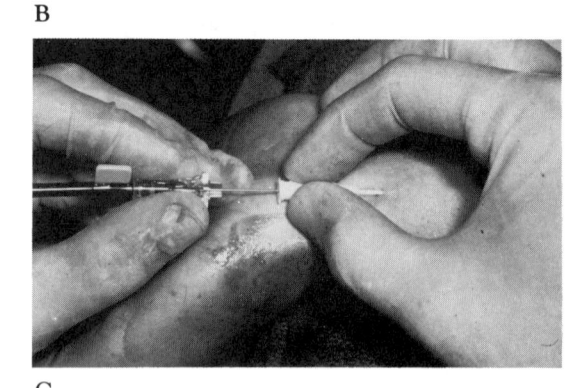

Fig. 4-9. A. An Arrow catheter-over-the-needle assembly with built-in spring guidewire. B. After entry into the radial artery, the unit is depressed to be in line with the course of the artery and the wire is advanced as shown. C. The catheter is then threaded over the wire as shown.

its fullest length. The guidewire and needle are then separated from the catheter and removed. Next, the catheter is attached to the transducer tubing for a pressure reading. The catheter can be sutured in place to ensure secure placement. It is advisable to use a small dab of an antiseptic such as povidone-iodine (Betadine) and to cover the site with a clear adhesive to protect against infection.

Other methods of radial artery placement can be achieved with the use of a regular catheter-over-the-needle technique. This is accomplished in two ways. In the first method the catheter and needle enter only through the anterior wall of the vessel. When blood flashback occurs, the catheter and needle are advanced another 1 to 2 mm and the catheter is then advanced separately into the vessel over the needle. In the second technique, the vessel is "transfixed," meaning the catheter-over-the-needle unit is advanced through both the anterior and posterior walls of the vessel. The needle is then removed and the catheter slowly withdrawn until the blood is seen to eject from the proximal end. The catheter is then advanced into the lumen of the vessel and secured in the usual way. The disadvantages of this method are that the needle travels a longer distance into the patient and may cause more pain and tissue damage. Touching the periosteum of the radius with the needle is very painful. The other disadvantage is that, instead of one, there are two openings into the vessel and hence the chance of hematoma is greater.

Femoral Artery Catheterization

There is no documented difference between the complication rate of radial artery and femoral artery cannulation, but it would be appropriate to avoid the femoral site in obese patients and in those with atherosclerosis. In obese patients it is difficult to maintain catheter hygiene and in patients with atherosclerosis the possibility exists of atheromatous embolization distally. A continuous heparin flush and use of nonthrombogenic material such as Teflon will keep the complication rate low [41].

The femoral artery is the second most commonly cannulated vessel after the radial. In many cases it is more easily detected and catheterized because the artery is large and more readily palpable, especially in patients with low arterial blood pressure. The disadvantages are that it is quite deeply situated in obese patients and the groin area is difficult to keep clean. The other problem is, because the artery is deep, regular-sized catheters (up to 2 in.) are not long enough for cannulation except in very thin individuals. Therefore, either a 4-in.-long Arrow catheter-over-the-needle unit or an 8 in., 17-gauge catheter-through-the-needle technique can be employed. In the latter, skin is prepared and draped in a manner similar to that of other techniques. Local anesthetic solution is instilled into the skin and a 17-gauge needle is inserted into the femoral artery. When blood spurts out from the proximal end, the needle hub is lowered slightly and the catheter inserted into the vessel through the needle. The needle is then withdrawn and the catheter sutured to the skin. The disadvantages of this technique include hematoma formation, the possibility of catheter shearing against the needle, arteriovenous (AV) fistula formation, atheromatous emboli to the periphery, and infection.

Axillary Artery Cannulation

Axillary artery cannulation can also be used for intraarterial monitoring [42]. This is the preferred method at some critical care units because it allows changing patient position without tubing entanglement and the catheter is in easy reach for nursing care. The disadvantage is that the catheter is too close to the central arteries and the ever-present danger exists of air and particulate emboli to the brain during catheter flushings. Since the insertion site is close to the axilla, it is also difficult to keep clean.

Occasionally, the dorsalis pedis artery is used when other vessels are not available due to trauma or burns.

Inaccuracies in Arterial Pressure Monitoring

It is important to understand that blood pressure readings may differ depending on the cannulation site (Figs. 4-10 and 4-11). Smaller peripheral arteries tend to have a larger wall–lumen ratio because of the amount of elastic tissue present in the vessel wall. This leads to a higher systolic and a lower diastolic pressure compared to the aortic root pressure, although the mean pressure decreases only slightly away from the heart.

Other factors also affect the monitored pressure. Lengthy, noncompliant, narrow tubing leads to

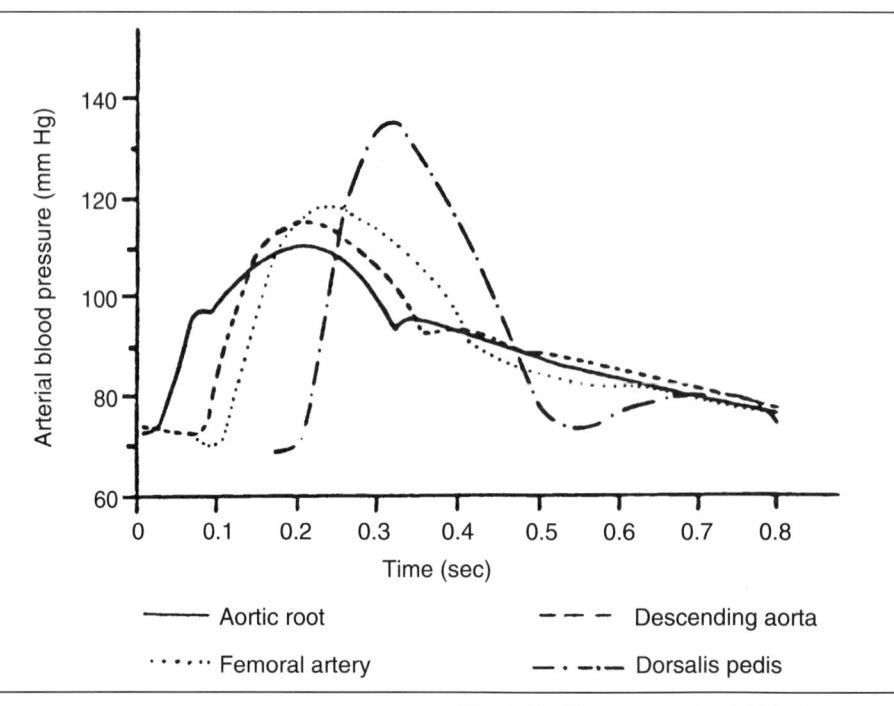

Fig. 4-10. Comparison of atrial blood pressure obtained at locations away from the heart.

falsely elevated systolic blood pressure. Typically, the tracing has a peaked, narrow, and pointed appearance, which can be corrected by inserting a "damper" in the system. An air bubble in the tubing will achieve the same result and dampen the "overshoot" that occurs with the systolic pressure. It is recommended that the number of stopcocks be reduced to minimum and that transducers be as close to the artery as possible for the most accurate readings.

Complications

Arterial cannulation is not without complications. Because of this, the decision to place arterial lines should be given careful prior consideration. Minor complications include pain associated with arterial cannulation, small hematoma formation related to catheter placement as well as its removal, and thrombosis or reduced blood flow. Thrombosis is common and occurs in more than 20 percent of patients. Factors associated with increased incidence of thrombosis are as follows:

1. *Duration of cannulation.* Bedford and Wollman [43] found that thrombosis is unlikely if the arterial catheter is left in place for less than 2 hours. It increases to 25 percent between 2 and 20 hours and to 50 percent thereafter.
2. *Catheter material.* Polyethylene catheters cause more thrombosis than Teflon catheters when catheters of the same size are used [41, 44].
3. *Size of the catheter.* Incidence of thrombosis is decreased when 20G instead of 18G catheters are used.
4. *Catheter style.* Tapered catheters tend to cause more thrombosis and decreased flow than non-tapered catheters [44].
5. *Arterial diameter.* Rate of occlusion is inversely proportional to the size of the artery [40].
6. *Wrist circumference.* Wrist circumference is inversely proportional to the incidence of thrombosis [45]. Weiss and Gattiker [46] found critical wrist circumference for a 20G catheter to be 15 cm.

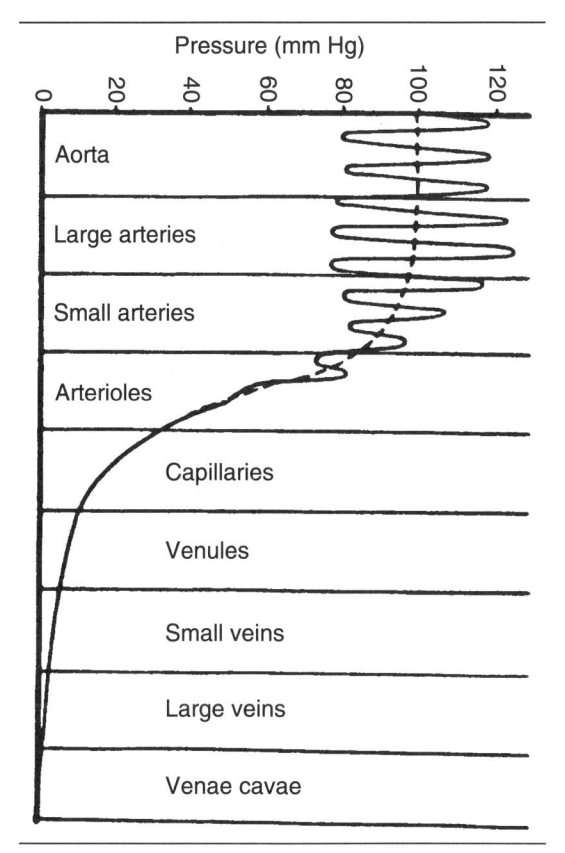

Fig. 4-11. Mean pressure in different vessels.

7. *Intermittent versus continuous heparin flush.* More frequent thrombosis occurs if intermittent irrigation is used as compared to a continuous flush with heparinized saline [47].
8. *Gender.* Slogoff and associates [39] showed a higher incidence of abnormal flow in female versus male patients after decannulation.

Thrombotic complications at the catheter site are increased when coexisting diseases, such as proximal emboli, hypoproteinemia, and prolonged shock, as well as the use of vasopressors, are present [48]. Abnormal flow after removal of catheters occurs in 25 percent of patients. It has been observed that when large vessels are used recanalization occurs within 4 to 7 days in 67 percent of patients, and when smaller vessels are cannulated the time to recanalize is prolonged [39]. It is possible to partially remove some thrombi during decannulation, by applying suction with a syringe while the catheter is being withdrawn [49]. A major complication [46, 48, 50] is severe curtailment of distal blood supply, occasionally progressing to necrosis and gangrene of the fingers or toes. Infection and emboli to the periphery, injury due to direct trauma during catheter insertion, or pressure compression due to hematoma are all possible. Migration of a severed catheter distally that required surgical exploration has also been reported. In experienced hands the complication rate is low and seems to be similar for radial and femoral catheterization.

Central Venous and Pulmonary Arterial Pressure Monitoring

Central Venous Pressure (CVP)

In the management of patients with unstable hemodynamics or when large fluid shifts are anticipated, it is important to have an accurate estimation of the patient's fluid status. This should be achieved by noninvasive means when possible, but in acute situations under anesthesia skin turgor and external jugular venous filling are not reliable indicators. Urine output is a good monitor of volume status but may be misleading in patients with acute trauma, in heart failure, in renal dysfunction, and in those who have received diuretics. In these cases one must have a measurable assessment of the patient's fluid status. In most cases measurement of the CVP is a satisfactory way to achieve this. However, Mangano [51] has shown that CVP is an accurate measure of right heart filling, but not left, when left ventricular ejection fraction decreases below 40 percent. Therefore, reliance on the CVP alone should only be considered when left ventricular function can be assumed to be normal.

When monitoring the CVP it is essential to verify that the catheter is indeed in the central vein, by chest x-ray or examination of the central venous wave forms on the monitor, or both. The CVP also displays respiratory fluctuations. The CVP can be measured using a water manometer, although it is not very convenient to use and has a slow response time. Furthermore, it is often difficult to ascertain the position of the central venous catheter by looking at the fluctuations of the water

Fig. 4-12. Central venous pressure tracing taken from a patient under anesthesia. a = atrial contraction; c = bulging of tricuspid valve; x = atrial relaxation; v = filling of blood in right atrium; y = opening of tricuspid valve and ventricular filling.

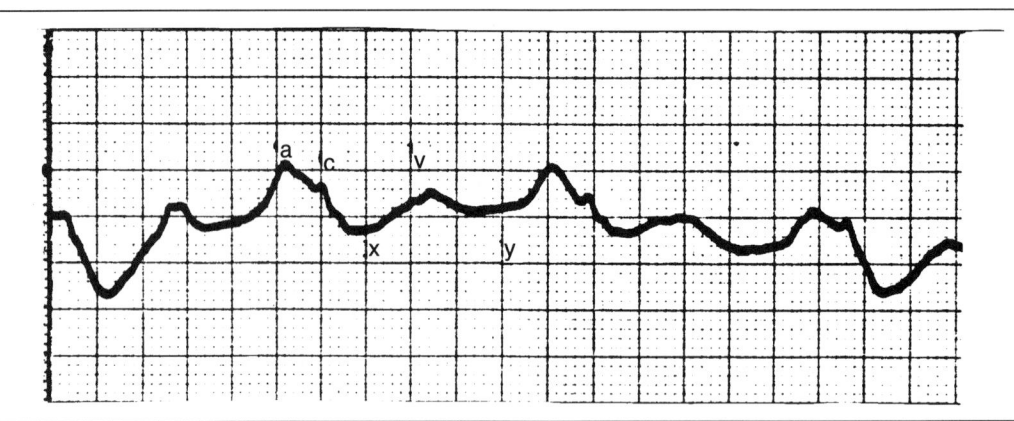

level. Transducer monitoring of CVP is the method of CVP measurement used today. It is convenient, easy to visualize, and accurate. The transducer setup must be carefully calibrated before use. With adequate enlargement of the trace on the monitor, it is possible to visualize waves with peaks and troughs related to the CVP (Fig. 4-12). The CVP tracing is characterized by an "a" wave produced by the arterial contraction, followed by a smaller "c" wave, which represents the initial bulging of the tricuspid valve (TV) into the atrium with the onset of ventricular systole. An "x" descent is attributed to the atrial relaxation and pulling down of the TV; a late positive "v" wave is seen due to accumulation of blood in the vena cava and right atrium with the TV closed. Lastly, a "y" descent occurs from the opening of the TV and right ventricular filling.

A hard-copy printout may be necessary for closer security of the wave form. In atrial fibrillation and other asynchronous AV contractions, the atrium contracts while the AV valve is closed, giving rise to a "giant" a wave, whereas a large v wave is seen in tricuspid incompetence. Normal mean venous pressure is between 5 and 10 mm Hg.

Sites of Venipuncture

Internal Jugular Vein (IJV). The IJV is the most direct route to the right heart. In experienced hands cannulation of the IJV is relatively safe. A common way to enter the IJV is via the anterior neck. All sterile precautions should be taken while an IJV catheter is being placed. It helps to have the patient in the Trendelenburg position. This fills the IJV and also prevents air emboli on insertion of the cannula into the vein. During right IJV puncture the head is turned to the left and the triangle made by the medial and lateral heads of the sternomastoid muscle on either side and the clavicle below is identified. After local anesthetic infiltration the apex of the triangle is entered with a 20-gauge finder needle. The needle is directed at a 60° angle to the skin and advanced along the lateral head of the sternomastoid muscle while gentle suction is applied on the syringe. A good blood flow will be established as soon as the needle enters the vein. An 18-gauge catheter-over-the-needle can then be inserted along the finder needle as its guide. Once the catheter is in place, it can be attached to the transducer to confirm its intravenous position and then a guidewire can be passed through the catheter. The catheter is subsequently removed and a larger cannula is inserted in the IJV over the guidewire (Seldinger technique) [52].

Subclavian Vein Approach. Since this approach is relatively easy and cannulation can be performed in a short time, it is the best route for central venous cannulation in emergencies. It is also a good approach in children. The patient is placed in the Trendelenburg position with the head turned to the opposite side. The area around the clavicle is prepared for the sterile procedure. Local anesthetic solution is instilled just under the clavicle at the junction between its medial two thirds and lateral one third. An 18-gauge 2½-in. needle is inserted just under the clavicle toward the sternal notch. Gentle suction is applied to the needle with a syringe as it is advanced into the patient. It is important to stay just under the clavicle, as a deeper course will lead to either lung injury or a subclavian artery puncture. When the needle is in good position, the Seldinger technique can be used to introduce a catheter into the subclavian vein. Recently, a new Raulerson syringe was introduced that allows passing of the wire directly through the plunger of the syringe, thereby eliminating the need to disconnect the syringe from the vein once blood return is seen.

Antecubital and Femoral Vein Approach. From both these veins a long catheter can be introduced into the central circulation. All catheters used for CVP should be radiopaque and their position should be confirmed both radiographically and by monitor tracing as described previously. It is important to rule out pneumothorax with the IJV and subclavian vein approaches.

The most common complications of CVP placement are inadvertent carotid or subclavian artery puncture and pneumothorax (Table 4-2). Inadvertent arterial puncture is dealt with in the section on pulmonary artery catheterization.

Pneumothorax occurs with moderate frequency with the subclavian approach (incidence 10%) and rarely with the IJV approach (<1%). If the chest x-ray findings show that there is a greater than 20 percent pneumothorax, a chest tube should be inserted on that side and connected to a water trap until it shows signs of resolving. A pneumothorax of less than 20 percent may be observed with serial chest x-rays while the clinical status of the patient is being assessed. If the pneumothorax increases in size radiologically or if the respiratory status of the patient deteriorates, a chest tube should be placed.

After a trace from the CVP catheter is obtained, it is important to interpret the data correctly. An incorrectly positioned and calibrated transducer will result in false CVP values, which could result in improper fluid or drug therapy. Older patients tolerate fluids poorly, especially if these individuals have associated renal dysfunction. In these patients fluid therapy should be instituted slowly and carefully even when the CVP is low. In patients with poor left ventricular function, there may be a discrepancy between the CVP and the pulmonary capillary wedge pressure (PCWP). Without the help of a pulmonary artery catheter, these patients could easily be fluid overloaded.

Pulmonary Artery Catheterization

In 1844, Claude Bernard was the first person to perform cardiac catheterization [53]. This was done in a retrograde fashion in a horse using the internal jugular and the carotid vessels to enter the right and the left sides of the heart, respectively. Werner Forsmann [54] is credited with being the first individual to catheterize the heart of a living human. He did this by inserting a catheter into his own arm vein and advancing it into the right atrium under fluoroscopic guidance. Dexter [55], in 1949, was instrumental in showing that pulmonary capillary wedge pressure was an accurate estimate of left atrial pressure. In 1970, a flow-directed pulmonary artery catheter [56] was developed and successfully used in humans by Swan and Ganz. The catheter was "floated" into the right ventricle and the pulmonary artery through a large vein, the direction of the catheter being guided along the blood flow by an inflated balloon much like a sail that propels a boat downwind. Today the catheter has become the most frequently used invasive monitoring device in high-risk patients.

The pulmonary artery catheter, with balloon-tipped floatation capability, allows the catheter to be placed in the pulmonary artery without the use of fluoroscopic equipment. This makes the device ideal for use by anesthesiologists in the operating room. Most anesthesiologists make use of the

Table 4-2. Complications associated with CVP monitoring

Inadvertent arterial puncture
Pneumothorax
Infection
Hematoma formation
Hemothorax
Catheter shearing
Nerve injury

catheter in the preinduction period, so that its use is maximized during the induction of anesthesia when the most severe hemodynamic changes are likely to occur. In the early 1970s when the catheters were relatively new, different venous accesses were utilized, such as the antecubital, femoral, internal jugular [57], and subclavian veins. Now anesthesiologists use the internal jugular and subclavian routes almost exclusively. The internal jugular route is most convenient for the anesthesiologist because if affords easy access and maneuverability of the catheter as needed. The second most frequently used site is the subclavian vein. This approach has a high success rate, but, as with subclavian CVPs, it is associated with an approximately 10 percent incidence of pneumothorax.

Another approach that is convenient, but associated with a smaller success rate, is the right external jugular vein. Unlike the IJV, which has a direct access to the right atrium, one has to negotiate a right-angle turn with the innominate vein before entering the superior vena cava (SVC). In order to achieve this, the Seldinger technique with a "J"-tip guidewire is essential [58]. In some instances it is impossible to negotiate the right-angle turn into the SVC, and catheter insertion is unsuccessful. Despite this, it is a helpful method when the IJV approach is contraindicated, for example, in carotid artery disease (when it is important to stay away from the artery to avoid inadvertent carotid puncture and cerebral emboli).

Indications for Use

Pulmonary artery catheters can yield a good amount of valuable information about the pulmonary circulation and left ventricular function—and, indirectly, myocardial ischemia. This is possible by obtaining pulmonary artery pressure and cardiac output measurements. The information can be used to provide pulmonary and systemic vascular resistances and aid in the pharmacologic treatment with vasoconstrictors, vasodilators, inotropes, and chronotropes. Despite this, no prospective, randomized study has been performed that attributed improvement in cardiovascular outcome to the use of pulmonary artery catheters. The use of the catheter has also come into scrutiny of late because of budgetary constraints and the desire to cut health care–related expenditure [59]. The cost of the catheter, introducer, and transducer is generally between $100 and $150, and the anesthesiologist's fee for insertion and interpretation of data derived from the catheter is up to $500. Critics of pulmonary artery catheters argue that in the absence of clear improvement in outcome, the use of these catheters should be significantly reduced. The proponents of the catheter claim that the hemodynamic information gained is important and helps in patient management. Since it is difficult to assess how many lives would be lost without the use of the catheter, the benefit of the doubt should tilt in favor of using it when indicated.

There are many indications for the use of the pulmonary artery catheter. Generally, the catheter can be used for patients with poor left ventricular function who are undergoing major surgical procedures. The more compromised the cardiovascular system and the more extensive the surgical procedure, the more compelling will be the reason for its use. Other indications include ischemic heart disease, septic shock, major trauma, and major vascular surgery.

Catheter Insertion Technique

The pulmonary artery catheter can be inserted from any of the sites described in the section on CVP monitoring; the best approach for the anesthesiologist is the IJV. The Seldinger technique is employed to insert a No. 8.5 French introducer into the central vein (Fig. 4-13). The pulmonary artery catheter is slipped through the protective sheath and the balloon is tested with air. Inflation should not be performed with more than 1.5 cc air. The catheter is inserted 20 cm into the central vein through the introducer and the balloon is inflated. The catheter is steadily advanced and should be in the right atrium between 30 and 35 cm. The right ventricle is usually reached between 35 and 40 cm and the pulmonary artery (PA) between 40 and 45 cm. The PCWP will be seen by advancing the catheter 5 cm beyond its entry into the pulmonary artery (Fig. 4-14). In the vast majority of patients, the PCWP is obtained when the catheter is 50 cm in the patient. If the catheter does not wedge at this length, it should not be advanced more than 2 to 3 cm further. If no wedge trace is obtained, the balloon should be deflated and the catheter pulled back to 50 cm and left there. The catheter will

4. Monitoring Cardiac Patients for Noncardiac Surgery   73

Fig. 4-13. Insertion of a pulmonary artery catheter using the internal jugular vein (IJV). After the IJV is located with a finder needle (A), an 18G catheter is inserted alongside it and the finder is removed (B). A wire is passed down the 18G catheter, and the catheter is then removed, leaving the wire. Next, an 8.5 introducer sheath is advanced over the wire using the Seldinger technique (C). A pulmonary artery catheter is then inserted through the introducer sheath (D).

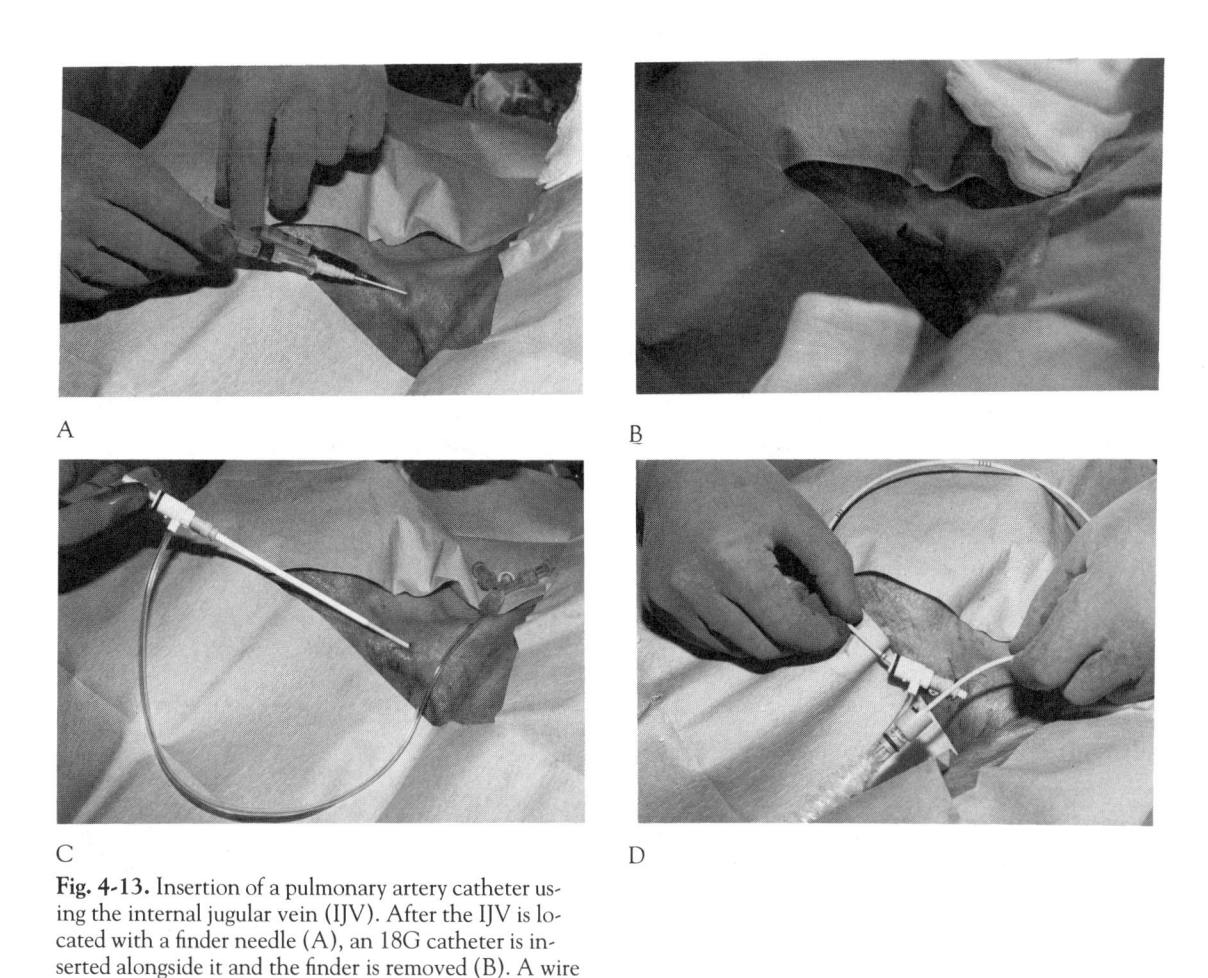

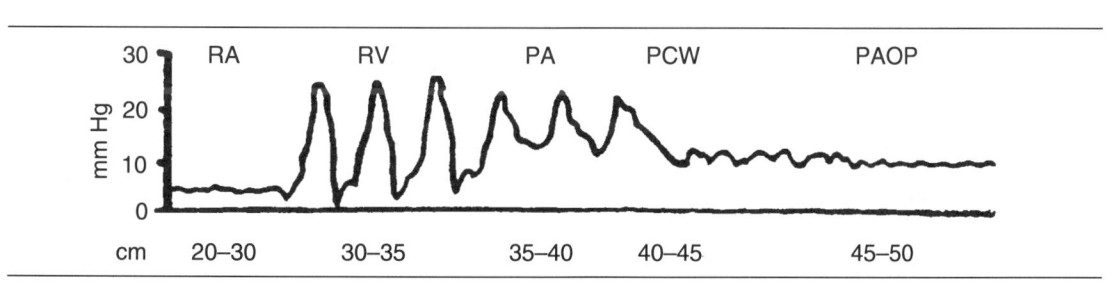

Fig. 4-14. Pressure wave forms as the pulmonary artery (PA) catheter is inserted into the PA. RA = right atrium; RV = right ventricle; PCW = pulmonary capillary wedge; PAOP = pulmonary artery occlusion pressure.

most likely advance a little with myocardial contraction and balloon occlusion will be possible. Temptation to advance the catheter beyond 55 cm should be avoided, because it could cause catheter knotting or pulmonary artery rupture. A common problem is difficulty in wedging the catheter when the PA pressure is elevated. In cases in which the PCWP is unobtainable, pulmonary artery diastolic pressure (PAD) can be used as a correlate of left atrial (LA) pressure. However, in certain disease states, such as mitral stenosis, there is poor correlation between PCWP and LA pressures.

Once in good position the catheter can be utilized to obtain thermodilution cardiac output determination. Table 4-3 discusses the various values that can be calculated using information derived from the pulmonary artery catheter.

Mixed Venous Oxygen Saturation (S$\bar{v}$O$_2$)

Approximately 10 years after the introduction of flow-directed pulmonary artery catheters, fiberoptic reflectance technology was incorporated into them, allowing clinicians to determine online S$\bar{v}$O$_2$ in addition to their other traditional uses [60]. In the beginning the expectation was that the S$\bar{v}$O$_2$ measurements would significantly reduce the number of arterial blood gas and cardiac output estimations. However, this has not been the case because S$\bar{v}$O$_2$ is not a reliable correlate of either arterial oxygenation or cardiac output. In addition, the increase in cost over regular pulmonary artery catheters has not justified their routine use in the operating room. They may, however, be more useful in critical care units for management of patients with multisystem failure [61, 62].

Mixed venous oxygen saturation technology is made possible by measuring light reflectance in a range of three different wavelengths. Using this technology oxyhemoglobin and total hemoglobin can be measured with accuracy. Methemoglobin and carboxyhemoglobin will interfere with the measurement since they fall in the same spectrum of wavelengths. Normal value for arterial oxygen saturation (SaO$_2$) is approximately 99 percent and, for S$\bar{v}$O$_2$, approximately 75 percent. Most anesthetic agents will decrease the basal metabolic rate, which will result in an increase in S$\bar{v}$O$_2$.

Oxygen Transport. Oxygen is transported in blood in two forms, as combined with hemoglobin (Hb; 20 ml/dl) and as dissolved in plasma (0.3 ml/dl). Since dissolved oxygen is an insignificant amount, it is generally excluded from calculations. Calculation of oxygen delivery (DO$_2$) is made as follows: 1 gm Hb carries 1.34 ml O$_2$ and 15 gm Hb has 1.34 × 15 = 20 ml O$_2$. This is the amount

Table 4-3. Derived hemodynamic values

Parameter	Formula	Normal values
Stroke volume (SV)	$SV = \dfrac{CO}{HR} \times 1{,}000$	60–90 ml/beat
Stroke index (SI)	$SI = \dfrac{SV}{BSA}$	40–65 ml/beat/m^2
LV stroke work index (LVSWI)	$LVSWI = \dfrac{1.36\,(MAP - PCWP)}{100} \times SI$	45–60 gm·m/m^2
RV stroke work index (RVSWI)	$RVSWI = \dfrac{1.36\,(PAP - CVP)}{100} \times SI$	5–10 gm·m/m^2
Systemic vascular resistance (SVR)	$SVR = \dfrac{MAP - CVP}{CO} \times 80$	900–1,500 dynes·sec/cm^5
Pulmonary vascular resistance (PVR)	$PVR = \dfrac{PAP - PCWP}{CO} \times 80$	50–150 dynes·sec/cm^5

CO = cardiac output; HR = heart rate; BSA = body surface area; LV = left ventricular; RV = right ventricular; MAP = mean arterial pressure; PCWP = pulmonary capillary wedge pressure; PAP = mean pulmonary artery pressure; CVP = central venous pressure.
Source: Modified from CC Hug, Monitoring. In RD Miller (ed), *Anesthesia* (2nd ed). New York: Churchill Livingstone, 1986, p. 453.

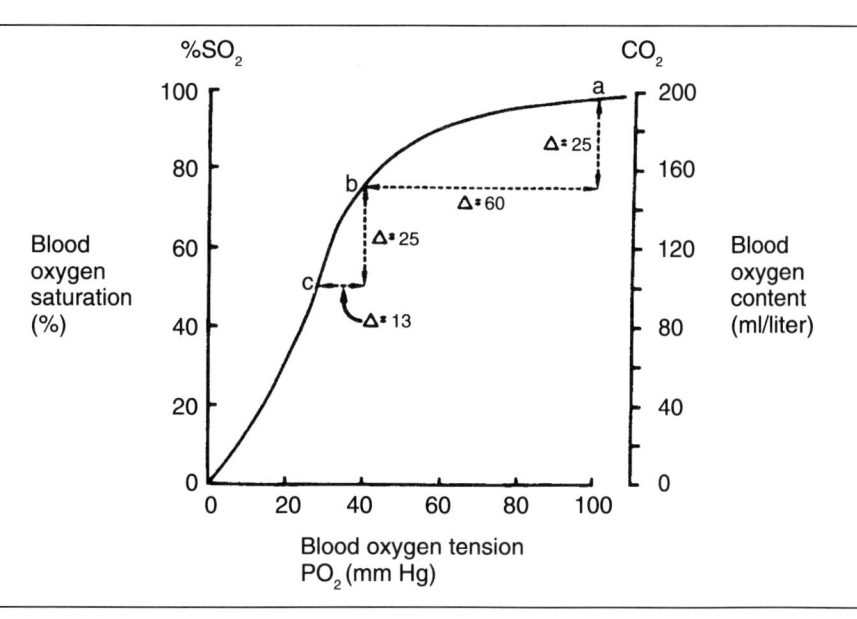

Fig. 4-15. The oxyhemoglobin dissociation curve showing importance of the sinusoidal shape of the curve and the ability to deliver a larger proportion of oxygen to the tissue at lower PO_2 (b–c when compared to a–b). (Reprinted with permission from DP Bernstein. In LM Capan, SM Miller, and H Turndorf (eds), *Trauma* (1st ed). Philadelphia: Lippincott, 1991.)

contained in 100 ml blood. When cardiac output is 5000 ml, 1000 ml oxygen is carried per minute.

Oxygen delivery is sufficient to meet the metabolic demands in healthy individuals. Oxygen consumption per unit time ($\dot{V}O_2$) can be measured indirectly by the following formula:

$$\dot{V}O_2 = CO \times (CaO_2 - CvO_2)$$

where $\dot{V}O_2$ = oxygen consumption, CO = cardiac output, CaO_2 = arterial oxygen content, and CvO_2 = venous oxygen content. Alternatively,

$$\dot{V}O_2 = CO \times Hb \times 13.8 \times (SaO_2 - S\bar{v}O_2)$$

Normal oxygen consumption = 230 ml oxygen per minute. However, when $\dot{V}O_2$ increases or DO_2 decreases beyond critical levels, anaerobic metabolism ensues, giving rise to lactic acidosis. In this circumstance the early warning may come from a drop in $S\bar{v}O_2$, which may alert the clinician of impending circulatory failure [63, 64].

There are three major determinants of DO_2: cardiac output, adequate arterial oxygen tension (PaO_2), and hemoglobin content. In clinical practice all three must be optimized when $S\bar{v}O_2$ shows a downward trend. It must be remembered that although decreased DO_2 will cause a decreased $S\bar{v}O_2$, $S\bar{v}O_2$ may also decrease because of a greatly increased oxygen demand, such as with hyperthermia, shivering, seizures, and so forth. When DO_2 is inadequate to meet metabolic needs, tissue extraction is enhanced by a decrease in tissue oxygen tension (PO_2) from 40 to 27 mm Hg, allowing 25 percent additional O_2 to be released to the tissues [65] (Fig. 4-15). A shift of the oxyhemoglobin dissociation curve to the right in an acid milieu also allows additional oxygen release by decreasing the affinity of hemoglobin for O_2. A minimum mandatory oxygen gradient is required for oxygen to diffuse to the mitochondria and oxygen availability is virtually zero below a PO_2 of 20 mm Hg.

Limitations of $S\bar{v}O_2$ Monitoring. Since $S\bar{v}O_2$ is measured from the pulmonary artery using a

Table 4-4. Causes of SṽO$_2$ changes

Causes of elevated SṽO$_2$	Causes of decreased SṽO$_2$

Increased O$_2$ delivery
  Increased FiO$_2$
  Increased hemoglobin
Decreased O$_2$ utilization
  Anesthesia
  Neuromuscular paralysis
  Sepsis (decreased utilization and increased arteriovenous shunt)
  Hypothermia
	Decreased O$_2$ delivery
	  Decreased hemoglobin
	  Decreased cardiac output
	  Hypoxemia
	Increased O$_2$ utilization
	  Hyperthermia
	  Shivering (including postoperative shivering)
	  Thyroid storm

FiO$_2$ = inspired oxygen concentration.

balloon-tipped catheter, it is important that the catheter not be in the "wedge" position to ensure a mixed venous and not an arterialized sample, which will erroneously elevate oxygen saturation [66]. Left-to-right shunts will also elevate SṽO$_2$, making determination of adequacy of DO$_2$ difficult. SṽO$_2$ is nonspecific in that it gives a global, not a local, indication of hypoxemia; therefore, it is possible to have normal SṽO$_2$ levels although an individual organ is undergoing ischemia, while others are supplied with a disproportionately high cardiac output [67]. In rare situations there may be a defect in oxygen extraction, such as generalized sepsis, which may paradoxically increase SṽO$_2$ although the oxygen demand has not been met and the cardiac index is within normal range. Anesthesia will also increase SṽO$_2$ secondary to decreased metabolic rate and decrease oxygen consumption (Table 4-4).

In conclusion, SṽO$_2$ catheters have a more important role in the intensive care unit, for patients in shock and multisystem failure, than in the operating room. However, their use should be encouraged when an ICU patient is scheduled for a surgical procedure.

Complications and Contraindications

Pulmonary artery catheters are associated with both minor and major complications [68]. Complications generally tend to be related to the insertion of the catheter. Minor complications are those that are transient and require no treatment, and major ones necessitate treatment and may cause harm if unrecognized or untreated. Minor complications are (1) premature atrial or ventricular contractions, or both, which occur in 85 percent of cases and generally require no treatment [69]; (2) small amounts of bleeding and hematoma at the insertion site; (3) carotid puncture [70] with a small-bore needle or an 18G catheter, which is usually harmless, occurs in approximately 5 percent of cases, and requires no treatment; (4) catheter kinking with inability to detect a pulmonary trace, which usually requires minor adjustment of the catheter or the introducer; and (5) catheter migration to the periphery with a permanent "wedge" tracing. The latter can be treated by pulling back on the catheter until a pulmonary artery trace appears on the screen. Leaving the catheter in the wedged position may lead to pulmonary infarct. Usually this condition requires no treatment, but in rare cases it may lead to pulmonary infection or bleeding. Additionally, if a pulmonary infarct occurs, it could lead to pulmonary fibrosis later. Another minor complication is that (6) pathogens may be cultured from the site of insertion or the tip of the catheter in a small percentage of cases. It is difficult to estimate how many of these develop into a full-blown infection. Pathogen growth from these locations increases when there is a break in the sterile technique and when the catheter is left in place for a prolonged period. The vast majority of positive cultures seems to be harmless and requires no treatment. When proper sterile technique is used and catheter change performed every 72 hours, the incidence of catheter contamination is greatly reduced.

Several major complications may also occur. Although carotid puncture [70] with a small-gauge needle or catheter occurs relatively frequently and needs no treatment, a large-bore dilator or introducer (No. 8.5 French) may on rare occasion inadvertently enter the carotid artery if proper precautionary steps are not taken. It is essential to transduce the 18G catheter when it is placed intravascularly before the insertion of the guidewire. This step reveals the catheter location when a CVP pressure tracing is displayed on the monitor. Only after a venous trace and pressure are confirmed should the operator proceed with the rest of the catheter insertion. Lack of an arterial tracing is not enough; the catheter or the needle may be in plaque, or kinked, and not give an arterial trace but still be in the artery.

There are other ways to confirm venous cannulation. Although obtaining oxygen tension from the catheter to distinguish between arterial and venous blood can be used, generally this is time-consuming and may yield equivocal results in patients with supplemental oxygen therapy, when venous PO_2 may be high, or in hypoxic patients, when the arterial PO_2 may be low. Looking at the color of blood is unreliable for the same reason. Blood flow change with respiration can be detected in the catheter and is one way to determine its location, but this method is not reliable in patients with increased venous pressure, making the transduced pressure the most reliable way to ensure the location of the catheter.

Even after proper precautions, there is a rare chance that the No. 8.5 French introducer sheath may be inadvertently inserted into the carotid artery, posing a management dilemma to the anesthesiologist as to the recommended course of action. Removal of the introducer from the carotid artery will invariably lead to a large hematoma, causing tracheal deviation and possibly pharyngeal edema. Since airway obstruction can compound the severity of complications, some physicians advocate tracheal intubation with the patient under anesthesia before the introducer is removed. The surgeon should be informed immediately in case the hematoma enlarges, requiring neck exploration. When the introducer is removed, pressure should be applied over the site for approximately 20 minutes. At this time proper assessment can be made as to the extent of the hematoma. If the patient is to undergo a surgical procedure that requires anticoagulation, it is best postponed until a later date. If surgery is of emergent nature or does not require anticoagulation, it can be performed with close observation of the neck. If the hematoma increases in size, surgical exploration may be required. It should be noted that the distal end of the dilator can also injure the carotid artery at a point below the initial puncture, leading to a hematoma or rarely to intrathoracic pseudoaneurysm formation.

Pulmonary artery rupture may occur as a result of excessive pressure caused by balloon inflation or catheter migration. Pulmonary artery rupture is the most significant complication of pulmonary artery catheterization and is associated with greater than 50 percent mortality [2, 71, 72]. This complication is more likely to occur in older patients with greater vessel fragility, in patients with increased pulmonary artery pressure (as in mitral stenosis or regurgitation), and in anticoagulated patients. It is recommended that the catheter balloon be inflated slowly, that inflations be discontinued once the "wedge" position is obtained, and that the inflation be of minimum duration and frequency. Balloon inflation should be avoided if possible in anticoagulated patients. Pulmonary rupture may cause massive bleeding, which is diagnosed when blood is seen in the endotracheal tube. Bleeding may be massive and result in decreased lung compliance and severe hypoxia. The treatment is to isolate the bleeding lung from the normal side. Since the pulmonary artery catheter more frequently floats to the right side, this may be assumed to be the site of bleeding. Insertion of a double-lumen tube, although ideal, may be very difficult or impossible due to lack of visibility from bleeding. If a double-lumen tube is unavailable or cannot be inserted successfully, a narrow, uncut, single-lumen endotracheal tube can be directed to the left main-stem bronchus by turning the patient's head to the right and pointing the concavity of the tube posteriorly while advancing the tube distally. If successful in isolating and ventilating the left lung, the anesthesiologist can then resuscitate the patient and reverse the anticoagulation. If bleeding stops, further surgical intervention may be avoided. Similar results may be achieved with a bronchial blocker inserted in the side that is bleeding. If bleeding does not cease, thoracotomy and pneumonectomy may be required.

In patients with left bundle-branch block, the introduction of a pulmonary artery catheter may produce right bundle-branch block, resulting in complete heart block [73]. It is recommended that pulmonary artery catheterization be either avoided in these cases or that pacing capability be available. This is discussed fully in Chap. 12.

In patients with an enlarged right atrium or right ventricle, or tricuspid regurgitation, the catheter tip may be deflected opposite to the intended direction during insertion. This can lead to knotting of the catheter, which in some cases may prevent its removal percutaneously, requiring surgical intervention.

If the introducer is not properly siliconized for lubrication, the catheter may get stuck during removal. This could cause it to break and travel toward the heart, requiring surgical removal. Although rare, this complication is sometimes seen in ICUs, where most of the pulmonary catheters inserted in the operating room are removed. Occasionally, during heart surgery, a suture may be taken through the right atrial cannulation site or a pacemaker wire and include the PA catheter in it. This may go unnoticed until the catheter removal is attempted at a later time and excessive resistance is met. Surgical removal of the right atrial suture will be necessary in order to free the catheter.

In conclusion, monitoring has increased our understanding of hemodynamics. It should be used carefully and with proper indications. In experienced hands the complication rate of most monitoring is acceptable, emphasizing the need for adequate training, and, if used appropriately, monitoring can enhance patient management.

REFERENCES

1. Rao, TK, Jacobs, KH, El-Etr, AA. Reinfarction following anesthesia in patients with myocardial infarction. *Anesthesiology* 59:499–505, 1983.
2. Muller, BJ, Gallucci, A. Pulmonary artery catheter induced pulmonary rupture in patients undergoing surgery. *Can Anesth Soc J* 32:258–264, 1985.
3. Cushing, HW. On the avoidance of shock in major amputations by cocainization of large nerve trunks preliminary to their division with observations on blood pressure changes in surgical cases. *Ann Surg* 36:321–345, 1902.
4. Cushing, HW. On routine determination of arterial tension in operation room and clinic. *Boston Med Surg J* 148:250–256, 1903.
5. Riva-Rocci, S. Un nuovo sfigmomanometro. *Gaz Med Torino* 47:981, 1906.
6. Korotkoff, NS. On the subject of methods of determining blood pressure. *Bull Imp Med Acad St. Petersburg* 11:365, 1905.
7. Zornow, MH, Schubert, A, Todd, MM. Intraoperative oscillometric arterial blood pressure monitoring using non-standard cuff locations. *Anesthesiology* 65: A135, 1986.
8. Geddes, LA, Voel, M, Combs, C, et al. Characterization of the oscillometric method for measuring indirect blood pressure. *Ann Biomed Engl* 10:271–280, 1982.
9. Hutton, P, Prys-Roberts, C. The oscillotonometer in theory and practice. *Br J Anesth* 54:581–591, 1982.
10. Showman, A. Hazards of automatic non-invasive blood pressure monitoring. *Anesthesiology* 55:717–718, 1981.
11. Sy, WP. Ulnar nerve palsy related to use of automatically cycled blood pressure cuff. *Anesth Anal* 60: 687–688, 1981.
12. Smith, NT, Werseling, KH, Dewit, B. Evaluation of two prototype devices producing non-invasive, pulsatile, calibrated blood pressure measurement from a finger. *J Clin Monit* 1:17–29, 1985.
13. Penaz, J. Photoelectric measurement of blood pressure, volume and flow in the finger. Dresden: *Digest of the 10th International Conference on Medical and Biological Engineering*, Vol 104, 1973.
14. Boehmer, RD. Continuous, real-time, non-invasive monitor of blood pressure. Penaz methodology applied to the finger. *J Clin Monit* 3:282–287, 1987.
15. Kurki, T, Smith, NT, Head, N, et al. Non-invasive continuous blood pressure measurement from the finger: Optimal measurement conditions and factors affecting reliability. *J Clin Monit* 3:6–13, 1987.
16. Slogoff, S, Keats, AS. Does perioperative myocardial ischemia lead to postoperative myocardial infarction? *Anesthesiology* 62:107–114, 1985.
17. London, MJ, Hollenberg, M, Wong, MG, et al. Intraoperative myocardial ischemia: Localization by continuous 12-lead electrocardiography. *Anesthesiology* 69:232–241, 1988.
18. London, MJ, Wong, MG, Hollenberg, M, et al. Electrocardiographic lead systems. *Anesthesiology* 70: 1027–1029, 1989.
19. Brazaral, MG, Norfleet, EA. Comparison of CB_5 and V_5 leads for intraoperative electrocardiographic monitoring. *Anesth Analg* 60:849–853, 1981.
20. Kotrly, KJ, Kotter, GS, Mortara, D, et al. Intraoperative detection of myocardial ischemia with an ST segment trend monitoring system. *Anesth Analg* 63: 343–345, 1984.
21. Frazin, L, Talano, JV, Stephanides, L, et al. Esophageal echocardiography. *Circulation* 54:102–108, 1976.
22. Pearlman, AS, Gardin, JM, Martin, RP, et al. Guidelines for optimal physician training in echocardiography: Recommendations of the American Society of Echocardiography Committee for Physician Training in Echocardiography. *Am J Cardiol* 60: 158–163, 1987.

23. Schuter, M, Lenganstein, BA, Polster, J, et al. Transesophageal cross-sectional echocardiography with phased array transducer system. Technique and initial clinical request. Br Heart J 48:67–72, 1982.
24. Konstadt, SN, Thys, D, Mindich, BP, et al. Validation of quantitative intraoperative transesophageal echocardiography. Anesthesiology 65:418–421, 1986.
25. Tennant, R, Wiggers, J. The effect of coronary occlusion on myocardial contraction. Am J Physiol 112:351–361, 1935.
26. Lieberman, AN, Weiss, JL, Jugdutt, BI, et al. Two-dimensional echocardiography and infarct size: Relationship of regional wall motion and thickening of the extent of myocardial infarction in the dog. Circulation 63:739–746, 1981.
27. Heger, JJ, Weyman, AE, Wann, LS, et al. Cross-sectional echocardiographic analysis of the extent of left ventricular asynergy in acute myocardial infarction. Circulation 61:1113–1118, 1980.
28. Eaton, LW, Weiss, JL, Bernadine, BH, et al. Regional cardiac dilatation after acute myocardial infarction. N Engl J Med 300:57–62, 1979.
29. Wohlgelernter, D, Jaffe, CC, Cabin, HS, et al. Silent ischemia during coronary occlusion produced by balloon inflation: Relation to regional myocardial dysfunction. J Am Coll Cardiol 10:491–498, 1987.
30. Smith, J, Cahalan, M, Benefiel, D, et al. Intraoperative detection of myocardial ischemia in high-risk patients: Electrocardiography versus two-dimensional transesophageal echocardiography. Circulation 72:1015–1021, 1985.
31. Matsumoto, M, Oka, Y, Strom, J, et al. Application of transesophageal echocardiograph to continuous intraoperative monitoring of left ventricular performance. Am J Cardiol 46:95–105, 1980.
32. Aschenberg, W, Schluter, M, Kremer, P, et al. Transesophageal two-dimensional echocardiography for the detection of left atrial appendage thrombus. J Am Coll Cardiol 7:163–166, 1986.
33. Cucchiara, RF, Nugent, M, Seward, JB, et al. Air embolism in upright neurosurgical patients: Detection and localization by two-dimensional transesophageal echocardiography. Anesthesiology 60:353–355, 1984.
34. Glenski, JA, Cucchiara, RF, Michenfelder, JD. Transesophageal echocardiography and transcutaneous O_2 and CO_2 monitoring for detection of venous air embolism. Anesthesiology 64:541–545, 1986.
35. Furuya, H, Okumura, F. Detection of paradoxical air embolism by transesophageal echocardiography. Anesthesiology 60:374–377, 1984.
36. Erbel, R, Borner, N, Steller, D, et al. Detection of aortic dissection by transesophageal echocardiography. Br Heart J 58:45–51, 1987.
37. Engberding, R, Bender, F, Gross-Heitmeyer, W, et al. Identification of dissection or aneurysm of the descending thoracic aorta by conventional and transesophageal two-dimensional echocardiography. Am J Cardiol 59:717–719, 1987.
38. Allen, EV. Thromboangiitis obliterans: Methods of diagnosis of chronic obstructive lesions distal to the wrist with illustrative cases. Am J Med Sci 178:237–244, 1929.
39. Slogoff, S, Keats, AS, Arlund, BS. On the safety of radial artery cannulation. Anesthesiology 59:42–47, 1983.
40. Bedford, RF. Radial arterial function following percutaneous cannulation with 18 and 20 gauge catheters. Anesthesiology 47:37–39, 1977.
41. Bedford, RF. Percutaneous radial-artery cannulation-increased safety using Teflon catheters. Anesthesiology 42:219–222, 1975.
42. Adler, DC, Bryan-Brown CW. Use of the axillary artery for intravascular monitoring. Crit Care Med 1:148–150, 1973.
43. Bedford, RF, Wollman, H. Complications of radial artery cannulation. Anesthesiology 38:228–236, 1973.
44. Downs, JB, Rackstein, AD, Klein, EF, et al. Hazards of radial artery catheterization. Anesthesiology 39:283–286, 1973.
45. Bedford, RF. Wrist circumference predicts the risk of radial arterial occlusion after cannulation. Anesthesiology 48:377–378, 1978.
46. Weiss, BM, Gattiker, RI. Complications during and following radial artery cannulation: A prospective study. Intens Care Med 12:424–428, 1986.
47. Downs, JB, Chapman, CL, Hawkins, IF. Prolonged radial-artery catheterization: An evaluation of heparinized catheters and continuous irrigation. Arch Surg 108:671–673, 1974.
48. Wilkins, RG. Radial artery cannulation and ischemic damage: A review. Anaesthesia 40:896–899, 1985.
49. Bedford, RF. Removal of radial artery thrombi following percutaneous cannulation for monitoring. Anesthesiology 46:430–432, 1977.
50. Chang, C, Dughi, J, Shitabata, P, et al. Air embolism and the radial arterial line. Crit Care Med 16:141–143, 1988.
51. Mangano, DT. Monitoring pulmonary arterial pressure in coronary-artery disease. Anesthesiology 53:364–370, 1980.
52. Seldinger, SI. Catheter placement of the needle in

percutaneous arteriography: A new technique. *Acta Radiol* 39:368–376, 1953.
53. Cournand, A. Cardiac catheterization: Development of the technique, its contributions to experimental medicine, and its initial application in mass. *Acta Med Scand* 579 (Suppl):3–32, 1975.
54. Forsmann, W. Die Sondierung dis rechtern Herzens. *Klin Wochenschr* 8:2085, 1929.
55. Hellems, HK, Hayes, FW, Dexter, L. Pulmonary "capillary" pressure in man. *J Appl Physiol* 2:24–29, 1949.
56. Swan, HJC, Ganz, W, Forrester, J, et al. Catheterization of a flow directed balloon-tipped catheter. *N Engl J Med* 283:447–451, 1970.
57. DeFalgue, RJ. Percutaneous catheterization of the internal jugular vein. *Anesth Analg* 53:116–121, 1974.
58. Blitt, CD, Wright, WA, Petty, WC, et al. Central venous catheterization via the external jugular vein: A technique employing the J wire. *JAMA* 229:817–818, 1974.
59. Pearson, KS, Gomez, MN, Carter, JG, et al. A cost/benefit analysis of randomized invasive monitoring in cardiac surgery. *Anesth Analg* 66:S138, 1987.
60. Shoemaker, WC, Montgomery, ES, Kaplan, E, et al. Physiologic pattern in surviving and nonsurviving shock patients. *Arch Surg* 106:630–636, 1973.
61. Jastremski, MS, Chelluri, L, Benay, KM, et al. Analysis of the effects of continuous on-line monitoring of mixed venous oxygen saturation on patient outcome and cost effectiveness. *Crit Care Med* 17:148–153, 1989.
62. Baele, PI, McMichan, JC, Marsh, HM, et al. Continuous monitoring of mixed venous oxygen saturation in critically ill patients. *Anesth Analg* 61:513–517, 1982.
63. Braunwald, E. Control of myocardial oxygen consumption: Physiologic and clinical consideration. *Am J Cardiol* 27:416–432, 1971.
64. Miller, MJ. Tissue oxygenation in clinical medicine: An historical review. *Anesth Analg* 61:527–535, 1982.
65. Lee, J, Wright, F, Barber, R, et al. Central venous oxygen saturation in shock: A study in man. *Anesthesiology* 36:472–478, 1972.
66. Shapiro, HM, Smith, G, Pribble, AH, et al. Errors in sampling pulmonary arterial blood with a Swan-Ganz catheter. *Anesthesiology* 40:291–295, 1974.
67. Suter, PM, Lindauer, JM, Failey, HB, et al. Errors in data derived from pulmonary artery blood gas values. *Crit Care Med* 3:175–181, 1975.
68. Shah, KB, Rao, TLK, Laughlin, S, et al. A review of pulmonary artery catheterization in 6,245 patients. *Anesthesiology* 61:271–275, 1984.
69. Royster, RL, Johnston, WE, Gravlee, GP, et al. Arrhythmias during venous cannulation prior to pulmonary artery catheter insertion. *Anesth Analg* 64:1214–1216, 1985.
70. Schwartz, AJ, Jobes, DR, Greenhow, DE, et al. Carotid artery puncture with internal jugular cannulation using the Seldinger technique: Incidence, recognition, treatment, and prevention. *Anesthesiology* 51:S160, 1979.
71. Hannan, AT, Brown, M, Bigman, O. Pulmonary artery catheter-induced hemorrhage. *Chest* 85:128–131, 1984.
72. Cohen, JA, Gravenstein, N, Blackshear, RH, et al. More frequent perforation by pulmonary artery catheters during hypothermia. *Anesth Analg* 68:A555, 1989.
73. Sprung, CI, Elser, B, Schein, RMH, et al. Risk of right bundle-branch block and complete heart block during pulmonary catheterization. *Crit Care Med* 17:1–3, 1989.

5
Ischemic Heart Disease

JOSE A. MELENDEZ
PAOLA MARINO

Ischemic heart disease (IHD) is the major cause of death in the United States. Updated statistics show that every year 550,000 deaths are attributable to coronary artery disease (CAD) and another six million individuals are newly diagnosed. Among the six million, one third to one half undergo anesthesia and surgery [1]. Despite the continually increasing numbers of patients with IHD exposed to surgical procedures, a consequence of an aging population, the perioperative ischemic death rates have declined in the last two decades. This is probably due to better understanding of the disease pathophysiology and improved medical therapy.

EPIDEMIOLOGY, MORBIDITY, AND MORTALITY

Epidemiologic studies have demonstrated an association between CAD and various factors. The Framingham Study [2] was the first to describe the risk factors in the United States. Men have a higher incidence of IHD than women. Although postmenopausal women have an equal risk of developing ischemic heart disease, both morbidity and mortality are higher in men. This is possibly related to a protective effect conferred by estrogens. Men may begin to experience symptoms of IHD between the ages of 35 and 44, and face a 35 percent risk of mortality by age 64. The other major risk factors for IHD are chronic cigarette smoking, hypertension, obesity, hyperlipidemia, and glucose intolerance. Smokers are 2.14 times more at risk of developing CAD than are nonsmokers [3]. The increase in the risk of CAD as a result of hypertension is continuous and graded, and, thus, there is no safe level of hypertension [4]. There is a linear relation between the cholesterol level and low-density lipoprotein (LDL), the primary atherogenic lipoprotein, and the risk of CAD [5]. Variations in serum cholesterol levels are related to 45 percent of the interpopulation variation in CAD mortality [6, 7]. The mechanism of CAD in patients with diabetes mellitus is multifactorial and may relate to altered platelet function or to increased red cell adhesion, or both, in addition to the frequent association of hypertension, obesity, and lipid abnormalities. A positive family history of CAD is an independent predictor of myocardial infarction [8]. Other minor risk factors of CAD are physical inactivity, stress, type A personality, hypercalcemia, hyperuricemia, cardiac transplantation, and elevated fibrinogen levels [9].

ETIOLOGY AND PATHOPHYSIOLOGY

Atherosclerosis of epicardial coronary arteries is the most common cause of myocardial ischemia. The precursor lesions of atherosclerosis are believed to be the fatty streak and diffuse intimal thickening. The typical advanced lesion is the fibrous plaque, which compromises blood flow. The plaque is often complicated by thrombosis, hemorrhage, and/or calcification. Fissures may develop, with consequent thrombosis, embolism, or aneurysmal dilatation, which may increase the dimension of the plaque with worsening of obstruction [10].

A fixed coronary lesion is not always necessary to produce ischemia. Subendocardial ischemia [11] may occur whenever the supply–demand ratio is reduced beyond the compensatory ability of the vasculature. It has been described in

1. Abnormally matched oxygen demand-supply (hypertensive ventricular hypertrophy, aortic stenosis, idiopathic hypertrophic subaortic stenosis)
2. Congenital abnormalities (arteriovenous fistulas, ductus arteriosus)
3. Reduction in oxygen-carrying capacity of the blood (anemia, carboxyhemoglobin)
4. Coronary artery embolism (infective, thrombotic)
5. Coronary spasm
6. Arteritis (luetic aortitis, polyarteritis nodosa)
7. Hematologic thrombosis (polycythemia vera, thrombocytosis)

The coexistence of multiple conditions, such as left ventricular hypertrophy in the presence of coronary spasm, is not uncommon.

The heart is an aerobic organ, and, thus, it can tolerate only a small oxygen debt. Oxygen supply is provided by coronary blood flow:

$$\text{Coronary } O_2 \text{ transport} = CBF \times CaO_2$$

where CBF = coronary blood flow and CaO_2 = arterial oxygen content. The latter is a function of hemoglobin concentration and arterial oxygen tension. Coronary blood flow depends on coronary perfusion pressure [aortic diastolic pressure − left ventricular end diastolic pressure (LVEDP)], coronary vascular resistance (controlled by autoregulation and sympathetic factors), and the duration of diastole. The normal vascular layer is capable of autoregulation, maintaining myocardial perfusion within a range of 140–120 mm Hg to 70–50 mm Hg. Below the critical pressure levels, loss of autoregulation occurs, with maximal coronary vascular dilatation and establishment of pressure-dependent flow. When obstructive coronary disease is present, coronary perfusion pressure is lower than aortic pressure. A reduction in the systemic pressure may result in lowering perfusion pressure below the critical level. This explains the need to prevent hypotension in patients with IHD.

There is a tight coupling between the coronary flow and myocardial oxygen demand ($M\dot{V}O_2$). The major factors affecting oxygen demand include intramyocardial wall tension, contractility, and heart rate. Wall tension is a direct function of radius and intraventricular pressure and is inversely related to wall thickness. The administration of inotropic agents to improve contractility results in the increased metabolic expenditure of the excitation-contraction mechanism for greater and faster Ca^{++} uptake. An acceleration of heart rate raises $M\dot{V}O_2$ by augmenting the frequency of tension development per unit time as well as increasing contractility. It has been suggested that with the increased energy expenditure by the heart there is a proportionally accelerated production of vasodilator metabolites, which in turn reduce coronary vascular resistance and raise coronary blood flow so that only small changes in oxygen extraction occur. Several mediators have been implicated, including oxygen and adenosine [12]. Normal coronary vessels have the ability to reduce flow resistance to 20 percent of basal levels as a response to increases in $M\dot{V}O_2$. A vessel stenosis of greater than 40 percent will result in poststenotic dilatation to maintain flow. An 80 percent reduction in the vessel diameter will produce maximal dilatation with maintenance of adequate perfusion at rest. Any degree of increase in $M\dot{V}O_2$ superimposed on this stenotic lesion will result in ischemia.

The subendocardium is most susceptible to ischemia. It has limited vasodilation reserve and a higher metabolic demand than the subepicardium.

Fig. 5-1. Cross section of myocardial wall during end diastole and end systole. Subendocardial susceptibility to ischemia is caused by the greater dependence on diastolic perfusion in addition to the greater degree of shortening during systole. (Reprinted with permission from JR Bell and AC Fox, Pathogenesis of subendocardial ischemia. Am J Med Sci 268:3, 1974.)

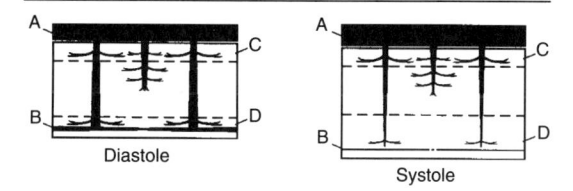

A - Epicardial artery
B - Subendocardial plexus
C - Subepicardium
D - Subendocardium

During systole, the subendocardium is subjected to a higher compression force that translates into a higher $M\dot{V}O_2$, as well as the redistribution of the coronary blood to the subepicardial layer (Fig. 5-1). This explains the higher incidence of subendocardial ischemia demonstrated by ST elevations on the electrocardiogram.

The clinical sequelae of myocardial ischemia may be the consequence of either an increase in $M\dot{V}O_2$ in the face of fixed obstruction or a reduction in myocardial oxygen supply resulting from coronary spasm or transient platelet aggregation. In the involved areas, metabolism switches from aerobic to anaerobic, with consequential loss of metabolic substrates and calcium entrapment. In addition, the perfusion impairment causes inadequate removal of metabolic by-products (inosine and hypoxanthine) along with potassium ions, prostaglandins, kinins, and acetate—which may lead to further vasodilatation and worsening hypoperfusion. Persistent ischemia will result in tissue death accompanied by paradoxical motion of the central ischemic area (dyskinesia), reduction of contractility of the adjacent areas (hypokinesis), and compensatory hyperfunction of uninvolved myocardium, resulting from local release of catecholamines and the Frank-Starling mechanism [13].

The functional effects of the injury are related to the extent of the lesion. Diastolic function becomes abnormal in the early phase of the ischemic event. If the loss of activity involves critical or large areas, the ventricular compliance is reduced, with a rise in end diastolic volume and end diastolic pressure further compromising coronary perfusion. This is followed by impairment of systolic function, with decrease of contractility and depression of stroke volume, cardiac output, and ejection fraction. Eventually, myocardial failure will be the result if the regional abnormalities overwhelm the compensatory activity of the uninvolved myocardium.

MYOCARDIAL ISCHEMIA
Chronic Stable Angina

Angina pectoris has been defined as "discomfort in the chest or adjacent areas caused by transient myocardial ischemia without necrosis" [14]. In order to distinguish the clinical manifestations of coronary artery disease, it is necessary to discern the characteristics of the pain pattern. Chronic stable angina has a prevalence of 90 percent in patients with CAD. The typical anginal pain is usually a frightening retrosternal discomfort, described as heaviness, pressure, or squeezing. The location of referred pain may be variable: ulnar surface of left arm, right arm, neck, jaw, throat, head, or epigastrium. Frequently associated symptoms are nausea, vomiting, sweating, and sometimes palpitations. Exertion and emotional stress are usual precipitating factors along with conditions increasing oxygen demand, such as cold exposure, fever, and hypoglycemia. Pain exacerbated by deep breaths or movements is unlikely to be of anginal origin. The patient is usually able to report the exact level of physical activity causing an anginal episode. Prompt improvement or relief of symptoms with rest or nitroglycerin administration, or both, provides useful diagnostic information. Indeed, pain lasting less than 5 minutes or more than 20 to 30 minutes is usually not of anginal origin.

In typical stable angina, the increase in $M\dot{V}O_2$, or the sudden fall of oxygen supply, results in ischemia of the area supplied by the obstructed epicardial coronary artery. The effects are related to the degree of the anatomic obstruction, to the effectiveness of the collateral layer (if present), and to the number and degree of vessels involved.

Unstable Angina

In order for a condition to be defined as unstable angina, the presence of CAD and the fulfillment of one or more of the following conditions are required: (1) changes in the characteristics of a preexisting chronic stable angina: more severe, more frequent, or more prolonged; (2) angina at rest with ST depression; and (3) angina of new onset (1–2 months) precipitated by light exertion. The pain is qualitatively similar to the typical anginal pain, but is prolonged, and nitroglycerin does not provide lasting relief. Unstable angina usually represents the acute worsening of atherosclerotic heart disease and carries a more grave prognosis if it is untreated. Events such as platelet aggregation, thrombosis, and spasm probably contribute to the precipitation of the ischemic episodes. Unstable angina of new onset can also be attributable to a vasoconstrictive component associated with a preexistent fixed obstruction of a single vessel [15].

Prinzmetal's Angina

Variant angina, first described by Prinzmetal [16], is characterized by its precipitation at rest associated with ST elevation. In order to differentiate it from unstable angina, it should be emphasized that this pain is not the evolution of a preexisting anginal syndrome. Exertion often has no impact on clinical features. The pain is usually experienced at night and can result in syncope, acute myocardial infarction, severe arrhythmias, and sudden death. Epidemiologic data reveal some peculiarities: Patients are younger than the average for coronary artery disease, and there is no male prevalence. Cigarette smokers seem to be at a higher risk, and an association with other vasomotility disorders, Raynaud's phenomenon among them, has been described.

The leading event is coronary artery spasm. The transient dramatic reduction of the diameter of an epicardial artery results in ischemia, even in the absence of increased $M\dot{V}O_2$. Usually the spasm is focal, often close to atheromatous plaques. The possible mechanisms include vascular hypercontractility, endothelial injury (with a paradoxical vasoconstrictive reaction to damage), and release of vasoconstrictive substances.

Left Main Coronary Artery Disease

Left main coronary artery disease is considered to have an ominous nature because a single event can cause infarction of a large quantity of myocardium. Left main lesions are life threatening; the mortality in medically treated patients is 29 percent at 18 months, 39 to 48 percent at 2 years, and 50 percent at 3 years [17], and depends on the degree of the stenosis (patients with a stenosis less than 50–70% have a better prognosis). Ischemic events are associated with large infarcts, onsets of heart block, and sudden death. Survivors of myocardial infarctions often progress to ventricular aneurysms.

Silent Myocardial Ischemia

Besides anginal events, patients with CAD often experience asymptomatic ischemic events. The incidence of silent ischemia was reported to be as high as 97 percent by Raby and associates [18] in a group of patients undergoing vascular surgery. Other studies have put this number between 70 and 85 percent [19]. The majority of silent ischemic episodes were unaccompanied by exertion or increase in heart rate. It is important to be able to detect perioperative silent ischemia because there is evidence to show that patients with ischemic episodes are more likely to have an undesirable cardiac event [20]. Also, the prognosis of patients with angina is similar to that of patients who have silent ischemia [21].

The clinical presentation of silent myocardial ischemia can be differentiated into three groups. Patients with type 1 have severe CAD that is completely asymptomatic; the prevalence is 2.5 to 10.0 percent. Patients with type 2 have myocardial infarction without any history of anginal pain; 20 to 30 percent do not experience any pain with myocardial infarction. Type 3 patients have a stable, unstable, or variant angina history associated with frequent silent episodes; at least 75 to 80 percent of ischemic events are asymptomatic and are diagnosed only on 24-hour Holter monitoring.

Silent myocardial ischemia is the most common type of perioperative ischemia. The pathogenesis of silent ischemic episodes is still not well understood. Some authors have suggested a reduced sensitivity to pain [17, 22], that is, a higher pain threshold, perhaps due to narcotic administration. A sensory neuropathy has been postulated in diabetic patients. In this group, subendocardial and transmural ischemia or myocardial infarction, or both, can occur without pain.

Myocardial Infarction

Myocardial infarctions are the result of total or near-total coronary artery obstruction. Thus, they represent the potential evolution of every episode of myocardial ischemia. Acute transmural infarctions are often caused by coronary thrombi close to the atherosclerotic plaque or may be precipitated by coronary artery embolism. The role of coronary spasm in the evolution of the episode is still not clear [13].

In subendocardial infarction, the necrosis involves only the subendocardium or the intramural myocardium, or both, without extension through the entire ventricular wall. The pathogenesis is often related to conditions that increase oxygen demand (pulmonary embolism, hypertension, hypotension, anemia) superimposed on narrowed but still patent vessels. In other instances, the cause is a thrombotic occlusion followed by early spontaneous thrombolysis.

The extent and the functional consequences of the acute myocardial infarction depend on anatomic and pathophysiologic factors (Table 5-1). This event is the end point of the imbalance between supply and demand; the result is necrosis of the myocardium and loss of functional activity. Acutely, left ventricular pump function is depressed, with decrease in cardiac output, stroke volume, and blood pressure. The scar that develops following the acute episode is fibrotic and may actually improve function because of its stiffness. This hypofunctioning area may decrease ventricular compliance but does not necessarily affect global left ventricular function. Myocardial cell dropout is a consequence of not only the infarcted area of tissue but also infarction expansion during postinfarction remodeling. This can result in larger volumes of injured tissue.

Right Heart Infarction

The occurrence of isolated right myocardial infarction is rare because of the lower oxygen requirements of the right ventricle. Furthermore, the more developed collateral system and the lower ventricular wall tension facilitate oxygen supply. Right ventricular infarction and failure are usually related to obstructive lesions of the right coronary artery. Often right ventricular involvement may result from a large inferior infarction. The presence of ST segment elevations on one or more of leads V_4R, V_5R, and V_6R is highly suspicious of a right ventricular infarct. Presence of pathologic states, such as pulmonary hypertension, that increase right ventricular work increase the risk. Echocardiographic interrogation will reveal right ventricular dilatation and wall motion abnormalities. The impaired right ventricular function often affects left ventricular performance; central venous pressure (CVP) and right atrial and right ventricular end diastolic pressures are increased while left filling pressures may be normal; however, cardiac output and arterial pressure are depressed.

Ventricular Dysfunction Secondary to Ischemic Heart Disease

Myocardial dysfunction is the direct consequence of the loss of tissue after a myocardial infarction or chronic persistent ischemia. Both acute and chronic events may lead to this anatomic alteration. Acute myocardial infarctions induce both systolic and diastolic abnormalities. The degree of both systolic and diastolic functional impairment depends on the percentage of myocardium affected: 10 percent of myocardium involved causes a decrease in ejection fraction, and a 15 percent involvement results in an increase in LVEDP and left

Table 5-1. Determining factors of injury extent after myocardial infarction

---
Location and severity of stenosis on coronary vessels
Size of vascular bed perfused by involved vessels
Oxygen needs of the injured myocardium
Effectiveness of collateral layer
Presence, site, severity of superimposed spasm
Limiting tissue factors
---

ventricular end diastolic volume (LVEDV). Congestive heart failure occurs after infarction of more than 25 percent of myocardium [13]. When the percentage of abnormal myocardium exceeds 40 percent, severe impairment of global function develops. This degree of involvement results in the deterioration of function in normal areas of myocardium, a probable consequence of volume overload [23]. Stretching of noncontractile myocardium results in aneurysmal dilatation. Left ventricular aneurysms have been reported to occur in 12 to 15 percent of patients who survive myocardial infarction. These are usually found anteriorly and/or apically. Functionally, ventricular aneurysms may exhibit either complete akinesis or dyskinetic systolic expansion of the ventricular wall with steal of some stroke volume. Incidence of symptomatic congestive heart failure in patients with ventricular aneurysm is 50 percent, while only 20 percent experience anginal pain [17].

Dysfunction of a papillary muscle has been noticed in 30 percent of patients with coronary artery disease who are undergoing coronary artery bypass surgery (CABG) [24]. Papillary muscles are perfused by the terminal division of the coronary tree; thus, they are very susceptible to ischemia. Necrosis or repeated ischemic episodes may lead to chronic papillary muscle dysfunction and acute mitral regurgitation. This will cause volume overload of the left ventricle and increased wall stress. Mitral regurgitation may also result from alterations in the spatial relationship between papillary muscles and chordae tendineae due to left ventricular dilatation.

Ventricular failure can also develop without evidence of previous infarction. This clinical entity has been termed *ischemic cardiomyopathy* [25]. In ischemic cardiomyopathy, dyspnea and heart failure, rather than angina, dominate the clinical presentation. Often these patients endure the typical course of congestive heart failure, with progressive respiratory distress, peripheral edema, decreased urinary output, hepatic congestion, and ascites. The etiology is still unclear, and several hypotheses have been formulated [26]. Multiple subclinical infarctions may cause subendocardial fibrosis involving large areas of ventricular myocardium [2]. In patients with silent ischemia, ischemic cardiomyopathy may develop without previous hints of CAD. A second type of ischemic cardiomyopathy can be described as a chronic low-flow condition, due to CAD, which is able to preserve viability but not function [27]. This situation, called the *hibernating myocardium*, is a reversible manifestation of ischemic cardiomyopathy. Indeed, noncontracting areas frequently are metabolically active. Another manifestation of ischemic cardiomyopathy is the stunned myocardium. After a short, transient occlusive episode, a prolonged but reversible functional depression may persist from several hours to days [17, 28]. This is partially due to decreased levels of adenosine triphosphate (ATP) in the myocytes and occurs after flow restoration [26]. The reperfusion injury is characterized by an increase in intracellular and mitochondrial Ca^{++} phosphate deposits and cellular swelling. Elevated levels of Ca^{++} cause conversion of xanthine dehydrogenase to xanthine oxidase and eventually the creation of free radicals. Their presence causes membrane lipid peroxidation and cellular degeneration [29, 30].

When ventricular dysfunction progresses beyond the capacity of the contractile reserve, congestive heart failure develops. Generalized adrenergic activation causes blood flow redistribution. The fall in cardiac output leads to renal hypoperfusion with activation of the renin-angiotensin-aldosterone system and vasopressin release. The result is salt and water retention. The pulmonary circulation becomes congested, followed by right ventricular involvement and eventually liver congestion and ascites.

DIAGNOSIS AND EVALUATION OF SEVERITY OF DISEASE

Physical Examination

The purpose of the preoperative diagnostic evaluation is to delineate the extent of ischemic heart disease and to assess its functional implications. The physical examination often provides little information, lacking both in specificity and sensitivity. However, some physical findings can be of predictive value. A displaced point of maximal impulse (PMI) or jugular venous distention, or both, indicates functional impairment and an ejection fraction (EF) of less than 50 percent. S_3 and S_4 heart sounds may denote decreased diastolic compliance and prior myocardial infarction (MI). In a phonocardiographic study Cohn and associates [31] reported that 42 of 93 patients with CAD had third or fourth sounds. A new apical holosystolic murmur due to papillary muscle dysfunction or valvular incompetence may be detected. If left ventricular function is profoundly impaired, dyspnea may be present or occur after mild exertion. Moist bilateral rales on inspiration, basal or diffused, may be demonstrated. Hepatomegaly, hepatojugular reflex, and peripheral edema are end-stage symptoms of congestive heart failure rarely seen in preoperative patients.

Although biochemical findings are usually not specific, they can provide information about risk factors; high levels of low-density lipoproteins, increased cholesterol levels, and elevated platelet aggregation are often related to underlying CAD. None of the typical markers of the myocardial infarction (creatine phosphokinase-MB [CPK-MB], lactic dehydrogenase, glutamic-oxaloacetic transaminase) are detectable 2 weeks after the ischemic injury. Thus, unless an acute event is witnessed, laboratory blood testing provides little in evaluation of IHD.

Chest X-ray

Of patients with an enlarged cardiac silhouette on chest radiography, 70 percent have ventricular dysfunction (EF < 0.50). This finding is even more significant when it is associated with signs of pulmonary interstitial fluid. Occasionally, calcium deposits within the coronary artery and in the aorta are detectable and considered predictive of coronary artery disease.

Electrocardiogram

The resting ECG is normal in 25 to 50 percent of patients with stable angina, although rarely in patients with significant ventricular dysfunction. Findings such as rare ventricular premature beats, conduction abnormalities, and ST segment and T-wave changes can be nonspecific. Premature ventricular contractions (PVCs) are the most common arrhythmias occurring in patients with chronic IHD. The arrhythmias that carry the greatest risks of sudden death include R on T phenomena, multiform repetitive PVCs, ventricular tachycardia, and fibrillation. Ventricular arrhythmias in the presence of a ventricular aneurysm markedly raise mortality [17]. Other conduction abnormalities that can predispose to perioperative events include complete heart block, Mobitz type II second-degree heart block, and bundle branch blocks. Patients with unstable angina may have transient depression or elevation of ST segments, and/or T-wave inversions. Findings such as ST segment elevation are common in patients experiencing variant angina. Abnormalities in the inferior leads are usually related to the involvement of a normal coronary artery, while anterolateral findings are probably related to spasm superimposed on a coronary artery plaque. After an acute myocardial infarction, the typical ECG pattern is not always present. Frequently, the first change is ST segment elevation in the leads facing the injury, with depression in the reciprocal leads. The spread of the ST elevation is related to the extent of the anatomic damage. The most diagnostic finding is a wide (0.04 seconds) and deep (25% of height of R) Q wave appearing within the first few hours. Classically, Q waves have been judged a specific marker of transmural injury, although autopsies have shown that subendocardial necrosis can sometimes be associated with Q waves. A pathologic Q wave is not always discernible and only 25 to 50 percent of patients with a history of an old MI have persistent Q waves. Q-wave loss after myocardial infarction may be related to a smaller infarction size and minimal ventricular impairment [32]. Atrioventricular (AV) block and other conduction abnormalities can result from myocardial infarction. Persistence of ST segment elevation in an area of infarction may suggest the presence of a ventricular aneurysm. ST segment elevation in V_4R-V_5R implies right ventricular infarction. If silent ischemia is suspected, Holter ECG (ambulatory ECG) can be of definitive diagnostic support.

Ambulatory ECG (AECG) [33–35] is an important diagnostic modality for detection of arrhythmias and ischemia. This method has been in use for many years, but its efficacy in ischemia detection was limited due to technical difficulties, which have since been resolved. The ECG monitor is applied to the patient for a duration of 24 hours, during which the subject is asked to perform normal daily activity. A note pad is provided so that specific events that induce a stress response can be chronologically entered for subsequent examination. This type of monitoring is beneficial in diagnosing silent ischemia.

Ambulatory ECG is also useful in the detection of arrhythmias. Because it is performed over a 24-hour period, the yield for arrhythmias is significantly higher than with the routinely performed 2-minute rhythm strips. The ability to detect PVCs is 85 percent on AECG, compared to 14 percent on a 2-minute ECG.

Ischemia detected on preoperative AECG and intraoperative ECG carries a worse prognosis when compared to the absence of such a finding. In 32 patients undergoing major vascular surgery who demonstrated ischemia during preoperative AECG, there was a 38 percent incidence of adverse cardiac outcome, whereas 144 patients with no ischemic episodes had less than a 1 percent incidence of adverse outcome [34]. Slogoff and Keats [20] have demonstrated a threefold increase in the postoperative infarction rate in patients with intraoperative ECG evidence of ischemia.

Stress Testing

Exercise ECG provides diagnosis and assessment of perioperative prognosis in patients with IHD. The morbidity and mortality associated with its performance is 24:100,000 and 10:100,000, respectively [36]. Exercise ECG is a very useful tool to diagnose IHD when the resting ECG is nondiagnostic. Positive findings (Table 5-2) correlate well with the incidence of perioperative myocardial infarction [37]. An indication of the propensity to ischemia can be obtained from the heart rate and blood pressure achieved during the test period. Recent reports have shown that heart rate adjustment of ST depression can provide an estimate of the extent of the obstruction to coronary blood flow [38, 39]. In addition, 10 percent of patients with IHD, previously studied by Holter monitoring (without evidence of arrhythmia), will only show evidence of serious arrhythmias during exercise stress testing. Exertion may result in Q waves that disappear at rest, a possible indication of ischemic cardiomyopa-

Table 5-2. Stress electrocardiography: positive findings for coronary artery disease

ST segment depression
  Downsloping, 2 mm, 0.06–0.08 sec after J point upsloping (very specific, 95%)
  Horizontal, at least 1 mm, 0.06–0.08 sec from J point (specificity, 85%)
  Upsloping, at least 1 mm, 0.08 sec from J point (specificity, 75–85%)
ST segment elevation (suggesting left main disease or severe triple-vessel disease)
Early positive ECG changes (within 7 min)
Heart rate < 120 bpm
Persistence of changes
Exertional hypotension (increase by 20 mm Hg or less, or decrease)

thy. In patients with variant angina, exercise ECG provides little information.

The need for "pharmacologic" stress testing becomes apparent because many patients with physical disabilities, such as claudication or advanced age, are poorly evaluated by standard exercise stress testing protocols. Much of the literature agrees that dipyridamole thallium-201 myocardial perfusion imaging is a good predictor of perioperative ischemic event in patients at risk [39, 40]. Dipyridamole induces maximal coronary vasodilatation, with resultant radionuclide perfusion defects. Upon the myocardial clearance of the drug, some defects will disappear as a result of thallium redistribution, which suggests the presence of hypoperfused viable myocardium, whereas persistent defects indicate scar. More recent data suggest that there may be areas of late redistribution that require a second dose of thallium in order to be distinguished from permanent perfusion deficits [41, 42]. This explains the incidence of ischemic events in patients thought to have fixed defects. Thallium stress testing may also provide information about the contractile reserve. Noncontracting but metabolically active areas may show improved function, with increase of ejection fraction after inotropic stimulation or afterload reduction.

Nuclear Imaging

Radionuclide angiography provides an evaluation of global cardiac function. In this test red blood cells are labeled with technetium (99m) and infused. A gated-pooled ventriculogram is then obtained. Ejection fractions obtained in this way correlate well with angiographic ejection fraction. The test can be performed both at rest and during exercise. Changes in ejection fraction and new dyskinesia with exercise can be quantitated.

Echocardiography

Two-dimensional and Doppler echocardiography provide a noninvasive functional assessment of abnormal cardiac anatomy and physiology, such as wall motion abnormalities, valvular regurgitation, aneurysms, and mural thrombi. While M-mode echocardiography has limited applications because it does not provide information about global heart function, two-dimensional echo has an excellent sensitivity and specificity rate (91%, 88%) for detection of wall motion abnormalities and ejection fraction, along with useful functional index derivations (Table 5-3). When one focuses on the coronary arteries, it is occasionally possible to detect the coronary obstruction [43]. Doppler evaluation can also be used to assess the diastolic function of the heart [44]. With the advent of transesophageal echocardiography, study limitations by technical difficulty or geometric considerations, or both, have been almost completely eliminated (see Chap. 4).

Table 5-3. Echocardiographic anatomic findings and derived functional indices in ischemic heart disease

---
Anatomic findings
Segmental wall motion abnormalities
Ventricular aneurysm
Pseudoaneurysm and mural thrombi
Ventricular septal defects
Valvular disease

Derived functional indices
Systolic function
 Ejection fraction
 Cardiac output by valvular Doppler
 Fractional shortening
Diastolic function
 Estimation of preload by LVEDV
 Indication of diastolic relaxation by Doppler E-A ratio
Afterload
 Wall stress

Cardiac Catheterization

Cardiac catheterization should only be reserved for patients in whom revascularization (either surgical correction or balloon angioplasty) procedures are considered before noncardiac surgery. Although highly invasive, it supplies the clinician with the accurate anatomic diagnosis and functional degree of the IHD. Ventriculography will accurately quantitate wall motion abnormalities. Coronary arteriography outlines the coronary arterial tree.

For variant angina the ergonovine test is very accurate, allowing the definitive diagnosis. The substance stimulates both α- and β-adrenergic receptors inducing coronary artery spasm. The test should be performed only after a careful evaluation of the coronary anatomy by coronary arteriography.

PERIOPERATIVE CARDIAC MORBIDITY

There is general agreement that the presence of cardiovascular disease substantially affects perioperative morbidity. Historically, the risk indices for quantifying perioperative predictors have been reported by the American Society of Anesthesiologists (ASA) [45], the New York Heart Association (NYHA) [46], and the Canadian Cardiovascular Society [47] (Table 5-4). In 1977, Goldman and associates [48] released a landmark study in which they preoperatively evaluated 1,001 patients and followed their postoperative cardiac outcome. They identified nine preoperative variables that independently predicted cardiac outcome and assigned them a relative predictive value. The variables and their point values are shown in Table 5-5. They placed patients in four cardiac risk index (CRI) categories based on their total perioperative variable score (Table 5-6). The CRI proved to have significant predictive potential. Since Goldman's landmark studies several investigators have evaluated the validity of the indices, widening the overview in this field with a large number of prospective and retrospective studies. Recently, Roizen [49] and Mangano [50] have reviewed the subject, and they have described the most accurate predicting factors of perioperative cardiac mortality (Table 5-7). While the results of these and other studies are still

Table 5-4. Classification of heart disease

Class	New York Heart Association	Canadian Cardiovascular Society
I	Patients with cardiac disease but without resulting limitations of physical activity. Ordinary physical activity does not cause undue fatigue, palpitation, dyspnea, or anginal pain.	Ordinary physical activity, such as walking and climbing stairs, does not cause angina. Angina with strenuous, rapid, or prolonged exertion at work or recreation.
II	Patients with cardiac disease resulting in slight limitation of physical activity. They are comfortable at rest. Ordinary physical activity results in fatigue, palpitation, dyspnea, or anginal pain.	Slight limitation of ordinary activity. Angina caused by walking or climbing stairs rapidly, walking uphill, walking or stair climbing after meals, in cold, in wind, or when under emotional stress, or only during the few hours after awakening. Also caused by walking more than two blocks on level ground and climbing more than one flight of ordinary stairs at a normal pace and in normal conditions.
III	Patients with cardiac disease resulting in marked limitation of activity. They are comfortable at rest. Less than ordinary physical activity causes fatigue, palpitation, dyspnea, or anginal pain.	Marked limitation of ordinary physical activity. Angina caused by walking one or two blocks on level ground and climbing one flight in normal conditions.
IV	Patients with cardiac disease resulting in inability to carry on physical activity without discomfort. Symptoms of cardiac insufficiency or of the anginal syndrome may be present even at rest. If any physical activity is undertaken, discomfort is increased.	Inability to carry on any physical activity without discomfort. Anginal syndrome may be present at rest.

somewhat controversial, generally, a history of recent myocardial infarction, patterns of unstable angina, left main disease with ST-T wave changes at rest, cardiomegaly on chest roentgenogram, and congestive heart failure are believed to affect the perioperative outcome.

The timing of a myocardial infarction correlates with perioperative morbidity. Tarhan and associates [51] reported a 6.6 percent incidence of reinfarctions if the previous episode had occurred more than 6 months before, 18 percent if it was 4 to 6 months before, and 37 percent if the infarction was as recent as 3 months or less. More recently Rao and colleagues [52] reported different results: A 4- to 6-month-old infarction had a 2.3 percent incidence of perioperative reinfarction, and 3 or fewer months raised the incidence to 5.8 percent. This decreased reinfarction rate was attributed to invasive monitoring and the aggressive hemodynamic management performed during the study.

Although there is general agreement that a recent history of a myocardial infarction is an independent predictor of perioperative cardiac morbidity (PCM), Foster and associates [53] emphasized the influence of the degree of ventricular dysfunction induced by the myocardial infarction. Congestive heart failure is a major cause of increased perioperative risk [54]. In individuals over 40 years of age, 6 percent of patients with controlled congestive heart failure and 16 percent with evident preoperative congestive heart failure developed cardiogenic pulmonary edema postoperatively [55]. Goldman and colleagues [48] considered an audible S_3 sound and orthopnea as univariate predictors of ominous outcome, while left ventricular wall motion scores were predictive using multivariate analysis.

The lack of consistent clinical–pathologic correlation in CAD [17] makes the use of clinical signs difficult in definitively assessing perioperative prognosis. Therefore, the identification of reliable testing predictors is essential to make a definitive estimation of risk. Stress ECG testing with its low costs and easy performance is still considered effective [56]. Cutler and associates [56] reported myocardial infarction in 37 percent of patients with a positive ischemia response, versus 1.5 percent of patients with a negative response. Exercise ECG can predict

Table 5-5. Computation of the cardiac risk index

Variable	Point value
History	
Age > 70 yr	5
MI in previous 6 mo	10
Physical examination	
S$_3$ gallop or JVD	11
Aortic stenosis	3
Electrocardiogram	
Rhythm other than sinus or PACs on last preoperative ECG	7
>5 PVCs/min documented at any time before operation	7
General status	
PO$_2$ < 60 or PCO$_2$ > 50 mm Hg	
K$^+$ < 3.0 or HCO$_3$ < 20 mEq/liter	
BUN > 50 or Cr > 3.0 mg/100 ml	
Abnormal SGOT, signs of chronic liver disease, or patient bedridden from noncardiac causes	3
Operation	
Intraperitoneal, intrathoracic, or aortic	3
Emergency	4
Total possible	53

JVD = jugular venous distention; PAC = premature atrial contractions; PO$_2$ = oxygen tension; HCO$_3$ = bicarbonate; BUN = blood urea nitrogen; Cr = creatinine; SGOT = serum glutamic oxaloacetic transaminase.
Source: Reprinted, by permission of the *New England Journal of Medicine.* From L Goldman, DL Caldera, SR Nussbaim, et al., Multifactorial index of cardiac risk in noncardiac surgical procedures. *N Engl J Med* 297:845, 1977.

Table 5-6. Cardiac risk index (CRI)

CRI class	Total predictive points	Risk of cardiac death (%)
I	0–5	0.2
II	6–12	2.0
III	13–25	2.0
IV	≥26	56.0

Source: Reprinted, by permission of the *New England Journal of Medicine.* From L Goldman, DL Caldera, SR Nussbaim, et al. Multifactorial index of cardiac risk in noncardiac surgical procedures. *N Engl J Med* 297:845, 1977.

Table 5-7. Perioperative cardiac morbidity: historical predictors

Roizen [49]	Mangano [50]
Age	Age (controversial)
Angina (NYHA and CCS evaluation); ST, T, QRS abnormalities	Angina (controversial)
Recent infarction (within 6 mo)	Previous MI
Congestive heart failure, history of cardiac heart failure, cardiomegaly	Congestive heart failure
Heart rhythm other than sinus, premature atrial contractions, more than 5 PVC/min	Dysrhythmias (PVC, rhythm other than sinus)
Aortic stenosis, mitral regurgitation	Valvular heart disease (predictive value of aortic or mitral is uncertain)
BUN > 50 mg/100 ml, K < 3.0 mEq/liter	Hypertension (controversial)
	Diabetes mellitus
	Peripheral vascular disease

NYHA = New York Heart Association; CCS = Canadian Cardiovascular Society.
Source: Modified from MF Roizen, Anesthetic Implications of Concurrent Diseases. In RE Miller (ed), *Anesthesia* (3rd ed). New York: Churchill Livingstone, 1990. Pp 793–893, and DT Mangano, Perioperative cardiac morbidity. *Anesthesiology* 72:153, 1990.

operative risk regardless of electrocardiographic findings. Gerson and colleagues [57] found that the inability to perform 2 minutes of exercise and achieve a heart rate of 100 beats per minute was the only independent predictor of adverse outcome in elderly patients undergoing major surgery. In a study by Pasternack and coworkers [58], gated-pooled radionuclide angiogram results correlated well with the incidence of perioperative myocardial infarction. Infarction occurrence was inversely related to the preoperative ejection fraction. No myocardial infarctions occurred if ejection fraction was between 56 and 83 percent, while ejection fractions of 36 to 55 percent and 35 percent or less were associated with an increased incidence of myocardial infarction (19 and 75%, respectively).

Dipyridamole thallium [59] has been legitimized as a valid predicting test for patients in the intermediate-risk categories. High sensitivity was attributed to the test when it was used to predict morbidity in patients undergoing vascular surgery. Fifty percent of patients with reversible defects experienced cardiac events, whereas patients without reversible defects suffered none. In another study [40] dipyridamole thallium imaging was used to stratify patients with positive clinical markers suggesting intermediate ischemic risk. The authors concluded that the test was safe, accurate, and cost effective for risk stratification in patients with evidence of congestive heart failure, angina, previous MI, or diabetes mellitus. More recently, other investigators demonstrated a low sensitivity of dipyridamole thallium testing, reporting failure in redistribution in 40 percent of patients with ischemic complications [60]. This may be due to either late thallium redistribution or low sensitivity in less severe coronary disease [61]. Therefore, some authors [62] do not regard this test as predictive.

A review of the Coronary Artery Surgery Study (CASS) [46] registry data in patients who subsequently underwent noncardiac surgery reveals that the presence of poor ventricular function was the only independent predictor of perioperative risk. Coronary anatomy was not an independent predictor of outcome. Ventricular function data can be obtained using noninvasive techniques, so that cardiac catheterization should be reserved for patients in whom preoperative revascularization is anticipated.

Strategy Evaluation

The high incidence of life-threatening complications associated with surgical procedures in patients with CAD mandates a careful evaluation of the strategy available. In patients at high risk for perioperative cardiac events, an alternative scheme must be employed to reduce the risk of cardiac complications. The choices include cancellation of the operative procedure, substitution for a lower-risk procedure, prophylactic revascularization, and combined intensive hemodynamic management and perioperative stress reduction [63].

Although cancellation of the operative procedure appears to be a viable alternative, this can only be done for nonessential surgery. However, many procedures planned on high-risk patients are emergent and life threatening, and cannot be canceled.

The magnitude of surgical intervention was shown by Goldman [64] to have predictive value in high-risk patients. In an attempt to reduce the perioperative risk, it would seem appropriate to attempt to substitute a low-risk procedure for a scheduled high-risk one. However, limited studies have failed to demonstrate any clear benefit to this approach. Comparison of high-risk patients undergoing abdominal vascular surgery with similar patients undergoing extraabdominal operation yielded a similar incidence of perioperative myocardial infarctions, 28 and 20 percent, respectively [65]. However, well-controlled prospective studies need to be performed before this approach is dismissed.

Prophylactic revascularization can be undertaken in patients at risk for perioperative infarction. Goldman CRI class I and II [48] patients have a total perioperative mortality, with or without prior cardiac surgery, of about 2.4 percent [51, 53]. Therefore, in this class of patients scheduled surgery should proceed without delay.

Coronary artery bypass grafting is indicated in severe left main coronary artery and multivessel disease. However, it is important to emphasize that this procedure carries a risk rate that is additive to the noncardiac surgical risk. In the CASS study [66], the perioperative mortality of CABG was 2.4 percent. Prior CABG decreases the mortality from 2.4 to 0.9 percent, the postsurgical angina incidence from 8.7 to 5.1 percent, and the incidence of postoperative myocardial infarction during noncardiac surgery from 6.0 to 1.1 percent [53, 67]. From these figures it would seem that the overall mortality would be lower for noncardiac surgery alone. Hertzer and associates [68] found a 5.3 percent mortality in 226 patients undergoing prophylactic CABG for severe correctable lesions. Others have reported a prohibitive mortality of 27 percent in patients undergoing sequential angiography, CABG, and vascular surgery [69]. Therefore, CABG may merely be a survival test for patients subsequently undergoing noncardiac surgery.

With the advent of percutaneous transluminal angioplasty (PTCA), the risk associated with coronary revascularization has been reduced. Minor and major complications occur in 7 and 4 percent of patients, respectively. The myocardial infarction rate is 2.6 percent, with a mortality close to zero [70]. The indications for PTCA include symptoms and evidence of worsening myocardial ischemia, vascular patients having a higher mortality risk during CABG, revascularization after post-CABG occlusion [71], early revascularization after acute myocardial infarction, and patients with severe systemic disease or advanced age, or both. PTCA has been successfully performed in patients experiencing variant angina [72]. However, not all lesions are amenable to PTCA and the effectiveness of PTCA as a risk-reducing option has not been studied.

Combined intensive hemodynamic management and perioperative stress reduction refers to a management strategy that includes invasive monitoring and aggressive hemodynamic manipulations in combination with an anesthetic technique that decreases the "stress response" of surgery and convalescence. Rao and associates [52] studied 733 patients with a history of a recent MI who were aggressively monitored in 5 days of intensive care stay after noncardiac surgery. They compared their 1.9 percent incidence of reinfarction with a 7.7 percent incidence in historical controls. The study involved the large expense of insertion of hemodynamic monitoring and intensive care stay. The investigators found that the incidence of reinfarction in study and control patients was zero in patients without angina or congestive heart failure (CHF). The inclusion of only patients with either angina or CHF in the study would have resulted in similar data at significantly lower cost. Using similar methodology, Wells and Kaplan [73] reported no reinfarctions in 48 patients operated on within 3 months of myocardial infarction, again crediting the astonishing results to the extensive monitoring, hemodynamic interventions, and special care unit stay for 2 to 3 days and, if needed, protracted intubation.

Perioperative stress reduction has recently become a popular concern to the anesthesiologist. Yeager and associates [74] reported a marked reduction of perioperative complications in patients anesthetized with a combination of general and epidural local anesthetic/narcotics. They compared "epigeneral" with standard general anesthetic techniques, and suggested that the favorable results were the consequence of sustained suppression of the stress response manifested by lower cortisol levels in the experimental group. The use of high-dose narcotic techniques common during cardiac surgery appears to not only have the advantage of hemodynamic stability but also stress suppression. Benefiel and colleagues [75] compared the effect of a high-dose sufentanil anesthetic with isoflurane. They reported a lower incidence of cardiac complications and attributed it to stress suppression manifested by lower plasma norepinephrine levels. Although many of these studies require well-controlled prospective corroboration, present data would suggest that a combination of aggressive hemodynamic management and a stress-reducing technique is the best way to handle high-risk patients.

PREOPERATIVE MEDICAL OPTIMIZATION

The anesthesiologist should carefully evaluate the patients' history and laboratory data searching for associated abnormalities in an attempt to further reduce the perioperative risk. Symptoms of CAD may easily be worsened by abnormalities of fluid and hemoglobin status, electrolyte imbalances, respiratory insufficiency, and drug effects. These abnormalities require quick diagnosis and proper intervention before surgery. Minimum blood testing should include electrolytes, glucose, and hemoglobin. In addition, many patients have significant pulmonary disease, making a baseline blood gas a requirement.

It is not unusual for this group of patients to be taking diuretics as part of their medical regimen. These patients can suffer electrolyte imbalances that may require supplementation. This is especially important in patients taking digoxin; in these individuals hypokalemia may lead to life-threatening arrhythmias.

Arrhythmias can carry a poor perioperative prognosis. Benign-appearing preoperative arrhythmias may become life threatening under anesthesia. The importance of any arrhythmia depends on the type of arrhythmia and its intrinsic prognosis, the hemodynamic consequence, the temporal relationship to perioperative stress, and the underlying heart disease [76]. The cause of the arrhythmia should be determined and treatment instituted before surgery.

Patients with IHD presenting for surgery often take a number of medications that may interact with anesthetics. Primarily, the preoperative administration of chronic medication must be directed at the pharmacologic optimization of the oxygen supply and demand ratio. The basic treatment of episodic stable angina includes the use of nitrates supplemented by either β-adrenergic blockers or Ca^{++} channel blockers, or both. The vasodilatory effects of nitrates diminish $M\dot{V}O_2$ by reducing wall tension and preload as well as increasing flow in myocardial arterioles. They should be continued through surgery.

Recent evidence suggests that cardiologists are treating an increasing number of patients suffering ischemic heart disease with calcium channel blockers rather than β-blockers. Ca^{++} channel blockers reduce smooth-muscle tone and the contractile state of the myocardium with prevention of vasospasm. They also cause dilatation of epicardial coronary vessels. Although, classically, Ca^{++} channel blockers can interact with anesthetics to increase the degree of AV block, they are administered up to and including the day of surgery [77].

β-Adrenergic blockers are the cornerstone in the treatment of ischemic heart disease. This group of drugs has been found more beneficial than Ca^{++} antagonists in severe exertional and rest angina. Their cardiovascular effects are related to the inhibition of β-adrenergic receptor stimulation by catecholamines. Therefore, they reduce $M\dot{V}O_2$ by lowering heart rate, blood pressure, and contractility. On the other hand their negative inotropic action causes an increase in end diastolic volume, which may result in deterioration of pump function in patients with left ventricular impairment. There is general agreement on the perioperative maintenance of β-blockade, in order to reduce the catecholamine response and avoid the possible rebound effects on angina pectoris, myocardial infarction, and hypertension [78]. Real consideration should be given to the supplementation of patients receiving Ca^{++} channel-blocking agents or nitrates, or both, with a β-adrenergic blocker perioperatively. Stone and associates [79] studied the protective effect of preoperative β-adrenergic blockers in untreated hypertensive patients. The administration of a single oral dose of labetalol, atenolol, or axprenolol in mildly hypertensive patients protects against hyperdynamic stress responses and myocardial ischemia during intubation and emergence from anesthesia. Use of β-adrenergic blockers such as metoprolol in patients with CHF is controversial, but is described by some authors as highly beneficial [80]. The anesthesiologist should be aware of the chance of significant interaction between Ca^{++} channel blockers and β-adrenergic blockers, particularly at decreasing AV conduction and reducing contractility. β-Adrenergic blockers used after a myocardial infarction may reduce incidence of sudden death and limit infarction size.

Digoxin is frequently used in the treatment of patients with CHF. This drug decreases heart rate and atrioventricular node conduction, increasing both force and velocity of contraction in the failing heart. LVEDP and LVEDV decrease, along with heart size and wall tension. The treatment should be continued until the time of surgery. This is especially true if CHF and atrial fibrillation or flutter with high ventricular rate are present. These patients must be kept well digitalized throughout the perioperative period.

In patients with a recent MI or evidence of congestive heart failure, or both, angiotensin-converting enzyme (ACE) inhibitors have been shown to provide significant benefits. Angiotensin II is a potent vasoconstrictor; the ACE inhibitors relax vascular smooth muscle and reduce both preload and afterload, without increasing heart rate or affecting $M\dot{V}O_2$. This reduces wall stress and improves left ventricular (LV) performance [19]. They also slow down the progression of postinfarction dilatation. Enalaprilat can be administered intraoperatively for rapid treatment of LV failure and prevention of ischemia [81] (Fig. 5-2). This group of drugs should be continued throughout the perioperative period.

Clonidine is a commonly used antihypertensive. It is a selective α_2 agonist that reduces central sympathetic outflow. Clonidine has been shown to reduce inhalation agent minimum alveolar concentration (MAC) and narcotic requirements during anesthesia. This drug should be continued, since sudden withdrawal can result in severe rebound hy-

5. Ischemic Heart Disease   95

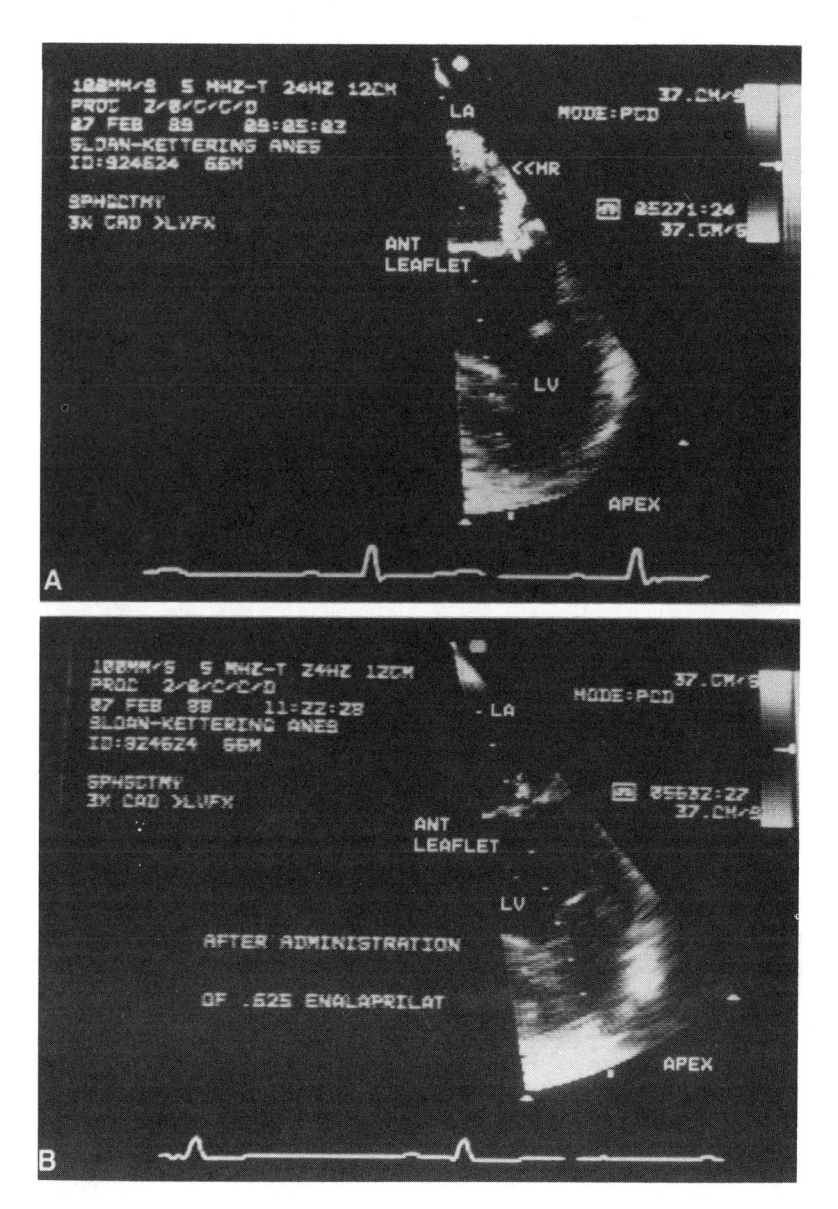

Fig. 5-2. Long-axis two-dimensional transesophageal echocardiographic view of the left ventricle with color-flow Doppler analysis. Mitral regurgitation (MR) is present in the first image (A), while it is absent in the second image, obtained 10 minutes after administration of enalaprilat (IV, 0.625 mg) (B). Structures from top to bottom are: left atrium (LA), mitral valve leaflets, left ventricular cavity (LV), left ventricular septum on left, and left ventricular free wall on right. (Reprinted with permission from the International Anesthesia Research Society. From GA Acampora, JA Melendez, DL Keefe, et al., Intraoperative administration of the intravenous angiotensin-converting enzyme inhibitor, enalaprilat, in a patient with congestive heart failure. *Anesth Analg* 69:833, 1989.)

pertension caused by markedly elevated circulating catecholamines.

ANESTHETIC MANAGEMENT
Premedication

Preoperative anxiety may lead to tachycardia, hypertension, ischemia, and possibly myocardial infarction. The preoperative visit should aim to establish rapport with the patient and attempt to ease concerns. At the completion of the interview, the patient should have a clear understanding of the procedures to be undertaken. The premedication should be tailored to the individual patient. In patients with reduced cardiac reserve, the doses of anxiolytics should be reduced. In most cases premedication should be accompanied by supplemental nasal oxygen. This can prevent the arterial desaturations sometimes seen following premedication.

Intraoperative Monitoring

The control of factors affecting perioperative cardiac morbidity is made possible by proper intraoperative monitoring. A more detailed description of intraoperative monitoring is presented in Chap. 4. Continuous ECG is routine. The standard leads II and V_5 provide information about the inferior and lateral myocardial wall. Changes recorded in these leads have been judged useful indicators of myocardial ischemia during surgery [82]. Computer ST segment analysis enables the identification of 70 to 90 percent of changes. Severity and duration of ST and T-wave changes can help to discriminate between nonspecific and specific alterations. However, the standard precordial ECG often fails in the detection of subendocardial ischemic events. Griffin and Kaplan [83] used computerized ST segment analysis to compare different lead systems, reporting the successful use of a single, bipolar, modified (CS_5 or CB_5) lead, substituting for V_5, in the detection of ischemic events, otherwise missed on the standard ECG. London and associates [84] checked a single-lead sensitivity using a 12-lead system. The most sensitive lead was V_5, followed by V_4; leads II and V_5 detected only 80 percent of episodes while V_4 and V_5 had a sensitivity of 90 percent.

Arterial monitoring of blood pressure is necessary to assure reliable measurements and enable repeated arterial blood sampling. The indwelling arterial catheter should be placed before the induction of anesthesia.

In patients exhibiting ventricular dysfunction, the intraoperative hemodynamic control should be aggressive, requiring reliable information about filling pressures, afterload, preload, contractility, and ventricular volumes. Thus, besides the routine monitoring techniques, placement of a pulmonary artery catheter (PAC) is suggested. Since the landmark study of Kaplan and Wells [85], the PAC has been used in the early detection of myocardial ischemia by recognizing decreases in left ventricular compliance. However, this conclusion has been criticized. It requires the ischemic area of myocardium to be large enough and dysfunctional enough to cause a significant change in the overall ventricular function since the surrounding well-supplied myocardium immediately takes over the function of the dysfunctional area, resulting in relatively unchanged hemodynamics [86]. However, elevations of pulmonary capillary wedge pressure (PCWP), a result of either ischemia or other factors such as volume overload, can certainly cause decreased coronary perfusion pressures, which can lead to ischemia and should be treated. It is undeniable that the PAC allows guidance to therapeutic choices with more complete assessment of pump function [52]. Recently, investigators have shown that the preoperative placement of PAC can lead to ECG ischemia, and it is important to remain aware of changes in ST segment morphology during any invasive procedure.

Transesophageal echocardiography (TEE) provides earlier and more sensitive indices of myocardial ischemia than the ECG, by displaying wall motion abnormalities [87, 88]. However, TEE has its limitations. Recently, London and associates [89] studied 156 patients undergoing noncardiac surgery. They observed segmental wall motion abnormalities in 20 percent of the patients, mostly characterized by hypokinesis and not always accompanied by significant hemodynamic changes. These findings were often discordant with ECG abnormality detections and were thought to be the result of limited specificity of the technique. Incoordinate contraction secondary to conduction abnormalities and the unmasking of old scar are two of the other causes of wall motion abnormalities detected by TEE. Additionally, studies cannot be performed during the critical phases, such as intubation and emergence from anesthesia [90]. Furthermore, failures in intraoperative myocardial ischemia detection have been described that are attributed to improper probe position [91].

Coronary lactate production is a result of myocardial ischemia. Its production can be quantitated by the placement of a coronary sinus catheter [92]. Although this procedure has been used in the operating room, it is still considered by most to be highly invasive and experimental.

Intraoperative Management

Throughout the intraoperative course the adequacy of respiratory performance should be verified to avert indirect myocardial depression due to hypoxemia, hypercarbia, or acidosis. Satisfactory blood volume and hemoglobin concentration should be maintained and electrolyte abnormalities resolved.

Anesthetic Choice

In an attempt to reduce the systemic effects of anesthetic drugs, regional anesthesia is often performed in patients with ischemic heart disease. Goldman and associates [55] reported that spinal anesthesia for general surgery was not associated with new or worsening heart failure, while general anesthesia resulted in 4 percent of new cases and 22 percent of worsening CHF. The sympathectomy provided by either spinal or epidural anesthesia leads to reductions of both preload and afterload, along with a decrease in contractility, probably due to drug activity and interruption of cardiac sympathetic innervation. Therefore, the risk of inducing an increase in $M\dot{V}O_2$ is decreased. One of the most appreciated advantages is certainly the pain control obtained through the use of local anesthetics without the adverse hypoxemia and pulmonary complications induced by narcotics [93]. On the other hand, many authors disagree with use of regional anesthesia in this patient population, partly because there is frequently a need for excess volume load to compensate for the sometimes unpredictable hypotension.

Treatment of hypotension may sometimes demand the use of vasoactive drugs. In patients with good left ventricular function (ejection fraction > 50%), phenylephrine can be used to maintain blood pressure and coronary perfusion pressure with minimal increase in $M\dot{V}O_2$ and without ejection fraction compromise or ventricular dilatation. However, in patients with marginal left ventricular function (ejection fraction < 35%) the use of a pure α-adrenergic agonist agent may produce increased LVEDV and LVEDP as a direct result of the inability of the compromised left ventricle, devoid of sympathetic stimuli, to handle the increase in afterload. These patients should probably receive a combined α-β–adrenergic agonist agent. This will cause an increase in coronary perfusion pressure while maintaining contractile status at the expense of an increase in $M\dot{V}O_2$. These hemodynamic parameters need careful control during regional anesthesia, as during general anesthesia; thus, invasive monitoring is a necessary part of a regional anesthetic technique in these patients.

Epidural anesthesia as an adjunct to general anesthesia has been described as a valuable technique. This combination can allow for the reduction in the amounts of parenteral drugs used and supplies excellent perioperative pain control. Yeager and associates [74] demonstrated more stable intraoperative hemodynamics due to the sensory blockade, the control of the adrenergic tone, and the systemic vasodilation with a reduction in afterload and preload. Postoperatively, pain control and a shorter endotracheal intubation period protected against pulmonary complications. The investigators observed CHF in 3.6 percent of patients when the technique was epidural plus light general anesthesia, with the associated use of postoperative epidural analgesia. In comparison, clinical signs of CHF were present in 40 percent of patients who underwent general anesthesia plus parenteral narcotic analgesia. Cortisol assays showed a diminution of the stress response after epidural anesthesia, which can represent a further protection for the ischemic myocardium. However, negative reports have appeared in the literature [94]. The hypotension caused by regional anesthesia is frequently treated with large volumes of fluid, which can be detrimental to the ischemic heart [95]. Additionally, the compensatory vasoconstriction occurring above the block may involve the cardiac sympathetic nerves, inducing coronary vasoconstriction [96].

Whether or not the choice of drugs and technique affects the outcome in patients with CAD is still controversial. Mangano [97] analyzed 27 studies of postanesthesia cardiac outcome and concluded that neither anesthetic drug choice nor anesthesia technique has a significant influence on the outcome of patients with underlying CAD. Indeed, 10 of 11 studies showed no difference between inhaled and opioid anesthesia, and no advantage has been postulated in the choice of either general or regional anesthesia. Only transurethral prostatectomy performed under spinal anesthesia and ophthalmologic procedures under local anesthesia seem to offer advantages in postoperative outcome [98]. Even in a population of high-risk patients, anesthetic technique appears to have much less influence on outcome than might be expected. Perhaps this is because careful clinical management with prompt treatment of hemodynamic alterations is the rule rather than the exception, and because these pharmacologic goals are met regardless of the anesthetic agent. In conclusion, even in the presence of severe ischemic heart disease, no one technique can substitute for clinical acumen and cautious anesthetic care.

Pharmacologic Strategy

The pharmacologic anesthetic strategy must achieve a balance between a reduction of workload and $M\dot{V}O_2$, and maintenance of effective pump function. The influence of anesthetic drugs on outcome has frequently been postulated. Despite their intrinsic hemodynamic effects, anesthetic drugs appear to contribute little to the outcome in high-risk patients when used cautiously. The effects of the various anesthetics on myocardial oxygen demand and supply are discussed in Chaps. 2 and 3.

The trauma induced by laryngoscopy and intubation can be the most stressful and potentially deleterious phase of anesthesia. The ideal induction agents should minimize the autonomic response to induction and intubation while maintaining hemodynamic stability. Barbiturates have been widely employed, although they cause myocardial depression, with a fall in the cardiac output and a rise in the heart rate, and consequential increase in $M\dot{V}O_2$. Etomidate has minimal cardiovascular effects, reducing $M\dot{V}O_2$ to 50 percent and increasing coronary sinus oxygen saturation by 20 to 30 percent [99]; hence, it is often considered the drug of choice in this group of patients. Benzodiazepines such as midazolam, at induction doses, are considered safe [100], although they produce slight decrease in blood pressure because of a reduction in systemic vascular resistance and mild negative inotropic effect. Additionally, the association of benzodiazepines with opioids and nitrous oxide (N_2O) may potentiate the hypotension [101]. Propofol causes decline both in oxygen supply and demand, thus not affecting the balance. On the other hand, inductive doses of propofol may cause significant hypotension and bradycardia, and may thus compromise coronary perfusion pressure, especially if used with opioids. When comparing induction using alfentanil with induction using thiopental, etomidate, and midazolam, alfentanil was found to be more cardiovascularly stable [102]. Even ketamine has been used in patients with IHD. When used in combination with a benzodiazepine, no difference was found, as compared to other drugs, in the incidence of induction ischemia [103]. However, most would exclude its use because of its well-known effects on $M\dot{V}O_2$, heart rate, and blood pressure.

In patients in whom postoperative ventilation is anticipated, induction can be executed using high-dose opioids, which provide a stable hemodynamic profile. A comparison between sufentanil, fentanyl, and morphine in prebypass patients undergoing cardiac surgery showed marked hemodynamic stability with the use of sufentanil and fentanyl and relative instability with morphine [104].

All inhalation agents, used for maintenance, cause a decrease in blood pressure. Halothane is the most potent myocardial depressant, followed by enflurane. In a nonimpaired left ventricle, the fall in cardiac work may be advantageous. Inhalation agents depress coronary blood flow and coronary perfusion pressure as well as $M\dot{V}O_2$. Indeed, in non–β-adrenergic blocked patients, these agents may depress the hyperdynamic response and have a protective effect. In β-adrenergic blocked patients, the negative inotropic effect is potentiated. Isoflurane seems to have the least myocardial depressant effect, but it is the most potent vasodilator (see Chap. 2). Although this combination may result in unchanged cardiac outputs, it may cause reflex tachycardia. Volatile agents used in patients with poor ventricular function or in patients with hemodynamics sustained by sympathetic activity may cause severe cardiovascular depression. Isoflurane, as well as halothane and enflurane, may further depress contractility in patients with CHF [105].

High-dose isoflurane has been implicated as a cause of intraoperative ischemic events. It has been postulated that a steal phenomenon attributable to isoflurane-induced redistribution of myocardial blood flow can occur at high doses in patients with steal-prone anatomy (Fig. 5-3). As a result of maximal coronary vasodilatation, the flow becomes higher in the normal arteries and correspondingly lower in the obstructed coronaries [106, 107]. This hypothesis is still controversial [108].

Potent agents have been recently implicated in two aspects of antianginal therapy not frequently considered intraoperatively. Sill and associates [109] have shown isoflurane to attenuate the effect of the mediators of coronary spasm in dogs. Intracoronary thrombi formation may be the most important etiology of ischemia in patients with unstable angina. Halothane, not isoflurane or enflurane, inhibits spontaneous and epinephrine-induced acute canine intracoronary thrombus formation [110]. The application to humans requires further study.

The use of nitrous oxide as supplement to general anesthesia is still debated. Although its use is common in clinical practice, nitrous oxide may cause sympathetic stimulation, and some authors described significant hemodynamic depression, with fall in coronary sinus blood flow, cardiac output [111], and worsening ischemia [112]. The use of nitrous oxide may also induce hemodynamic changes, partly as a result of the reduction in inspired oxygen concentration (F_{IO_2}) [113]. Therefore, in patients with a marginal respiratory reserve, the avoidance of nitrous oxide should be considered.

Opioids are generally exempt from direct myocardial depressant effects. They enhance parasympathetic tone, causing bradycardia (sufentanil, fentanyl), and may cause hypotension due to his-

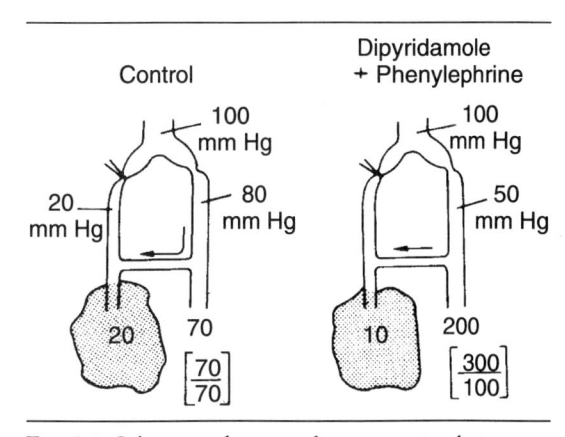

Fig. 5-3. Schematic diagram of coronary circulation, showing proposed mechanism for dipyridamole-induced coronary steal. The coronary artery divides in two branches, one completely occluded, the other stenosed and providing collaterals to the first. Control situation (*left*): The gradient across the stenosis is small and the flow in the distribution of the stenotic vessel is 70 ml/min/100 gm and is equally distributed to the subendocardium (lower value in the bracket) and in the subepicardium (upper value). The flow in the ischemic area (darker area) is 20 ml/min/100 gm and is determined by the difference between pressure in the bed supplying collaterals (80 mm Hg) and the ischemic bed (20 mm Hg). Dipyridamole administration (*right*): Pressure is maintained constant by phenylephrine. Flow in the nonischemic area increases to 200 ml/min/100 gm but is maldistributed between subendocardium and subepicardium. The pressure distal to the stenosis falls to 50 mm Hg and, therefore, the flow to the ischemic region decreases to 10 ml/min/100 gm. (Reprinted by permission of the American Heart Association, Inc. From LC Becker, Conditions for vasodilator-induced coronary steal in experimental myocardial ischemia. *Circulation* 57:1103, 1978.)

tamine release (morphine). On the other hand they are able to maintain adequate myocardial oxygen supply and can be successfully employed in this group of patients. High doses are sometimes required to avoid pain-related cardiovascular responses. As sole anesthetics, even at high dosages, opioids do not protect against hypertension and tachycardia, which result from extremely painful stimuli [114]. Additionally, recall after use of high-dose narcotics has been described when benzodiazepines were not also administered.

Muscle relaxants have a variety of effects when administered in clinical doses. The rapid administration of curare, and, to a lesser extent, metocurine and atracurium can cause hypotension resulting from histamine release, ganglionic blockade, and prostacycline release. It is important that, if these muscle relaxants have been chosen, they be administered slowly with attention to the patient's fluid status. On the other hand, the steroidal-type muscle relaxants, such as pancuronium, have muscarinic blocking effects. The vagolytic effect of pancuronium can be used advantageously to counteract the bradycardiac effect of the synthetic narcotics. Vecuronium is devoid of hemodynamic effects when administered in clinical doses (<300.0 μg/kg). Although this drug would seem to be ideal, its short action may require multiple dosing during protracted procedures. Pipercuronium and doxocurium, two newer long-acting muscle relaxants, also have minimal cardiovascular effects.

Myocardial Protection

Hemodynamic fluctuations are common during anesthesia; however, their occurrence must be controlled in order to avoid detrimental effects on the myocardial equilibrium. Anesthesia per se has a stabilizing action on the ischemic heart. For example, potent agents have been shown to reduce the incidence of ischemia during rapid atrial pacing. However, whether the ischemia is silent or hyperdynamically induced, anesthesia often provides inadequate protection. Some authors have suggested the use of a perioperative prophylactic nitroglycerin infusion [115]. The fall in blood pressure can be antagonized with fluid infusion, head-down position, or phenylephrine in patients without evidence of CHF. The choice is guided by central monitoring. Intracoronary nitroglycerin infusion increases the stenotic diameter of coronary vessels. It also reduces platelet aggregation, one of the mechanisms believed to be responsible for unstable angina and possibly silent ischemia. The drug also improves coronary flow by reducing preload and to some extent afterload, decreasing ventricular filling. However, n.any investigators have been unable to show any benefits to prophylactic nitroglycerin except for a decrease of perioperative hypertension. Yousif and associates [116] administered intravenous isosorbide dinitrate to 100 patients before surgery. Although they noted a decrease in the incidence of perioperative ischemic events, no difference was found in the number of postoperative myocardial infarctions. Additionally, nitroglycerin may be responsible for myocardial ischemia due to vasodilation causing excessive drop in coronary perfusion pressure. Intravenous nitroglycerin therapy has also been associated with hypoxemia secondary to the creation of a ventilation-perfusion mismatch, and methemoglobin.

Since tachycardia is commonly a consequence of stress and pain, deepening anesthesia may often be the only intervention required. A persistently high heart rate will increase oxygen consumption and reduce diastolic time and oxygen delivery. In some instances tachycardia may be the result of hypovolemia, hypotension, hypoxemia, and/or hypercarbia. If correction of these derangements does not resolve tachycardia, and there is evidence that the tachycardia may be of hyperdynamic origin, the administration of a β-adrenergic blocker may be indicated. Some studies suggest that the intraoperative administration of β-adrenergic blockers during the hyperdynamic state can reduce the incidence of perioperative infarctions. Esmolol, the short-acting $β_1$-selective-adrenergic blocker, is an ideal drug that can be administered as either a bolus or a continuous infusion titrated to effect.

Although there is no proof that intraoperative arrhythmias predict postoperative morbidity [52], these episodes should be treated immediately to avoid increases in oxygen demand and damaging effects on contractility. Many changes, such as respiratory alkalosis, hypoxemia, hypercarbia, and hypokalemia, cause alterations of the normal heart rhythm. PVCs as frequent as six or more per minute should be controlled with lidocaine. Atrial fibrillation requires control of ventricular response or cardioversion (see Chap. 10).

Hypertension is often associated with ischemic events. The rise in wall tension results in increased demand, and the rise in ventricular end diastolic pressure decreases coronary perfusion pressure. Nitroprusside is a nonspecific vasodilator that induces nonselective coronary dilatation. Its use in the control of hypertension in patients with CAD is plagued by unwanted effects, and may result in coronary steal [117]. The drug also reduces diastolic pressure, worsening coronary perfusion, and may lead to a reflex tachycardia. Nitroglycerin may be a more useful drug for the management of intraoperative hypertension in these patients.

In the presence of a coronary lesion, a severe fall in arterial diastolic pressure below the limits of autoregulation reduces coronary blood flow. Some investigators [52, 118] identify hypotension as a predictor of perioperative myocardial infarction, while others [119] disagree. Generally, a fall in blood pressure lasting less than 10 minutes that does not exceed 33 percent of preoperative values and/or a sudden drop of less than 50 percent below preoperative values are considered unlikely to produce ischemia. Anesthetic-induced hypotension usually responds to fluid replacement. If pharmacologic intervention is required, and the patient has evidence of good EF, phenylephrine can be used [120]. If low blood pressure is associated with high PCWP and low cardiac output (CO), the management may require the improvement of ventricular function with inotropic drugs.

In patients with severe pump failure, pump function improves following the use of inotropic agents only if there is a contractile reserve (Fig. 5-4). Drugs such as dobutamine and dopamine, which increase intracellular Ca^{++} ions, can be used in combination with vasodilators to improve myocardial performance before surgery. If ventricular dysfunction is refractory to standard therapy, amrinone, a phosphodiesterase inhibitor, should be considered. Biventricular failure may require preload increase combined with arterial dilatation to improve cardiac output.

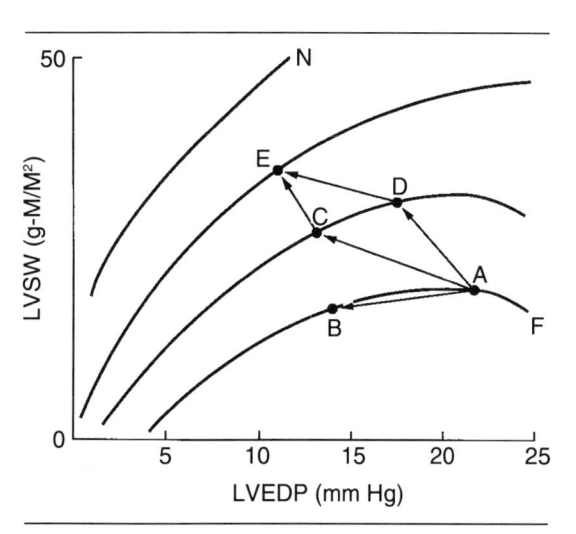

Fig. 5-4. Modification of left ventricular performance in heart failure (F) and after drug therapy. A: failure; B: diuretics decrease left ventricular end diastolic pressure (LVEDP) although left ventricular stroke work (LVSW) does not increase; C: vasodilators may increase stroke work and decrease left ventricular filling pressure, especially if combined (E) with inotropes (D); N: normal performance.

Postoperative Management

Postoperative observation in the postanesthesia care unit (PACU) is mandatory for patients with ischemic heart disease. Myocardial reinfarction is often asymptomatic and has a poor prognosis (>50% mortality) [118]. Historically, high-risk patients have been monitored for up to 5 days following surgery. Charlson and associates [121] suggested continuous ECG monitoring in the first 2 days, with subsequent CPK (creatine phosphokinase) and lactic dehydrogenase (LDH) isoenzymes if ECG changes were detected. This design provided positive findings, 58 percent of which would have been missed with the traditional occasional monitoring. Rao and colleagues [52] showed that myocardial infarction and mortality in high-risk patients could be reduced when the aggressive operative monitoring was extended into the postoperative period for 5 days. More recent data suggest that myocardial ischemia is more common in the postoperative (rather than intraoperative) period [53]. Silent ECG ischemia accounts for the overwhelming majority of postoperative ischemic events. Only in a subgroup of patients is ischemia associated with an increase in heart rate. Although the peak demand on the myocardium occurs in the hours immediately following the operation, the increased incidence of ischemia occurs not only in the early postoperative period but also in the late (up to 10 days, with a peak on second to third day) postoperative period. Early diagnosis and treatment of postoperative ischemia may result in better outcome in high-risk patients.

The control of respiratory function may need to be continued in order to avoid deleterious effects on the oxygen supply-demand relationship. The patient is not to be extubated until he or she is able to produce satisfactory levels of negative inspiratory pressure, tidal volume, vital capacity, saturation, and normocarbia on low FiO_2 (<50%). In patients with signs of left ventricular failure, additional caution is required in the evaluation of weaning criteria. Not only is respiratory function affected by the failing heart, but use of positive pressure ventilation may mislead the evaluation of preload; therefore, one must consider the possibility of an abrupt increase in preload following the reestablishment of spontaneous ventilation.

Many of the events that occur in the postoperative phase affect oxygen consumption. An important goal in the postoperative course is prevention of abrupt increases in oxygen consumption that may be detrimental to the already marginal condition of the cardiac patient. Hypothermia and shivering increase oxygen consumption, carbon dioxide production, and metabolic rate, and this must be avoided. The treatment of postoperative pain should be a major concern. Following surgery, pain may result in hypertension and arrhythmias with an increased MVO_2. If narcotics have not been administered during anesthesia, their requirement becomes evident early in the postoperative period. Morphine is usually administered with observation of respiratory function. Epidural narcotics grant stable levels of analgesia at lower doses; nonetheless, respiratory depression can occur. Patient-controlled analgesic pumps allow psychological relief, constant plasma levels, and lower dosages. Hypertension and tachycardia may also be the result of respiratory imbalances, electrolyte derangements, or fluid overload. If correction of these conditions fails to resolve hypertension, small doses of labetolol may be indicated. If nitroprusside or trimethaphan is employed to control hypertension, a β-adrenergic blocker will most likely be required. β-Adrenergic blockade can be initiated with either propranolol or esmolol. Pasternack and associates [122] showed that the use of β-adrenergic blocking agents after aortic aneurysm repair reduced infarction rate from 18 to 3 percent.

Hypotensive episodes should be minimized to reduce the chances of diminished coronary flow. Hypotension may indicate blood and third-space fluid loss or an impending myocardial infarction. Treatment will require rapid assessment with the aid of invasive monitoring. Hypotension associated with a low PCWP will require fluid administration, while association with a high PCWP may necessitate catecholamine or nitroglycerin infusion, or both.

Emergency Surgery

From a review of several studies, emergency surgery appears to increase the risk of perioperative myocardial infarction two- to fivefold [44, 123, 124]. Only Rao and associates [52] found no significant increase in reinfarction risk during emergency surgery. Much of the risk added by emergency situations in the management of a patient with IHD is related to the lack of information relative to the cardiac functional reserve. If allowed by time constraints and emergency nature, a preoperative cardiac assessment should be attempted to identify other predictors of perioperative morbidity.

Some emergency situations, such as ruptured aortic aneurysm, have an inescapable urgency. However, most patients are not in shock; their minimal laboratory data should include hemoglobin, electrolytes, creatinine, glucose, an ECG and a chest roentgenogram. Special considerations pertain to digitalized patients who are hypokalemic. Although K^+ replacement is dangerous and does not affect intracellular levels, it may stabilize irritable myocardial membranes. For all cases other than peripheral superficial surgery where fluid shifts are not anticipated, invasive central monitoring is mandatory and TEE may be useful. If cardiac dysfunction exists, central venous pressure does not provide any useful information. Therefore, a reliable source of data, such as PAC, should be obtained as soon as possible.

Induction should result in minimal hemodynamic fluctuations. Maintenance should be designed to avoid or limit the magnitude of events such as tachycardia, hypertension, hypotension, and fluid overload. Once again, the known side effects of anesthetic drugs should guide the choice of pharmacologic approach. The judicious use of vasodilators and inotropes may be required to maintain cardiac output.

REFERENCES

1. Mangano, DT. Preoperative Assessment of the Patient with Ischemic Heart Disease. In DT Mangano (ed), *Preoperative Cardiac Assessment*. Philadelphia: Lippincott, 1990. Pp 1–47.

2. Kannel, WB, McGee, D, Gordon, T. A general cardiovascular risk profile. Framingham Study. *Am J Cardiol* 38:46, 1976.
3. Shapiro, S, Weinblatt, E, Frank, CW, et al. Incidence of coronary disease in a population insured for medical care (HIP): Myocardial infarction, angina pectoris and possible myocardial infarction. *Am J Publ Health* 59 (Suppl):1, 1969.
4. Stamler, J, Stamler, R, Lui, KJ. High Blood Pressure. In WE Connor, JD Bristow (ed), *Coronary Artery Disease. Prevention, Complications and Treatment*. Philadelphia: Lippincott, 1985.
5. Simons, LA. Interrelations of lipids and lipoproteins with coronary artery disease mortality in 19 countries. *Am J Cardiol* 57:5, 1986.
6. Cohn, PF, Gabbay, SI, Weglicki, WB, et al. Serum lipid levels in angiographically defined coronary artery disease. *Ann Intern Med* 84:241, 1976.
7. Simons, LA. Interrelations of lipids and lipoproteins with coronary artery disease mortality in 19 countries. *Am J Cardiol* 57:5G, 1986.
8. Friedlander, Y, Kark, JD, Stein, Y. Family history of myocardial infarction as an independent risk factor for coronary heart disease. *Br Heart J* 53:382, 1985.
9. Gotto, AM, Farmer, JA. Risk Factors for Coronary Artery Disease. In E Braunwald (ed), *Heart Disease. A Textbook of Cardiovascular Medicine* (3rd ed). Philadelphia: Saunders, 1988. Pp 1153–1190.
10. Ross, R. The Pathogenesis of Atherosclerosis. In E Braunwald (ed), *Heart Disease. A Textbook of Cardiovascular Medicine* (3rd ed). Philadelphia: Saunders, 1988. Pp 1135–1152.
11. Bell, JR, Fox, AC. Pathogenesis of subendocardial ischemia. *Am J Med Sci* 268:2, 1974.
12. Braunwald, E, Sarnoff, SJ, Case, RB, et al. Hemodynamic determinants of coronary flow: Effect of changes in aortic pressure and cardiac output on the relationship between myocardial oxygen consumption and coronary flow. *Am J Physiol* 192:157, 1958.
13. Pasternack, RC, Braunwald, E, Sobel, BE. Acute Myocardial Infarction. In E Braunwald (ed), *Heart Disease. A Textbook of Cardiovascular Medicine* (3rd ed). Philadelphia: Saunders, 1988. Pp 1222–1313.
14. Mathews, MB, Julian, DG. Angina Pectoris: Definition and Description. In MB Mattews and DG Julian (eds), *Angina Pectoris* (2nd ed). New York: Churchill Livingstone, 1985. Pp 2–25.
15. Victor, MF, Likoff, MJ, Mintz, GS, et al. Unstable angina pectoris of new onset: A prospective clinical and arteriographic study of 75 patients. *Am J Cardiol* 47:228, 1981.
16. Prinzmetal, M, Kennamer, R, Merliss, R, et al. A variant form of angina pectoris. *Am J Med* 27:375, 1959.
17. Rutheford, JD, Braunwald, E, Cohn, PF. Chronic Ischemic Heart Disease. In E Braunwald (ed), *Heart Disease. A Textbook of Cardiovascular Medicine* (3rd ed). Philadelphia: Saunders, 1988. Pp 1314–1378.
18. Raby, KE, Goldman, L, Creager, MA, et al. Correlation between perioperative ischemia and major cardiac events after peripheral vascular surgery. *N Engl J Med* 321:1296–1300, 1989.
19. Roy, WL, Edelist, G, Gilbert, B. Myocardial ischemia during non-cardiac surgical procedures in patients with coronary artery disease. *Anesthesiology* 51:393–397, 1979.
20. Slogoff, S, Keats, AS. Does perioperative myocardial ischemia lead to postoperative myocardial infarction? *Anesthesiology* 62:107–114, 1985.
21. Deedwania, PC, Carbajal, EV. Silent ischemia during daily life as an independent predictor of mortality in stable angina. *Circulation* 81:748–756, 1990.
22. Maseri, A, Chierchia, S, Davies, G, et al. Mechanism of ischemic cardiac pain and silent myocardial ischemia. *Am J Med* 79(IIIA):7, 1985.
23. Pfeffer, MA, Braunwald, E. Ventricular remodeling after myocardial infarction: Experimental observations and clinical implications. *Circulation* 81:116, 1990.
24. Gahl, K, Sutton, R, Pearson, M, et al. Mitral regurgitation in coronary artery disease. *Br Heart J* 39:13, 1977.
25. Burch, GE, Giles, TD, Colcolough, HL. Ischemic cardiomyopathy. *Am Heart J* 79:291, 1970.
26. Kloner, RA. Ischemic cardiomyopathy: A manifestation of stunned myocardium? *Heart Failure* 7:5, 1991.
27. Rahimtoola, SH. The hibernating myocardium. *Am Heart J* 117:211, 1989.
28. Braunwald, E, Kloner, RA. The stunned myocardium, prolonged postischemic ventricular dysfunction. *Circulation* 66:1146, 1982.
29. Chambers, DE, Parks, DA, Petterson, G. Xanthine oxidase as a source of the radical damage in myocardial ischemia. *J Mol Cell Cardiol* 17:145, 1985.
30. McCord, JM. Oxygen derived free radicals in post-ischemic tissue injury. *N Engl J Med* 312:159, 1985.
31. Cohn, PF, Vokonas, PS, Williams, RA, et al. Diastolic heart sounds and filling waves in coronary artery disease. *Circulation* 44:196, 1971.
32. Coll, S, Betriu, A, de Flores, T, et al. Significance of Q-wave regression after transmural acute myocardial infarction. *Am J Cardiol* 61:739, 1988.

33. Holter, NJ. New method for heart studies. Continuous electrocardiography of active subjects over long periods is now practical. *Science* 134:1214–1220, 1961.
34. Kennedy, HL, Wiens, RD. Ambulatory (Holter) electrocardiography and myocardial ischemia. *Am Heart J* 17:164–176, 1989.
35. Knoebel, SB, Crawford, MH, Dunn, MI, et al. Guidelines for ambulatory electrocardiography. *Circulation* 79:206–215, 1989.
36. Rochmis, P, Blackburn, H. Exercise tests. A survey of procedures, safety and litigation experience in approximately 170,000 tests. *JAMA* 217:1061, 1971.
37. Cutler, BS, Wheeler, HB, Paraskos, JA, et al. Assessment of operative risk with electrocardiographic exercise testing in patients with peripheral vascular disease. *Am J Surg* 137:484, 1979.
38. Kligfield, P, Ameisen, O, Okin, PM. Heart rate adjustment of ST segment depression for improved detection of coronary artery disease. *Circulation* 79:245, 1989.
39. Okin, PM, Kligfield, P, Ameisen, O, et al. Identification of anatomically extensive coronary artery disease by the exercise ECG ST/HR slope. *Am Heart J* 115:1002, 1988.
40. Eagle, KA, Coley, CM, Newell, JB, et al. Combining clinical and thallium data optimizes preoperative assessment of cardiac risk before major vascular surgery. *Ann Intern Med* 110:859, 1989.
41. Josephson, MA, Brown, BG, Hecht, HS, et al. Noninvasive detection and localization of coronary stenoses in patients: Comparison of resting dipyridamole and exercise thallium-201 myocardial perfusion imaging. *Am Heart J* 103:1008, 1982.
42. Dilsizian, V, Rocco, TP, Freedman, NMT, et al. Enhanced detection of ischemic but viable myocardium by the reinfusion of thallium after stress redistribution imaging. *N Engl J Med* 323:141, 1990.
43. Rink, LD, Feigenbaum, H, Goldley, RW, et al. Echographic detection of left main coronary artery obstruction. *Circulation* 65:719, 1982.
44. Labovitz, AJ, Pearson, AC. Evalution of left ventricular diastolic function: Clinical relevance and recent Doppler echographic insights. *Am Heart J* 114:836, 1987.
45. American Society of Anesthesiologists. New classification of physical status. *Anesthesiology* 24:111, 1963.
46. Criteria Committee of the NYHA. *Diseases of the Heart and Blood Vessels: Nomenclature and Criteria for Diagnosis* (6th ed). Boston: Little, Brown, 1964.
47. Coronary Artery Surgery Study (CASS). *Manual of Operations II: Data Collection and Storage. Collaborative Studies in Coronary Artery Surgery.* Washington, DC: National Heart, Lung and Blood Institute. Prepared by the CASS Coordinating Center, University of Washington, Seattle, 1978.
48. Goldman, L, Caldera, DL, Nussbaim SR, et al. Multifactorial index of cardiac risk in noncardiac surgical procedures. *N Engl J Med* 297:845, 1977.
49. Roizen, MF. Anesthetic Implications of Concurrent Diseases. In RE Miller (ed), *Anesthesia* (3rd ed). New York: Churchill Livingstone, 1990. Pp 793–893.
50. Mangano, DT. Perioperative cardiac morbidity. *Anesthesiology* 72:153, 1990.
51. Tarhan, S, Moffitt, EA, Taylor, WF, et al. Myocardial infarction after general anesthesia. *JAMA* 220:1451, 1972.
52. Rao, TK, Jacobs, KH, El-Etr, AA. Reinfarction following anesthesia in patients with myocardial infarction. *Anesthesiology* 59:499, 1983.
53. Foster, ED, Davis, KB, Carpenter, JA, et al. Risk of noncardiac operation in patients with defined coronary disease: The Coronary Artery Surgery Study (CASS) registry study. *Am Thorac Surg* 41:42, 1986.
54. Goldman, L, Marshall, AW, Braunwald, E. General Anesthesia and Noncardiac Cardiac Surgery in Patients with Heart Disease. In E Braunwald (ed), *Heart Disease. A Textbook of Cardiovascular Medicine* (3rd ed). Philadelphia: Saunders, 1988. Pp 1693–1705.
55. Goldman, L, Caldera, DL, Southwick FS, et al. Cardiac risk factors and complications in non-cardiac surgery. *Medicine* 57:357, 1978.
56. Cutler, BS, Wheeler, HB, Paraskos, JA, et al. Applicability and interpretation of ECG stress testing in patients with peripheral vascular disease. *Am J Surg* 141:501, 1981.
57. Gerson, MC, Hurst, JM, Hertzberg, VS, et al. Cardiac prognosis in noncardiac geriatric surgery. *Ann Intern Med* 103:832, 1985.
58. Pasternack, PF, Imparato, AM, Riles, TS, et al. The value of the radionuclear angiogram in the prediction of perioperative myocardial infarction in patients undergoing lower extremity revascularization procedures. *Circulation* 72:11–13, 1985.
59. Boucher, CA, Brewster, DC, Darling, C, et al. Determination of cardiac risk by dipyridamole thallium imaging before peripheral vascular surgery. *N Engl J Med* 312:389, 1985.
60. McEnroe, CS, O'Donnel, TF, Jr, Yeager, A, et al. Comparison of ejection fraction and Goldman risk factor analysis to dipyridamole–thallium 201 studies in the evaluation of cardiac morbidity after aortic aneurysm surgery. *J Vasc Surg* 11:497, 1990.

61. Gould, MD. Quantitative imaging in nuclear cardiology. *Circulation* 66:1141, 1982.
62. Coriat, P. Dipyridamole-thallium imaging—no routine test prior to vascular surgery. Society of Cardiovascular Anesthesiologists, 13th Annual Meeting, 1991.
63. Thomson, IR. Personal communication, 1989.
64. Goldman, L. Multifactorial index of cardiac risk in noncardiac surgery: Ten year status report. *J Cardiothorac Anesth* 1:237, 1987.
65. Arous, EJ, Baum, PL, Cutler, BS. The ischemic exercise test in patients with peripheral vascular disease: Implications for management. *Arch Surg* 119:780, 1984.
66. Myers, WO, Davis, K, Foster, ED, et al. Surgical survival in the Coronary Artery Surgery Study registry. *Ann Thorac Surg* 40:245, 1985.
67. Reul, GJ, Cooley, DA, Duncan, M, et al. The effect of coronary bypass on the outcome of peripheral vascular operations in 1093 patients. *J Vasc Surg* 3:788, 1986.
68. Hertzer, NR, Beven, EG, Young, JR, et al. Coronary artery disease in peripheral vascular patients: A classification of 1000 coronary angiograms and results of surgical management. *Ann Surg* 199:223, 1984.
69. Leppo, J, Boucher, CA, Okada, RD, et al. Serial thallium-201 myocardial imaging after dipyridamole infusion: Diagnostic utility in detecting coronary stenoses and relationship to regional wall motion. *Circulation* 66:649, 1982.
70. Bredlau, CE, Roubin, GS, Leimgruber, PP, et al. In-hospital morbidity and mortality in patients undergoing elective coronary angioplasty. *Circulation* 72:1044, 1985.
71. Kahn, JK, Rutherford, BD, McConahay, DR, et al. Early postoperative balloon coronary angioplasty for failed coronary artery bypass grafting. *Am J Cardiol* 66:943, 1990.
72. Corcos, T, David, PR, Bourassa, MG, et al. Percutaneous transluminal coronary angioplasty for the treatment of variant angina. *J Am Coll Cardiol* 5:1046, 1985.
73. Wells, PH, Kaplan, JA. Optimal management of patients with ischemic heart disease for noncardiac surgery by complementary anesthesiologist and cardiologist interaction. *Am Heart J* 102:1029, 1981.
74. Yeager, M, Glass, D, Neff, R, et al. Epidural anesthesia and analgesia in high-risk surgical patients. *Anesthesiology* 66:729, 1987.
75. Benefiel, DJ, Roizen, MF, Lampe, GH, et al. Morbidity after aortic surgery with sufentanil vs isoflurane anesthesia. *Anesthesiology* 65:A516, 1986.
76. Clark, NJ, Stanley, TH. Anesthesia for Vascular Surgery. In RD Miller (ed), *Anesthesia* (3rd ed). New York: Churchill Livingstone, 1990. P 1527.
77. Slogoff, S, Keats, AS. Does chronic treatment with calcium entry blocking drugs reduce perioperative myocardial ischemia? *Anesthesiology* 68:676, 1988.
78. Nattel, S, Rangno, RE, Van Loon, G. Mechanism of propranolol withdrawal phenomenon. *Circulation* 59:1158, 1979.
79. Stone, JG, Foex, P, Sear, JW, et al. Myocardial ischemia in untreated hypertensive patients: Effect of a single small oral dose of a beta-adrenergic blocking agent. *Anesthesiology* 68:495, 1988.
80. Waagstein, F, Caidahl, K, Wallentin, I, et al. Long term beta blockade in dilated cardiomyopathy: Effects of short and long term metoprolol treatment followed by withdrawal and readministration of metoprolol. *Circulation* 80:551, 1989.
81. Acampora, GA, Melendez, JA, Keefe, DL, et al. Intraoperative administration of the intravenous angiotensin-converting enzyme inhibitor, enalaprilat, in a patient with congestive heart failure. *Anesth Analg* 69:833, 1989.
82. Kaplan, JA, King, SB. The precordial electrocardiographic lead (V5) in patients who have coronary artery disease. *Anesthesiology* 45:570, 1976.
83. Griffin, RM, Kaplan, JA. Myocardial ischemia during non-cardiac surgery. *Anaesthesia* 42:155, 1987.
84. London, NJ, Hollenberg, M, Wong, MG, et al. SPI Research Group. Intraoperative myocardial ischemia. Localization by continuous 12-lead electrocardiography. *Anesthesiology* 69:232, 1988.
85. Kaplan, JA, Wells, PH. Early diagnosis of myocardial ischemia using the pulmonary arterial catheter. *Anesth Analg* 60:789, 1981.
86. Van Daele, M, Sutherland, GR, Mitchell, MM, et al. Do changes in pulmonary capillary wedge pressure adequately reflect myocardial ischemia during anesthesia? *Circulation* 81:865, 1990.
87. Wohlgelernter, D, Cleman, M, Highman, H, et al. Regional myocardial dysfunction during coronary angioplasty: Evaluation by two-dimensional echocardiography and 12 lead electrocardiography. *J Am Coll Cardiol* 7:1245, 1986.
88. Hauser, AM, Gangadharan, V, Ramos, R, et al. Sequence of mechanical, electrocardiographic and clinical effects of repeated coronary artery occlusion in human beings: Echocardiographic observations during coronary. *J Am Coll Cardiol* 59:193, 1985.
89. London, MJ, Tubau, JF, Wong, MG, et al. The natural history of segmental wall motion abnormalities in patients undergoing noncardiac surgery. SPI Research Group. *Anesthesiology* 73:644, 1990.
90. McCloskey, G, Barash, PG. Transesophageal echo-

cardiography is not the gold standard for detection of myocardial ischemia. *J Cardiothorac Anesth* 3:372, 1989.
91. Chung, F, Seyone, C, Rakowski, H. Transesophageal echocardiogram may fail to diagnose perioperative myocardial infarction. *Can J Anaesth* 38:98, 1991.
92. Gertz, EW, Wisneski, JA, Neese, R, et al. Myocardial lactate metabolism: Evidence of lactate released during net chemical extraction in man. *Circulation* 63:1273, 1981.
93. Rawal, N, Sjostrand, U, Christoffersson, E, et al. Comparison of i.m. and epidural morphine for postoperative analgesia in the grossly obese: Influence on postoperative ambulation and pulmonary function. *Anesth Analg* 63:583, 1984.
94. Reinhart, K, Foehring, U, Kersting, T, et al. Effects of thoracic epidural anesthesia on systemic hemodynamic function and systemic oxygen supply-demand relationship. *Anesth Analg* 69:360, 1989.
95. Shenaq, SA, Epidural anesthesia is not a valuable adjunct to general anesthesia for abdominal vascular surgery. *J Cardiothorac Anesth* 3:509, 1989.
96. Krantz, EM, Viljoen, JF, Gilbert, MS. Prinzmetal's variant angina during extradural anesthesia. *Br J Anaesth* 52:945, 1980.
97. Mangano, DT. Anesthetics, coronary artery disease, and outcome: Unresolved controversies. *Anesthesiology* 70:175, 1989.
98. McGowen, SW, Smith, GFN. Anesthesia for transurethral prostatectomy: A comparison of spinal intradural analgesia with two methods of general anaesthesia. *Anaesthesia* 35:847, 1980.
99. Larsen, R, Rathgeber, J, Bagdahn, A, et al. Effects of propofol on cardiovascular dynamics and coronary blood flow, in geriatric patients. A comparison with etomidate. *Anesthesia* 435:25, 1988.
100. Reves, JG. Benzodiazepines are not contraindicated as induction agents for coronary artery surgery. *J Cardiothorac Anesth* 2:844, 1988.
101. Reves, JG, Croughwell, N. Valium-Fentanyl Interaction. In JG Reves, KD Hall (eds), *Common Problems in Cardiac Anesthesia.* Chicago: Year Book, 1987. Pp 356–361.
102. Nauta, J, Stanley, TH, de Lange, S, et al. Anesthesia induction with alfentanil: Comparison with thiopental, midazolam, etomidate. *Can Anaesth Soc J* 30:53, 1983.
103. Tuman, KJ, McCarthy, RJ, Speiss, BD, et al. Does choice of anesthetic agents significantly affect outcome after coronary artery surgery. *Anesthesiology* 70:199, 1989.
104. Benthuysen, JL, Foltz, BD, Smith, NT, et al. Prebypass hemodynamic stability of sufentanil-O_2, fentanyl-O_2, morphine-O_2 anesthesia during cardiac surgery: A comparison of cardiovascular profiles. *J Cardiothorac Anesth* 2:749, 1988.
105. Kemmatsu, O, Hashimoto, Y, Shimasato, S. Inotropic effects of isoflurane on mechanics of contraction in isolated cat papillary muscles from normal and failing hearts. *Anesthesiology* 39:470, 1973.
106. Reiz, S, Balfors, E, Sorensen, V, et al. Isoflurane—a powerful coronary vasodilator in patients with coronary artery disease. *Anesthesiology* 59:91, 1983.
107. Priebe, HJ. Isoflurane and coronary hemodynamics. *Anesthesiology* 71:960, 1989.
108. Becker, L. Is isoflurane dangerous for the patient with coronary artery disease? (editorial). *Anesthesiology* 66:259, 1987.
109. Sills, JC, Bove, AA, Nugent, M, et al. Effects of isoflurane on coronary arteries and coronary arterioles in the intact dog. *Anesthesiology* 66:273, 1987.
110. Bertha, BG, Folts, JD, Nugent, M, et al. Halothane but not isoflurane or enflurane protects against spontaneous and epinephrine exacerbated acute thrombus formation in stenosed dog coronary arteries. *Anesthesiology* 71:96, 1989.
111. Moffitt, EA, Scovil, JE, Barker, RA, et al. The effects of nitrous oxide on myocardial metabolism and hemodynamics during fentanyl or enflurane anesthesia in patients with coronary diseases. *Anesth Analg* 63:1071, 1984.
112. Cason, BA, Datias, KA, Mazer, CD, et al. Effects of nitrous oxide on coronary pressure and regional contractile function in experimental myocardial ischemia. *Anesth Analg* 72:604, 1991.
113. Michaelis, I, Kay, H, Barash, P. Does nitrous oxide or a reduced FiO_2 alter hemodynamic function during high dose fentanyl anesthesia? *Anesthesiology* 57:A44, 1982.
114. Waller, JL, Hug, CC, Nagle, DN, et al. Hemodynamic changes during fentanyl oxygen anesthesia for aorto-coronary bypass operations. *Anesthesiology* 55:212, 1981.
115. Coriat, P, Harari, A, Daloz, M, et al. Clinical predictors of intraoperative myocardial ischemia in patients with coronary artery disease undergoing noncardiac surgery. *Acta Anaesth Scand* 26:287, 1982.
116. Yousif, H, Davies, G, Westaby, S, et al. Preoperative myocardial ischaemia: Its relation to perioperative infarction. *Br Heart J* 58:9, 1987.
117. Becker, LC. Conditions for vasodilator-induced coronary steal in experimental ischemia. *Circulation* 57:1103, 1978.

118. Steen, PA, Tinker, JH, Tarhan, S. Myocardial reinfarction after anesthesia and surgery. *JAMA* 239: 2566, 1978.
119. Nachlas, MM, Abrams, SJ, Goldberg, MM. The influence of arteriosclerotic heart disease on surgical risk. *Am J Surg* 101:447, 1961.
120. Smith, ER, Redwood, DR, McCarron, WE, et al. Coronary artery occlusion in the conscious dog. Effects of alterations in arterial pressure produced by nitroglycerin, hemorrhage, and alpha-adrenergic agonists on the degree of myocardial ischemia. *Circulation* 47:51, 1973.
121. Charlson, ME, MacKenzie, CR, Ales, K, et al. Surveillance for postoperative myocardial infarction after noncardiac operations. *Surg Gynecol Obstet* 167:407, 1988.
122. Pasternack, PF, Imparato, AM, Baumann, FG, et al. The hemodynamics of β-blockade in patients undergoing abdominal aortic aneurysm repair. *Circulation* 76 (Suppl):III–1, 1987.
123. Larsen, SF, Olesen, KH, Jacobsen, E, et al. Prediction of cardiac risk in non cardiac surgery. *Eur Heart J* 8:179, 1987.
124. Djokovic, JL, Hedley-White, J. Prediction of outcome of surgery and anesthesia in patients over 80. *JAMA* 242:2301, 1979.

6
Aortic Valve Disease

Joseph I. Simpson

The safe anesthetic management of the patient with aortic valve disease can be challenging. Patients frequently present to the operating room electively with aortic stenosis or aortic regurgitation of insufficient magnitude to warrant an aortic valve replacement, yet of sufficient magnitude to complicate their anesthetic management for an elective noncardiac procedure.

Occasionally, patients with critical aortic stenosis or severe aortic regurgitation present for emergency noncardiac surgery before their aortic valve replacement. In this chapter we discuss the anesthetic management of these patients. The anesthetic management of the patient with idiopathic hypertrophic subaortic stenosis or hypertrophic cardiomyopathy is discussed in detail in the chapter on cardiomyopathies (Chap. 9).

ANATOMY

The aortic valve consists of three semilunar cusps that surround the aortic orifice and are attached to the wall of the aorta at its junction with the left ventricle. These include the right coronary cusp, left coronary cusp, and noncoronary cusp, so named because the ostia of the left and right coronary arteries lie behind their corresponding aortic valve leaflets. This relationship is important to understand, as coronary blood flow occurs largely when the aortic valve is in the closed position (diastole) and the coronary sinuses are open and unobstructed to blood flow. Additionally, coronary blood flow depends on diastolic pressure in the aortic root, which is primarily generated by a competent, closed aortic valve during diastole.

The left ventricular (LV) outflow tract through which all of the blood directed out the aortic valve must travel consists of the superior membranous and muscular left ventricular septum and the anterior mitral leaflet apparatus (Fig. 6-1).

AORTIC STENOSIS

Epidemiology

Isolated aortic stenosis is usually congenital or degenerative in origin. Congenital aortic stenosis is usually caused by a congenitally abnormal aortic valve that, over a period of many years, undergoes fibrosis, scarring, and calcification, and ultimately becomes stenotic [1]. Congenitally abnormal valves that predispose to later development of aortic stenosis include the congenitally bicuspid valve, the tricuspid valve with unequal cusp size, and a valve with partially fused commissures (Fig. 6-2).

110 The Adult Patient

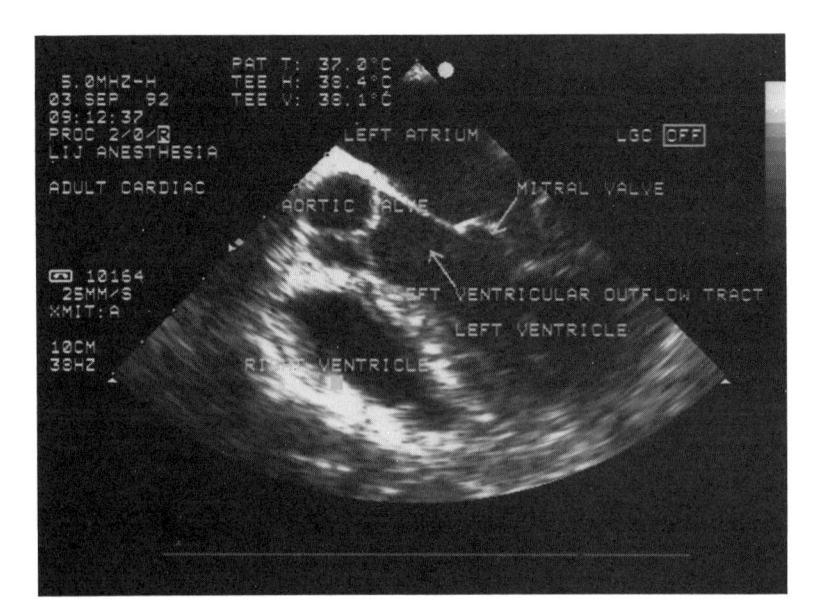

Fig. 6-1. Transesophageal echocardiographic image of the heart in diastole. Note the three cusps of the aortic valve and the left ventricular outflow tract bounded by the septum and anterior mitral leaflet.

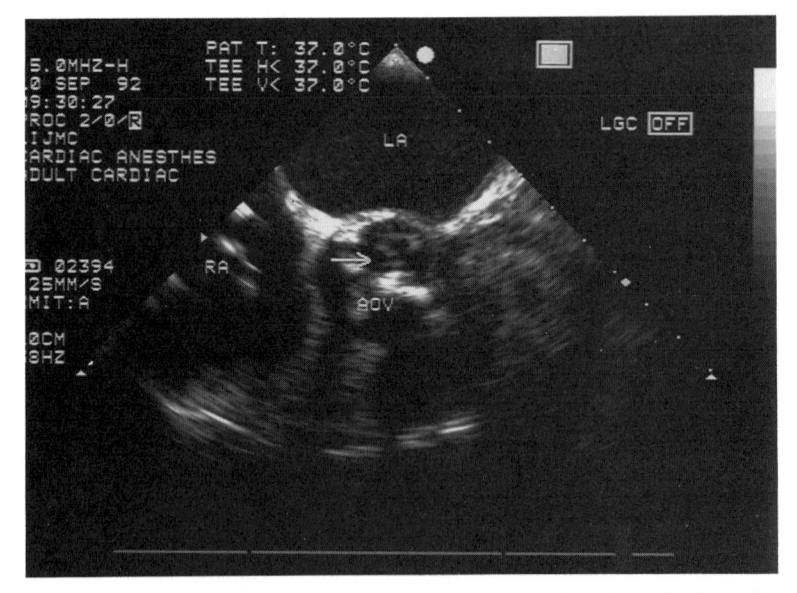

Fig. 6-2. Transesophageal echocardiographic view of a stenotic aortic valve. This congenitally bicuspid valve had an effective valve area of 0.5 cm^2. Note the thickened calcium-laden cusps and the small opening during systole (*arrow*). LA = left atrium; RA = right atrium; AOV = aortic valve.

Table 6-1. Causes of valvular aortic stenosis

Cause	Percent of cases
Congenital valve defect (bicuspid, etc.)	25–50
Degenerative calcification	25–50
Rheumatic myocarditis	25
Other	< 5

Idiopathic degenerative aortic stenosis seen in the elderly is usually calcific in nature and develops over many years [2]. Diabetes appears to be a risk factor for this type of aortic valve degeneration [3].

Rheumatic aortic stenosis is almost always seen in combination with rheumatic mitral valve disease. Commissural fusion is common. Isolated aortic stenosis is rare in this setting and the majority of patients with rheumatic aortic stenosis exhibit aortic regurgitation as well. Table 6-1 lists the most common causes of valvular aortic stenosis.

Natural History

Despite severe aortic stenosis, patients may remain symptom free for many years (Fig. 6-3). The classic triad of symptoms—angina, syncope, and congestive heart failure—do not occur until late in the disease process. When the patient finally does become symptomatic, survival is immediately affected. Patients who have angina and syncope survive 2 to 3 years (without surgical correction), while patients who have congestive heart failure only survive 1 to 2 years [4]. These patients are at risk for sudden death, probably caused by cerebral hypoperfusion or cardiac arrhythmias, or both [5].

It is important to remember that because these patients remain symptom free for so long, they may have a very high pressure gradient, high ventricular systolic pressure, and decreased myocardial perfusion, and still be asymptomatic. Therefore, an asymptomatic patient with aortic stenosis should be given similar consideration as one who is symptomatic.

Pathophysiology

Aortic stenosis leads to severe left ventricular hypertrophy (Fig. 6-4). As opposed to aortic regurgitation, the hypertrophy is concentric, that is, there is an increase in muscle mass without an increase in chamber size [6]. With parallel sarcomere replication this concentric hypertrophy is a compensatory response that normalizes wall tension in the face of increased intracavitary pressures [7]. Con-

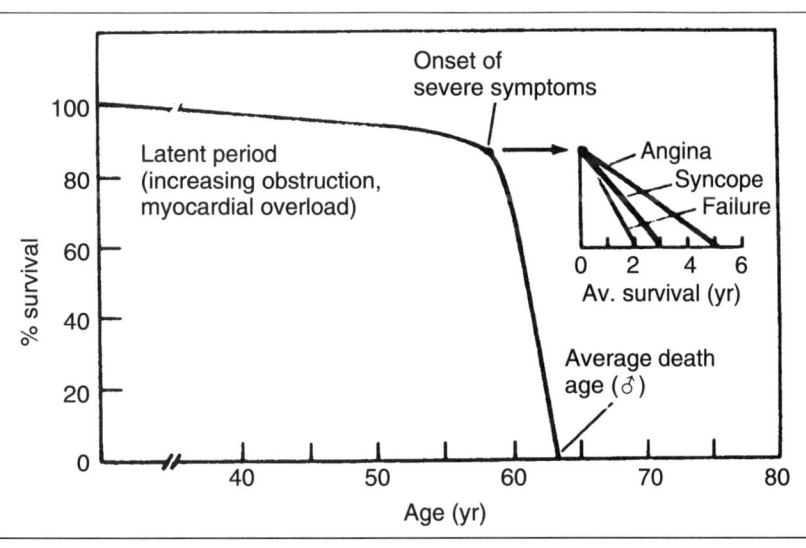

Fig. 6-3. The natural history of aortic stenosis. (Reprinted with permission from J Ross, Jr and E Braunwald, Aortic stenosis. *Circulation* 38 (Suppl V):61, 1968.)

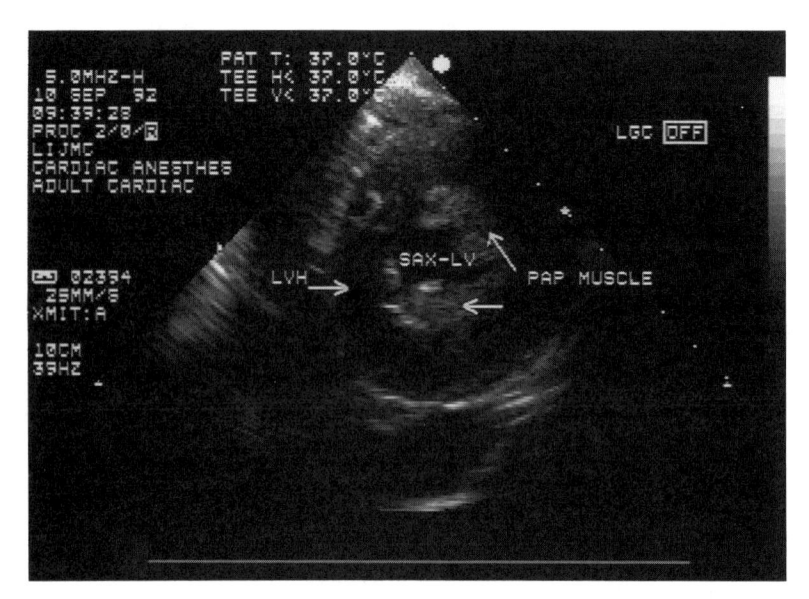

Fig. 6-4. Transesophageal short-axis view of the left ventricle (SAX-LV) at the midpapillary (PAP) muscle level. Note the severely hypertrophied ventricular wall (LVH).

tractility and systolic function are well maintained until very late in the disease process [8]. The normal aortic valve area is 2.5 to 3.5 cm². When the functional valve area decreases below 1 cm², most patients become symptomatic and severe aortic stenosis exists. At less than 0.5 cm² valve area, critical aortic stenosis is present and the incidence of sudden death is high. The severity of aortic stenosis can often be followed by the changing magnitude of the peak systolic gradient between the left ventricle and the aorta. A gradient greater than 50 mm Hg is considered to be severe obstruction (Fig. 6-5).

Systolic Function

As stated earlier, systolic function as measured by ejection fraction and contractility is usually well preserved until very late in the disease process. When ejection fraction does decline, it is usually a result of subendocardial or transmural ischemia or of inadequate concentric hypertrophy to overcome the outflow obstruction [9, 10].

It is important to note that late in the disease, systolic dysfunction may occur secondary to fibrosis. When this occurs, LV dilatation follows, with a resultant decrease in stroke volume and systolic flow. Thus, the gradient at this point may actually decline while the stenosis is in fact worsening (Fig. 6-6). Therefore, calculated valve area may be a better indicator of severity of aortic stenosis in this type of patient.

Diastolic Function

Patients with aortic stenosis have decreased ventricular compliance, caused predominantly by the concentric hypertrophy and in some cases by a chronic low level of subendocardial ischemia [11]. Because of this decrease in compliance, the atrial kick becomes much more important, in terms of the contribution of atrial systole to diastolic ventricular filling. In patients with aortic stenosis, atrial systole can contribute up to 40 to 50 percent of cardiac output, whereas in normal patients it only contributes 15 to 20 percent. Thus, maintenance of sinus rhythm is very important in terms of maintaining adequate cardiac output. The sudden appearance of junctional rhythms, atrial fibrillation, and so forth may lead to precipitous hemodynamic deterioration, out of proportion to that which the same rhythm would cause in a patient

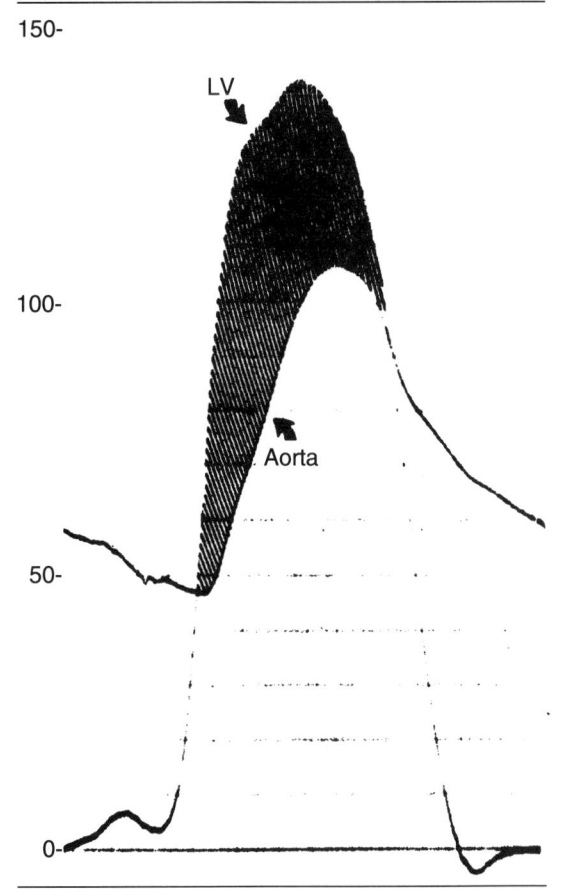

Fig. 6-5. Simultaneous pressure tracings in the left ventricle (LV) and aortic root in a patient with aortic stenosis. Note the pressure gradient between the two (*shaded area*). (Reprinted with permission from AK Ream and RP Fogdall, *Acute Cardiovascular Management: Anesthesia and Intensive Care*. Philadelphia: Lippincott, 1982.)

without aortic stenosis. Additionally, to obtain an adequate left ventricular end diastolic volume (LVEDV), relatively high left ventricular end diastolic pressure (LVEDP) is needed. Without the atrial kick, high mean left atrial pressure is required and consequently pulmonary edema can develop.

The patient with aortic stenosis is already using his or her preload reserve to generate the high LVEDP needed. Further increases in preload in an attempt to increase LVEDV may greatly increase LVEDP and cause pulmonary edema. Figure 6-7 illustrates schematically the physiologic consequences of aortic stenosis.

Myocardial Ischemia

Patients with aortic stenosis have an imbalance of myocardial oxygen supply and demand [12]. Fifty percent of patients with severe aortic stenosis have symptoms of angina. Of these, only half have demonstrable coronary lesions on angiography, while the other half have normal coronary anatomy [13, 14].

There is an increased myocardial oxygen demand ($M\dot{V}O_2$) in aortic stenosis. Reasons for this include the greatly increased muscle mass (concentric hypertrophy), increased left ventricular systolic pressure work [15], and increased wall stress, especially in patients in whom the stenosis is so severe that the hypertrophy is inadequate and wall stress rises (Table 6-2).

Myocardial oxygen supply is diminished relative to demand. The reasons for this are multifactorial. There is some evidence that coronary arteries to not enlarge and increase in number in proportion to the increase in muscle mass [12]. Also, the abnormally high LVEDP will inhibit subendocardial blood flow (back pressure) as well as lower overall coronary perfusion pressure [16]. Since most coronary perfusion to the left ventricle occurs during diastole, there is again a limitation in myocardial oxygen supply because of the abnormally long ejection phase during systole (in aortic stenosis), which is at the expense of diastolic time (Table 6-3).

Increasing the heart rate in a patient with aortic stenosis is therefore detrimental for several reasons. First, increasing heart rate will greatly increase myocardial oxygen demand in an already precarious situation. Second, since increasing heart rate shortens diastolic time more than systolic time [17], increasing heart rate will allow less time for coronary perfusion, which occurs primarily during diastole.

Decreasing afterload will do little to improve ventricular function since the ventricular afterload is fixed at the stenotic valve, but may significantly reduce coronary perfusion by decreasing aortic diastolic pressure.

Right ventricular pressures are often elevated in patients with aortic stenosis, even in the absence

114   The Adult Patient

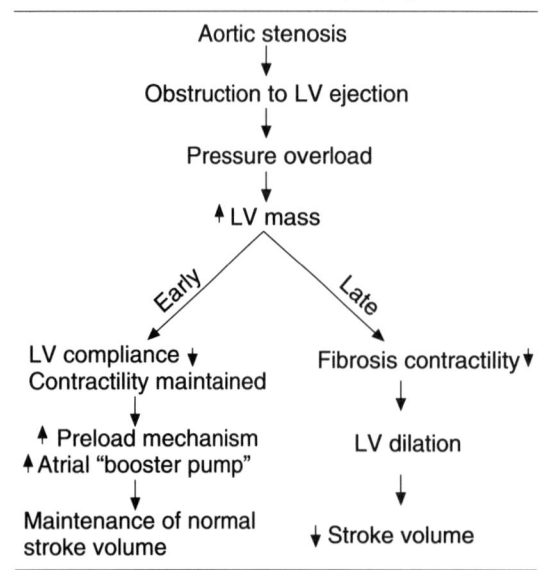

Fig. 6-6. Aortic flow versus aortic-LV pressure gradient for a variety of aortic valve areas. Note that at smaller valve areas (more severe aortic stenosis) the flow generating a given gradient is greatly reduced secondary to late systolic dysfunction; thus, gradient alone may be an inadequate predictor of the severity of the aortic stenosis (i.e., a gradient of 200 mm Hg may represent a valve area of 0.8 cm^2 and a systolic flow of 550 ml/sec systole, or the same gradient of 200 mm Hg may represent a valve area of 0.2 cm^2 with a systole flow of 100 ml/sec systole). (Reprinted with permission from AK Ream and RP Fogdall, *Acute Cardiovascular Management: Anesthesia and Intensive Care*. Philadelphia: Lippincott, 1982.)

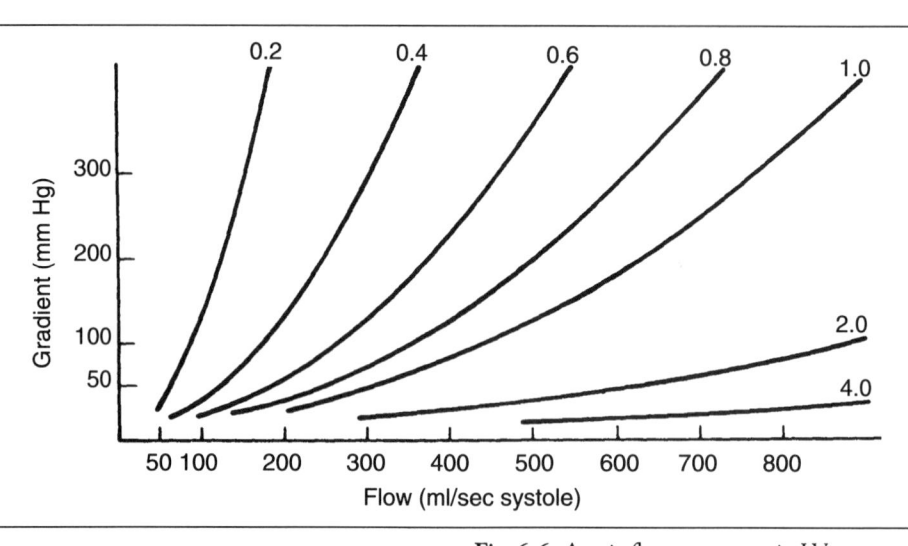

Fig. 6-7. The physiologic consequences of aortic stenosis. (Reprinted with permission from *International Anesthesiology Clinics*. From SJ Thomas and E Lowenstein, Anesthetic management of the patient with valvular heart disease. *Int Anesth Clin* 17:67, 1979.)

Aortic stenosis
↓
Obstruction to LV ejection
↓
Pressure overload
↓
↑ LV mass
   Early ↙   ↘ Late
LV compliance ↓   Fibrosis contractility ↓
Contractility maintained   ↓
   ↓   LV dilation
↑ Preload mechanism   ↓
↑ Atrial "booster pump"   ↓ Stroke volume
   ↓
Maintenance of normal
stroke volume

Table 6-2. Causes of increased myocardial oxygen demand in aortic stenosis

Increased myocardial mass
Increased pressure work
Increased left ventricular ejection time
Increased left ventricular wall stress

Table 6-3. Causes of decreased myocardial oxygen supply in aortic stenosis

Decreased diastolic time
Inadequate coronary artery hypertrophy and proliferation
Increased transmural pressure (coronary compression)
Increased LVEDP (decreased coronary perfusion pressure)

of left ventricular failure [18, 19]. This is especially true when the transaortic gradient exceeds 120 mm Hg [20]. Possible mechanisms for this include chronically elevated LVEDP causing elevated pulmonary pressures and low-grade right ventricular failure.

History and Physical Examination

Symptoms

The most common initial complaint is dyspnea especially on exertion. This is caused primarily by increasing pulmonary artery pressures secondary to elevations in LVEDP, especially with the increasing heart rate seen with exertion. As stated earlier, increasing the heart rate may not allow adequate time for ejection and may worsen an already precarious myocardial oxygen supply-demand problem causing ischemia, which will further elevate LVEDP and consequently pulmonary pressures. Although this scenario may not occur until late in the disease process, as stated earlier, most patients are asymptomatic and unaware of their pathology until this point.

Syncope is an ominous sign in the patient with aortic stenosis. The cause of this syncope may be transient arrhythmias caused by ischemia or baroreceptor malfunction [21, 22]. As discussed earlier, angina, even in the absence of coronary disease, is the other common complaint in the patient with symptomatic aortic stenosis.

Physical Examination

The jugular pulse usually has prominent "a" waves and the carotid pulse has a slow delayed upstroke. There may be a thrill over the second intercostal space transmitted into the neck. S_1 is normal and S_4 is loud. S_2 may be single (since prolongation of LV ejection may make A_2 and P_2 coincide) or may be paradoxically split. There is a crescendo-decrescendo systolic murmur that peaks in midsystole and ends before A_2 (when it is heard). It is heard best at the base of the heart (although it can also be heard at the apex), and radiates into the neck. An aortic stenosis murmur that becomes softer may be a sign of worsening obstruction as flow across the valve decreases (Fig. 6-8, Table 6-4).

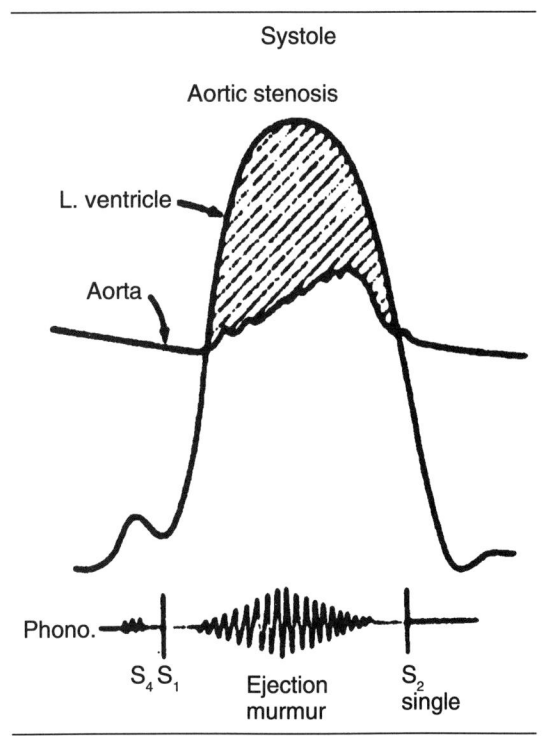

Fig. 6-8. Pressure tracing of the aorta and left ventricle in aortic stenosis during systole with simultaneous phonocardiogram. The shaded area is the pressure gradient between the left ventricle and the aorta. Note the S_4, crescendo-decrescendo murmur and the single S_2 on the phonocardiogram. (Reprinted with permission from PB Beeson, W McDermott, and J Wyngaarden, *Textbook of Medicine* (15th ed). Philadelphia: Saunders, 1979.)

Table 6-4. Auscultatory findings in aortic stenosis

Loud S_4
Single S_2
   Late A_2
   P_2 buried in murmurs
Crescendo-decrescendo systolic murmur
   Ending before S_2

ECG

The most common ECG finding in aortic stenosis is left ventricular hypertrophy (LVH). ST segment depression in a "strain" pattern and T-wave inversion are also common. Left atrial enlargement is also present in many patients with aortic stenosis [23]. The degree of LVH does not correlate with the severity of the aortic stenosis.

Chest X-ray

Most patients with aortic stenosis will have concentric hypertrophy and only a minimally enlarged heart on chest x-ray (CXR). Poststenotic dilatation of the aorta is sometimes seen (Fig. 6-9). There is usually calcification around the aortic annulus and the absence of calcifications in the adult patient makes the presence of significant aortic stenosis unlikely [24]. There may also be evidence of pulmonary congestion in advanced disease.

Echocardiography

Doppler echocardiography allows calculation of the ventricular to aortic gradient [25]. These figures have been shown to correlate well with those determined by cardiac catheterization [26]. Two-dimensional echocardiography can evaluate the valve leaflets and LV wall thickness, as well as other possible coexisting valvular abnormalities.

Preoperative Evaluation

The preoperative evaluation of the patient with aortic stenosis should take into account all of the previously mentioned pathophysiologic considerations. In the case of emergency noncardiac surgery, the influence of the emergency presentation on the aortic stenosis must be taken into account. Is the patient tachycardic and hypertensive because of pain, fever, or another condition? Is the afterload and coronary perfusion pressure decreased secondary to sepsis? Wherever possible the patient's cardiovascular status should be optimized.

Information about valve area, gradient, and history of congestive heart failure, syncope, and angina can give some indication about severity of disease, and is essential in planning the anesthetic management of the patient with severe or critical aortic stenosis. Similarly, the presence or absence of coexistent coronary lesions is important information. As with all patients with valvular or congenital heart disease, antibiotic prophylaxis is indicated (see Chap. 17).

Fig. 6-9. Transesophageal image of the aortic valve and ascending aorta. Note the poststenotic dilatation in the anterior part of the ascending aorta. AO = aorta; AOV = aortic valve.

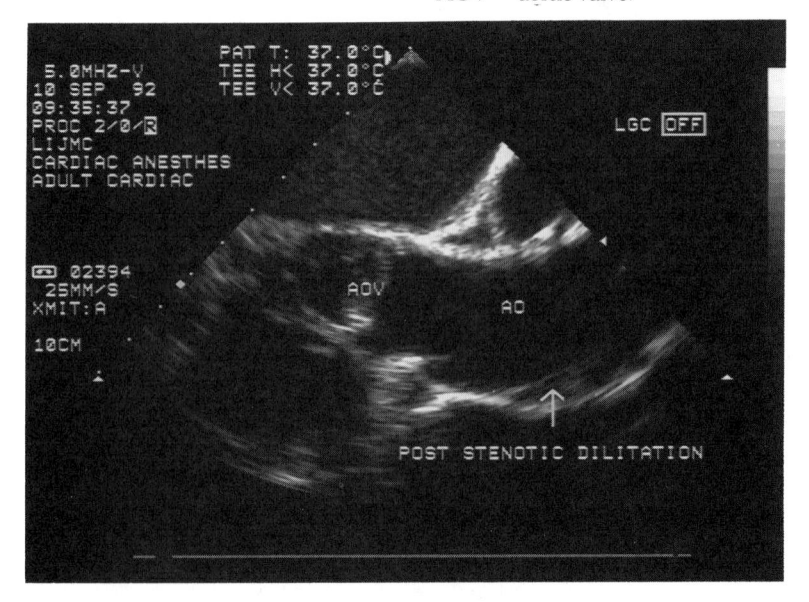

Hemodynamic Goals

Heart Rate
Heart rate is the most important variable to control. In general a rate of 60 to 80 beats per minute is beneficial. A slower rate will decrease cardiac output and cause hypotension and potentially ischemia. A more rapid rate will not allow for ejection and will increase $M\dot{V}O_2$ and the likelihood of acute myocardial ischemia.

Rhythm
Maintenance of normal sinus rhythm is absolutely essential. Loss of sinus rhythm will cause a rapid and precipitous fall in cardiac output and blood pressure, with resultant ischemia and hemodynamic collapse. A synchronized defibrillator should always be available to treat supraventricular and atrial tachyarrhythmias (see Chap. 10).

Afterload
Afterload should be maintained at near normal levels. This will not have a significant impact on left ventricular afterload as this is essentially fixed by the valvular stenosis. Allowing the afterload to decrease will decrease coronary perfusion pressure (CPP) and lead to the rapid onset of myocardial ischemia.

Preload
Maintenance of adequate preload is important in a patient with a noncompliant left ventricle. These patients require elevated filling pressures to maintain their normally elevated LVEDP. Venodilatation and preload reduction will be marked by rapid decreases in cardiac output and hemodynamic collapse. On the other hand rapid elevations in filling pressure above baseline will result in an increase in LVEDP and consequently a reduction in CPP. Coronary perfusion pressure is defined by the following equation:

$$CPP = \text{aortic diastolic pressure} - LVEDP$$

Decreases in coronary perfusion pressure by either a decrease in aortic diastolic pressure or an increase in LVEDP are poorly tolerated in the patient with aortic stenosis.

Table 6-5. Hemodynamic goals in aortic stenosis

Maintain heart rate at 60–80 bpm
Maintain afterload and coronary perfusion pressure (CPP)

Maintain preload at baseline
  Decreased preload = decreased cardiac output
  Increased preload = decreased CPP

Maintain sinus rhythm
Monitor for and aggressively treat ischemia

Ischemia
As discussed earlier, patients with aortic stenosis have an ever-present risk of developing myocardial ischemia. This is due to the chronic imbalance of myocardial oxygen supply-demand (see previous text). It is of utmost importance to maintain CPP. Signs of ischemia must be looked for throughout the perioperative period. Invasive ischemic monitoring is usually indicated (see below).

If ischemia develops it must be managed aggressively. Management of ischemia includes the usual treatment with nitrates (nitroglycerin), β-blockers (esmolol), and other coronary vasodilators. Additionally, in the patient with aortic stenosis, CPP must be returned to normal if it is low. This is usually accomplished by the use of an α-adrenergic agonist such as phenylephrine to increase aortic diastolic pressure and nitroglycerin to decrease LVEDP. Care must be taken not to reduce aortic diastolic pressure with the nitrates as this may worsen the ischemia. The only possible exception to this is when the ischemia is precipitated by hypertension and tachycardia. The hemodynamic goals for the patient with aortic stenosis are summarized in Table 6-5.

Anesthetic Management

Premedication
In the stable patient with aortic stenosis who is not in heart failure, adequate premedication is helpful. Premedication may help avoid the anxiety-related hypertension and tachycardia that can be so detrimental to the patient with aortic stenosis. As usual care must be taken not to oversedate. Hypercarbia can cause tachycardia and hypertension, and hy-

poxia can worsen ischemia. Additionally, venodilatation, sometimes seen with heavy premedication, may cause an acute decrease in preload that may not be well tolerated (see previous text). To help avoid the possibility of hypoxia, all patients should receive supplemental nasal oxygen after premedication.

Monitoring

All patients should have two-lead ECG monitoring (II and V_5) to maximize the ability to detect ischemia [27]. End-tidal carbon dioxide and pulse oximetry monitoring should be standard. Most patients will benefit from the use of a pulmonary artery (PA) catheter. A PA catheter is useful both in ischemia detection [28] and in an adequate evaluation of left ventricular preload, both of which are important issues in this patient population. One reason to avoid a PA catheter is the possibility of inducing arrhythmias, particularly supraventricular or junctional arrhythmias, on insertion. As discussed earlier maintenance of sinus rhythm is of utmost importance and loss of the atrial kick is poorly tolerated. Furthermore, it is important to keep in mind that if a patient does indeed develop a junctional rhythm on placement of a PA catheter, pacing the ventricle alone will not be enough and a standard paceport PA catheter will not be helpful. Rather, if possible, a pacing catheter or an atrioventricular (AV) sequential paceport catheter should be used, so that the atrial kick can be maintained during pacing. In general, except for the most minor surgical procedures, the potential benefits of a PA catheter will outweigh the risks.

In most cases arterial pressure should be monitored invasively. The possibility of rapid changes in cardiac output and blood pressure makes the use of an arterial line very helpful. Transesophageal echocardiography (TEE) can be very useful for evaluation of ventricular function [29] and helpful in detection of ischemia. New wall motion abnormalities that appear intraoperatively may alert the clinician to the possible development of new ischemia before it is seen on the PA catheter or ECG [30, 31]. However, the use of TEE is somewhat limited by the cost of the equipment and the need for specially trained clinicians to properly interpret real-time images.

Anesthetic Agents

Volatile Inhalation Agents (see Chap. 2). Although the volatile agents can be used in patients with aortic stenosis, several problems exist. All of the volatile agents are vasodilators, reducing both preload and afterload [32, 33]. This may compromise CPP and a preload-dependent cardiac output. Isoflurane is particularly known for its effects on afterload. Additionally, isoflurane may cause coronary steal [34, 35] and worsen ischemia if it is present (see Chap. 2).

Most of the inhalational agents are known to produce junctional rhythms. Halothane, especially in combination with pancuronium, is the worst offender in this regard [36]. This loss of the atrial kick will not be well tolerated in the patient with aortic stenosis. Additionally, the negative inotropic effects of the various inhalational agents [37, 38] can impede the ability of the ventricle to generate the high intracavitary systolic pressures necessary in aortic stenosis.

Taking all of these factors into account, one can see that great care must be exercised when the volatile agents are used in this patient population, with careful monitoring of rhythm, preload, cardiac output, and signs of ischemia.

Nitrous Oxide (see Chap. 2). Nitrous oxide (N_2O) has been reported to both cause [39, 40] and not cause myocardial ischemia [41]. It is also known for its potential to produce junctional rhythms [42]. Nevertheless, N_2O is usually well tolerated in the patient with aortic stenosis. The mild tachycardia usually seen with N_2O is not present when it is used in combination with narcotics or benzodiazepines.

Narcotics and Benzodiazepines (see Chap. 3). Fentanyl, sufentanil, and midazolam are usually well tolerated in the patient with aortic stenosis. They do not cause myocardial depression and may only mildly decrease preload [42]. Care should be taken when benzodiazepines are added to high doses of narcotics, as this may precipitate hypotension, with its attendant decrease in CPP. Narcotics frequently slow the heart rate, and one must avoid very low heart rates, as this will interfere with cardiac output.

Other Intravenous Agents (see Chap. 3). Barbiturates can decrease preload and depress the myocardium [43] and should be used with extreme caution. Droperidol can cause unpredictable decreases in afterload and CPP, and should be avoided [44]. Propofol, like the barbiturates, can decrease preload and afterload and cause a decrease in cardiac output [45]. It should be used with extreme caution. Ketamine will cause tachycardia and hypertension. It can precipitate ischemia in a patient with aortic stenosis and should be avoided [46].

Muscle Relaxants. Most of the newer muscle relaxants are well tolerated in the patient with aortic stenosis [47]. Vecuronium, pipecuronium, and doxacurium are preferred because they do not affect heart rate. Atracurium can cause histamine release and hypotension, and should be used with caution. Pancuronium can cause tachycardia, with its attendant increase in myocardial oxygen consumption. In the presence of narcotics, the effects of pancuronium on heart rate are diminished. Succinylcholine is thought to be safe in this patient population but may cause junctional arrhythmias (see previous text).

Regional Anesthesia
General anesthesia is usually preferred over regional anesthesia. The sympatholysis, with its attendant decreases in both preload and afterload, commonly seen with spinal or epidural anesthesia, can cause acute ischemia and hemodynamic collapse in patients with aortic stenosis. Nevertheless, where clearly indicated, for example, in a patient with severe asthma for an emergency procedure on a lower extremity, a slowly titrated epidural anesthetic may be safe. Careful hydration and monitoring of preload are essential. Hypotension must be rapidly and vigorously treated with an α-adrenergic agonist such as phenylephrine. It should be kept in mind that regional anesthesia does not obviate the need for invasive hemodynamic monitoring. On the contrary monitoring of blood pressure and preload is even more important when a major regional anesthetic is used.

AORTIC REGURGITATION
Epidemiology

Aortic regurgitation (AR) can be caused by both abnormalities of the valve itself or abnormalities of the aortic root (Table 6-6). Of patients with AR, 75 percent are male and 25 percent are female. Valvular lesions are often caused by rheumatic heart disease. In rheumatic disease fibrous tissues infiltrate the valve cusps, causing the valve to leak. Rheumatic AR frequently exists in combination with mitral valve disease. Congenitally malformed valves such as a bicuspid aortic valve may degenerate into a leaking valve. Other valvular causes of AR include endocarditis and trauma.

Aortic regurgitation can also be caused by aortic root dilatation. Aortic root dilatation causes failure of the cusps to coapt and, consequently, valvular regurgitation. Causes of aortic root dilatation include Marfan's syndrome, Ehlers-Danlos syndrome, and other connective tissue disorders. Aortic regurgitation is also associated with immunologic disorders such as lupus and arthritis [48]. Syphilitic aortitis is becoming increasingly less common as a cause of AR.

Trauma to the aorta such as that seen with a deceleration injury may produce acute AR. Aortic dissection with retrograde extension into the valve is another cause of acute AR.

Table 6-6. Causes of aortic regurgitation

Valvular
    Congenital valvular abnormalities, e.g., bicuspid
    Rheumatic
    Endocarditis
    Trauma
Aorta
    Trauma
    Dissecting aortic aneurysm
    Connective tissue disorders, e.g., Marfan's syndrome
    Aortitis, e.g., syphilitic
    Autoimmune disorders, e.g., rheumatoid arthritis

Natural History

Acute aortic regurgitation is usually caused by trauma or endocarditis. Acute AR is a life-threatening event with patients presenting in fulminant pulmonary edema and usually requires emergency aortic valve replacement [49]. These patients almost never present for noncardiac surgery.

Chronic aortic regurgitation usually remains asymptomatic for a long time. Symptoms generally do not develop until much myocardial damage has ensued. Before that, the only symptoms a patient may have are those related to occasional arrhythmias and the wide pulse pressure, so that the patient may complain of palpitations, head bobbing, and head pounding. When symptoms do finally develop, they are usually those of congestive heart failure, such as dyspnea on exertion, paroxysmal nocturnal dyspnea, orthopnea, and finally dyspnea at rest. Unlike the situation with aortic stenosis, development of symptoms is not related to imminent death. Patients may go on to live up to 10 years with untreated symptomatic AR [50]. Also, severity of symptoms correlates poorly with severity of myocardial damage, and the degree of ventricular dysfunction is hard to estimate from the history alone.

Late in the disease process, angina may develop with or without the presence of coronary artery lesions (see later in text). Nocturnal angina in the presence of normal coronaries is also occasionally seen with AR. Unlike aortic stenosis, sudden death is rare with aortic regurgitation. However, death usually occurs within 3 to 4 years after the development of angina in patients with untreated AR.

Pathophysiology

Chronic volume overloading of the left ventricle results in eccentric hypertrophy [51], an increase in muscle mass accompanied by an increase in ventricular chamber size with series sarcomere replication. Overall left ventricular mass is greatly elevated, perhaps more so than in any other valvular heart disease. Aortic regurgitation occurs during diastole. The extent of the regurgitation is dependent on the aortic diastolic pressure, the ventricular diastolic pressure, the size of the valve opening during diastole (normally 0), and on the amount of time the heart spends in diastole.

Systolic Function

Systolic function is usually well preserved until end-stage AR develops. Stroke volume is increased, as the stroke volume now equals the sum of the effective forward stroke volume and the volume regurgitated back into the ventricle. Low aortic diastolic pressure presents a low afterload picture to the left ventricle and facilitates systolic function and emptying.

As AR worsens, systolic function is maintained by progressively increased utilization of the preload reserve. Eventually, left ventricular dilatation increases myocardial wall tension, as the heart tries to maintain the same level of systolic function. As the ventricle begins to fail (often before symptoms develop), systolic wall tension further increases, and the preload reserve is exhausted. Ultimately, ejection fraction and forward stroke volume decrease at rest, leading to the onset of symptoms of congestive heart failure (CHF). It is important to reemphasize that symptoms are not a good indication of the contractile state of the left ventricle, and significant ventricular deterioration can occur before significant symptoms develop.

Diastolic Function

The primary compensatory mechanism in early AR is an increase in LVEDV, utilizing the preload reserve, without an increase in LVEDP [6]. Thus, ventricular compliance is increased. During diastole, regurgitation occurs and left ventricular pressure equalizes, with aortic diastolic pressure late in diastole (Fig. 6-10). Left ventricular filling pressures may not be an accurate representation of volume and relatively large changes in volume can occur without changes in pressure. However, there is a steep portion of the compliance curve, and rapidly increasing filling pressures are usually an indication of volume overload. As the left ventricle ultimately fails, compliance decreases and LVEDP rises with corresponding rises in left atrial pressure and pulmonary capillary wedge pressure (PCWP) and the development of CHF. Until end-stage AR develops, the atrial kick is not as major a contrib-

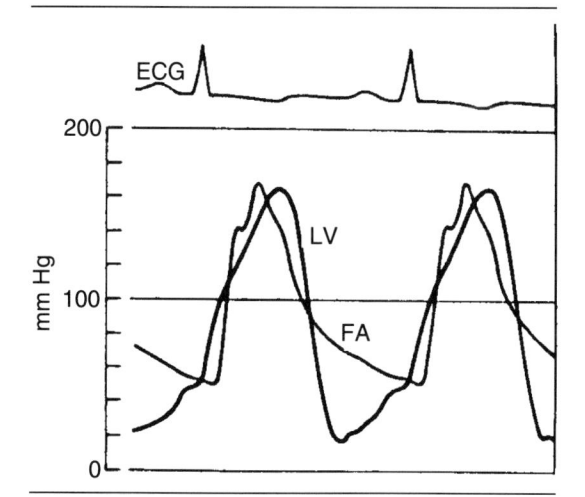

Fig. 6-10. Femoral artery (FA) and left ventricular (LV) pressure curves in severe aortic regurgitation. Note the wide pulse pressure in the FA tracing and the equalization of pressures between FA and LV late in diastole. (Reprinted with permission from E Braunwald, *Heart Disease. A Textbook of Cardiovascular Medicine* (4th ed). Philadelphia: Saunders, 1992.)

Table 6-7. Alterations in myocardial oxygen supply and demand in aortic regurgitation

Increased demand
  Increased myocardial mass
  Increased wall stress (minimal)
  Increased ventricular work
Decreased supply
  Low aortic diastolic pressure
  High LVEDP
    Early in acute AR
    Late in chronic AR

uting factor to ventricular filling as that seen with aortic stenosis. In end-stage AR as the preload reserve is exhausted the atrial kick again takes on its importance in ventricular filling.

Myocardial Ischemia

Patients with aortic regurgitation are at increased risk for the development of myocardial ischemia (Table 6-7), even in the absence of coronary artery disease, although this is not as common as in aortic stenosis. The huge increase in muscle mass and moderate increase in wall tension cause an increase in MVO_2. Coronary perfusion pressure is low, both because of the low aortic diastolic pressure and the mildly elevated LVEDP (especially late in the disease). Coronary vascular reserve is also compromised [52].

Although myocardial ischemia can create problems, it usually does not interfere with hemodynamic function until very late in the disease. Much of the increased ventricular work in AR (especially early in the disease) is by increased fiber shortening, a process that causes relatively little increase in MVO_2.

Acute Aortic Regurgitation

With acute aortic regurgitation there is a sudden increase in ventricular volume without the compensatory effects of eccentric hypertrophy and increased ventricular compliance. There is a rapid rise in LVEDP and a fall in forward flow. Acute ventricular distention may cause mitral regurgitation, and CHF develops early. Myocardial ischemia occurs frequently, as a result of the increased wall stress as well as the acutely increased LVEDP. Figures 6-11 and 6-12 describe the pathophysiology of AR.

History and Physical Examination

Patients frequently complain of head bobbing, palpitations, dyspnea, orthopnea, and occasionally chest pain. Carotid, brachial, and femoral pulses are usually bounding and have been described as "water-hammer," with a rapid sharp rise and a sudden collapse. Auscultation over the femoral arteries reveals "pistol-shot sounds." A bisferiens pulse, that is, a double-peaked pulse, can be palpated in the carotid, brachial, and femoral arteries. The systolic pressure is high and the diastolic pressure is low, leading to a widened pulse pressure (see Fig. 6-10). Magnitude of the pulse pressure is not always an indication of severity of disease, as late in the disease process aortic diastolic pressure may actually rise because of a rising LVEDP, leading to a narrower pulse pressure. Cardiac auscultation reveals a

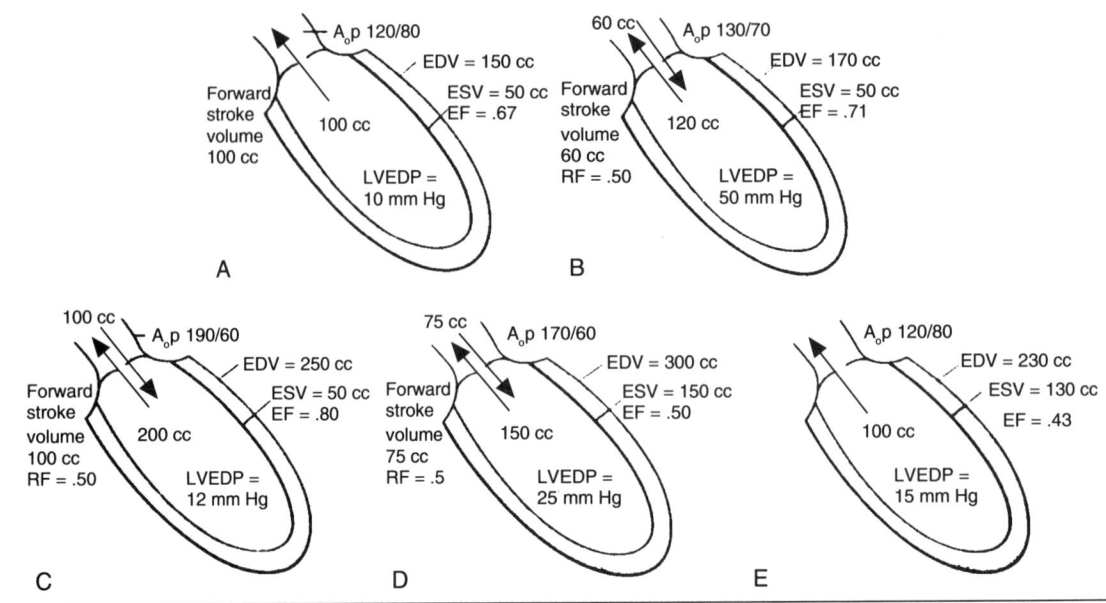

Fig. 6-11. Hemodynamics of aortic regurgitation. A. Normal. B. Acute aortic regurgitation. Note high LVEDP. C. Chronic compensated aortic regurgitation. Note low LVEDP and normal forward stroke volume. D. Chronic decompensated aortic regurgitation. Note elevation of LVEDP and fall in ejection fraction and forward flow. E. Immediately after aortic valve replacement. AP = aortic pressure; EDV = end diastolic volume; ESV = end systolic volume; EF = ejection fraction; LVEDP = left ventricular end diastolic pressure; RF = regurgitation fraction. (Reprinted with permission from BA Carabello, Aortic Regurgitation: Hemodynamic Determinants of Prognosis. In LH Cohn and VJ Disesa (eds), *Aortic Regurgitation: Medical and Surgical Management*. New York: Marcel Dekker, 1986. By courtesy of Marcel Dekker, Inc.)

soft S_1; A_2 may be absent or very soft, and P_2 may be obscured by the murmur. S_3 is frequently present and S_4 is occasionally present. There is frequently a loud systolic ejection sound caused by the sudden dilatation of the aorta.

The murmur of AR is high pitched, blowing, decrescendo, and diastolic (Fig. 6-13). It is heard best at the third left intercostal space. It begins after A_2 and is frequently holodiastolic, especially in severe AR. Severity of regurgitation correlates better with duration than with intensity of the murmur. The patient may also have a short mid-systolic murmur caused by the increased ejection rate and volume. An Austin Flint murmur (mid- to late diastolic rumble) may be present because of the rapid flow across the mitral valve (Table 6-8).

Patients with acute AR often present in hemodynamic collapse, with fulminant pulmonary edema, tachycardia, and vasoconstriction. They have a soft or absent S_1 and a near normal pulse pressure. The murmur is early diastolic, soft, and short. The Austin Flint murmur is usually not present.

ECG

The ECG in acute AR will not be much different from normal. Nonspecific ST-T wave changes may be present. In chronic AR the ECG will show signs of left ventricular hypertrophy with "strain." Late

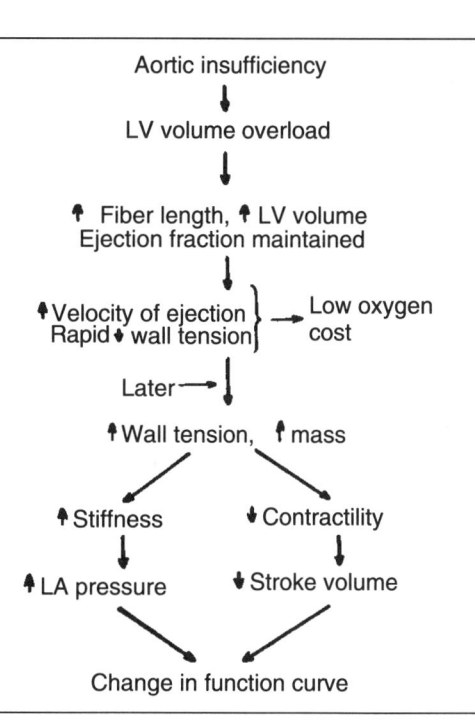

Fig. 6-12. The physiologic consequences of aortic insufficiency. LV = left ventricular; LA = left atrial. (Reprinted with permission from *International Anesthesiology Clinics*. From SJ Thomas and E Lowenstein, Anesthetic management of the patient with valvular heart disease. *Int Anesth Clin* 17:67, 1979.)

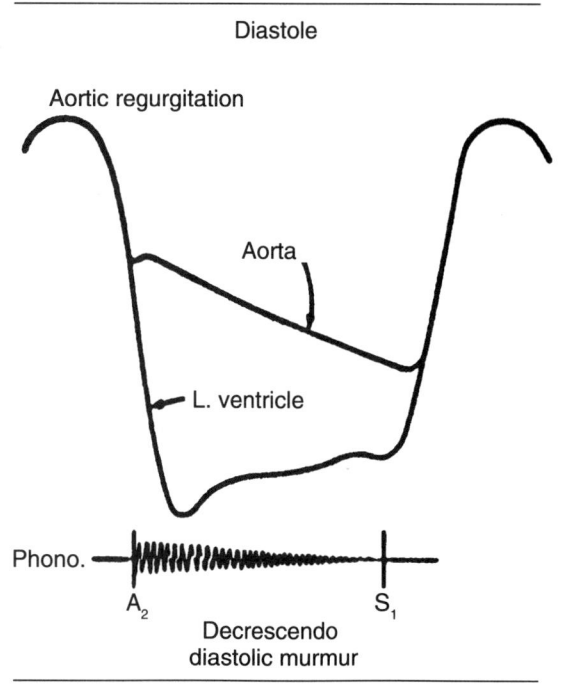

Fig. 6-13. Pressure tracing of the aorta and left ventricle during diastole with simultaneous phonocardiogram. Note rapidly falling aortic diastolic pressure and increasing ventricular diastolic pressure until they are both equal at end diastole. The decrescendo murmur decreases in amplitude as the diastolic gradient between the aorta and ventricle diminishes. (Reprinted with permission from PB Beeson, W McDermott, and J Wyngaarden, *Textbook of Medicine* (15th ed). Philadelphia: Saunders, 1979.)

in the disease, left ventricular conduction abnormalities will develop.

CXR

Patients with acute AR usually have a normal heart size on CXR and evidence of pulmonary edema. In chronic AR, the heart size is massively enlarged. The heart is displaced in a leftward direction. Left atrial size is usually not enlarged and dilatation of the ascending aorta is frequently present. Pulmonary edema is usually not seen except in end-stage decompensated chronic AR.

Echocardiography

Two-dimensional echocardiography can give an assessment of ventricular function by looking at end systolic and end diastolic diameters. Doppler echocardiography, particularly color-flow Doppler, can give a good representation of the severity of the re-

Table 6-8. Auscultatory findings in aortic regurgitation

Soft S_1
Soft or absent A_2, soft or absent P_2
S_3
$\pm S_4$*
Decrescendo holodiastolic murmur (shorter in acute AR)
Systolic ejection sound*
Austin Flint murmur*
Early soft systolic murmur*

*May be absent in acute AR.

gurgitation. Echocardiography can also look at the valve leaflets, aorta, and aortic root, and thus possibly help determine the cause of the AR [53].

Preoperative Evaluation

The preoperative evaluation should take into account all of the previously mentioned pathophysiology. An accurate assessment of the severity of the AR or the amount of ventricular dysfunction present is often difficult from the history alone. Results of angiography and echocardiography may be helpful in this regard. If the patient presents for emergency noncardiac surgery, the influence of the other medical condition, such as sepsis, pain, fever, or tachycardia, should be considered (see later in text).

Patients may be receiving a variety of medications, including digoxin, angiotensin-converting enzyme (ACE) inhibitors, nitrates, hydralazine, and these may affect anesthetic management. As with aortic stenosis, antibiotic prophylaxis should be administered where indicated (see Chap. 17).

Hemodynamic Goals (Table 6-9)

Heart Rate

Heart rates below 65 beats per minute should be avoided. Bradycardia will increase diastolic time, thus increasing the regurgitant fraction. This in turn will increase ventricular volume and will ultimately increase ventricular systolic wall tension, which will increase $M\dot{V}O_2$. An increase in LVEDP will decrease CPP.

Increasing the heart rate will decrease the amount of time the heart spends in diastole and the volume of regurgitation, and will increase cardiac output. However, increasing heart rate is a double-edged sword. At higher heart rates the $M\dot{V}O_2$ increases, making an already precarious situation worse, and ischemia can develop (considering low CPP as discussed earlier). Heart rates of 75 to 95 beats per minute are probably optimal [54].

Rhythm

Sinus rhythm is not as important in AR as in aortic stenosis. The only exception to this is when the patient has end-stage AR with severely elevated LVEDP. Junctional rhythms are usually well tolerated, but very rapid rhythms, such as poorly controlled atrial fibrillation, junctional tachycardia, or paroxysmal supraventricular tachycardia (PSVT), are not (see previous text).

Afterload

Increasing afterload will usually increase the regurgitant fraction, and is detrimental. The only exception is during ischemia, when increasing afterload will increase CPP. In acute AR decreasing afterload is helpful and vasodilators are the mainstay of therapy. Decreasing afterload in acute AR will improve forward flow and decrease the regurgitant fraction [55]. In chronic AR decreasing afterload is only helpful in end-stage disease. Those patients who have diminished forward flow and a high LVEDP will benefit from diminished afterload. Patients with a normal or increased forward flow and a normal or moderately increased LVEDP may actually do worse with afterload reduction, primarily because of the decrease in CPP and preload (see below) that goes along with the decreased afterload.

Preload

Decreasing preload will decrease LVEDP and increase the aortic-to-ventricular diastolic gradient. This will worsen the regurgitation and decrease forward flow. It should be recalled that increasing ventricular preload is the major compensatory mechanism to maintain forward flow. Increasing preload too much will increase LVEDP and potentially worsen CPP, which can result in ischemia. As a general rule LVEDP should be left at baseline (usually, PCWP = 15–20 mm Hg) in chronic well-compensated AR. Reduction may be helpful in acute and chronic decompensated AR (usually starting with PCWP at 20–30 mm Hg).

Table 6-9. Hemodynamic goals in aortic regurgitation

Maintain modest tachycardia (80–90 bpm)
Decrease afterload but not at expense of CPP
Maintain preload at baseline (reduce in acute AR)
Maintain sinus rhythm (less important than in aortic stenosis)
Ischemia less of an issue than in aortic stenosis

Treatment of Hypotension

In general hypotension is better treated with a mixed alpha-beta agonist such as ephedrine than a pure vasoconstrictor like phenylephrine. The only exception is when acute ischemia has developed secondary to the hypotension, in which case increasing CPP is the primary goal. In chronic and more so in acute AR, increasing afterload will usually worsen regurgitation.

As always the most appropriate treatment for hypotension is to treat the cause. The most common causes for hypotension under anesthesia are hypovolemia, decreased contractility (both poorly tolerated in AR), and vasodilatation (tolerated in moderation). Although the immediate therapy for hypotension may require ephedrine or phenylephrine, immediate volume replacement should restore the preload to baseline. In severe hypotension the use of a beta agonist infusion such as dopamine (low dose) or dobutamine may be needed to increase cardiac output and blood pressure.

Ischemia

As discussed earlier ischemia is an important issue, though not as important as in aortic stenosis. In well-compensated AR ischemia is usually not a problem so long as CPP is maintained and $M\dot{V}O_2$ is not greatly increased (such as by very rapid heart rates). In acute AR ischemia may play a role in the hemodynamic collapse as the very high LVEDP will decrease CPP, and the greatly increased wall tension (and tachycardia) will increase $M\dot{V}O_2$.

Anesthetic Management

Premedication

As a general rule light premedication is indicated in most of these patients. It should be recalled that severity of disease and ventricular function are difficult to estimate from the clinical examination and history. Patients with acute AR should not be given any sedative premedication.

Monitoring

All patients should have two-lead ECG monitoring (II and V_5) to maximize the detection of ischemia [27]. End-tidal CO_2 and pulse oximetry monitoring should be standard. Most patients will benefit from the use of a PA catheter, which will be helpful for preload estimation and in ischemia detection [28]. Patients with AR may have diffuse carotid pulsations in the neck, making insertion of a PA catheter via the internal jugular route more dangerous. Drawing the patient's "Starling curve" by measuring cardiac output at various different filling pressures (PCWP) will help determine the optimal preload for a given patient.

In acute AR there may be premature closure of the mitral valve because of high left ventricular diastolic pressures or mitral regurgitation because of acute ventricular dilatation. Thus, the PCWP may, respectively, under- or overestimate the true ventricular filling pressures.

As with aortic stenosis, invasively monitoring arterial pressure is usually helpful. Transesophageal echocardiography may be useful in helping to estimate ventricular volumes, amount of regurgitation, and the appearance of new wall motion abnormalities indicative of ischemia [30, 31].

Anesthetic Agents

Volatile Inhalational Agents (see Chap. 2). The volatile inhalational agents are all myocardial depressants [56] and vasodilators [32, 33]. Isoflurane, sevoflurane, and desflurane are potent afterload reducers [57] and thus may be well tolerated in chronic compensated AR. Halothane and enflurane produce more myocardial depression and slowing of the heart rate [58] and, thus, may not be tolerated as well. As stated earlier the severity of ventricular dysfunction in AR is hard to estimate by history alone and significant myocardial dysfunction may exist. This can be worsened by the negative inotropic effects of the volatile agents. Thus, these agents should be used with caution in these patients.

In acute AR the volatile agents should be avoided. The ventricle is already stressed and operating at maximum ability. These hearts will not tolerate a negative inotropic agent.

Nitrous Oxide (see Chap. 2). The mild tachycardia seen with N_2O is sometimes helpful in AR [59]. Nitrous oxide can cause myocardial depression, especially in combination with the potent inhalation agents [60]. Therefore, in patients with well-compensated chronic AR, N_2O is usually well tolerated. It must, however, be used with extreme caution in acute AR or in decompensated chronic AR.

Narcotics and Benzodiazepines (see Chap. 3). Fentanyl, sufentanil, midazolam, and diazepam are usually well tolerated in patients with AR. Narcotics generally do not depress contractility and only minimally affect hemodynamics. Two problems exist with the use of narcotics. First, high-dose potent narcotics can cause bradycardias when used alone. Bradycardia will be poorly tolerated in the patient with AR, chronic or acute. Second, narcotics occasionally decrease preload and may have mild effects on decreasing afterload. This is especially true with sufentanil [61]. Therefore, heart rate may need to be maintained with pancuronium or atropine and preload increased with fluids when high-dose narcotics are used.

Benzodiazepines can decrease preload and blood pressure, especially in combination with high-dose narcotics (see Chap. 3). This may cause a precipitous fall in cardiac output in the patient with AR, and care should be taken to optimize preload and afterload before benzodiazepines are added to a high-dose narcotic anesthetic.

Other Intravenous Agents (see Chap. 3). Barbiturates can decrease preload and depress the myocardium [43]. While they can be safely used in small doses in chronic compensated AR, they can cause hemodynamic collapse in decompensated or acute AR.

While droperidol will decrease afterload [44] and thus can potentially be helpful in AR, the drop in afterload can be unpredictable in magnitude and relatively long lasting. Therefore, droperidol should be used in very low doses with extreme caution, if at all. Propofol, like the barbiturates, can decrease preload and depress the myocardium [45] and should be avoided. Ketamine will cause tachycardia [46], which can be both useful and detrimental in this patient population. Ketamine will also cause hypertension and increased afterload, which is counterproductive in AR. In acute AR, ketamine used in small doses may be safe as long as the patient is not catecholamine depleted, as this would unmask ketamine's intrinsic negative inotropy.

Muscle Relaxants. Pancuronium, vecuronium, doxacurium, pipecuronium, and mivacurium are usually well tolerated in AR. Pancuronium, with its attendant increase in heart rate, may be especially useful in AR. Atracurium, when used in high doses, may release histamine and thus reduce afterload, which may be helpful in AR so long as preload is maintained. Succinylcholine is safe. However, when it is combined with a high-dose narcotic, significant bradycardias may develop, which may be detrimental to the patient with AR.

Regional Anesthesia. While general anesthesia is usually preferred, regional anesthesia (spinal, epidural) may be safe and useful because of the decrease in afterload. While the decreased afterload is helpful, the decreased preload that frequently goes along with it is not. It cannot be overemphasized that the use of regional anesthesia is not an excuse to forgo invasive monitoring of preload and invasive arterial pressure monitoring. On the contrary, preload, afterload, and blood pressure may change rapidly and drastically in the patient with AR who receives a regional anesthetic. Maintaining adequate preload is of utmost importance.

Another possible problem associated with the use of regional anesthesia is the possibility of bradycardia (detrimental in AR) when high levels of sympathectomy are attained. Thus, the sympathetic level should be monitored closely and atropine/ephedrine should be readily available.

REFERENCES

1. Braunwald, E, Goldblatt, A, Aygen, MM, et al. Congenital aortic stenosis: Critical and hemodynamic findings in 100 patients. *Circulation* 27:426, 1963.
2. Passik, CS, Ackermann, DM, Pluth, JR, et al. Temporal changes in the causes of aortic stenosis: A surgical pathologic study of 646 cases. *Mayo Clin Proc* 62:119, 1987.
3. Deutscher, S, Rockette, HE, Krishnaswami, V. Diabetes and hypercholesterolemia among patients with calcific aortic stenosis. *J Chron Dis* 37:407, 1984.
4. Kelly, TA, Rothbart, RM, Cooper, M, et al. Comparison of outcome of asymptomatic to symptomatic patients older than 20 years of age with valvular aortic stenosis. *Am J Cardiol* 61:123, 1988.

5. Klein, RC. Ventricular arrhythmias in aortic valve disease: Analysis of 102 patients. Am J Cardiol 53: 1079, 1984.
6. Kennedy, JW, Twiss, RD, Blackmon, JR. Quantitative angiography. III. Relationships of left ventricular pressure volume and mass in aortic valve disease. Circulation 38:838, 1968.
7. Hood, WP, Rackley, CE, Rolett, EL. Wall stress in the normal and hypertrophied human left ventricle. Am J Cardiol 22:550, 1968.
8. Sasayama, S, Franklin, D, Ross, J. Hyperfunction with normal inotropic state of the hypertrophied left ventricle. Am J Physiol 232:H418, 1977.
9. Ross, J. Left ventricular function and the timing of surgical treatment in valvular heart disease. Ann Intern Med 94:498–504, 1981.
10. Gunther, S, Grossman, W. Determinants of ventricular function in pressure overload hypertrophy in man. Circulation 59:679, 1979.
11. Hanrath, R, Mathey, DG, Siegert, R, et al. Left ventricular relaxation and filling pattern in different forms of left ventricular hypertrophy: An echocardiographic study. Am J Cardiol 45:15–23, 1980.
12. Bertrand, ME, LaBlanche, JM, Tilmant, PY, et al. Coronary sinus blood flow at rest and during isometric exercise in patients with aortic valve disease. Mechanism of angina pectoris in presence of normal coronary arteries. Am J Cardiol 47:199, 1981.
13. Vandeplas, A, Willems, JL, Piessens, J, et al. Frequency of angina pectoris and coronary artery disease in severe isolated valvular aortic stenosis. Am J Cardiol 62:117, 1988.
14. Hakki, AH, Kimbiris, D, Iskandrian, AS, et al. Angina pectoris and coronary artery disease in patients with severe aortic valvular disease. Am Heart J 100: 441, 1980.
15. Marcus, ML. Effects of Cardiac Hypertrophy on the Coronary Circulation. In ML Marcus (ed), The Coronary Circulation in Health and Disease. New York: McGraw-Hill, 1983.
16. Vinten-Johansen, J, Weiss, HR. Oxygen consumption in subepicardial and subendocardial regions of the canine left ventricle—the effect of experimental acute valvular aortic stenosis. Circ Res 46:139, 1980.
17. Boudoulas, H, Rittgers, SE, Lewis, RP, et al. Changes in diastolic time with various pharmacologic agents. Implications for myocardial perfusion. Circulation 60:164–169, 1979.
18. Smulyan, H, Obeid, AI, Eich, RH. Right ventricular dysfunction in aortic stenosis. Circulation 42 (Suppl IV):220, 1973.
19. Langille, BL, Jones, DR. Mechanical interaction between the ventricles during systole. Can J Physiol Pharmacol 55:373–380, 1977.
20. Boldt, J, Zickmann, B, Ballesteros, M, et al. Right ventricular function in patients with aortic stenosis undergoing aortic valve replacement. J Cardiothorac Vasc Anesth 6:287–291, 1992.
21. Grech, ED, Ramsdale, DR. Exertional syncope in aortic stenosis: Evidence to support inappropriate left ventricular baroreceptor response. Am Heart J 121:603, 1991.
22. Selzer, A. Changing aspects of the natural history of valvular aortic stenosis. N Engl J Med 317:91, 1987.
23. Gooch, AS, Calatayud, JB, Rogers, PA, et al. Analysis of the P wave in severe aortic stenosis. Dis Chest 49:459, 1966.
24. Siegel, RJ, Maurer, G, Navatpumin, T, et al. Accurate noninvasive assessment of critical aortic valve stenosis in the elderly. J Am Coll Cardiol 1:639, 1983.
25. Agatston, AS, Chengot, M, Rao, A, et al. Doppler diagnosis of valvular aortic stenosis in patients over 60 years of age. Am J Cardiol 56:106, 1985.
26. Currie, PJ, Hagler, DJ, Seward, JB, et al. Instantaneous pressure gradient: A simultaneous Doppler and dual catheter correlative study. J Am Coll Cardiol 7:800, 1986.
27. London, MJ. Intraoperative myocardial ischemia: Localization by continuous 12-lead electrocardiography. Anesthesiology 69:232–241, 1988.
28. Kaplan, J, et al. Early diagnosis of myocardial ischemia using the pulmonary arterial catheter. Anesth Analg 60:789–793, 1981.
29. Bennett, DH, Evans, DW, Raj, MVJ. Echocardiographic left ventricular dimensions in pressure and volume overload: Their use in assessing aortic stenosis. Br Heart J 37:971–977, 1975.
30. Clements, FM, et al. Perioperative evaluation of regional wall motion by transesophageal two-dimensional echocardiography. Anesth Analg 66:249–261, 1987.
31. Smith, JS, Cahalan, MK, Benefiel, DJ, et al. Intraoperative detection of myocardial ischemia in high-risk patients: Electrocardiography versus two-dimensional transesophageal echocardiography. Circulation 73:1015–1021, 1985.
32. Priebe, HJ. Differential effects of isoflurane on regional right and left ventricular performances, and on coronary, systemic, and pulmonary hemodynamics in the dog. Anesthesiology 66:262–272, 1987.
33. Gelman, S, Fowler, KC, Smith, LR. Regional blood flow during isoflurane and halothane anesthesia. Anesth Analg 63:557–565, 1984.

34. Buffington, CW, Romson, JL, Levine, A, et al. Isoflurane induces coronary steal in a canine model of chronic coronary occlusion. *Anesthesiology* 66:280–292, 1987.
35. Priebe, HJ. Isoflurane and coronary hemodynamics. Review article. *Anesthesiology* 71:960–976, 1989.
36. Scheffer, GJ, Jonges, R, Holley, S, et al. Effects of halothane on the conduction system of the heart in humans. *Anesth Analg* 69:721–726, 1989.
37. Lynch, C, III. Effects of halothane and isoflurane on isolated human ventricular myocardium. *Anesthesiology* 68:429–432, 1988.
38. Pagel, PS, Kampine, JP, Schmeling, WT, et al. Influence of volatile anesthetics on myocardial contractility in vivo: Desflurane versus isoflurane. *Anesthesiology* 74:900–907, 1991.
39. Nathan, HJ. Nitrous oxide worsens myocardial ischemia in isoflurane-anesthetized dogs. *Anesthesiology* 68:407–415, 1988.
40. Leone, BJ, Philbin, DM, Lehot, JJ, et al. Gradual or abrupt nitrous oxide administration in a canine model of critical coronary stenosis induces regional myocardial dysfunction that is worsened by halothane. *Anesth Analg* 67:814–822, 1988.
41. Cahalan, MK, Prakash, O, Rulf, ENR, et al. Addition of nitrous oxide to fentanyl anesthesia does not induce myocardial ischemia in patients with ischemic heart disease. *Anesthesiology* 67:925–929, 1987.
42. Roizen, MF, Plummer, GO, Lichtor, JL. Nitrous oxide and dysrhythmias. *Anesthesiology* 66:427–431, 1987.
43. Eckstein, JW, Hamilton, WK, McCammond, JM. The effect of thiopental on peripheral venous tone. *Anesthesiology* 22:525–528, 1961.
44. Reves, JG, McKay, RD. Cardiovascular Therapy. In P. Newfield and JE Cottrell (eds), *Handbook of Neuroanesthesia: Clinical and Physiologic Essentials*. Boston: Little, Brown, 1983.
45. Brussel, T, Theissen, JL, Vigfusson, G, et al. Hemodynamic and cardiodynamic effects of propofol and etomidate: Negative inotropic properties of propofol. *Anesth Analg* 69:35–40, 1989.
46. Traber, DL, Wilson, RD. Involvement of the sympathetic nervous system in the pressor response to ketamine. *Anesth Analg* 48:248–252, 1969.
47. Larach, DR, Hensley, FA, Martin, DE, et al. Hemodynamic effects of muscle relaxant drugs during anesthetic induction in patients with mitral or aortic valvular heart disease. *J Cardiothorac Vasc Anesth* 5:126–131, 1991.
48. Chartash, EK, Lans, DM, Paget, SA, et al. Aortic insufficiency and mitral regurgitation in patients with severe systemic lupus erythematosus and the antiphospholipid syndrome. *Am J Med* 86:407, 1989.
49. Perloff, JK. Acute severe aortic regurgitation: Recognition and management. *J Cardiovasc Med* 8:209, 1983.
50. Smith, HJ, Neutze, JM, Roche, AHG, et al. The natural history of rheumatic aortic regurgitation and the indications for surgery. *Br Heart J* 38:147, 1976.
51. Grossman, W, Jones, D, McLaurin, LP. Wall stress and patterns of hypertrophy in the human left ventricle. *J Clin Invest* 56:56, 1975.
52. Eastham, CL, Doty, DB, Hiratzka, LF, et al. Volume-overload left ventricular hypertrophy impairs coronary reserve in humans. *Circulation* 64 (Suppl IV):26, 1981.
53. DePace, NL, Nestico, PF, Kotler, MN, et al. Comparison of echocardiography and angiography in determining the cause of severe aortic regurgitation. *Br Heart J* 51:36, 1984.
54. Latson, WL, Lappas, DG. Use of a pacing catheter to control heart rate in a patient with aortic insufficiency and coronary artery disease. *Anesthesiology* 63:712–715, 1985.
55. Miller, RR, Vismara, LA, DeMaria, AN, et al. Afterload reduction therapy with nitroprusside in severe aortic regurgitation. Improved cardiac performance and reduced regurgitant volume. *Am J Cardiol* 38:564, 1976.
56. Brown, BB, Crout, JR. A comparative study of the effects of five general anesthetics on myocardial contractility. *Anesthesiology* 34:236–245, 1971.
57. Pagel, PS, Kampine, JP, Schmeling, WT, et al. Comparison of the systemic and coronary hemodynamic actions of desflurane, isoflurane, halothane, and enflurane in the chronically instrumented dog. *Anesthesiology* 74:539–551, 1991.
58. Calverley, RK, Smith, NT, Prys-Roberts, C, et al. Cardiovascular effects of enflurane anesthesia during controlled ventilation in man. *Anesth Analg* 57:619–628, 1978.
59. Smith, NT, Eger, EI, Stoetting, RK, et al. The cardiovascular and sympathomimetic responses to the addition of nitrous oxide to halothane in man. *Anesthesiology* 32:410–421, 1970.
60. Eisele, JH, Smith, NT. Cardiovascular effects of 40 percent nitrous oxide in man. *Anesth Analg* 51:956, 1972.
61. Stanley, TH, de Lange, S. Comparison of sufentanil-oxygen and fentanyl-oxygen anesthesia for mitral and aortic valvular surgery. *J Cardiothorac Anesth* 1:6–11, 1987.

7
Mitral Valve Disease

Sheldon Goldstein
Michael S. Taragin

Safe anesthetic management of patients with mitral valve disease is quite challenging. A careful history and physical examination provide helpful clues to the severity of the patient's valvular and myocardial function. The electrocardiogram, chest x-ray, or special studies may offer insight into the severity of the patient's condition, which in the compensated patient may not be apparent from the history and physical examination.

During both general and regional anesthesia, patients may receive numerous drugs that may have varying hemodynamic effects. Patients with mitral valve disease often require precise management of preload, afterload, heart rate, and contractility. Preoperative assessment focuses on determining the severity of the patient's underlying disease process. Perioperative care includes placement of necessary monitors and choosing and maintaining an appropriate anesthetic technique. Planning for the postoperative period requires the anesthesiologist to predict which patients will need extended care and what problems are likely to be encountered.

ANATOMY AND PHYSIOLOGY
Anatomy of the Mitral Valve

The mitral valve apparatus consists of the annulus, valve leaflets, chordae tendineae, and anteromedial and posterolateral papillary muscles. Working in unison they ensure normal mitral valve function by preventing regurgitation during systole, yet allowing diastolic passage of blood (preload) into the left ventricle without a pressure gradient across the valve [1]. Abnormalities of these structures, whether congenital or acquired, may contribute to mitral stenosis (MS), mitral regurgitation (MR), or mitral valve prolapse (MVP). Supporting musculature of the left atrium and ventricle are also important for proper function of the valve complex. Atrial dilation will most commonly affect mitral valve function because of associated arrhythmias. Left ventricular hypertrophy (LVH) and dilatation as seen in the hypertensive patient can result in MR, both by preventing the annulus from decreasing in size during systole and by alteration of the anatomic relationships of the papillary muscles [2]. Ventricular dilatation due to alcohol abuse or scarring due to infarction may also affect valve function adversely. The papillary muscles extend from the ventricular wall into the ventricle and attach to chordae tendineae, which in turn are attached to cusps of the mitral valve. Coaptation of the leaflets of the mitral valve occurs before the time when significant tension has developed in the papillary muscles. The papillary muscles apply tension to the valve during systole. This serves to prevent prolapse of the leaflets into the left atrium while

Fig. 7-1. The normal pressure-volume loop of the cardiac cycle. (Reprinted with permission from PG Barash and CJ Kopriva, Cardiac Pump Function and How to Monitor It. In SJ Thomas (ed), *Manual of Cardiac Anesthesia.* New York: Churchill Livingstone, 1984. P 7.)

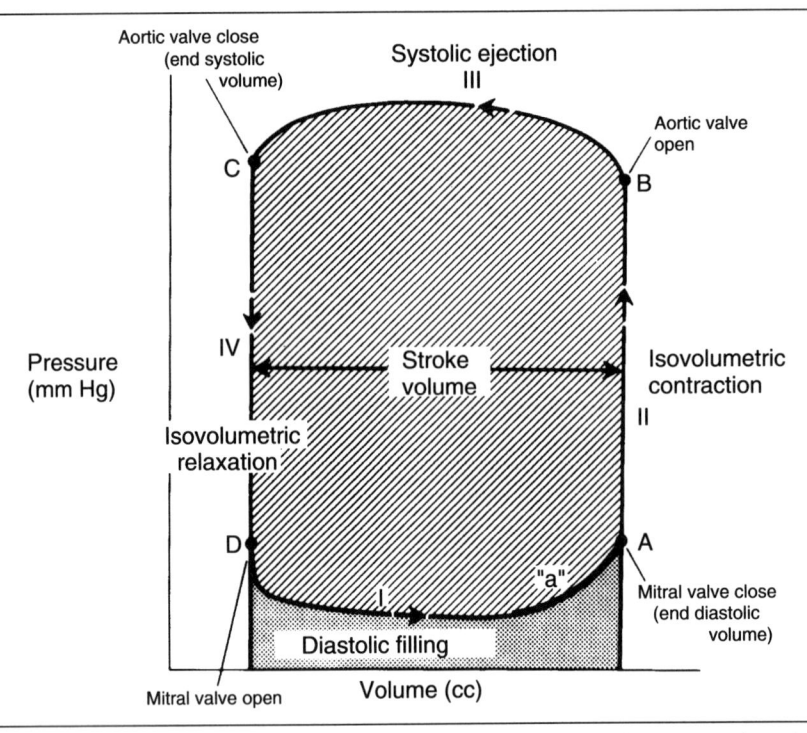

the forces of systole impinge on the mitral valve. Therefore, regurgitation due to papillary muscle dysfunction occurs after valve closure and is due to failure to maintain closure of the valve during systole. However, abnormal ventricular function may need to be present as well, in order for MR to result. Papillary muscle dysfunction occurs as a result of ischemia, infarction, or surgical damage to a papillary muscle and the adjacent ventricular myocardium. In order to understand echocardiographic images, it should be appreciated that the anterior leaflet of the mitral valve is a portion of the left ventricular outflow tract.

Physiology of the Mitral Valve

If we think of the mitral valve as the path via which left ventricular preload enters, as well as the gate that must be closed during systole to ensure forward cardiac output, it becomes easy to appreciate why patients with mitral valve disease may be critically ill. Mitral valve function can be understood by examining the normal ventricular pressure-volume loop, created by plotting points on a curve representing ventricular pressure at varying volumes during a single cardiac cycle. Such a diagram helps visualize the contribution of various filling pressures to stroke volume and is depicted in Fig. 7-1.

Phase I occurs during ventricular filling and depicts ventricular preload before systole. From early to mid-diastole, ventricular filling depends on the gradient between left atrial and left ventricular pressure, therefore occurring both rapidly and passively. In late ventricular diastole atrial systole occurs. This "atrial kick" may account for 15 to 20 percent of ventricular preload in a normal patient and may contribute even more to cardiac output in patients with moderate to severe mitral stenosis [3] or those with decreased ventricular compliance. However, this benefit may not be realized in patients who are tachycardic. It is clear that the underlying cardiac rate and rhythm also contribute to normal function of the mitral valve.

The normal left ventricle is compliant, accommodating large increases in preload with small changes in diastolic pressure. Phase II of the pressure-volume loop displays the isovolumetric period of systole, during which large increases in intraventricular pressure occur. However, intraventricular volume remains unchanged because (1) no atrioventricular flow occurs since the high ventricular pressure maintains the mitral valve in the closed position and (2) the aortic valve has not yet opened. Phase III represents that portion of systole when the intraventricular pressure exceeds that in the aorta, thus opening the aortic valve. Aortic valve closure, which marks the end of phase III, is the end systolic pressure-volume coordinate and reflects the inotropic state of the myocardium.

MITRAL STENOSIS

Epidemiology

Mitral stenosis is almost always rheumatic in origin [4]. If only the chordae tendineae are involved, pure MS may occur, but usually involvement of the leaflets prevents their normal coaptation, resulting in combined stenosis and regurgitation. It is more common in women than men and only about half the patients with rheumatic mitral stenosis recall having had the disease [5].

Though a calcified mitral annulus usually results in mitral regurgitation, if the calcification involves the valvular or subvalvular region stenosis may occur [6]. Similarly, the presence of an atrial myxoma can impede flow across the mitral valve apparatus [7]. Although this may result in functional MS, it may also result in complete obstruction of the annulus and sudden hemodynamic collapse. Despite the differences in pathophysiology, management of these forms of mitral stenosis is similar to that of rheumatic stenosis.

Congenital stenosis of the mitral valve is rarely seen in adults and is usually associated with other cardiac abnormalities. Infants and young children with this lesion tend to do poorly because of difficulties in repairing such a small valve and the associated pulmonary hypertension. Still, some children do survive to an age when mitral valve replacement is feasible, although they may need serial surgical procedures as they increase in size. Those who survive frequently have return of their pulmonary artery (PA) pressures and pulmonary vascular resistance (PVR) to near normal levels. If surgery is not performed, it is unlikely that a patient with congenital MS will survive until adulthood [8].

Natural History

Mitral stenosis results when the leaflets and chordae tendineae become scarred and contracted during the healing process of acute rheumatic fever. Adhesions frequently form between the two leaflets [9]. Combined MS and MR will occur when the leaflets become so adherent that the valve can no longer open or close normally [10].

Rheumatic fever usually occurs between the ages of 8 and 14. The mitral valve area will progressively decrease in size until it is small enough to cause symptoms. The most common presenting symptom will be dyspnea with exertion, occurring during exercise, sexual activity, bronchitis, atrial fibrillation, or pregnancy. With time these same events may precipitate pulmonary edema. Dyspnea with exertion often occurs around age 30, or at least 10 years after the acute process [5]. Progressive increases in left atrial and pulmonary arterial pressures will eventually lead to pulmonary edema, pulmonary hypertension, and right-sided heart failure [11, 12]. In about one third of patients with MS, pulmonary vasoconstriction will develop early in the course of their disease. Though right-sided failure and cor pulmonale will develop, these patients will have some degree of protection against pulmonary edema [13]. If not treated, the patient with MS will likely die at approximately 40 years of age. Rarely, symptoms of severe MS may occur as quickly as 2 years after the acute disease. In particular, the disease process advances more rapidly in tropical climates, where severe MS may occur in adolescence [14].

Atrial fibrillation initially occurs intermittently, but with time frequently becomes chronic and may contribute to systemic or pulmonary emboli, which may cause death [15]. Thromboemboli are a serious consequence of mitral stenosis. Before the development of surgical treatment, emboli developed in approximately 20 percent of patients at some time during the disease and 10 to 15 percent of these patients died because of systemic or pulmonary embolization [16]. The occurrence of emboli correlates directly with the patient's age and size of the left atrial appendage (but not the valve area) and inversely with the cardiac output. Of those patients in whom systemic emboli develop, 80 percent are in atrial fibrillation. Right atrial thromboses may result in pulmonary emboli and severe right-sided heart failure [15].

Pathophysiology

The pathophysiology of mitral stenosis is best understood by considering its effects on different areas of the cardiovascular system. Those areas affected by mitral stenosis include the left ventricle, left atrium, conduction system, pulmonary circulation, and the right side of the heart.

Mitral stenosis presents conditions of volume underloading to the left ventricle while increasing the pressure in the left atrium. Left ventricular loading is usually maintained by increases in left atrial pressure. However, this may jeopardize the pulmonary circulation and ultimately the right ventricle.

Exercise, pregnancy, or other stressful activities cause shortness of breath due to associated tachycardia. Since diastole decreases proportionately more than systole during tachycardia, increases in heart rate compromise diastolic filling time of the left ventricle. The decrease in time spent in diastole results in less time available for flow across the valve, thereby elevating left atrial pressure. The transvalvular gradient is dependent on the flow rate, so that a stress-produced tachycardia that increases flow rate by a factor of two will increase the transvalvular gradient by a factor of four. That the transvalvular gradient will increase as the square of the increase in flow is described by Gorlin's formula, which states that

$$\text{Valve area} = \int K \times CO/\sqrt{PG}$$

where CO = cardiac output and PG = pressure gradient. It is apparent that when cardiac output increases or diastolic filling decreases, the gradient across the valve will vary by the square of the change [17]. It is therefore easy to understand why tachycardia will significantly increase left atrial pressure in patients with moderate or severe mitral stenosis [18]. In patients with moderate MS, cardiac output and left atrial pressures are often reasonable even if atrial fibrillation results in loss of the atrial kick as long as the ventricular rate is slow. If a rapid ventricular rate ensues, an increase in left atrial pressure will occur [19]. The severity of the rise of left atrial pressure will depend on other factors besides heart rate, specifically left atrial size and compliance. Although the atrial contraction of sinus rhythm helps minimize the mean left atrial pressure, as the disease worsens diastolic filling time becomes more important than atrial systole in preserving forward flow. That a slower heart rate is more beneficial than the atrial contribution to preload is demonstrated when propranolol decreases left atrial pressure in patients with atrial fibrillation, resulting in an increase in cardiac output [20].

The normal adult mitral valve has an area of 4 to 6 cm^2. A decrease of 2 cm^2 requires an increase in the transvalvular pressure gradient to maintain normal blood flow. Mild disease exists with an area of 1.5 to 2.5 cm^2. Moderate disease exists with an area of 1.1 to 1.5 cm^2. Critical mitral stenosis exists when the valve area decreases to 0.6 to 1.0 cm^2 [11]. When the valve area is approximately 2 cm^2, passage of left ventricular preload depends on a small pressure gradient. When the valve area has decreased to approximately 1 cm^2 the gradient between the atrium and ventricle needed to maintain ventricular preload is approximately 20 mm Hg. Since normal left ventricular diastolic pressure is 5 mm Hg, this will result in a mean left atrial pressure (LAP) of approximately 25 mm Hg, and when an elevated left ventricular diastolic pressure exists, an elevated mean left atrial pressure will be required to maintain the transvalvular gradient necessary for diastolic passage of left ventricular preload. Such high left atrial pressures frequently result in pulmonary edema. The increase in left atrial pressure results in an increased pressure in the pulmonary veins and capillaries. Pulmonary edema is likely to occur when the pulmonary capillary pressure is greater than 25 mm Hg, which is the normal oncotic pressure of plasma. This is especially true if the mean LAP rises suddenly. However, if LAP rises gradually, lymphatic drainage from the lungs increases and capillary basement

Table 7-1. Causes of elevated LVEDP in patients with mitral stenosis

Mitral regurgitation
Aortic stenosis
Aortic regurgitation
Hypertension
Coronary artery disease
Myocardial disease

membranes thicken so that patients may tolerate left atrial pressures greater than 25 mm Hg without the development of pulmonary edema [21]. It is therefore apparent that there is minimal margin of error in these patients regarding both intravascular volume and systemic vascular resistance. Either can significantly affect the transvalvular gradient and even small differences in left atrial pressure can move the patient from a state of decreased left ventricular filling and forward cardiac output to pulmonary edema.

Left ventricular end diastolic pressures and volumes generally remain normal in patients with pure MS because ventricular compliance and diastolic function are usually not changed significantly. If they are elevated, the presence of one of the disease processes listed in Table 7-1 should be suspected. Rather, the underlying problem in pure MS is that preload reserve is limited. However, not only do high left atrial pressures place the patient at risk of developing pulmonary edema, but raising the filling pressures even higher does not necessarily cause a significant increase in left ventricular end diastolic volume (LVEDV) due to the gradient across the mitral valve. Patients with severe MS may have decreased systemic perfusion because of a decreased cardiac output. This is a result of a decreased ejection fraction secondary to an increased afterload and no compensatory increase in preload [22]. Despite this these patients may have normal indices of contractility.

The Left Atrium in Mitral Stenosis

Mitral valve disease and inflammation due to rheumatic carditis result in dilatation of the atrium and disorganization and fibrosis of the atrial wall. The result is conduction abnormalities, which initially will manifest as premature atrial contractions but with time frequently cause atrial fibrillation. These patients often have high left atrial pressures because with loss of the atrial kick, elevated left atrial pressures help to maintain ventricular filling. Ventricular filling can be augmented by increasing the length of diastole and therefore a slow heart rate may be crucial in such patients and tachycardia may be quite detrimental, resulting in a significant decrease in left ventricular preload. For these reasons, it is important to maintain a slow ventricular response in atrial fibrillation. This can be accomplished with agents such as β-blockers, some calcium channel blockers, and digoxin. Patients with atrial fibrillation may also have a decreased cardiac output, as the atrial kick supplies up to 33 percent of ventricular preload in some patients with MS, as compared to 15 to 20 percent in patients with normal hearts [23].

The Left Ventricle in Mitral Stenosis

The pressure-volume loop for mitral stenosis with normal left ventricular (LV) function is depicted in Fig. 7-2. The curve is similar to the normal curve because left ventricular function is usually normal in pure MS. It is apparent that decreased preload results in a lower LVEDP and stroke volume. In turn systolic blood pressure is usually decreased in patients with MS.

Though rheumatic myocardial inflammation and subsequent fibrosis are frequent in patients with MS [24], there are varying opinions regarding whether abnormalities of left ventricular contrac-

Fig. 7-2. Pressure-volume loop for mitral stenosis. LV = left ventricular. (Reprinted with permission from JM Jackson, SJ Thomas and E Lowenstein, Anesthetic management of patients with valvular heart disease. *Semin Anesth* 1:244, 1982.)

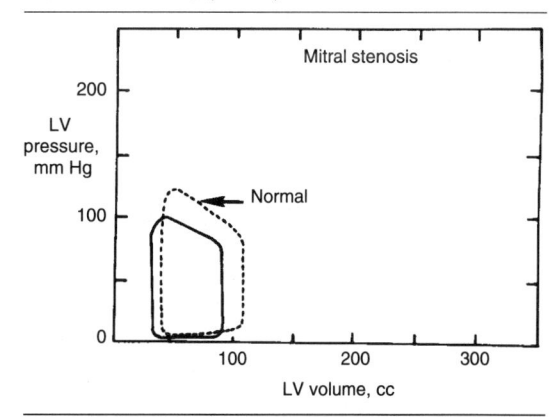

tion are present. Regional hypokinesis has been attributed to scar tissue that extends from the mitral valve into the posterobasal myocardium, resulting in immobilization of that portion of the heart [25]. Similarly, Bolen and associates [26] reported that fibrosis of the myocardium secondary to rheumatic fever in the posterobasal region of the ventricle may be responsible for segmental wall motion abnormalities and decreased systolic function. During isometric exercise, which increases heart rate only a small amount, LVEDVs are similar in normal patients and patients with MS, but end systolic volumes are greater in patients with MS. They attributed this abnormality of ventricular contractility to fibrosis, which has been described as a common finding on autopsy in patients with MS [27].

The left ventricle's altered load, along with secondary or compensatory responses to this altered load, may explain significant differences between the patient's symptoms and underlying inotropic state. For example, while myocardial contractility is frequently normal in patients with MS [22] they may be symptomatic because of poor systemic perfusion. Gash and associates [22] attributed the decreased LV ejection performance in patients with MS to changes in loading conditions caused by either decreased end systolic LV wall thickness or increased systemic vascular resistance. Because the stenotic valve diminishes filling, Starling's mechanism cannot compensate for the increased afterload. However, these authors found LV muscle function to be normal in most patients with MS [22]. In some patients, the underloaded ventricle's fixed stroke volume activates a reflex sympathetic response and increases systemic vascular resistance, thereby depressing ejection phase indices [22]. Systolic function is depressed because the inotropically normal myocardium is simultaneously underloaded (stenotic mitral valve) and afterload stressed (high systemic vascular resistance), that is, afterload mismatched.

Pulmonary and Right Ventricular Function in Mitral Stenosis

Dyspnea in patients with severe MS may be due to pulmonary abnormalities. Vital capacity is decreased secondary to engorged pulmonary vessels and interstitial edema. In addition, pulmonary blood flow is redistributed from the bases to the apices, resulting in a significant ventilation-perfusion mismatch [28, 29]. Lung volumes and flow rates decrease over time as the PA pressure and PVR rise. These patients may have significantly decreased lung compliance, resulting in an increased work of breathing. Shortness of breath may be due to the increased work required of the respiratory muscles [30]. There is a good correlation between the pulmonary abnormalities and the severity of the MS, such that a decreased vital capacity may predict the occurrence of congestive heart failure in the near future [31]. Resting blood gases may show normocarbia or mild hypocarbia as well as hypoxia that worsens as MS progresses. With significant MS, diffusion capacity may be impaired as well.

In patients with a short history of MS, transmission of the increased LAP to the pulmonary veins will occur. Pulmonary artery pressures in these patients will be reversibly elevated but pulmonary vascular resistance will remain within the normal range. Early on, right ventricular function will be normal. With time the pulmonary vasculature will become abnormal, developing histologic changes that result in increased pulmonary vascular resistance (PVR). Reactive pulmonary hypertension is caused by left atrial and pulmonary venous hypertension [32]. Chronic obliterative changes secondary to recurrent pulmonary emboli may occur as well.

Severe chronic pulmonary hypertension will eventually result in right ventricular failure. This produces what can be referred to as a second stenosis, representing the increased afterload against which the right ventricle (RV) must pump. Since the RV is better able to handle volume than pressure, an afterload mismatch occurs, and with time the RV will fail. These patients will display the usual clinical signs associated with right ventricular failure, including jugular venous distention, hepatomegaly, and lower-extremity edema. Still, right ventricular contractile function is normal in most patients with MS, even those with moderate pulmonary hypertension [33]. If right heart failure develops, episodes of pulmonary edema may become less frequent. This is due to decreased filling of the left heart secondary to RV failure [13]. Patients such as these who present for noncardiac surgery are extremely difficult to manage. On the other hand, patients who have undergone mitral valve replacement frequently have a decrease in their PVR after surgery [34, 35].

History and Physical Examination

Patients with mitral stenosis may develop symptoms that are related to increased left atrial pressure or decreased tissue perfusion, or that are complications of embolization. These symptoms are listed in Table 7-2. If cor pulmonale and right-sided failure develop, the signs and symptoms of these disorders will be present as well. They are listed in Table 7-3. The presentations of cor pulmonale and right ventricular failure are different than that of left ventricular failure. When increased left atrial pressure backs up into the lungs, patients become acutely distressed. In contrast, symptoms develop insidiously in many patients with cor pulmonale and right-sided failure. Frequently, the progression of symptoms over time is attributed to the primary disorder, in this case mitral stenosis. Only at right heart catheterization will the elevated pulmonary artery pressure and central venous pressure make the diagnosis apparent.

When dyspnea and orthopnea occur in patients with MS, the left atrial pressure is usually in the range of 25 mm Hg. Although the symptoms are generally attributed to rising left atrial pressure, the possibility that they may be caused by pulmonary abnormalities should be considered as well. Generalized fatigue may be present as a result of poor systemic perfusion. Forty percent of patients with mitral stenosis have at least one episode of hemoptysis. Severe hemorrhage is unusual, but it can be present early in the course of the disease, even be-

Table 7-2. Symptoms that occur in patients with mitral stenosis

---
Orthopnea
Dyspnea
Paroxysmal nocturnal dyspnea
Pulmonary edema
Hemoptysis
Palpitations
Syncope
Neurologic changes (due to systemic embolization)
Chest pain

Table 7-3. Signs and symptoms that occur in cor pulmonale and right-sided heart failure

---
Jugular venous distention
Hepatomegaly
Peripheral edema
Cough
Fatigue
Dyspnea on exertion
Cyanosis with exercise
---

fore the onset of dyspnea. This is because bronchial veins form collateral vessels that allow blood to travel from the high-pressure pulmonary veins to the low-pressure systemic veins. Early on, these anastomotic collaterals carry a large amount of blood, and rapid elevations in left atrial pressure or coughing may disrupt them. As systemic venous pressures increase over time, cardiac output decreases and massive hemorrhage is less likely to occur. Still, pink frothy secretions may occur even late in the disease, especially during episodes of pulmonary edema [36].

The murmur of MS is low pitched and heard best at the apex, with the patient in the left lateral decubitus position. It is frequently described as a mid-diastolic rumble, and is due to turbulent flow across the mitral valve. S_1 may be increased. Because the increased left atrial pressure keeps the valve wide open at the beginning of ventricular contraction, it closes over a wider excursion than is normal. Early on, a loud S_1 may be the only auscultatory finding. The opening snap (OS) of mitral stenosis occurs early in diastole, producing a short high-pitched sound after A_2. The time interval from A_2 to the opening snap reflects the abnormal pressure gradient across the mitral valve. As the stenosis worsens, atrial pressure increases and the valve is open progressively longer in diastole, with the opening snap moving closer to A_2. There is therefore an inverse relationship between the A_2-OS interval and the severity of the stenosis such that the smaller the A_2-OS interval, the worse the MS and the higher the left atrial pressure. However, since this physical finding depends on elevation of left atrial pressure the A_2-OS interval may not be short in a patient with a large, compliant left atrium who does not have significantly elevated left atrial pressure. Cal-

Table 7-4. Auscultatory findings in mitral stenosis

Accentuated first heart sound
Opening snap
Mid-diastolic rumbling murmur
Presystolic accentuation of the murmur

cification of the valve may make the opening snap inaudible and the leaflets may become so adherent that they are unable to close, thus leading to combined mitral stenosis and regurgitation and sometimes the absence of S_1 [10]. In many patients a presystolic accentuation of the murmur immediately precedes the S_1 because of the increased flow with left atrial contraction, and is usually lost when atrial fibrillation develops. Auscultatory findings in mitral stenosis are listed in Table 7-4.

Other physical findings of mitral stenosis may be present. The classic "mitral facies" is characterized by a malar flush and cyanosis of the lips, but is not frequently seen. In a patient with pure mitral stenosis, increased jugular venous pressure is a sign of right-sided failure, due to secondary pulmonary hypertension. Because left ventricular diastolic pressure is normal, the apical impulse is normal. A parasternal heave suggests the presence of right ventricular hypertrophy (RVH) due to pulmonary hypertension. Thus, the physical examination in mitral stenosis includes a diastolic low-pitched rumbling at the apex, increased jugular venous pressure, mitral facies, and parasternal heave (suggesting pulmonary hypertension and RVH).

Chest Pain in the Patient with Mitral Stenosis

Chest pain is a frequent complaint among patients with mitral valve disease, regardless of the type of lesion. The possibility that the patient has coronary disease in addition to mitral valve disease should be considered. If patients have coronary artery disease (CAD), it is important to keep in mind that the low blood pressure that patients with MS often manifest combined with possibly elevated left ventricular end diastolic pressure (LVEDP) due to CAD will result in decreased coronary perfusion pressure. It is therefore quite helpful to have angiographic documentation of coronary anatomy before patients with MS and anginal symptoms are anesthetized. Mattina and associates [37] reported that among patients with mitral stenosis, angina had a sensitivity of 37 percent and a specificity of 84 percent for significant CAD, which was defined as at least a 70 percent obstruction of a major coronary artery or at least 50 percent obstruction of the left main coronary artery. Not only does this support the fact that CAD frequently coexists with MS but it also points out that it is often silent [37]. Therefore, while approximately 15 percent of patients with MS complain of chest pain that is indistinguishable from that due to ischemia [38], many patients have atypical chest pain, and the possibility of CAD should be considered in these patients as well. While some patients certainly have concomitant atherosclerotic coronary disease [39], many of these individuals do not have any obvious cause of their pain.

The Chest X-ray in Mitral Stenosis

The chest x-ray may show straightening of the left heart border that is caused by left atrial enlargement and an increased angle at the carina due to displacement of the left main-stem bronchus. If pulmonary hypertension is present, right ventricular enlargement may be noted as well. If the patient is acutely compromised, signs of congestive heart failure will be seen. A chest x-ray of a patient with a straight heart border, indicating left atrial enlargement, is depicted in Fig. 7-3.

Fig. 7-3. Chest x-ray of a patient with a straight heart border indicating left atrial enlargement.

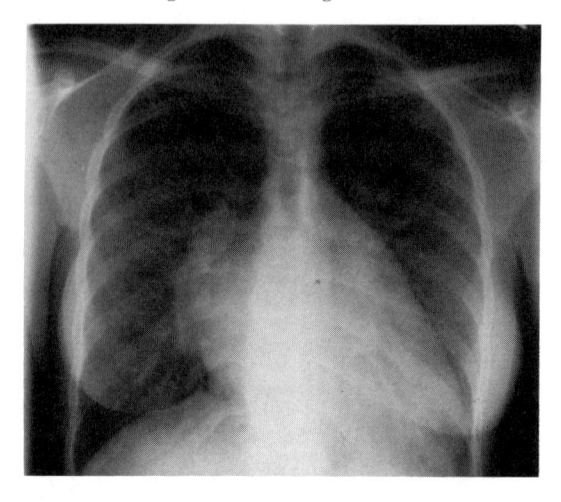

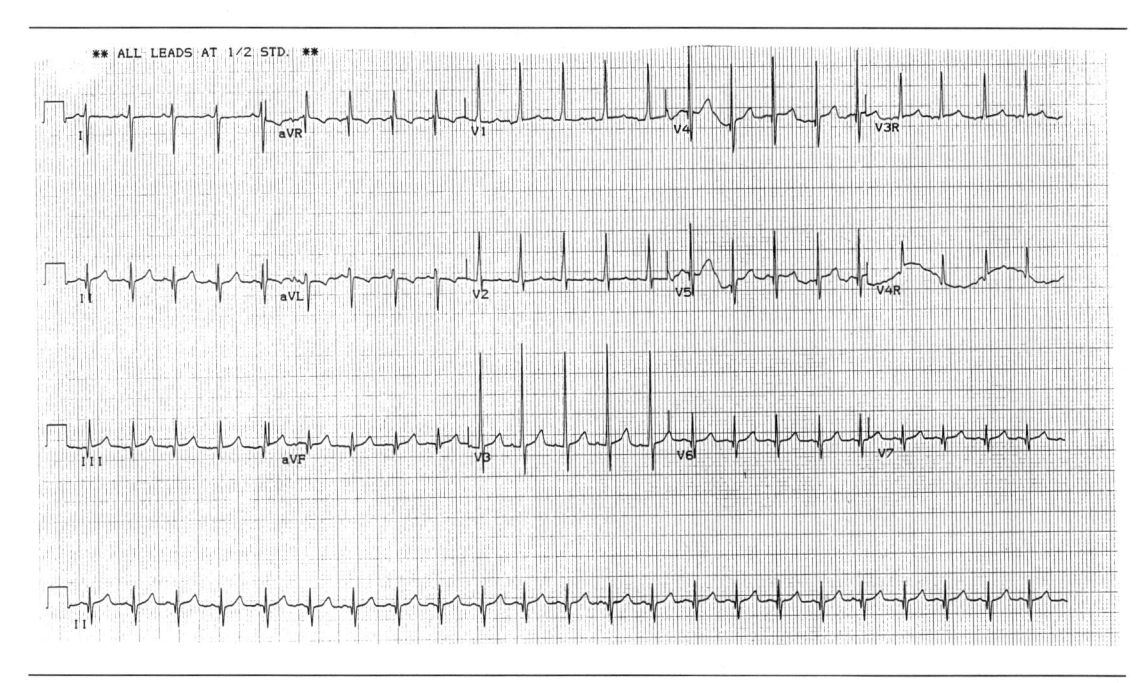

Fig. 7-4. Electrocardiogram showing right ventricular hypertrophy.

The Electrocardiogram in Mitral Stenosis

If the patient is in sinus rhythm, large biphasic P waves (P mitrale) are indicative of left atrial enlargement. P mitrale manifests wide, notched P waves in limb leads I and II, with biphasic or inverted P waves in lead III, although notching of the P waves is occasionally best appreciated in the midprecordial leads. The presence of P mitrale or atrial fibrillation with right-axis deviation strongly supports the diagnosis of MS. The presence of atrial fibrillation and right-axis deviation in a patient less than 40 years of age is almost pathognomonic for MS [40]. The presence of right ventricular hypertrophy on the ECG, as seen in Fig. 7-4, implies that there has been chronic stress on the right ventricle, and such patients may have an increased perioperative risk. Right ventricular hypertrophy is indicated by a significant R wave in lead V_1 and a large S wave in lead V_6, as well as right-axis deviation of +90 degrees or greater. If the RVH is severe, the R wave in lead V_2 may be prominent as well. Repolarization changes, such as ST depression and T-wave inversion, in leads V_1 and V_2 may also occur. The large R-wave voltages seen in lead V_1 and possibly lead V_2 are due to movement of the mean wave of depolarization toward the right ventricle. It is important to understand that although the presence of these changes implies the existence of RVH, their absence does not rule it out. This is because biventricular hypertrophy may be present and if the left ventricular muscle mass is still significantly greater than the right ventricular muscle mass, the mean wave of depolarization will still be seen as moving toward the left ventricle.

The Echocardiogram in Mitral Stenosis

The echocardiogram is uniquely suited to evaluate valvular heart disease. While M-mode echo (Fig. 7-5) obtains quality images of valve motion,

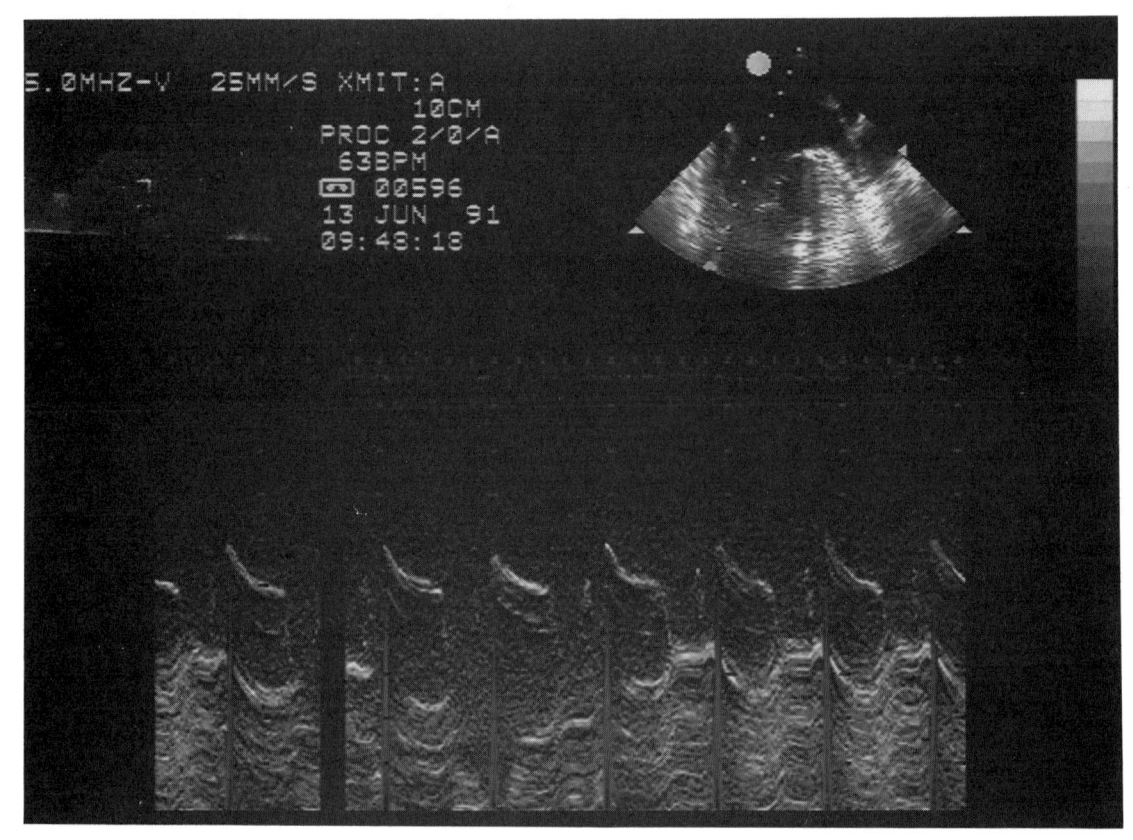

Fig. 7-5. Normal M-mode echocardiogram of the mitral valve.

two-dimensional echo allows us to visualize the shape of the valves during the cardiac cycle, as well as the surrounding tissues. Doppler echo allows us to determine flow across the valves. Finally, transesophageal echocardiography (TEE) allows us to visualize the heart intraoperatively without interfering with the surgical field.

On M-mode echocardiography the normal anterior leaflet closes shortly after opening, with a peak at the E point. In patients with MS early diastolic closure either does not occur or occurs at a much slower rate, that is, the mid-diastolic closing velocity of the valve is significantly attenuated [41, 42]. Normally, blood empties rapidly from the left atrium to the ventricles so that by mid-diastole relatively little mitral flow occurs and the valve tends toward closure. With MS, however, flow across the valve is slowed, with the valve being maintained in the open position because of the gradient between the left atrium and left ventricle. Thus, the M-mode echocardiographic findings that occur in patients with MS include decreased diastolic closing (E-F) slope, abnormal motion of the posterior mitral valve leaflet, and thickening of the mitral valve leaflets.

If M-mode echocardiography is unable to make the diagnosis of MS, the presence of diastolic doming on two-dimensional echo will. Doming is due to the fact that the valve is unable to accommodate all the blood that must cross it in order to enter the left ventricle. Two-dimensional echo is also useful for quantitating the degree of mitral stenosis by measuring the valve area [43, 44]. The addition of Doppler technology gives the physician the ability to assess transvalvular flow and quantify the pressure gradient across the valve [45, 46]. One group of patients in whom echocardiography may not be accurate are those who have had a commissurotomy, as the orifice is no longer elliptical and it may therefore be difficult to properly define the edges of the orifice. The echocardiogram can be used to measure the size of the left atrium and document the presence of thrombus formation.

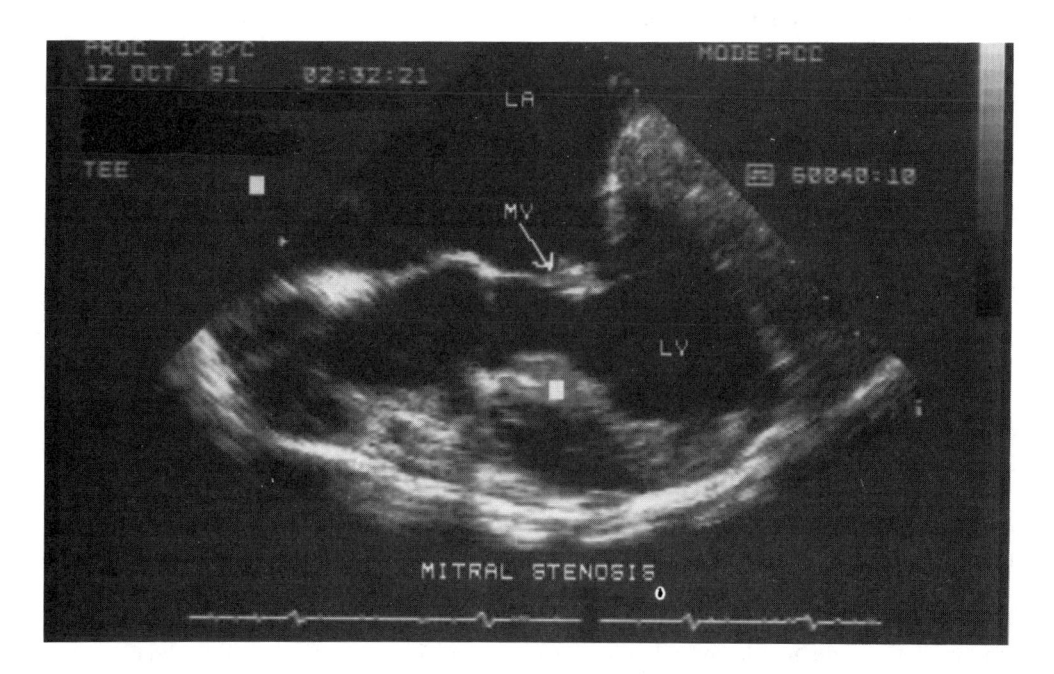

Fig. 7-6. Mitral stenosis as seen by transesophageal echocardiography. Note the thickened anterior leaflet and the abnormally small opening during diastole.

Left atrial dimensions in patients with mitral valve disease correlate with rhythm and embolic phenomena, so that patients with larger atria have a higher incidence of these complications [47]. Echocardiography in MS may also reveal paradoxical septal motion due to more rapid filling of the RV as compared to the LV in early diastole [48]. The use of TEE is becoming more common in the operating room. Today's devices combine various echo modalities with color-flow Doppler and are excellent tools for assessing the hemodynamic state of the critically ill patient with MS. Their only drawback is that a fair amount of experience is required on the part of the clinician to accurately interpret the information and translate it into appropriate clinical decisions. Figure 7-6 shows the appearance of MS using TEE.

Angiography in Mitral Stenosis

Echocardiography often offers sufficient information about the mitral valve and ventricular function so that angiography is often not required. Exceptions would include patients in whom symptoms suggest the presence of coexisting CAD, or in whom dyspnea seems to be more severe than that explained by the valve lesion. In the latter case measurement of PVR is important, especially if the coronary arteries are free of disease and pulmonary function tests do not explain the symptoms. Finally, in patients with severe dyspnea unexplained by MS, coronary disease, or pulmonary disease, consideration should be given to studying the pulmonary arteries angiographically, especially if signs or symptoms suggest the presence of pulmonary emboli. Any patient catheterized for MS should have his or her PVR calculated during the procedure. It is important to note that if the gradient across the mitral valve is less than 5 mm Hg there may be significant error in calculation of the mitral valve area (MVA).

The normal mitral valve area is between 4 and 6 cm^2. The severity of mitral stenosis can be defined by the MVA, and general guidelines for expected hemodynamic findings can be made. Mild disease is defined as an area between 1.5 and 2.5 cm^2. At rest these patients will have normal values for left atrial (LA) pressure, PA pressure, and cardiac output (CO), while all three will increase with exertion. Moderate MS is defined as a mitral valve area between 1.1 and 1.5 cm^2. At rest these patients will have elevations of LA and PA pressures, but cardiac output will remain normal. With exertion, LA and PA pressures will increase further than baseline, and cardiac output will increase as well. Severe MS is defined by a mitral valve area of 0.6 to 1.0 cm^2. Left atrial pressure will be increased at rest, and PA pressure will be increased moderately or severely. These patients usually manifest a decrease in cardiac output with exertion, and this decrease may be severe [11].

Still, many variations of hemodynamic parameters occur in patients with MS. In some patients with valve orifices as small as 1.0 to 1.5 cm^2, cardiac output may be normal at rest and may elevate normally with exercise. However, such patients display prominent increases in left atrial and pulmonary capillary pressures. Therefore, with exercise there will be a large transvalvular gradient that will produce pulmonary congestion. If CO does increase in patients with severe MS during exercise, they usually have only minimal elevations of cardiac output. This results in a lower pulmonary venous pressure and fewer symptoms of pulmonary congestion than would be present if the output increased normally. Calculation of the valve area is necessary to document the severity of disease in these patients. When the valve area is less than 1 cm^2, cardiac output is usually decreased at rest and fails to rise during exercise, especially if PVR is increased. These patients usually complain of weakness and fatigue even at rest, symptoms that are explained by their decreased cardiac output.

Preoperative Evaluation

The history and physical examination will help identify those patients with significant lesions. Exercise tolerance, such as the ability to engage in vigorous physical activity, quite reliably rules out the presence of significant mitral stenosis. Clinical judgment is required for those patients with a decrease in exercise tolerance or vague symptoms such as mild fatigue or dyspnea. Although such a history combined with the murmur suggests the necessity of a preoperative echocardiogram, the murmur is not always easy to hear and auscultation for this lesion should take place in a quiet area. It is important to realize that the presence of symptoms such as dyspnea or fatigue does not necessarily mean that the contractility of the ventricle is compromised. Altered loading conditions or tachycardia may result in pulmonary edema even with normal ventricular function, and 25 percent of patients with MS will have a decreased ejection fraction, likely due to decreased preload and increased afterload [22], which may result in fatigue. Still, most patients with MS will manifest an increased ejection fraction and decreased end systolic volume during physical exercise [49]. Hemodynamic studies in patients with MS may be particularly helpful when obtained during exercise. Due to the associated increase in flow across the mitral valve and the decrease in time spent in diastole, the pressure gradient across the valve increases, resulting in symptoms of pulmonary congestion. Even patients with mild MS may manifest enough increase in left atrial pressure with exercise to cause symptoms.

Evidence of cor pulmonale on the preoperative electrocardiogram as well as abnormal values on arterial blood gases may warn of the presence of pulmonary hypertension. In patients in whom severe symptoms raise doubts about their ability to withstand the perioperative period, angiography or pulmonary artery catheterization, or both, with measurement of hemodynamic parameters, may be helpful in deciding if the patient will tolerate the stress of the perioperative period. Some patients with cor pulmonale due to hypoxemia may manifest a reduction in their PA pressures with chronic oxygen therapy, and such treatment should be considered in preparing patients with cor pulmonale for elective surgery.

Patients who have mild or moderate MS with normal pulmonary vascular resistance will have PA pressures that are normal or only minimally increased at rest. Still, even those with normal PA pressures at rest may have them increase with exercise, resulting in dyspnea on exertion. Patients with significantly elevated PVR or severe MS will have increased PA pressures at rest, with further increases of left atrial and PA pressures occurring with exercise or increased heart rates. Right ventricular failure may ensue when PA systolic pressures exceed 70 mm Hg [33]. This will be manifested as elevated right ventricular end diastolic and right atrial pressures on right heart catheterization. These patients are likely to have signs of right-sided heart failure such as jugular venous distention, peripheral edema, and hepatomegaly, which are important to recognize preoperatively.

If the history, physical examination, and routine

studies do not provide an adequate assessment of the patient with MS, echocardiography will offer information about both the mitral valve area and ventricular function. When deemed necessary, angiography can also be performed to assess the presence and severity of any CAD.

Monitoring the Patient with Mitral Stenosis

Patients with mild MS who offer a history of good exercise tolerance usually are adequately monitored with a Foley catheter. Patients with moderate disease or those with decreased exercise tolerance should probably be monitored with an arterial line and at least a central venous catheter, since tachycardia may cause a precipitous rise in left atrial pressure in these patients. If they have severe stenosis, a PA catheter will be helpful. The arterial line will be useful to assess the hemodynamic consequences of arrhythmias and to detect the development of an increased A-a gradient. The central venous pressure (CVP) may reflect an increase in right-sided pressures transmitted from the left side of the heart via the pulmonary circulation. For patients with severe MS or moderate MS with known decreased ventricular function, a pulmonary artery catheter will be very helpful for perioperative management. If a patient with less severe MS develops pulmonary edema or borderline blood pressure, or both, intraoperatively, a PA catheter should be inserted at that time. One finding that is frequently noted on the CVP tracing of patients with MS is an increased A wave. This represents increased diastolic flow during atrial contraction and displays the importance of the atrial kick in maintaining ventricular preload. It is usually assumed that pulmonary capillary wedge pressure (PCWP) reflects left atrial pressure. This may not be the case in patients with MS and even greater error may be introduced if the patient has chronic pulmonary hypertension. As a rule, the PCWP will underestimate left ventricular end diastolic pressure and therefore filling pressure and volume in patients with MS. Though left ventricular end diastolic volume is normal in many patients with MS, it will be reduced in those with severe stenosis. This may suggest the need to administer fluid to a hypotensive patient with MS despite an "elevated" PCWP. In some patients with MS, especially those with high PA pressures (PAP), it may be difficult to wedge the catheter at all. To be sure a proper wedge is being measured, the mean PCWP should be less than the mean PAP and blood drawn from the wedged position should be at least 95 percent saturated with oxygen, or equal to the saturation of the arterial blood. This confirms that the tip of the catheter is wedged because these measurements assure that blood has been drawn from the left side of the heart. The PA catheter may have to be passed further in patients with pulmonary hypertension than in normal patients to obtain the wedge position, a difference noted to be approximately 5 cm via the right internal jugular approach [50]. Great care should be taken to monitor for inadvertent maintenance of the wedge position, as patients with pulmonary hypertension probably have a greater risk than the general population for catheter-induced pulmonary artery perforation and rupture [50–52].

Hemodynamic Goals and Intraoperative Concerns

The most important concept to bear in mind when caring for a patient with mitral stenosis is the avoidance of tachycardia since it produces two problems. Diastolic filling time is important in order to maintain left ventricular preload. Tachycardia results in decreased diastolic filling, and therefore stroke volume and blood pressure will decrease. Second, tachycardia will cause left atrial pressure to rise and place the patient at risk for development of pulmonary edema. Tachycardia can therefore paradoxically result in the simultaneous occurrence of a decrease in LV preload and pulmonary edema. Assuming the heart rate is controlled, it is also important to maintain intravascular volume in patients with MS, as they require some elevation of left atrial pressure in order to maintain filling across the stenotic valve. Finally, care should be taken to avoid maneuvers that would increase PAP. It is often suggested that afterload should be maintained normally. However, some patients with MS have a chronically elevated systemic vascular resistance (SVR), and decreasing this abnormally high resistance may result in sudden hypotension. It is best to avoid depression of myocardial contractility, as some patients with severe stenosis will be dependent on contractility to maintain cardiac output. Patients with MS usually do well with heart rates (HR) between 70 and 90 beats per minute.

Heart rates above this should be controlled pharmacologically. Despite these recommendations a rare patient will decompensate with a slow heart rate and improve with a faster heart rate. This may be due to an increase in CO associated with the increase in HR, or perhaps the patient improves because of the presence of coincident mitral regurgitation. If PVR is critically elevated and RV systolic function is poor, decreasing PVR will help increase RV cardiac output. This must be done carefully, as essentially all the agents used to decrease PVR (i.e., nitroglycerin, nitroprusside, amrinone, prostaglandin E_1, tolazoline, etc.) will cause some degree of systemic vasodilation as well. Inhaled nitric oxide, a new agent undergoing research trials, may be the exception, that is, it may decrease PVR while not significantly lowering systemic blood pressure. It is also important in patients with MS to avoid maneuvers that will increase PVR, that is, avoid hypoxia, hypercarbia, and acidosis. Hemodynamic goals for the patient with mitral stenosis are summarized in Table 7-5.

A defibrillator should be available and prepared for all patients with MS who are brought to the operating room, due to their propensity for development of supraventricular arrhythmias. All routine monitors should be in place. The decision to use more invasive monitors, such as an arterial line, central venous catheter, or pulmonary artery catheter, should be based on information obtained from the preoperative evaluation.

Patients with pure MS have increased pressures proximal, but not distal, to the valve, so that LVEDP is usually not significantly elevated. However, as discussed earlier (see Table 7-1), patients with MS may have an elevated LVEDP due to the presence of other disease processes. Subendocardial perfusion is dependent on coronary perfusion pressure. Since patients with moderate to severe MS frequently have decreased blood pressure, if they also have an elevated LVEDP they are at risk for decreased coronary perfusion. Patients with significant MS and coronary artery disease are therefore at increased risk of developing myocardial ischemia and should be carefully monitored in the perioperative period.

In an occasional patient with MS who is in normal sinus rhythm, a supraventricular arrhythmia will develop for the first time in the perioperative period. If the patient is hemodynamically unstable, synchronous cardioversion should be performed. A short run of supraventricular tachycardia should not place the patient at risk for thrombus formation. However, an occasional patient will present for surgery who recently developed new-onset, hemodynamically stable atrial fibrillation that reverted to sinus rhythm, either spontaneously or secondary to pharmacologic therapy or cardioversion. Alternatively, the patient may offer a history of atrial fibrillation in the more distant past. If the patient was in atrial fibrillation for a significant amount of time, the possibility of thrombus formation exists, and if such a patient presented to the operating room in sinus rhythm and developed a perioperative supraventricular tachycardia that required cardioversion due to hemodynamic instability, the attendant risk of embolization should be appreciated. Although there is no specific known amount of time, once a patient has been in atrial fibrillation for 24 to 48 hours, there is concern that thrombus formation may have occurred and may result in an embolic event during cardioversion. This is important to remember if a patient who is cardioverted intraoperatively does not awaken appropriately. Obviously, in an emergent perioperative setting, the luxury of anticoagulating the patient before proceeding with cardioversion does not exist.

Use of Pharmacologic Therapy

Anesthetic management is based on maintaining the hemodynamic goals described previously, and a variety of anesthetic agents are available that will permit one to do so. However, in patients with moderate or severe MS anesthetic agents alone

Table 7-5. Hemodynamic goals for the patient with mitral stenosis

---

Maintain adequate preload

Maintain the heart rate between 70 and 90 beats per minute

Maintain afterload in the normal range (SVR may need to be maintained elevated in those with chronic elevation of the SVR)

Do not depress myocardial contractility

In critically ill patients monitor SVR and PVR and adjust accordingly

---

may be unable to maintain hemodynamic parameters as preferred. It is therefore often necessary for the anesthesiologist to administer nonanesthetic pharmacologic therapy, that is, with β-blockers, vasodilators, inotropes, and so forth. Pharmacologic agents used in patients with MS are usually limited to those that slow the heart rate or decrease PAPs. The importance of slowing the heart rate has been discussed previously. Although propranolol has been the classic agent used, esmolol may be particularly suited to emergent situations, as its short half-life makes it easy to titrate. When a stable state has been achieved, a continuous infusion can be begun. Calcium channel blockers or digitalis preparations can be used as well.

Even early in the disease, an exponential rise in transmitral gradient occurs when cardiac output or heart rate increases, such as is seen in patients with fever, stress, or hyperthyroidism. The use of propranolol to decrease heart rate and cardiac output in patients with mild MS with normal sinus rhythm results in an improvement in symptoms, which at this stage are due to left atrial and pulmonary venous hypertension [53]. Meister and associates [53] documented decreases in mitral diastolic gradient, pulmonary wedge pressure, and pulmonary artery pressure in patients with pure MS treated with propranolol.

Nitroprusside is a good choice to control systemic and pulmonary artery pressures in patients with mitral stenosis. However, cardiac index may increase only when severe pulmonary hypertension or some mitral regurgitation, or both, are present. Still, in some patients with severe pulmonary hypertension and mitral stenosis nitroprusside may increase cardiac index remarkably [54]. The importance of replacing preload in patients placed on vasodilators must be stressed, and in a study by Stone and associates [55], patients who arrived in the operating suite with high systemic vascular resistance and borderline cardiac indices were markedly improved by the combination of nitroprusside and crystalloid infusion. Decreasing pulmonary vascular resistance with nitroprusside may be beneficial in these patients, as decreased RV afterload will result in improved LV preload [54]. Increased wedge pressures in patients with poor ventricular function and MS will be decreased by nitroprusside, which may be useful in those patients in whom increases in afterload can be detrimental to cardiac output. However, unless pulmonary hypertension or gross LV failure [26] exists, afterload reduction with nitroprusside in patients with isolated MS does not necessarily result in a significant increase in cardiac index or decrease in wedge pressure. Lack of an increase in cardiac index in some patients with MS may be explained by the fact that the limiting factor in cardiac output is preload, which is being limited by the MS.

Pulmonary vascular resistance may decrease significantly more in patients treated with amrinone than in those treated with nitroprusside [56]. In patients with mitral stenosis and pulmonary hypertension, amrinone may be particularly effective in decreasing PAPs [57]; however, the same requirement to maintain preload exists as with nitroprusside. The main problem encountered with the use of amrinone is the associated decrease in SVR. We sometimes use a simultaneous infusion of norepinephrine to maintain SVR and systemic blood pressure while administering amrinone. Norepinephrine used in this manner must be carefully titrated, as an inadvertent increase in the dose administered to a patient with severe MS can precipitate florid pulmonary edema.

Anesthetic Management

Since hypercarbia, hypoxia, and acidosis may elevate pulmonary vascular resistance, premedication must be used cautiously in patients with MS. Although morphine sulfate, 0.05 to 0.1 mg/kg intramuscularly, with scopolamine, 0.004 mg/kg IM, will usually provide acceptable premedication, in those patients who are critically ill, 1 or 2 mg morphine sulfate IM may be all the premedication that will be tolerated. Other alternatives include diazepam, 0.035 mg/kg by mouth, or midazolam, 0.03 mg/kg IM. It is imperative that all patients with MS receive oxygen from the time of their premedication until arrival in the operating room. While we prefer to err on the side of minimal premedication, as soon as an intravenous line is placed we administer additional sedation for placement of invasive monitors, as this may be painful or cause anxiety, both of which could result in a deleterious tachycardia. If ventilatory difficulties do ensue at that time, at least it is under the supervision of the anesthesiologist and not during transfer to the operating suite. When placing invasive monitoring lines, consideration should be given to minimizing the Trendelenburg position, as it may precipitate pulmonary edema.

Reductions in SVR due to anesthetic agents may cause sudden and severe hypotension in patients with MS. Alternatively, vasoconstriction may result in dangerous increases in SVR and PAP. At first glance one might consider the use of ephedrine to treat hypotension, as it offers both increased inotropy and pulmonary vasodilation via its β-agonist effects. Still, hypotension in patients with MS is probably best treated with phenylephrine, as the beta effects of ephedrine may result in a deleterious elevation of heart rate. Phenylephrine may raise the PAPs and the increased afterload may compromise forward cardiac output [57]. Still, phenylephrine is likely to maintain or slow the heart rate, and when used in small increments it is usually tolerated for maintenance of blood pressure that has decreased due to an anesthetic-induced reduction in SVR. Light anesthesia may lead to increases in systemic and pulmonary artery pressures, as well as tachycardia, and should be avoided. If a patient with MS develops severe tachycardia intraoperatively, such as that due to a supraventricular tachycardia, and blood pressure is compromised, he or she should be synchronously cardioverted.

Anticholinergic agents may result in hemodynamic compromise due to reductions in diastolic filling time and some prefer to avoid them. However, if their use is judged to be warranted, as, for example, before a fiberoptic intubation, scopolamine or glycopyrrolate should be chosen, as they have less of a chronotropic effect than atropine.

Severe increases in PA pressures can limit filling of the left side of the heart and result in systemic hypotension. Right ventricular failure may ensue as well. Although several agents are available to reduce PA pressure, they have some systemic vasodilating effect and therefore compromise systemic blood pressure as well. These agents include nitroglycerin, nitroprusside, amrinone, prostaglandin E_1, and tolazoline. A new agent, nitric oxide, which is administered by inhalation, is showing significant promise as a selective pulmonary vasodilator and may offer a true advance in the management of these patients [58].

General Anesthesia in the Patient with Mitral Stenosis

Inhalation Anesthetics. The volatile inhalational agents are likely to be tolerated in patients with mild MS. They will probably also be tolerated in patients with moderate disease as long as the heart rate does not increase. For this reason it may be best to avoid isoflurane in these patients. For increases in heart rate associated with surgical stimulation, small doses of halothane or enflurane could be used to deepen the anesthetic and help slow the heart rate.

Nitrous Oxide. The use of nitrous oxide may be risky in patients with mitral stenosis. Hilgenberg and associates [59] studied 11 patients scheduled for elective mitral valve replacement (MVR). The patients were premedicated with morphine and scopolamine. Compared with awake control measurements while breathing 50 percent oxygen in nitrogen, HR, cardiac index (CI), systemic and pulmonary pressures, SVR, and systolic blood pressure remained unchanged after administration of 50 percent nitrous oxide for 10 minutes. The only significant change was an increase in PVR from 159 dynes/sec/cm^5 before nitrous oxide inhalation to 213 dynes/sec/cm^5 during nitrous oxide inhalation. Nitrous oxide increases PVR in patients with preexisting pulmonary hypertension. In this study this increase was not associated with alterations in other measured or calculated hemodynamic variables. Although these authors concluded that it may not be necessary to avoid nitrous oxide in these patients, in patients with moderate or severe mitral stenosis or known pulmonary hypertension, it may be preferable to limit the use of nitrous oxide to those who have a PA catheter in place. If the PA pressure does rise, it usually returns to normal shortly after the nitrous oxide is discontinued.

Narcotics. Opioids are associated with bradycardia due to a central vagotonic effect [60] and they blunt the sympathetic responses associated with intubation and surgery. They are therefore useful agents for patients with mitral stenosis. However, in patients who are critically ill, increased afterload may be supporting blood pressure, and decreased sympathetic tone secondary to narcotics may precipitate hypotension. This is more likely to occur with sufentanil than with other opioids. It may be best to initially titrate opioids in small doses until the patient's response to their administration is evaluated.

Barbiturates. The primary hemodynamic effect of barbiturates is venodilation [61]. Since patients with MS require increased preload to maintain filling, barbiturates may result in a significant decrease in stroke volume. Barbiturates can also cause an increase in heart rate when blood pressure decreases, due to the baroreceptor reflex. This can further elevate left atrial pressure and be deleterious in the patient with MS. Still, patients with mild or moderate disease will usually tolerate barbiturates quite well. However, they probably should be avoided in patients with severe MS.

Nonbarbiturate Intravenous Anesthetics. Benzodiazepines may depress myocardial contractility when combined with narcotics and they should likewise be carefully titrated in patients with critical disease. For patients with severe MS who present to the operating suite in hemodynamic distress, consideration should be given to avoiding both nitrous oxide and benzodiazepines. A good alternative is intravenous scopolamine, which will provide amnesia and, if titrated in small doses, is unlikely to elevate the heart rate. Ketamine should be avoided as the associated increase in heart rate will compromise ventricular filling. Although small doses of droperidol may be tolerated, it should be used cautiously in patients with severe disease, as α-blockade associated with its use may result in a precipitous drop in afterload and thereby produce hypotension.

Although small doses of propofol may be tolerated, it is not likely to be a good choice of primary anesthetic for patients with severe stenosis, as induction doses may decrease systolic blood pressure by as much as 40 percent [62]. This is due to a decrease in SVR as well as a direct myocardial depressant effect that decreases cardiac index [62]. Even maintenance doses may decrease blood pressure up to 30 percent and may not be tolerated in these patients. Interestingly, PCWP decreases, implying a decrease in preload as well [63].

Etomidate offers the advantage of hemodynamic stability. Induction with 0.3 mg/kg causes minimal changes in systemic blood pressure, pulmonary artery pressure, central venous pressure, PCWP, systemic vascular resistance, and cardiac index. A small increase in heart rate and decrease in PVR may occur [64]. Minimal hemodynamic changes have also been confirmed when an induction dose of 0.45 mg/kg was used [65]. Cardiovascular stability has also been noted during induction with etomidate and during maintenance as part of a balanced technique in patients with valvular heart disease [66].

Muscle Relaxants. Muscle relaxants are perhaps best chosen for patients with mitral stenosis based on their effects on heart rate. Vecuronium or pipecuronium is perhaps a better choice than pancuronium, which may increase heart rate as a result of its vagolytic effect, or atracurium, which may decrease blood pressure secondary to histamine release. Pipecuronium, a new long-acting, nondepolarizing neuromuscular blocking agent, is devoid of significant cardiovascular effects [67]. Doxacurium, another new long-acting, nondepolarizing agent, has been shown to be essentially devoid of cardiovascular effects in doses up to three times its ED95 [68]. For long procedures, doxacurium or pipecuronium may provide muscle relaxation for a period of time similar to that of pancuronium, but without the adverse hemodynamic effects. Succinylcholine can be used if preferred for rapid-sequence induction.

Regional Anesthesia in the Patient with Mitral Stenosis

Regional anesthesia presents a formidable problem in the patient with MS because it decreases both preload and afterload. Spinal anesthesia, with its attendant rapid decrease in sympathetic tone, can cause a sudden, severe decrease in stroke volume and therefore blood pressure. However, the technique may be useful when other considerations increase the risk of a general anesthetic. Performance of a saddle block, for example, may be acceptable if adequate preload is administered before the block is performed.

Epidural anesthesia can be used for patients with mild MS, but becomes more difficult to administer with more severe disease, due to hemodynamic considerations. However, in certain situations its use may be preferred. For example, an asthmatic patient who presents for an emergent appendectomy but is actively wheezing could be managed with an epidural anesthetic as long as preload is maintained. (Clearly, we would administer appropriate therapy for the patient's pulmonary disease.) This becomes more difficult to do with severe MS, as the administration of large amounts of fluid combined with the return of sympathetic tone as the anesthetic wears off, may precipitate pulmonary edema. The risks and benefits of the different anesthetics obviously need to be assessed on a case-by-case basis. In a situation of severe asthma, the ability to avoid manipulation of the airway may provide a safer anesthetic despite possible hemodynamic fluctuations secondary to the epidural anesthetic. One must remember that regional anesthesia does not obviate the need for invasive monitoring. On the contrary, accurate measurement of preload and SVR may be even more important when a spinal or epidural anesthetic is chosen.

Epidural analgesia is useful for control of pain in patients with MS as it prevents the increase in heart rate and SVR secondary to pain. Preload will need to be maintained during administration of an epidural local anesthetic. Low concentrations of anesthetics such as 0.1 percent bupivacaine (Marcaine) combined with fentanyl may provide adequate postoperative pain relief with minimal hemodynamic effect. Mitral stenosis is a common valvular lesion in parturients and epidural analgesia is useful during labor for the reasons described. Again, preload will need to be augmented before performance of the regional block. Epidural analgesia and anesthesia for the parturient with heart disease are discussed in Chap. 14.

Postoperative Concerns in the Patient with Mitral Stenosis

Postoperative concerns in the patient with MS are the same as those during the course of surgery. Adequate intravascular volume and prevention of tachycardia are important to maintain appropriate left ventricular and left atrial pressures and to ensure adequate cardiac output and tissue perfusion. The role of hypoxia and hypercarbia in the exacerbation of pulmonary hypertension makes it imperative to extubate after appropriate criteria have been met and to monitor these patients in the recovery room with pulse oximetry and end-tidal carbon dioxide. Changes in pulmonary vasculature that result in decreased lung compliance and increased work of breathing may place these patients at increased risk of postoperative pulmonary complications. Due to the increased work of breathing, mechanical ventilation may be required in the postoperative period. Patients with severe mitral stenosis can decompensate rapidly and if they undergo major surgery may warrant several days of close hemodynamic monitoring in an intensive care setting. Postoperative hypercarbia, hypoxemia, or pain may cause increases of systemic and/or pulmonary artery pressures or tachycardia, which may result in pulmonary edema or right-sided failure, or both. Epidural analgesia can be useful in these patients postoperatively for pain control as it may prevent tachycardia and will assist in coughing and deep breathing. However, the decreased systemic resistance may compromise the patient if preload is not adequately maintained. As noted previously, low concentrations of local anesthetic combined with narcotic may offer the patient adequate pain relief while avoiding significant sympathetic blockade.

Summary

While it may be difficult to document an increase in perioperative complications due to MS, numerous problems place these patients at risk. These include abnormalities of loading conditions and heart rhythm, the risk of pulmonary edema, and abnormalities of pulmonary function. Management of these problems requires preoperative evaluation in order to properly choose monitoring and anesthetic techniques that best serve these patients. Maintaining appropriate care through the postoperative period will help increase the likelihood that these patients will have a positive anesthetic experience.

MITRAL REGURGITATION
Epidemiology

Mitral regurgitation is most commonly due to rheumatic heart disease. It occurs more frequently in men than in women. It may be due to shortening and deformity of one or both cusps of the mitral valve or abnormalities of the papillary muscles or chordae tendineae. Though rheumatic disease may initially cause MS, when fusion and contraction of the chordae tendineae occur, MR results and is often worse than the stenosis, thereby producing a combined lesion. It is not uncommon for patients to have more than one valve involved as rheumatic disease affects all the valves. The mitral valve is most commonly affected, the aortic valve next most frequently, followed by the tricuspid and then the pulmonic valve. Other causes of mitral regurgitation are listed in Table 7-6 and include torn leaflets, annular dilatation, destruction of the valve ring as occurs with endocarditis or trauma, damage to supporting structures such as the chordae tendineae, or papillary muscle dysfunction, which is most commonly due to ischemia. It is interesting that patients with MR on an ischemic basis tend to have lower PVR than do those with rheumatic-based disease. Presumably, this is due to the shorter time course of the disease [69].

The mitral annulus circumference measures approximately 10 cm in the adult. Contraction of surrounding LV muscle during systole contributes to the seal the valve provides. Thus, significant dilatation of the ventricle on any basis may lead to regurgitation [70], although regurgitation on this basis tends to be less severe than that due to valvular disease [71]. Idiopathic calcification of the mitral valve annulus is usually of minimal functional significance [72]. However, when severe it can cause significant MR. This form of MR is more common in women than men. Calcification may impair opening in diastole as well as closure during systole, but MR is a much more frequent occurrence than MS. Still, with severe calcification, the diastolic effects may impair LV filling while the systolic effects may aggravate MR. Approximately half of the patients with severe mitral annular calcification will also have calcification of the aortic valve, but this does not usually lead to stenosis. Patients with severe mitral calcification may also have ventricular or atrioventricular impairment of conduction [73]. Calcium deposits may even extend into the coronary arteries and result in ischemic heart disease. Degenerative calcification of the mitral annulus may occur more rapidly in the presence of hypertension, aortic stenosis, diabetes, and chronic renal failure with secondary hyperparathyroidism [74].

Chordal rupture may be spontaneous secondary to a congenital abnormality, or may be due to rheumatic fever, endocarditis, trauma, or connective tissue abnormalities, such as those seen in myxomatous proliferation or osteogenesis imperfecta [71, 75, 76]. It may also occur as a result of chronic stress secondary to mitral valve prolapse [77]. In one large series mitral valve prolapse was the second most common cause of regurgitation, accounting for 25 percent of cases. Furthermore, when patients with isolated mitral regurgitation were considered, mitral valve prolapse was the most common cause of regurgitation, accounting for 38 percent of cases. Of the 31 patients operated on in this series, MVP was responsible for the regurgitation in 48 percent [78].

Ischemia of the papillary muscles is an important cause of MR. Although MR occurs in about 65 percent of patients suffering an acute myocardial infarction, severe MR due to ischemic rupture of a papillary muscle is quite rare. When it does occur, it usually happens 2 to 7 days after infarction. Usually, one or several heads of the muscle are disrupted, although occasionally an entire trunk will tear. Though silent ischemia usually occurs in patients with symptoms of angina, it should also be considered in a patient being evaluated for a new regurgitant murmur. Papillary muscle ischemia may fluctuate with myocardial oxygen balance so that regurgitation comes and goes related to episodes of ischemia. Tachycardia from any etiology may result in papillary muscle ischemia due to the increased myocardial oxygen demand, especially if underlying coronary insufficiency or significant LVH ex-

Table 7-6. Causes of mitral regurgitation

Mitral valve prolapse
Rheumatic heart disease
Dilation of mitral valve annulus (LV dilation)
Papillary muscle ischemia
Endocarditis
Trauma
Prosthetic valve malfunction
Systemic lupus erythematosus
Scleroderma
Calcification of the mitral valve annulus

ists. If papillary muscle ischemia persists, it may result in scarring and thereby cause chronic MR. The papillary muscles are particularly at risk for ischemia because the end arteries that perfuse them must first pass through the thickness of the ventricular wall. The posterior papillary muscle receives its oxygen supply from the posterior descending coronary artery, so that obstruction of the right coronary artery alone can cause posterior papillary muscle ischemia. It is therefore more prone to ischemia and infarction than the anterior papillary muscle, which is supplied by diagonal branches of the left anterior descending coronary artery as well as marginal branches of the circumflex coronary artery. For ischemia of the anterior papillary muscle to occur, usually both the left anterior descending and circumflex coronary arteries would need to be obstructed. Other causes of papillary muscle ischemia include severe anemia, shock, coronary arteritis, and an anomalous left coronary artery [71]. Mitral regurgitation is also a frequent occurrence in patients with healed infarcts when dyskinesis of the left ventricular myocardium is present at the base of a papillary muscle [71, 79]. In fact some amount of MR is present in one third of patients who undergo coronary bypass surgery. This is caused by papillary muscle damage secondary to ischemia or dilation of the valve ring, or both [80]. Table 7-6 lists the most common causes of mitral regurgitation.

Natural History

The natural history of MR varies greatly between patients. It depends on both the severity of the regurgitation and the underlying etiology. While patients with severe regurgitation due to destruction of the valve by endocarditis may rapidly become hemodynamically unstable, patients with mild MR secondary to rheumatic disease may be asymptomatic for many years. Regurgitation also tends to progress more quickly in patients with connective tissue disease than in patients with rheumatic heart disease [71]. In one study of patients with severe regurgitation who were not treated because surgical therapy was not yet common, about 80 percent survived 5 years beyond diagnosis and almost 60 percent of patients were alive 10 years after the diagnosis of MR was made [11]. However, among patients with combined MS and MR only one third were alive after 5 years and just 30 percent after 10 years. For patients with severe MR, fewer than half survive 5 years with medical therapy [81].

Pathophysiology

The pressure-volume loop of chronic mitral regurgitation shown in Fig. 7-7 displays the situation that occurs in patients with a compliant left atrium. It should be noted that LVEDP does not increase significantly until end diastolic volumes are significantly elevated. The right-sided portion of the curve is somewhat abolished because isovolumetric systole hardly exists, as regurgitation into the LA begins almost immediately with ventricular contraction.

In patients with MR left ventricular ejection can occur via two paths: the aortic valve or the mitral valve. The volume emptying into the left atrium depends on the resistance to forward ejection, and this is increased by high systemic resistance and especially the presence of aortic stenosis. The amount of regurgitation depends on both the size of the orifice and the pressure difference between the left atrium and ventricle. Since both of these are affected perioperatively, they can be adjusted pharmacologically by the anesthesiologist and can therefore affect patient outcome. Increased preload

Fig. 7-7. Pressure-volume loop of a patient with chronic mitral regurgitation. (Reprinted with permission from JM Jackson, SJ Thomas and E Lowenstein, Anesthetic management of patients with valvular heart disease. Semin Anesth 1:248, 1982.)

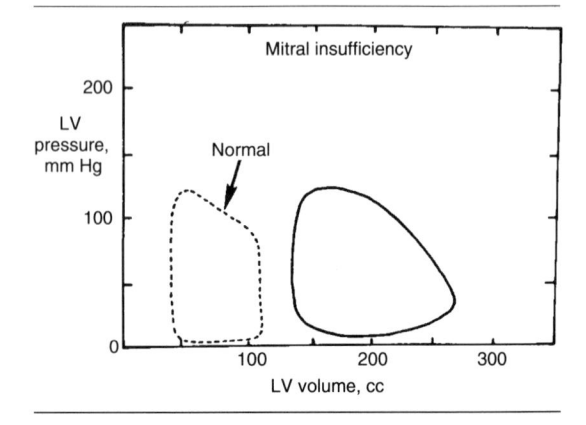

or afterload, or a reduction in contractility, can all result in left ventricular distention and enlargement of the mitral annulus, thereby increasing the regurgitant fraction [82]. Although the left ventricle may increase total output initially to compensate for acute MR [83], left ventricular end diastolic volume will eventually increase, with a concomitant increase in wall tension.

Radionuclide ventriculography documents total LV output to be increased until late in the disease process. Forward cardiac output is usually reduced in patients with significant symptoms [84], and it is only via increasing preload due to Starling's mechanism that these patients maintain adequate forward flow. As preload increases wall tension increases as does myocardial oxygen demand. The increased wall tension associated with longstanding mitral regurgitation may significantly compromise pump function. Although measures of myocardial contractility, such as ejection fraction, velocity of circumferential fiber shortening, and fractional fiber shortening, may be increased in MR, it should be understood that these often reflect measurements in compensated patients who have increased preload and decreased afterload [85]. The end systolic volume is a more useful preoperative indicator of outcome than end diastolic volume, end diastolic pressure, or ejection fraction, and predicted patients at high risk of perioperative cardiac death, with all such deaths occurring in patients with end systolic volumes greater than 60 ml/sq m [84, 86]. It may be difficult to apply data generated in patients undergoing mitral valve replacement to those undergoing noncardiac surgery, as the former group are stressed by a significant increase in afterload postrepair caused by the "competent" prosthetic valve.

Clinical symptoms and prognosis in MR are related to the compliance of the left atrium. Patients can be divided into one of three groups. Most commonly, compliance is moderately increased. These patients can function fairly well even in the face of chronic, severe MR. They have varying amounts of left atrial pressure elevation, which will be somewhat related to the increase in size of the chamber. The second group includes patients with normal or decreased left atrial compliance. These patients have minimal increase in left atrial dimensions. This results in marked elevation of mean left atrial pressure and therefore these patients tend to have symptoms of pulmonary congestion. They also tend to have significant increases of the V wave on the PCWP tracing. Many of these patients are those in whom MR occurred suddenly, such as that due to infarction of a papillary muscle or rupture of chordae tendineae. These patients "operate" in the steep area of the pressure-volume curve. When sinus rhythm is maintained, enlargement and hypertrophy of the atrium may allow contraction to significantly contribute to LV filling by permitting a larger increase in preload while preventing a severe rise in left atrial pressure [87]. However, despite these adaptive changes a toll is taken and with time thickening of the pulmonary veins and proliferative changes in the pulmonary vascular bed develop, often within a year, resulting in pulmonary hypertension. The third group of patients are those with longstanding MR who have a massive increase in left atrial size. Their left atrial pressure tends to be normal or only minimally increased. Pulmonary artery pressure and PVR are normal or only slightly increased. Atrial fibrillation and a decreased cardiac output are commonly present [88]. Most often, these patients tend to complain of weakness due to low cardiac output, rather than symptoms of congestive failure.

In patients with severe mitral regurgitation who have symptoms of decreased cardiac reserve or congestive heart failure, cardiac output is frequently below normal, mean left atrial pressure is elevated, and V waves are particularly tall [88]. In such patients the PA pressure is frequently increased proportionately more than left atrial pressure due to elevations of pulmonary vascular resistance. In this group of patients, clinical signs of right-sided heart failure are not uncommon [89, 90]. In several reported series, there have been one or two patients who manifested decreased cardiac reserve and left atrial enlargement, but who had LA or PCW pressures that were normal. It has been suggested that in some patients with chronic mitral regurgitation length tension characteristics of the left atrium may be altered so that it is more compliant [88].

Although patients with papillary muscle rupture require urgent mitral valve replacement and will almost never present for noncardiac surgery, this disease process represents a good model for acute MR and is discussed for the purpose of completeness.

Patients in whom rupture of the papillary muscle develops secondary to a myocardial infarction, are at risk of dying. Optimal therapy is surgical replacement of the mitral valve. As with MR of any etiology, an increase in systemic resistance will lower the cardiac index and raise the pulmonary capillary wedge pressure, thereby producing an A-a gradient. These patients require careful titration of the SVR in order to maintain forward flow [91]. Papillary muscle rupture with severe MR places an acute volume load on the LV and an acute pressure load on the RV, as the LA is unable to accommodate the acute increase in pressure and volume to which it is subjected. The results are LV failure, pulmonary edema, pulmonary hypertension, and right ventricular failure. Mitral regurgitation causes a decrease in LV afterload, but increases LV preload, with a reflex increase in both heart rate and contractility. An imbalance occurs because myocardial oxygen demand is increased by the tachycardia and increased preload, while at the same time oxygen delivery is curtailed by hypotension and to a small extent by hypoxemia. Patients with papillary muscle rupture frequently die secondary to left ventricular failure or infarction, or both [92], though death can also be caused by pulmonary edema or right ventricular failure.

History and Physical Examination

The symptoms in patients with MR depend not only on the severity of the lesion but also the PA pressure, and whether other valve lesions or associated coronary artery disease are present. In patients with chronic MR, symptoms often do not develop until the LV fails so that the time of symptom onset may be 20 years or more. Acute pulmonary edema is a less frequent occurrence than in MS and is probably due to a lower incidence of precipitous increases in left atrial pressure [38]. These patients tend to complain more of weakness or fatigue due to the decreased cardiac output. In fact patients with mild MR may be asymptomatic their entire life [93] unless regurgitation worsens as a result of rupture of chordae tendineae [94], papillary muscle ischemia, or endocarditis. Interestingly, patients with MR may report that they have less dyspnea with exertion. This is due to decreased SVR and tachycardia, which may accompany exercise; they decrease the regurgitant fraction and, therefore, mean left atrial pressure.

The murmur of isolated mitral regurgitation is systolic and best heard at the apex, with radiation to the axilla. An increase in intensity of the murmur with hand grip is consistent with MR. Alternatively, if cuffs are inflated on both upper or lower extremities, the severity of the murmur will increase if the underlying cause is MR. The murmur of MR is usually associated with a soft or absent S_1 and a loud S_3. The S_3 may be followed by a short diastolic rumble due to excessive flow across the valve, but this is a rare finding and is more commonly associated with MS. The compensatory chamber enlargement can often be felt by palpation as a gentle rocking motion, at the fifth or sixth left intercostal space between the midclavicular and anterior axillary lines. A thrill may be palpable at the apex. When examining patients with mitral valve disease, it is important to listen for findings consistent with other valvular lesions, since multiple-valve lesions may be present.

In patients with chronic severe MR with a very large LA and only minimal increases in left atrial pressure, clinical signs of right heart failure are often present. These include lower-extremity edema, distended neck veins, hepatomegaly, and ascites. These signs may also be seen in acute MR if the patient has elevated PVR.

In some patients with MR, severe or irreversible LV dysfunction may have occurred by the time symptoms develop, and they may represent too great a risk for the patient to undergo mitral valve replacement. These patients are very difficult to care for if they present for emergent noncardiac surgery. Frequently, signs and symptoms of both MR and congestive heart failure are present simultaneously and it may not be possible to determine which was the initial event.

The Chest X-ray in Mitral Regurgitation

Patients with chronic MR will usually have cardiomegaly on the chest x-ray, due to left ventricular enlargement. Left atrial enlargement is often present as well. However, since there may be no correlation between left atrial pressure and size, this finding does not necessarily add information beyond that found on physical examination. Although it is less common to find changes in the lung fields with MR than with MS, patients with acute MR or increasing left ventricular failure will often manifest interstitial edema or Kerley B lines, or both.

When patients have both MS and MR, it may be difficult to determine which is more significant, right or left ventricular enlargement. While it is not always possible to know which lesion is more significant by chest x-ray, MS is often manifested by milder cardiomegaly, with straightening of the left heart border consistent with left atrial enlargement and the presence of signs of pulmonary congestion. Alternatively, MR is suggested as the predominant lesion when severe cardiomegaly is present with minimal or no changes in the lung fields. Aneurysmal dilatation of the left atrium almost always indicates that chronic MR is the predominant lesion. Calcification of the mitral valve does not support any particular diagnosis, as it may occur in patients with regurgitation, stenosis, or both. In fact, it may be present in the elderly in the absence of significant valvular pathology.

The Electrocardiogram in Mitral Regurgitation

There are no specific findings on electrocardiography that make the diagnosis of MR, but there are particular findings that may relate to the etiology of the MR. If the MR has occurred as a result of ischemic heart disease, ST segment changes or Q waves secondary to infarction may be present. If MR has occurred secondary to dilation of the left ventricle, criteria for LVH may be met. Since chronic MR results in left atrial enlargement as well, the size of the P waves in lead V_1 may be increased [95]. If the patient's underlying rhythm is atrial fibrillation, a coarse fibrillatory pattern suggests the presence of left atrial enlargement [96].

The Echocardiogram in Mitral Regurgitation

M-mode echocardiography in the patient with MR may reveal left atrial enlargement and, since there is not a strong sustained flow of blood antegrade into the aorta, gradual closure of the aortic valve during systole. The interventricular septum moves abnormally as well [97]. Downward diastolic motion of the aorta in diastole may occur earlier than usual [98]. There is a significant decrease in left ventricular diameter in the preejection period because the incompetent valve essentially prevents the occurrence of the isovolumetric phase of contraction [99], a finding that is confirmed by loss of the isovolumetric contraction phase, as seen on the pressure-volume loop for MR shown in Fig. 7-7.

Transesophageal echocardiography can assess the distance the jet travels past the valve orifice as well as the width of the jet, as seen in Fig. 7-8. The etiology of the MR can be seen as well, such as the torn chordae depicted in Fig. 7-9. Occasionally, catheter-induced mitral regurgitation will be seen on angiography. TEE is useful in this setting as it can confirm normal valve function or the presence of MR. It is important to note that a small amount of "functional" regurgitation may be a normal finding. Pulsed Doppler echocardiography can detect high-velocity turbulent flow in the left atrium [100, 101], as well as systolic flow reversal in the pulmonary veins in patients with MR. However, systolic flow reversal may be seen in patients with MS who are in sinus rhythm and therefore is not a reliable criterion for MR in this setting. Echocardiography may also be useful in defining papillary muscle dysfunction [102].

Mitral regurgitation may occur in patients who have had mechanical or porcine prosthetic valve replacements, and echocardiography is useful to detect both regurgitation through the valve orifice and paravalvular leak. Doppler echocardiography is probably the best technique to detect regurgitation in a patient with a prosthetic valve [103]. In addition to a regurgitant jet, echocardiography may also detect dehiscence of the valve or a rocking motion that takes the valve past its normal excursion. Alternatively, volume overload of the left ventricle may be a sign of regurgitation in a patient with a prosthetic valve.

Patients with endocarditis who have vegetations detected by echocardiography are at risk of embolization, congestive heart failure, and death. However, patients with aortic vegetations seem to be at a higher risk, as Buda and associates [104] reported in a study in which all patients with mitral vegetations survived, whereas five with aortic vegetations died [104].

Angiography in Mitral Regurgitation

Hemodynamic performance in patients with chronic, severe MR may be reported as normal by

152 The Adult Patient

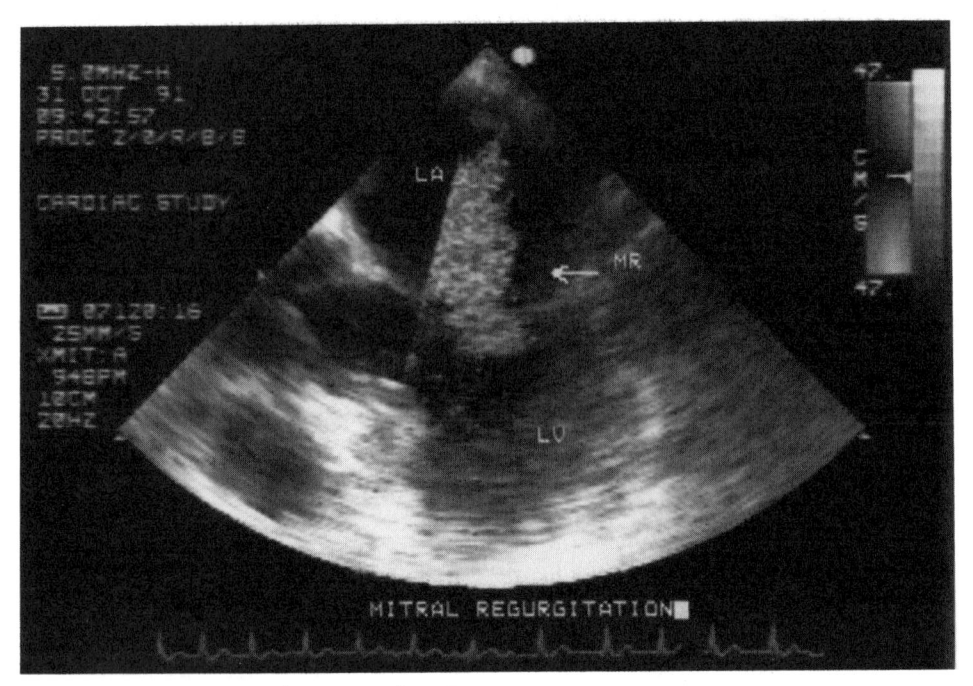

Fig. 7-8. Mitral regurgitation as seen by transesophageal echocardiography.

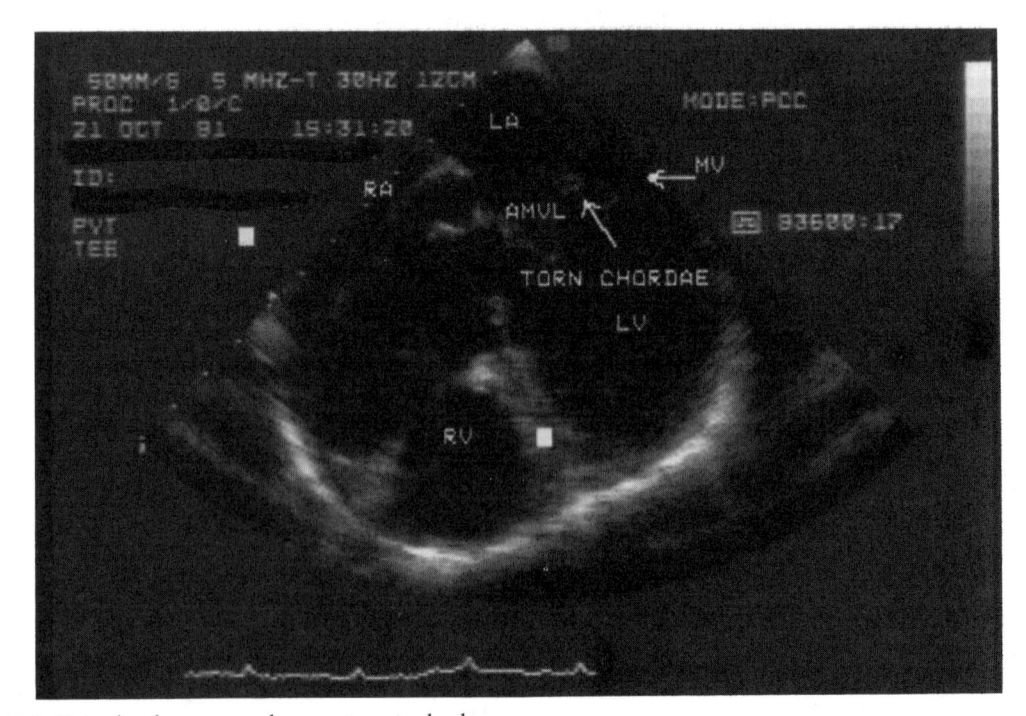

Fig. 7-9. Torn chordae seen on the anterior mitral valve leaflet are the cause of mitral regurgitation in this patient.

noninvasive assessment of ejection fraction (EF). Similarly, angiography may report preserved contractility. Factors that may account for this include increased end diastolic volume (EDV) and decreased afterload. Although patients with chronic, severe MR begin LV contraction with augmented EDV, their end systolic volume (ESV) is unusually large, suggesting that a normal EF in these patients does not indicate normal contractility [105]. Angiography detects MR by showing the appearance of contrast in the left atrium almost immediately after it is injected into the left ventricle. The regurgitant volume can be calculated as the difference between total stroke volume and Fick determination of effective forward stroke volume. Mitral regurgitation due to rheumatic disease usually manifests a centrally placed regurgitant jet and thickened leaflets with decreased motion. In contrast, in MR due to ruptured chordae or papillary muscles, or calcification or dilatation of the annulus, the jet may not be centered and the valves may be seen as thinned structures with increased motion. This pathophysiology may be confirmed by TEE.

Angiography in patients with MR is performed to assess the severity of regurgitation, left ventricular function, and the extent of any coronary disease. Assessment of mitral regurgitation by angiography can be made qualitatively on a scale of 1+ to 4+, or quantitatively by calculating regurgitant fraction. It should be understood that calculation of the regurgitant fraction depends on measurement of an average beat. The information derived may be particularly inaccurate if the patient is in atrial fibrillation. Accuracy is improved by measuring and averaging several beats. To some extent the actual regurgitant flow in liters will correlate with the 1+ to 4+ classification [106]. This qualitative assessment is determined by the amount of opacification of the left atrium due to regurgitation of dye through the insufficient mitral valve. 1+ (mild) regurgitation is noted when the atrium clears with each beat and never becomes fully opaque. 2+ regurgitation (moderate) does not clear with one beat yet faintly opacifies the whole atrium after several beats. With 2+ regurgitation the left atrium appears less opaque than the left ventricle. 3+ regurgitation (moderately severe) is noted when the left atrium becomes completely opacified and is just as opaque as the left ventricle. 4+ regurgitation (severe) describes the occurrence of left atrial opacification within one beat. The opacification intensifies with each beat, and during ventricular systole, contrast is noted to reflux into the pulmonary veins [107].

It is important in all patients with mitral valve disease to measure right atrial pressure to help rule out right ventricular failure, to measure PA pressure to rule out pulmonary hypertension, and to examine the wedge tracing for the presence of a significant V wave. Left heart catheterization should measure gradients across the mitral and aortic valves. In addition, measurement of LVEDP is important, as in the presence of MR it is usually much less than LA or mean PCWP. A nitroprusside infusion can be used to measure cardiac output with a lower afterload. Total stroke volume will not change, but with lower aortic impedance forward stroke volume may increase and regurgitant stroke volume will decrease by the same amount [107].

Preoperative Evaluation

Some patients with MR are not easily fatigued but may complain of dyspnea on exertion. This may be due to volume overload of the left ventricle and may be better detected with exercise. Many of these patients will be unable to increase forward cardiac output. Alternatively, some patients will increase cardiac output normally, but at the expense of a large increase in PCWP and the development of large V waves on the pulmonary capillary wedge tracing. Exercise angiography is especially helpful in those patients who are comfortable at rest but are dyspneic or weak with exertion. If the cardiac output with exercise increases less than 80 percent of predicted, it is likely that the symptoms are cardiac in origin. In addition, the wedge pressure will usually increase to 35 mm Hg or greater within 4 to 5 minutes of exercise if cardiac pathology accounts for the dyspnea [107]. Interestingly, some patients with MR will report less dyspnea with exertion than at rest, perhaps due to the associated reduction in SVR and increase in heart rate.

Patients with MR may appear to offer a confusing history as they may be severely symptomatic yet have normal indices of contractility. It should be understood that such patients are severely ill and, if presenting for noncardiac surgery, should undergo invasive monitoring despite documentation of "normal" contractility studies. In addition, patients in obvious congestive failure may have only slightly reduced indices of contractility [85, 108]. These misleading values may be due to the fact that contractility indices are extremely sensitive to afterload at the time of assessment [109]. Finally, it should be appreciated that while an ejection fraction of 40 or 50 percent probably represents some amount of myocardial dysfunction in patients with MR, an EF less than 40 percent is consistent with severe myocardial dysfunction and these patients are at increased perioperative risk [110]. This is because calculation of ejection fraction does not take into account the fact that a significant portion of the stroke volume that exits the ventricle does so retrograde into the low-pressure left atrium (as compared to the aorta).

Preoperative contractile performance of left ventricular myocardium can be assessed by end systolic volume. Since impairment of the myocardium may be present despite overall good cardiac performance, preoperative evaluation of myocardial contractility is helpful, especially in chronically overloaded ventricles such as occur with mitral regurgitation. In these patients increases of PCWP and depression of forward cardiac output usually occur as late consequences of left ventricular failure [111, 112]. This is because increases in left ventricular end diastolic pressure and volume are dependent on ventricular compliance, the degree of regurgitation, and myocardial function, and, therefore, LVEDP may not accurately reflect the contractile state of the myocardium [113, 114]. In addition, the ejection fraction, augmented by the markedly increased preload delivered to the ventricle, may remain normal despite significant left ventricular dysfunction [105]. Preoperative end systolic volume may predict those patients at high risk for perioperative cardiac mortality because it depends on the contractile state of the ventricle and not preload [86]. It is important to remember that in patients with mitral regurgitation the presence or absence of symptoms may not correlate with the severity of the disease process [115]. Nevertheless, patients with significant symptoms should probably be monitored invasively despite a "normal" ejection fraction.

The question of associated CAD in patients with mitral valve disease is an important one. Many of these patients complain of palpitations and, not infrequently, chest pain. The pain is sometimes of an atypical nature but should not be disregarded. Baxter and associates [116] reported that 33 percent of patients with mitral valve disease were believed to have angina, and of those who had angina and mitral valve disease 67 percent had significant CAD, which was defined as reduction of the lumen of a coronary vessel by more than 50 percent.

Monitoring the Patient with Mitral Regurgitation

Patients with mild disease and a good exercise tolerance probably do not require any additional monitors other than those necessary for the surgical procedure. For patients with mild symptoms, a central venous catheter is probably sufficient. However, any large increase in CVP should be considered as possibly reflecting an increase in left atrial pressure and therefore insertion of a pulmonary artery catheter should be considered at that time. Finally, for those patients with poor exercise tolerance, easy fatigability, or a history of congestive failure, a PA catheter should be inserted, except perhaps for short simple procedures.

The A wave of atrial contraction in the left atrial pressure tracing is large, though not as prominent as in MS. The V wave is often much taller in MR than in MS because it occurs during systole at a time when the left atrium is filled with blood from the pulmonary veins antegrade as well as the left ventricle retrograde. Patients with pure MR will have a rapid y descent in early diastole because the distended left atrium empties suddenly.

Interpretation of the PA values must be based on understanding the pathophysiology of the lesion. Because the PA pressure will usually be greater than the LA pressure, especially if pulmonary hypertension exists, one should not rush to treat elevations of the PA pressure. It is helpful to know whether the patient with MR has a large V wave in the wedge pressure tracing. The V wave that is present in both the left atrial and PCWP tracings represents filling of the left atrium during left ventricular systole, when the mitral valve is closed. A small V wave is normal, is seen in all patients, and is associated with filling of the left atrium from the pulmonary veins during systole. Giant V waves, the peak of which is more than twice the mean wedge pressure, may be seen in patients with acute mitral regurgitation who have steep pressure-volume curves due to the noncompliant left atrium, which has had no time to dilate [117]. Some patients with MS will have a noncompliant atrium and will manifest a V wave. Decreased compliance of the myocardium may also result in production of a V wave in the PCWP tracing. Since ischemia can worsen compliance, a large V wave may represent ischemia in some patients in the absence of MR. Still, as a rule, a V wave more than twice mean left atrial or PCW pressure suggests the presence of MR, while a measurement three times LA or PCW pressure virtually confirms the diagnosis of severe MR [107]. Two situations occur in which severe MR may be present without a prominent V wave. First, if the left atrium has dilated slowly over a long period it may be highly compliant and a prominent V wave may be absent even in the presence of severe MR [118]. Secondly, the presence of a prominent V wave depends not only on the severity of regurgitation, but also on the direction and reversal of flow in the pulmonary veins, which may not always occur [119]. The severity of mitral regurgitation may be aggravated by an increase in afterload [120]. Therefore, if a patient's MR seems to be worsening intraoperatively, consideration should be given to decreasing afterload, perhaps by deepening the anesthetic. Measurement of the SVR before and after this is done and reassessment of the MR will help determine if an increased afterload contributed to the increased amount of regurgitation. As discussed previously, a V wave does not always signify regurgitation and Pichard and associates [121] have reported that the percentage of patients with large V waves who in fact have MR is approximately 63 percent [118]. Because the mitral valve lines up nicely with the Doppler beam, transesophageal echocardiography with color-flow Doppler may be a particularly useful tool to monitor the amount of MR on a beat-to-beat basis in the intraoperative setting.

Hemodynamic Goals

Decreasing the size of the regurgitant orifice will help maintain forward flow in patients with MR. This goal can be achieved by maintenance of a decreased preload and an increased heart rate. Patients with mitral regurgitation usually do well when the heart rate is a bit fast, usually 85 to 95 beats per minute, though some patients may have a smaller regurgitant fraction when the heart rate is even faster. When the ventricle is dilated, more regurgitation tends to occur. Therefore, the preload should be kept normal or on the low side. Nitroglycerin can be useful to accomplish this goal. The afterload should be kept on the low side as this will decrease the impedance to ejection and therefore promote forward flow. It is important not to impair contractility, as decreased ability to pump can result in ventricular distention and acute pulmonary edema. The PA usually is greater than the LA with MR, so that a pulmonary artery diastolic pressure (PAD) of 15 or 20 in a patient who is doing well does not necessarily indicate the need for diuretics or vasodilators. In this situation an arterial blood gas is often useful. If the A-a gradient is unchanged from a preoperative measurement, it offers reasonable evidence that pulmonary edema has not developed (personal observation).

Use of Pharmacologic Agents

With severe mitral regurgitation the use of invasive monitoring, vasodilators, and adjustment of intravascular volume may so improve forward cardiac output as to make the difference between mortality and a good outcome. Effective measures to decrease the size of the regurgitant orifice include preload reduction, such as with nitroglycerin, and afterload reduction with arterial dilators, such as nitroprusside or hydralazine. Inotropes, by increasing cardiac contractility, when used with preload and afterload reducers, may also help shrink the ventricle and therefore the size of the mitral annulus. Reduction in the amplitude of the V wave on the PCWP tracing may provide some evidence for a decrease in regurgitant volume. Similarly, changes in the amount of MR can easily be seen by TEE with color-flow Doppler. Patients with severe mitral regurgitation may need treatment for severe congestive heart failure, such as nitrates, vasodilators, and perhaps even an intraaortic balloon pump, the use of which has been reviewed in more detail elsewhere [122]. Even patients with mitral regurgitation who are not in congestive failure have a decreased ventricular volume and regurgitant fraction when nitroprusside is used to decrease afterload [123]. Other beneficial effects include decreases in right and left ventricular filling pressures, pulmonary artery pressures, and PVR. The decrease in regurgitant fraction may be due to improved valvular competence, attributable to both improved function of valvular components when the LV is smaller as well as relief of myocardial ischemia and papillary muscle ischemia [124].

If a vasoconstrictor is used to raise blood pressure, the left ventricle may fail, both because of its inability to pump against the increased afterload and the increased oxygen demand associated with the increased afterload. If only the wedge pressure is high, nitroglycerin (NTG) has been the drug of choice. For patients with simultaneous elevation of PCWP and systemic vascular resistance, use of sodium nitroprusside is appropriate, as it dilates the arterial as well as the venous side of the circulation. Intravenous nitroglycerin uniformly decreases wedge pressure but will not always increase cardiac output in severe congestive heart failure (CHF) [125]. However, NTG probably does decrease the size of the regurgitant orifice [126, 127]. Dobutamine is effective therapy for patients with MR and CHF. It may decrease the regurgitant orifice as a result of a combination of increasing contractility and reducing SVR. Since it may be more effective in patients with large regurgitant volumes than in patients with small ones, its adjustment of ventricular geometry and anatomy of the orifice may be its more important effect [128]. However, some patients with CHF have a decreased responsiveness to dobutamine. Presumably this is due to desensitization of myocardial beta receptors in patients with chronic CHF and elevated norepinephrine levels [129].

Furosemide can also be used to decrease the wedge pressure by venodilation. As diuresis ensues intravascular volume decreases and then the wedge pressure will decrease further. An increase in cardiac output compensates for the decrease in SVR, so that there may be no change in blood pressure. Patients with MR who will undergo aortic crossclamping (as for abdominal aortic aneurysm surgery) may benefit from the decreased SVR and increased contractility associated with amrinone [130].

Anesthetic Management

Patients with MR can be quite ill and may present a true challenge to the anesthesiologist. The hemodynamic goals described should be borne in mind when choosing an anesthetic technique. For patients with mild MR, this can be as simple as choosing isoflurane for the primary anesthetic agent. Nitrous oxide should be tolerated well by essentially all patients with mild MR. Indeed, the mild increase in sympathetic tone will help maintain the heart rate. While narcotics can be used, their central vagotonic effect may make it necessary to add agents such as isoflurane to maintain a faster heart rate, or to choose an agent such as pancuronium for muscle relaxation. Propofol, with its preload and afterload reducing effects, may be well tolerated in patients with mild MR, but in those with more severe disease it may decrease preload and afterload to an extent that will result in significant hypotension. Additionally, it may worsen the MR by decreasing myocardial contractility. Halothane may not be a good choice for patients with moderate or severe disease, as the combination of a slow heart rate with myocardial depression may compromise the patient.

Patients with MR and coronary artery disease present a dilemma in terms of preferred hemodynamic parameters, that is, a fast heart rate versus a slow heart rate. If ischemia results in ventricular dilatation, MR will worsen. Fortunately, nitroglycerin is an excellent agent for both these processes. In patients in cardiogenic shock due to acute or severe chronic mitral regurgitation, with or without concurrent ischemia, intraaortic balloon counterpulsation may be lifesaving and may decrease both LVEDP and the V wave on the wedge tracing [122].

If a patient has more than one valve lesion, it is helpful to determine preoperatively which is the more severe lesion. Usually, the best results will be obtained by maintaining a hemodynamic profile consistent with good outcome for the more severe lesion. However, what may be the more severe lesion on angiography may not behave so clinically, and on rare occasions the hemodynamic profile that supports the patient best is the one consistent with the less severe lesion. The bivalvular combination that is most frequent and of the most concern is probably mitral regurgitation and aortic stenosis. Mitral regurgitation is best managed with a decreased or adequate preload, a decreased afterload, and an increased heart rate. However, a decreased afterload and fast heart rate may be quite detrimental for the patient with aortic stenosis (see Chap. 6) and can lead to acute ischemia. It is therefore best to assess the severity of valvular lesions preoperatively. If an aortic murmur is heard, it is helpful to examine the ECG for evidence of LVH. LVH is the heart's response to try and overcome the pressure gradient imposed on the left ventricle by a stenotic aortic valve. While it is possible that a patient with mitral regurgitation may have LVH due to concurrent hypertension, if LVH is not present it is unlikely that the patient has significant aortic stenosis (AS). However, since the patient with MR may have LVH, the presence of LVH does not guarantee that the murmur represents AS. The carotid pulsations may be decreased in patients with aortic stenosis and almost certainly will be if the aortic stenosis is severe. Although the murmur of aortic stenosis is fairly characteristic, being systolic and radiating to the carotids, it may actually decrease as the stenosis worsens. Fortunately, the history helps to assess the severity of aortic stenosis, as patients with significant disease usually have angina, syncope, or CHF. The severity correlates somewhat with the symptoms, as the time to death without valvular correction is approximately 5 years from the onset of angina, 3 years from the onset of syncope, and 2 years from the onset of congestive failure [131]. In patients with significant symptoms, it may be best to obtain preoperative echocardiographic or angiographic studies as indicated, to assess the severity of the valvular pathology. Although aortic stenosis has been used as an example, the same thought process should be used any time a patient has more than one valve lesion, that is, an attempt should be made to determine which is the most severe lesion and to adjust hemodynamics to best treat that lesion.

Narcotics and Benzodiazepines in the Patient with Mitral Regurgitation

Narcotics in general are well tolerated in patients with MR. They do not depress the myocardium. However, they do decrease sympathetic tone and in patients with critical disease may cause hypotension. Their vagotonic effect may not be appropriate for patients with MR, but when combined with other agents, as for example isoflurane or pancuronium, they can be the basis for a balanced technique. Benzodiazepines will cause some myocardial depression, especially when administered to patients who are also receiving narcotics. However, they are usually tolerated when carefully titrated and can be used to provide the amnestic component of a balanced anesthetic.

Inhalation Anesthetics in the Patient with Mitral Regurgitation

All inhalation anesthetics will produce some myocardial depression. They may be chosen based on other characteristics. Halothane produces slowing of the heart rate and may cause the most significant myocardial depression of the three agents commonly available; therefore, it would not be a preferred choice. Isoflurane maintains forward flow by decreasing systemic vascular resistance and causing reflex tachycardia, both of which are ideal for the patient with MR. Enflurane may cause tachycardia but does not decrease SVR as significantly as does isoflurane.

Intravenous Anesthetics in the Patient with Mitral Regurgitation

Droperidol, at least in small doses, will be tolerated by patients with MR. It should be titrated carefully, however, in patients with severe disease, as its dilating effects may result in significant hypotension. Ketamine is not a good choice for these patients. Although tachycardia is acceptable, the increase in circulating catecholamines will increase both preload and afterload and may precipitate acute pulmonary edema. Propofol may be tolerated as it decreases afterload, but it also decreases preload and decreases myocardial contractility and the combination may produce profound hypotension. Etomidate may be a useful agent for induction in patients with severe MR. It has been shown to have minimal hemodynamic effects in patients with valvular heart disease [66]. Its cardiovascular effects have been reviewed in the section on MS and in Chap. 3.

Barbiturates in the Patient with Mitral Regurgitation

The myocardial depression associated with the barbiturates may not be tolerated by patients with severe MR and significant hypotension may result. For patients with mild disease, barbiturates are likely to be well tolerated. However, the possibility of an associated decrease in preload and reflex tachycardia should be borne in mind.

Muscle Relaxants in the Patient with Mitral Regurgitation

Although agents such as vecuronium and pipecuronium are acceptable, it may be more useful to choose a muscle relaxant that will promote tachycardia. The obvious choice would be pancuronium. If a patient with severe MR presented to the operating room for emergency surgery, such as an appendectomy or cholecystectomy, a fentanyl-based anesthetic might be chosen in order to prevent myocardial depression. Pancuronium can be used if the heart rate decreased secondary to the narcotic. Alternatively, short-acting nonvagolytic muscle relaxants can be used, and glycopyrrolate can be titrated in small doses to elevate the heart rate as needed.

Postoperative Concerns in the Patient with Mitral Regurgitation

Postoperative concerns in patients with MR are essentially those that raise the possibility of damaging hemodynamic effects. Pain may produce an increase in circulating catecholamines and thereby result in an elevation in SVR and pulmonary edema. Epidural analgesia can prevent this rise in SVR. Fluid overload may also precipitate pulmonary edema. Since epidural analgesia decreases sympathetic tone, preload will decrease, resulting in a decrease in regurgitant fraction. Serial physical examinations and appropriate use of diuretics to prevent elevation of filling pressures when third-space fluids mobilize are in order.

Summary

Management of patients with MR may vary from simple to complex. Patients may have minimal symptoms preoperatively, yet have significantly decreased ventricular function. When MR has progressed to the point of causing significant ventricular dysfunction, these patients often require invasive monitoring and careful attention to their hemodynamic determinants of cardiac output. Careful preoperative evaluation will help identify those patients at increased risk.

MITRAL VALVE PROLAPSE

Mitral valve prolapse (MVP) has been given various names, including the click-murmur syndrome, floppy-valve syndrome, and Barlow's syndrome, after the physician who demonstrated that the midsystolic click and late systolic murmur were of cardiac origin, often associated with prolapse of the valve and regurgitation [132]. Barlow and his colleagues described what is best termed a billowing valve, which represents an exaggeration of the normal slight systolic billowing of the mitral valve into the left atrium. A floppy valve reflects more movement of the valve into the atrium. Mitral valve prolapse is the term that describes the condition in which the valve leaflets do not coapt, thereby resulting in regurgitation. A flail valve refers to one in which the prolapse is due to chordal rupture. Various criteria have been devised to ascertain the diagnosis of MVP and indeed various reported incidences may vary according to the diagnostic criteria employed.

The criteria to diagnose MVP by echocardiography vary significantly in different laboratories [133]. Posterior bowing of the valve may lead to a falsely high incidence of diagnosis. Wann and associates [134] have suggested that extension of leaflet tissue cephalad to the plane of the annulus would offer a criterion that would prevent overdiagnosis of the syndrome. Patients with holosystolic prolapse present a challenge in terms of interpretation of the echo, and this has led to a very high incidence of MVP diagnosis by echocardiography in these patients [135]. Also, many patients will demonstrate echocardiographic findings only on the performance of provocative maneuvers. This explains the variations in the reported incidence of the disease.

Epidemiology

Procacci and associates [136] reported that MVP is present in about 6 to 10 percent of the population, while Markiewicz and colleagues [137] reported a greater than 10 percent incidence of MVP detected by echocardiography in asymptomatic college students. Kowalski [138] reported that there is a genetic predisposition and Malcolm [139] reported that MVP may be transmitted in an autosomal

Table 7-7. Conditions causing or associated with mitral valve prolapse

Marfan's syndrome
Rheumatic endocarditis
Coronary artery disease (papillary muscle dysfunction)
Myocarditis
Systemic lupus erythematosus
Ehlers-Danlos syndrome
Muscular dystrophy
Thoracic skeletal abnormalities
Hyperthyroidism
von Willebrand's syndrome
Anxiety neurosis
Congenital prolonged QT syndrome
Athlete's heart
Turner's syndrome
Noonan's syndrome
Atrial septal defect
Ventricular septal defect
Patent ductus arteriosus
Ebstein's anomaly
Congenital heart disease

Source: Adapted with permission from WA Pocock, Mitral Leaflet Billowing and Prolapse. In JB Barlow, Perspectives on the Mitral Valve. Philadelphia: Davis, 1987. P 61.

dominant fashion. Although MVP does occur in young healthy patients, it is often associated with other conditions, some of which are listed in Table 7-7. There tends to be a particular relationship between MVP and disorders of connective tissue, such as myxomatous proliferation of the valve, Marfan's syndrome, Ehlers-Danlos syndrome, osteogenesis imperfecta, pseudoxanthoma elasticum, and others [71].

In some patients MVP occurred for the first time after they suffered an acute infarction [140]. Mitral valve prolapse itself may cause ischemia by increasing tension on the involved papillary muscle [141], and this may be the mechanism by which patients with MVP suffer infarction despite normal coronary arteries. It has also been suggested that prolapse-induced ischemia may cause angina, arrhythmias, or sudden death [142]. Gottdiener and associates [143] reported that MVP may occur following surgical commissurotomy of the valve.

Natural History

Most patients with MVP are asymptomatic [144]. Others complain of fatigue, palpitations, or chest pain. Although the chest pain described is sometimes of anginal character, usually it is of a sharp or stabbing quality and not related to exertion. The symptoms may be due to autonomic dysfunction [145, 146], increased circulating concentrations of catecholamines that result in abnormal amounts of vasoconstriction, and papillary muscle ischemia [145]. Many patients suffer symptoms that interfere with their daily lifestyle and their work. Patients who are found to have MR on Doppler study may have a greater incidence of arrhythmias. Shah and associates [147] reported that among patients with MVP, those with MR detected by pulsed-wave Doppler had a higher prevalence of ventricular arrhythmias (61%) as compared to those without detectable MR (22%).

Although the diagnosis of the syndrome is common, it has various clinical presentations. Though many patients are asymptomatic, others suffer life-threatening arrhythmias and even sudden death. Complications associated with MVP are listed in Table 7-8. Nevertheless, most patients with MVP are asymptomatic for many years. One in seven patients will have worsening MR over 10 to 15 years. These patients tend to be those who have both a click and a murmur, and MVP is a common underlying etiology of MR requiring mitral valve replacement [78].

Table 7-8. Complications associated with mitral valve prolapse

Mitral regurgitation
Infective endocarditis
Ruptured chordae tendineae
Transient ischemic attacks and cerebrovascular accidents
Cardiac dysrhythmias—ventricular premature beats
Ventricular tachycardia
Atrioventricular heart block
ST segment and T-wave changes
Sudden death (extremely rare)

Source: Adapted with permission from Valvular Heart Disease. In RK Stoelting, SF Dierdorf, and RL McCammon (eds), Anesthesia and Co-Existing Disease (2nd ed). New York: Churchill Livingstone, 1988. P 52.

Anatomy

Normal mitral valve function requires proper function of the leaflets, chordae tendineae, annulus, left atrium, papillary muscles, and left ventricular wall, and MVP involves all of these components. Specific anatomic abnormalities of the structures that comprise the mitral valve have been described in association with MVP [148]. Mitral valve cusps, chordae tendineae, and the valve annulus may all develop myxomatous degeneration. Although the term used to describe the histopathologic abnormality in mitral valve prolapse is myxomatous degeneration, in fact the primary finding is degeneration of collagen within the leaflets [149]. When large amounts of "myxomatous tissue" are present, the valve leaflets become abnormal to gross examination and abnormal collagen is displayed by electron microscopy. Chordal rupture with worsening of regurgitation has been postulated as related to two etiologies. First, collagen degeneration within the chordae may weaken them and result in tearing. Second, the chordae may be under increased tension due to the increased area of the valve cusps [150].

History and Physical Examination

Although many patients with MVP are asymptomatic, others have symptoms. They include chest pain, dyspnea, fatigue, light-headedness, dizziness, palpitations, syncope, and transient neurologic events or cerebrovascular accidents due to cerebral emboli [151]. Classic anxiety attacks may occur and several studies have documented a high incidence of MVP in patients who suffer panic attacks [152]. Sudden death has been reported as well [153]. Some of the symptoms have been theorized to be due to dysfunction of the autonomic nervous system and may be related to decreased vagal responsiveness or chronically elevated α-adrenergic activity. Plasma norepinephrine levels are increased, possibly as a mechanism to compensate for a decreased circulating intravascular volume. This theory is supported by the fact that these patients have decreased plasma volume and do not have an elevated cardiac output [153].

Patients with MVP vary from those with no evidence of regurgitation to those with severe regurgitation. The usual signs of MR, including the characteristic murmur and thrill, may be present. A mid- to late systolic murmur may be seen even in the absence of clinically significant regurgitation, and may be crescendo in character. If the murmur is soft, short, and late in systole, the MR is usually not significant. With worsening MR the murmur begins earlier in systole and may even become holosystolic. Classically, these patients have a mid-systolic click that is detected by phonocardiography at least 0.14 seconds after S_1, but some patients have multiple clicks, possibly due to sudden tensing of the chordae and the prolapsed leaflets. The findings may be quite variable, so that both the click and murmur are present simultaneously, only one at a time, or neither, and the findings may vary from time to time in a given patient. Some patients may demonstrate findings consistent with MVP only after experiencing emotional stress [154]. Indeed, examination for MVP entails maneuvers to increase the possibility of detecting these findings. Since there may be no prolapse with a large ventricle, it may be easier to detect the click or murmur, or both, after the Valsalva maneuver, especially if the patient then suddenly assumes the supine position, which is known to increase both the intensity and duration of the murmur. This will move the click/murmur earlier in systole. On the other hand, maneuvers that increase the size of the left ventricle, such as changing from the standing to the prone position, will result in the click/murmur occurring later in systole. When the murmur is delayed, its duration and severity are usually attenuated due to the concomitant reduction in severity of the prolapse. The pressure generated in the ventricle also affects the amount of regurgitation and therefore the intensity of the murmur. Amyl nitrate decreases the size of the left ventricle and therefore causes the click to occur earlier in systole and the murmur to be of longer duration. However, amyl nitrate also results in a lower left ventricular systolic pressure and this in turn results in less regurgitation. The end result is that the intensity of the murmur decreases. On the other hand, phenylephrine will increase the size of the ventricle, and therefore the click and the murmur will occur later in systole. However, the elevated left ventricular systolic pressure will aggravate the regurgitation and thereby increase the intensity of the murmur. Sometimes the clicks will be heard well at the lower left sternal border. As a rule, when examining the patient for findings consistent with MVP, changes in the loudness of the murmur are not as important as those related to the timing of the click [71].

The Chest X-ray and Electrocardiogram in Mitral Valve Prolapse

Most patients who are asymptomatic will have a normal electrocardiogram. A small percentage of asymptomatic patients and many patients with typical symptoms of MVP will have inverted or biphasic T waves as well as nonspecific ST changes in the inferior leads, and occasionally in the anterolateral leads [71]. Arrhythmias that may occur include atrial and ventricular premature beats, AV block, bradyarrhythmias, and supraventricular and ventricular arrhythmias [71]. The sudden onset of supraventricular tachycardia is the most common arrhythmia seen in patients with MVP. There is an increased incidence of left-sided bypass tracts in these patients and this is important because digitalis preparations or calcium channel blockers, which can be useful in arrhythmias of reentry etiology, may be dangerous in the presence of antegrade conduction over an atrioventricular bypass tract. An increased incidence of QT prolongation in patients with MVP may predispose to ventricular arrhythmias [155]. Kligfield and associates [156] have suggested that sudden death may be related in some patients to the presence of MVP, and that patients at increased risk are those with significant MR, complex ventricular arrhythmias, a history of syncope, complaints of palpitations, or prolongation of the QT interval. Boudoulas and colleagues [157] reported nine patients with MVP who suffered a cardiac arrest, and ventricular fibrillation was recorded in eight patients, of whom seven were successfully resuscitated.

The Echocardiogram in Mitral Valve Prolapse

Echocardiography is frequently used to confirm the auscultatory diagnosis of MVP. M-mode echocardiography reveals posterior displacement of the posterior or anterior and posterior leaflets during midsystole. In some patients the prolapse of one or both leaflets will be present throughout systole.

Mitral valve prolapse has been detected by two-dimensional echocardiography in some patients in whom it was not detected by M-mode echo. Echocardiography may be especially helpful in detecting patients at increased risk of developing significant regurgitation or endocarditis, as these patients will display thickened or redundant valve leaflets [158]. Moderate to severe regurgitation is detected in up to 10 percent of patients with MVP when using color-flow Doppler, and is usually found in men over the age of 50 years [159]. Some patients will have a click on examination but no evidence of MVP on echocardiographic study. It is unclear whether this reflects the dynamic state of a lesion in that perhaps MVP would be found in the same patient under different hemodynamic and loading conditions. In addition to bowing and displacement of the valve, posterior displacement of the point where the leaflets coapt has been described as a criterion for diagnosis of MVP [160]. Bending of the septum toward the left ventricle has been described as well [161].

Angiography in Mitral Valve Prolapse

Extension of the leaflets of the mitral valve posterior and inferior to their point of attachment to the annulus supports the diagnosis of MVP. Redundant tissue may be seen as scalloped edges on the leaflets [162]. Although angiography may detect an increased rate of circumferential fiber shortening when significant regurgitation is present, this is not a specific finding, as it is present in MR of other etiologies as well [163]. Other findings that may be seen in MVP on angiography include dilatation of the annulus, calcification of the annulus, decreased contraction of the basal region of the left ventricle, and decreased systolic contraction [163]. Performance of coronary angiography is helpful to assess patients who have complaints of chest pain, for in general, even when chest pain occurs on a chronic basis, patients who have normal coronary arteries have a better prognosis than those with CAD [164].

Preoperative Evaluation

Preoperative evaluation should focus on symptoms and signs that imply the presence of arrhythmias or severe regurgitation. Patients whose symptoms could be explained by arrhythmias, such as those with palpitations or syncope, should probably undergo stress testing and Holter monitoring. Patients with prolongation of the QT interval should be similarly studied. A prior history of palpitations or syncope may warn of life-threatening ventricular arrhythmias. Certainly, any patient who had experienced a past cardiac arrest should be considered at risk for a ventricular arrhythmia and all resuscitation drugs and equipment should be immediately at hand. Antiarrhythmic therapy may be warranted in these patients as guided by Holter and electrophysiologic (EP) evaluation.

Preoperative stress testing may offer useful information, as premature ventricular contractions (PVCs) may be initiated by exercise [165], and ST segment depression consistent with ischemia has been documented in MVP during exercise in the absence of coronary artery disease [166]. Stress testing may be especially helpful because many patients with atypical chest pain will have no chest pain during exercise-induced ischemic-type ST changes, supporting the contention that the ST changes in these patients are occurring on the basis of the MVP and that the chest pain reflects tension on the papillary muscles and not ischemia related to coronary artery disease. Although chest pain may occur during the test, it frequently does not occur simultaneously with the ST changes. If ECG stress testing is not conclusive, it is best to evaluate such patients with a thallium stress test. Lack of evidence of exercise-induced ischemia supports the diagnosis of isolated MVP, without underlying coronary artery disease. Some patients with MVP do not increase ejection fraction with exercise, even when no associated MR is present, a finding that may be detected on a stress echocardiogram. This supports the contention that these patients may also have an underlying cardiomyopathy [167].

Arrhythmias in the Patient with Mitral Valve Prolapse

As with studies of other aspects of MVP, those reviewing rhythm disturbances report varying data because of different criteria used to define the syndrome. Still, it is generally accepted that patients with MVP do suffer from an increased incidence of arrhythmias. A short discussion of this topic follows, but it has been extensively reviewed elsewhere [168, 169].

Patients with MVP may develop tachyarrhythmias, such as atrial flutter, atrial fibrillation, and AV nodal reentry tachycardia; bradyarrhythmias, such as sinus bradycardia and sinus exit block; ventricular tachycardia; and ventricular fibrillation. Mechanisms proposed for the arrhythmias include autonomic dysfunction, accessory atrioventricular bypass tracts, and AV node reentry. The presence of collagen in the endocardium of the atrium [170] and fatty infiltration near the sinoatrial and atrioventricular nodes [171] may predispose these patients to development of supraventricular arrhythmias. In addition, abnormalities of ventricular endocardium have been documented to be increased in patients with MVP [170, 172] and may predispose these patients to ventricular arrhythmias. Many patients with MVP have been documented to have a prolonged QT interval. However, whether there is a primary association between these two processes, or MVP is simply documented in many patients with the prolonged QT syndrome, because of the frequency with which MVP occurs in the general population is unknown. Still, as long as a patient displays a QT interval corrected for heart rate that is greater than 0.44 seconds, the patient may be at increased risk of sudden death. β-Blockade is probably the best choice of therapy in patients with a prolonged QT interval and a history of ventricular arrhythmias [168]. Occasionally, other antiarrhythmic agents will need to be added. The patient should have serial ECGs to ensure that the antiarrhythmic therapy has not prolonged the QT interval further. It should be noted that the risk of sudden death in patients with MVP is greater in those with severe MR and left ventricular dysfunction [173].

Patients who present to the operating room in sinus rhythm and have no history of arrhythmias are unlikely to have significant intraoperative arrhythmias. However, if the electrocardiogram reveals supraventricular or ventricular ectopy it is wise for patients to be evaluated by a cardiologist, and often they have been in the past. Detailed consultation with the patient's cardiologist may be quite beneficial. If there is a history of syncope or presyncope, the patient may have undergone electrophysiologic studies (EPS), the results of which should be made available to the anesthesiologist preoperatively.

For patients undergoing emergency surgery, antiarrhythmic therapy may be required intraoperatively. It is important that an electrocardiogram be performed on these patients preoperatively to look for the presence of Wolff-Parkinson-White (WPW) syndrome or a prolonged corrected QT interval. If the history and physical examination support the diagnosis of MVP and the patient has no symptoms of LV dysfunction but has frequent supraventricular or ventricular ectopy, we prefer to titrate intravenous propranolol, until the heart rate is between 70 and 80 beats per minute. Careful titration of low doses is especially important in patients who are already anesthetized, as additive or synergistic effects with anesthetics may result in severe bradycardia. Verapamil slows AV conduction and therefore may slow or prevent a supraventricular tachycardia. In addition, the negative inotropic effect is useful in the management of patients with MVP. If patients continue to have frequent ectopy after propranolol, we sometimes administer verapamil as well in increments of 0.015 mg/kg every 3 to 5 minutes, to a total dose of 0.07 mg/kg. We usually limit therapy to low doses, again because of concern for significant slowing of the heart rate in patients who are anesthetized. However, we have occasionally used higher doses of both propranolol and verapamil. Although we have had good results in prevention and control of arrhythmias in patients with MVP using propranolol and sometimes propranolol and verapamil, there are no controlled studies to support such treatment prophylactically in the patient with MVP in the perioperative period. However, oral propranolol has been shown to decrease the frequency of PVCs and paroxysmal ventricular tachycardia [174], though it may not be efficacious in all patients.

There is a concern that verapamil may result in rapid conduction through an accessory pathway in patients with WPW syndrome and atrial fibrillation, although this is unusual. Still, if WPW syndrome is documented and the patient is in atrial fibrillation, propranolol is clearly a better choice. In addition, β-adrenergic blocking agents probably decrease the incidence of life-threatening arrhythmias in patients with MVP, and decrease the occurrence of chest pain and palpitations as well [174].

They are also useful to treat ischemia if CAD is present [175], especially since preload reduction from nitrates may aggravate prolapse. Digitalis should not be used in the presence of WPW syndrome and atrial fibrillation, since it will result in rapid atrioventricular conduction in approximately one third of patients [176].

Monitoring and Hemodynamic Goals for the Patient with Mitral Valve Prolapse

The level of monitoring required for patients with MVP varies with the level of functional impairment. Asymptomatic patients with normal exercise tolerance and no evidence of regurgitation should have their hemodynamics adjusted similarly as for a patient with MS, that is, appropriately full intravascular volume and a slow heart rate, with a somewhat elevated SVR. However, in contrast to MS, as long as baseline left ventricular function is not significantly decreased, patients with MVP may do better with agents that depress the myocardium. This is because the ventricle will tend not to empty and therefore the mitral valve leaflets will have a lesser tendency to prolapse. As in patients with idiopathic hypertrophic subaortic stenosis (IHSS) (see Chap. 9), an elevated SVR may be preferred. Decreases in left ventricular volume may cause or aggravate regurgitation. Increases in contractility should be avoided as this may shrink the ventricle and worsen prolapse and MR. Invasive monitoring is probably not warranted for mild MVP/mild MR unless dictated by the surgical procedure itself. Signs and symptoms of significant MR may be justification for invasive monitoring as well as adjusting therapy toward that appropriate for MR rather than MS. Still, since many patients will develop MR specifically as prolapse worsens, the primary maneuver should be to maintain the preferred hemodynamics for MVP. If there is less prolapse, there should be less MR. TEE may be especially useful in this situation as the amount of MVP and MR can be documented during various hemodynamic maneuvers. Patients with a history of arrhythmias should have a large-bore intravenous or perhaps central access line placed. In patients with a history of supraventricular or ventricular arrhythmias, an arterial line is helpful to gauge the severity of hemodynamic impairment during any intraoperative arrhythmias. The electrocardiogram is best monitored with leads II and V_5 in order to detect the presence of both arrhythmias and ischemia.

Anesthetic Management

There are no specific problems with any anesthetic agents and no favored agents for patients with MVP, as long as the hemodynamic determinants of preload and afterload are kept where preferred for the lesion at hand. It should be appreciated that most patients with MVP will have had minimal symptoms before being diagnosed by echocardiography. Many of these patients will inform the anesthesiologist of their diagnosis but on examination may have no findings to support it. Others will have a murmur or click, or both. Only an occasional patient will have a murmur that supports the diagnosis of significant MR. Therefore, anesthetic management of patients with MVP needs to be tailored to the individual patient. As a rule, the hemodynamic rules that apply to MS should be used, as a patient who is maintained "slow and full" with a somewhat elevated SVR has less chance of developing significant prolapse and associated mitral valvular regurgitation. The distinction from MS is made regarding contractility, which is preferably maintained as is or perhaps even decreased in patients with good left ventricular function. It is clearly preferable for contractility not to be increased as this will shrink the ventricle and may worsen prolapse and MR. Still, if a patient with MVP develops significant MR during anesthesia, as determined by a clear change in the murmur or TEE, or is followed by a cardiologist and known to have chronic MR that is confirmed by the presence of a murmur of MR, it may be preferable to adjust the hemodynamic parameters to those preferred for MR, that is, decreased preload and afterload and an increased heart rate. It should be understood that the preference to depress or maintain contractility in the patient with MVP assumes normal baseline LV function. In patients with compromised LV function or known CAD, the risk associated with further depression of myocardial function may not be worth the possible decreased chance of prolapse, and in patients with MVP and LV failure inotropic therapy may be required.

For the discussion at hand, we refer to those patients who do not currently have MR. Halothane is a useful agent for patients with MVP without MR, as it slows the heart rate and decreases contractility. Enflurane can be used as well. Isoflurane is not a good choice of anesthetic for these patients due to the associated tachycardia and decreased afterload. Ketamine should probably be avoided, as the associated release of endogenous catecholamines may increase the risk of arrhythmias, to which these patients are already prone, as well as the increased contractility, which can worsen or cause MR. Narcotics can be used safely and offer some slowing of the heart rate. Propofol may not be a good choice as the decrease in preload and afterload may predispose to MR. Etomidate is likely to be well tolerated by these patients.

Regional anesthesia can be used in these patients, but it may be difficult to maintain the preferred hemodynamics and care must be taken to ensure that this is done. Adequate preload needs to be maintained and though this can be achieved with appropriate use of crystalloid and colloids there is concern regarding their return to the central circulation when the epidural is discontinued. Although sympathetic blockade offers the advantage of a slow heart rate, it also decreases the SVR and this may be associated with an increase in CO, thereby precipitating prolapse and MR.

Overall, most patients with MVP are asymptomatic and the majority of patients with MVP do well. Even patients who manifest arrhythmias preoperatively usually do well with appropriate management.

Postoperative Concerns in the Patient with Mitral Valve Prolapse

The postoperative concerns for patients with MVP are essentially the same as those during the intraoperative period. Most patients should be treated to obtain the same hemodynamic parameters set forth for MS, that is, maintained intravascular volume and a slow heart rate. Pain control is therefore important in these patients. While good pain relief will help avoid possibly detrimental increases in heart rate, the use of postoperative epidural analgesia will require maintenance of preload. The use of intravenous patient-controlled analgesia (PCA) with an agent with predominantly vagal effects may be preferable. Morphine sulfate is a good choice. This will provide a reasonable amount of pain relief and help maintain a slow heart rate, without causing a large decrease in SVR. Still, preload will need to be maintained due to venodilation and histamine release.

Antibiotic Prophylaxis

Antibiotic prophylaxis is recommended for patients with valvular heart disease who are undergoing most surgical procedures. Specific recommendations have been reviewed elsewhere [177] and adherence to such a protocol may significantly decrease the risk of developing infective endocarditis (IE) (see Chap. 17).

While there has been no question about the necessity for prophylaxis in patients with rheumatic heart disease, some patients with MVP require prophylaxis as well. Antibiotic prophylaxis is certainly in order when mitral regurgitation is present in patients with MVP. MacMahon and associates [178] reported that the risk of developing endocarditis was 35 times greater for patients with MVP and a systolic murmur than for patients with MVP who do not have a systolic murmur, and that prophylactically treating those with a murmur would include over 90 percent of patients with MVP in whom infectious endocarditis would develop. In a report of 25 patients who developed infective endocarditis on a prolapsing mitral valve after using an oral irrigation device, all had a holosystolic murmur, while none manifested a click without a murmur [179], and Corrigall and colleagues [180] have recommended that patients with evidence of MVP and a murmur indicating MR should receive antibiotic prophylaxis for procedures that constitute a risk of IE.

Since patients with MVP who display echocardiographic evidence of valve thickening or redundancy are at increased risk for development of IE [181], it is preferable for echocardiography to be performed preoperatively in order to identify those patients at risk. Consultation with the cardiologist interpreting the echo should focus on whether the patient should receive prophylactic antibiotics. Most physicians believe that antibiotic prophylaxis would not be required in a patient who has a click but does not have a murmur of MR or echocardiographic evidence of MVP.

Patients with mitral valve disease vary from those with minimal cardiovascular dysfunction to those with severe disease. Preoperative evaluation will help identify patients who require invasive monitoring. Patients who are severely ill will require careful tailoring of their anesthetic, and preoperative identification of these patients will permit time to plan for a postoperative intensive care setting. There are no strict rules governing which anesthetics can be administered to a patient with any given lesion, and in fact most patients can receive one of several anesthetics with good results as long as appropriate care is taken to maintain the determinants of cardiac output in an appropriate range for the particular lesion. While the variety of mitral valve diseases offers many variables to the anesthesiologist, thereby making them a true challenge to manage, safe care of these patients is therefore quite satisfying as well.

REFERENCES

1. Silverman, ME, Hurst, WJ. The mitral complex. Interaction of the anatomy, physiology and pathology of the mitral annulus, mitral valve leaflets, chordae tendineae, and papillary muscles. *Am Heart J* 76: 399, 1968.
2. Perloff, JK, Roberts, WC. The mitral apparatus. Functional anatomy of mitral regurgitation. *Circulation* 46:227, 1972.
3. Thompson, ME, Shaver, JA, Leon, DF. Effect of tachycardia on atrial transport in mitral stenosis. *Am Heart J* 94:297, 1977.
4. Olson, LJ, Subramanian, R, et al. Surgical pathology of the mitral valve: A study of 712 cases spanning 21 years. *Mayo Clin Proc* 62:22, 1987.
5. Rowe, JC, Bland, EF, et al. The course of mitral stenosis without surgery: Ten and twenty year perspectives. *Ann Intern Med* 52:741, 1960.
6. Osterberger, LE, Goldstein, S, et al. Functional mitral stenosis in patients with massive mitral annular calcification. *Circulation* 64:472, 1981.
7. Nasser, WK, Davis, RH, Dillon, JC, et al. Atrial myxoma. I. Clinical and pathologic features in nine cases. *Am Heart J* 83:694, 1972.
8. Nugent, EW, Plauth, WH, et al. The Pathology, Abnormal Physiology, Clinical Recognition, and Medi-

cal and Surgical Treatment of Congenital Heart Disease. In JW Hurst, RC Schlant, et al (eds), *The Heart, Arteries and Veins* (7th ed). New York: McGraw-Hill, 1990. Pp 655–794.
9. Rackley, CE, Edwards, JE, Karp, RB. Mitral Valve Disease. In JW Hurst, RC Schlant, et al (eds), *The Heart, Arteries and Veins* (7th ed). New York: McGraw-Hill, 1990. Pp 820–851.
10. Wells, B. The assessment of mitral stenosis by phonocardiography. *Br Heart J* 16:261, 1954.
11. Rapaport, E. Natural history of aortic and mitral valve disease. *Am J Cardiol* 35:221, 1975.
12. Selzer, A, Cohn, KE. Natural history of mitral stenosis: A review. *Circulation* 45:878, 1972.
13. Valvular Heart Disease. In MC Fishman, AR Hoffman, et al, *Medicine* (2nd ed). Philadelphia: Lippincott, 1985. Pp 40–52.
14. Chopra, P, Tandon, HD, et al. Comparative studies of mitral valves in rheumatic heart disease. *Arch Intern Med* 143:661, 1983.
15. Jordon, RA, Scheifley, CH, Edwards, JE. Mural thrombosis and arterial embolism in mitral stenosis: A clinicopathologic study of fifty-one cases. *Circulation* 3:363, 1951.
16. Nielson, GH, Galea, EG, Houssack, KF. Thromboembolic complications of mitral valve disease. *Aust NZ J Med* 8:372, 1978.
17. Gorlin, R, Gorlin, SG. Hydraulic formula of the area of stenotic mitral valve, other cardiac valves and central circulatory shunts. *Am Heart J* 41:1, 1951.
18. Nakhjavan, FK, Katz, MR, et al. Analysis of influence of catecholamines and tachycardia during supine exercise in patients with mitral stenosis and sinus rhythm. *Br Heart J* 31:753, 1969.
19. Selzer, A. Effects of atrial fibrillation upon the circulation in patients with mitral stenosis. *Am Heart J* 59:518, 1960.
20. Jackson, J. Valvular Heart Disease. In SJ Thomas (ed), *Manual of Cardiac Anesthesia*. New York: Churchill Livingstone, 1984. Pp 231–258.
21. Valvular Heart Disease. In RK Stoelting, SF Dierdorf, and RL McCammon, *Anesthesia and Co-Existing Disease* (2nd ed). New York: Churchill Livingstone, 1988. Pp 37–55.
22. Gash, AK, Carabello, BA, et al. Left ventricular ejection performance and systolic muscle function in patients with mitral stenosis. *Circulation* 67:148, 1983.
23. Woods, AM, and Difazio, CA. Maternal-fetal Monitoring in Obstetrics. In CL Lake (ed), *Clinical Monitoring*. Philadelphia: Saunders, 1990. Pp 345–407.
24. Feigenbaum, H, Campbell, RW, et al. Evaluation of the left ventricle in patients with mitral stenosis. *Circulation* 34:462, 1966.

25. Heller, SJ, Carleton, RA. Abnormal left ventricular contraction in patients with mitral stenosis. *Circulation* 42:1099, 1970.
26. Bolen, JL, Lopes, MG, et al. Analysis of left ventricular function in response to afterload changes in patients with mitral stenosis. *Circulation* 52:894, 1975.
27. Grant, RP. Architectonics of the heart. *Am Heart J* 46:405, 1953.
28. Friedman, BL, Macias, DJ, Yu, PN. Pulmonary function studies in patients with mitral stenosis. *Am Rev Tuberc* 79:265, 1959.
29. Wood, TE, McLeod, P, et al. Mechanics of breathing in mitral stenosis. *Am Rev Respr Dis* 104:52, 1971.
30. DeTroyer, A, Estenne, M, Yernault, JC. Disturbance of respiratory muscle function in patients with mitral valve disease. *Am J Med* 69:867, 1980.
31. Kannel, WB, Seidman, JM, Fercho, W. Vital capacity and congestive heart failure: The Framingham Study. *Circulation* 49:1160, 1974.
32. Halperin, JL, Brooks, KM, et al. Effect of nitroglycerin on the pulmonary venous gradient in patients after mitral valve replacement. *J Am Coll Cardiol* 5:34, 1985.
33. Wroblewski, E, James, F, et al. Right ventricular performance in mitral stenosis. *Am J Cardiol* 47:51, 1981.
34. Braunwald, E, Braunwald, NS, et al. Effects of mitral-valve replacement on the pulmonary vascular dynamics of patients with pulmonary hypertension. *N Engl J Med* 273:509, 1965.
35. Dalen, JE, Matloff, JM, et al. Early reduction of pulmonary vascular resistance after mitral-valve replacement. *N Engl J Med* 277:387, 1967.
36. Hemoptysis. In MC Fishman, AR Hoffman, et al, *Medicine* (2nd ed). Philadelphia: Lippincott, 1985. Pp 150–153.
37. Mattina, CJ, Green, SJ, et al. Frequency of angiographically significant coronary arterial narrowing in mitral stenosis. *Am J Cardiol* 57:802, 1986.
38. Reichek, N, Shelburne, JC, Perloff, JR. Clinical aspects of rheumatic valvular disease. *Prog Cardiovasc Dis* 15:491, 1973.
39. Reis, RN, Roberts, WC. Amounts of coronary arterial narrowing by atherosclerotic plaques in clinically isolated mitral valve stenosis: Analysis of 76 necropsy patients older than 30 years. *Am J Cardiol* 57:1117, 1986.
40. Miscellaneous Conditions. In HJL Marriott, *Practical Electrocardiography* (7th ed). Baltimore: Williams & Wilkins, 1983. Pp 456–477.
41. Edler, I, Gustafson, A. Ultrasonic cardiogram in mitral stenosis. *Acta Med Scand* 159:85, 1957.
42. Segal, BL, Likoff, W, Kingsley, B. Echocardiography:

Clinical application in mitral stenosis. JAMA 195: 161, 1966.
43. Marino, P, Zanolla, L, et al. Interpretative reproducibility of two-dimensional echocardiographic images. Analysis of intraobserver, interobserver, and beat-to-beat reproducibility of the mitral valve orifice. Eur Heart J 4:733, 1983.
44. Glover, MU, Warren, SE, et al. M-mode and two-dimensional echocardiographic correlation with findings at catheterization and surgery in patients with mitral stenosis. Am Heart J 105:98, 1983.
45. Kalmanson, D, Veyrat, C, et al. Non-invasive recording of mitral valve flow velocity patterns using pulsed Doppler echocardiography: Application to diagnosis and evaluation of mitral valve disease. Br Heart J 39:517, 1977.
46. Holen, J, Simonsen, S. Determination of pressure gradient in mitral stenosis with Doppler echocardiography. Br Heart J 41:529, 1979.
47. Sherrid, M, Clark, R, Cohn, K. Echocardiographic analysis of left atrial dimensions pre and postoperatively in mitral disease (abstract). Am J Cardiol 43: 406, 1979.
48. Weyman, AE, Heger, JJ, et al. Mechanism of paradoxical early diastolic septal motion in patients with mitral stenosis: A cross-sectional study. Am J Cardiol 40:691, 1977.
49. Johnston, DL, Kostuk, WJ. Left and right ventricular function during symptom-limited exercise in patients with isolated mitral stenosis. Chest 89:186, 1986.
50. Johnston, WE, Royster, RL, et al. Influence of balloon inflation and deflation on location of pulmonary artery catheter tip. Anesthesiology 67:110, 1987.
51. Lemen, R, Jones, JG, Cowan, G. A mechanism of pulmonary-artery perforation by Swan-Ganz catheters. N Engl J Med 292:211, 1975.
52. Barash, PG, Nardi, D, et al. Catheter-induced pulmonary artery perforation: Mechanisms, management and modifications. J Thorac Cardiovasc Surg 82:5, 1981.
53. Meister, SG, Engel, TR, et al. Propranolol in mitral stenosis during sinus rhythm. Am Heart J 94:685, 1977.
54. Stone, JG, Hoar, PF, et al. Nitroprusside and mitral stenosis. Anesth Analg 59:662, 1980.
55. Stone, JG, Hoar, PF, et al. Afterload reduction and preload augmentation improve the anesthetic management of patients with cardiac failure and valvular regurgitation. Anesth Analg 59:737, 1980.
56. Hess, W. Effects of amrinone on the right side of the heart. J Cardiothorac Anesth 3 (Suppl 2):38, 1989.
57. Hess, W, Arnold, B, Veit, S. The haemodynamic effects of amrinone in patients with mitral stenosis and pulmonary hypertension. Eur Heart J 7:800, 1986.
58. Frostell, C, Fratacci, M-D, et al. Inhaled nitric oxide: A selective pulmonary vasodilator reversing hypoxic pulmonary vasoconstriction. Circulation 83:2038, 1991.
59. Hilgenberg, JC, McCammon, RL, Stoelting, RK. Pulmonary and systemic vascular responses to nitrous oxide in patients with mitral stenosis and pulmonary hypertension. Anesth Analg 59:323–326, 1980.
60. Bovill, JG, Sebel, PS, Stanley, TH. Opioid analgesics in anesthesia: With special reference to their use in cardiovascular anesthesia. Anesthesiology 61: 731, 1984.
61. Eckstein, JW, Hamilton, WK, McCammond, JM. The effect of thiopental on peripheral venous tone. Anesthesiology 22:525, 1961.
62. Claeys, MA, Gepts, E, Camu, F. Haemodynamic changes during anaesthesia induced and maintained with propofol. Br J Anaesth 60:3, 1988.
63. Aun, C, Major, E. The cardiorespiratory effects of ICI 35 868 in patients with valvular heart disease. Anaesthesia 39:1096, 1984.
64. Gooding, JM, Corssen, G. Effect of etomidate on the cardiovascular system. Anesth Analg 56:717, 1977.
65. Criado, A, Maseda, J, et al. Induction of anaesthesia with etomidate: Haemodynamic study of 36 patients. Br J Anaesth 52:803, 1980.
66. Lindeburg, T, Spotoft, H, et al. Cardiovascular effects of etomidate used for induction and in combination with fentanyl pancuronium for maintenance of anaesthesia in patients with valvular heart disease. Acta Anaesth Scand 26:205, 1982.
67. Larijani, GE, Bartkowski, RR, et al. Clinical pharmacology of pipecuronium bromide. Anesth Analg 68:734, 1989.
68. Stoops, CM, Curtis, CA, et al. Hemodynamic effects of doxacurium chloride in patients receiving oxygen sufentanil anesthesia for coronary artery bypass grafting or valve replacement. Anesthesiology 69:365, 1988.
69. Baxley, WA, Kennedy, JW, et al. Hemodynamics in ruptured chordae tendineae and chronic rheumatic mitral regurgitation. Circulation 48:1288, 1973.
70. Boltwood, CM, Tei, C, et al. Quantitative echocardiography of the mitral complex in dilated cardiomyopathy: The mechanism of functional mitral regurgitation. Circulation 68:498, 1983.
71. Braunwald, E. Valvular Heart Disease. In EB Braunwald (ed), Heart Disease: A Textbook of Cardiovascular Medicine (4th ed). Philadelphia: Saunders, 1992. Pp 1007–1077.

72. Bloor, CM. Valvular heart disease in the elderly. *J Am Geriatr Soc* 30:466, 1982.
73. Takamoto, T, Popp, RL. Conduction disturbances related to the site and severity of mitral annular calcification: A 2-dimensional echocardiographic and electrocardiographic correlative study. *Am J Cardiol* 51:1644, 1983.
74. Nestico, PF, DePace, NL, et al. Calcium phosphorus metabolism in dialysis patients with and without mitral annular calcium. Analysis of 30 patients. *Am J Cardiol* 51:497, 1983.
75. Oliveira, DBG, Dawkins, KD, et al. Chordal rupture. I: Aetiology and natural history. *Br Heart J* 50:312, 1983.
76. Hickey, AJ, Wilcken, DEL, et al. Primary (spontaneous) chordal rupture: Relation to myxomatous valve disease and mitral valve prolapse. *J Am Coll Cardiol* 5:1341, 1985.
77. DiNardo, JA. Anesthesia for Valve Replacement in Patients with Acquired Valvular Heart Disease. In JA DiNardo, MJ Schwartz (eds), *Anesthesia For Cardiac Surgery*. Norwalk: Appleton & Lange, 1990. Pp 85–115.
78. Guy, FC, MacDonald, RPR, Fraser, DB, Smith, ER. Mitral valve prolapse as a cause of hemodynamically important mitral regurgitation. *Can J Surg* 23:166, 1980.
79. Izumi, S, Miyatake, K, et al. Mechanism of mitral regurgitation in patients with myocardial infarction: A study using real-time two-dimensional Doppler flow imaging and echocardiography. *Circulation* 76:777, 1987.
80. Balu, V, Hershowitz, S, et al. Mitral regurgitation in coronary artery disease. *Chest* 81:550, 1982.
81. Munoz, S, Gallardo, J, et al. Influence of surgery on the natural history of rheumatic mitral and aortic valve disease. *Am J Cardiol* 35:234, 1975.
82. Yellin, EL, Yoran, C, et al. Dynamics of Acute Experimental Mitral Regurgitation. In MI Ionescu, LH Cohn (eds), *Mitral Valve Disease: Diagnosis and Treatment*. London: Butterworth, 1985. Pp 11–26.
83. Corin, WJ, Monrad, ES, et al. The relationship of afterload to ejection performance in chronic mitral regurgitation. *Circulation* 76:59, 1987.
84. Boucher, CA, Bingham, JB, et al. Early changes in left ventricular size and function after correction of left ventricular volume overload. *Am J Cardiol* 47:991, 1981.
85. Ross, J, Jr. Left ventricular function and the timing of surgical treatment in valvular heart disease. *Ann Intern Med* 94:498, 1981.
86. Borow, KM, Green, LH, et al. End-systolic volume as a predictor of postoperative left ventricular performance in volume overload from valvular regurgitation. *Am J Med* 68:655, 1980.
87. Kihara, Y, Sasayama, S, et al. Role of the left atrium in adaptation of the heart to chronic mitral regurgitation in conscious dogs. *Circ Res* 62:543, 1988.
88. Braunwald, E, Awe, WC. The syndrome of severe mitral regurgitation with normal left atrial pressure. *Circulation* 27:29, 1963.
89. Ross, J, Jr, Braunwald, E, Morrow, AG. Clinical and hemodynamic observations in pure mitral insufficiency. *Am J Cardiol* 2:11, 1958.
90. Bentivoglio, L, Uricchio, JF, Likoff, W. The paradox of right ventricular enlargement in mitral insufficiency. *Am J Med* 24:193, 1958.
91. Stone, JG, Faltas, AN, Hoar, PF. Sodium nitroprusside therapy for cardiac failure in anesthetized patients with valvular insufficiency. *Anesthesiology* 49:414, 1978.
92. Nishimura, RA, Schaff, HV, et al. Papillary muscle rupture complicating acute myocardial infarction: Analysis of 17 patients. *Am J Cardiol* 51:373, 1983.
93. Stapleton, JF. Natural History of Chronic Valvular Disease. In WS Frankl, AN Brest (eds), *Cardiovascular Clinics. Valvular Heart Disease: Comprehensive Evaluation and Management*. Philadelphia: Davis, 1986. Pp 105–148.
94. Roberts, WC, Braunwald, E, Morrow, AG. Acute severe mitral regurgitation secondary to ruptured chordae tendineae. Clinical, hemodynamic and pathologic considerations. *Circulation* 33:58, 1966.
95. Bentivoglio, LG, Uricchio, JF, et al. An electrocardiographic analysis of mitral regurgitation. *Circulation* 18:572, 1956.
96. Peter, RH, Morris, JJ, Jr, McIntosh, HD. Relationship of fibrillatory waves and P waves in the electrocardiogram. *Circulation* 33:599, 1966.
97. Fujino, T, Ito, M, et al. Echocardiographic abnormal motion of the interventricular septum in mitral insufficiency. *J Cardiogr* 6:613, 1976.
98. Reeves, WC, Nanda, NC, Gramiak, R. The relationship between aortic valve closure and aortic root motion. *Radiology* 127:751, 1978.
99. Chandraratna, PAN, Vlahovich, G, Aronow, WS. Echocardiographic study of significance of left ventricular minor axis shortening during the preejection phase of systole. *Br Heart J* 41:392, 1979.
100. Abbasi, AS, Allen, MW, et al. Detection and estimation of the degree of MR by range-gated pulsed Doppler echocardiography. *Circulation* 61:143, 1980.
101. Veyrat, C, Ameur, A, et al. Pulsed Doppler echocardiographic indices for assessing mitral regurgitation. *Br Heart J* 51:130, 1984.

102. Hayakawa, M, Inoh, T, et al. Two-dimensional echocardiographic findings of patients with papillary muscle dysfunction. *J Cardiogr* 12:137, 1982.
103. Ferrara, RP, Labovitz, AJ, et al. Prosthetic mitral regurgitation detected by Doppler echocardiography. *Am J Cardiol* 55:229, 1985.
104. Buda, AJ, Zotz, RJ, et al. Prognostic significance of vegetations detected by two-dimensional echocardiography in infective endocarditis. *Am Heart J* 113:1291, 1986.
105. Eckberg, DL, Gault, JH, et al. Mechanics of left ventricular contraction in chronic severe mitral regurgitation. *Circulation* 47:1252, 1973.
106. Croft, CH, Lipscomb, K, et al. Limitations of qualitative angiographic grading in aortic or mitral regurgitation. *Am J Cardiol* 53:1593, 1984.
107. Grossman, W. Profiles in Valvular Heart Disease. In W Grossman, DS Baim (eds), *Cardiac Catheterization, Angiography and Intervention* (4th ed). Philadelphia: Lea & Febiger, 1991. Pp 557–581.
108. Kontos, GJ, Jr, Schaff, HV, et al. Left ventricular function in subacute and chronic mitral regurgitation: Effect on function early postoperatively. *J Thorac Cardiovasc Surg* 98:163, 1989.
109. Wisenbach, T. Does normal pump function belie muscle dysfunction in patients with chronic severe mitral regurgitation. *Circulation* 77:515, 1988.
110. Osbakken, MD, Bove, AA, Spann, JF. Left ventricular regional wall motion and velocity of shortening in chronic mitral and aortic regurgitation. *Am J Cardiol* 47:1005, 1981.
111. Braunwald, E. Mitral regurgitation: Physiologic, clinical, and surgical considerations. *N Engl J Med* 281:425, 1969.
112. Goldberg, H, Bakst, AA, et al. The dynamics of aortic valvular disease. *Am Heart J* 47:527, 1954.
113. Cohn, KE, Rao, BS, Russell, AG. Force generation and shortening capabilities of left ventricular myocardium in primary and secondary forms of mitral regurgitation. *Br Heart J* 31:474, 1969.
114. Tyrrell, MJ, Ellison, RC, et al. Correlation of degree of left ventricular volume overload with clinical course in aortic and mitral regurgitation. *Br Heart J* 32:683, 1970.
115. Ross, J, Jr. Afterload mismatch in aortic and mitral valve disease: Implications for surgical therapy. *J Am Coll Cardiol* 5:811, 1985.
116. Baxter, RH, Reid, JM, et al. Relation of angina to coronary artery disease in mitral and in aortic valve disease. *Br Heart J* 40:918–922, 1978.
117. Ganz, P, Swan, HJC, Ganz, W. Balloon-Tipped Flow-Directed Catheters. In W Grossman and DS Baim (eds), *Cardiac Catheterization and Angiography* (4th ed). Philadelphia: Lea & Febiger, 1991. Pp 91–102.
118. Fuchs, RM, Heuser, RR, et al. Limitations of pulmonary wedge V waves in diagnosing mitral regurgitation. *Am J Cardiol* 49:849, 1982.
119. Weiss, SJ, Savino, JS. Relationship of V-waves and pulmonary vein blood flow to mitral regurgitation. Abstracts of Annual Meeting of the Society of Cardiovascular Anesthesiologists, 1991. P 137.
120. Harshaw, CW, Grossman, W, et al. Reduced systemic vascular resistance as therapy for severe mitral regurgitation of valvular origin. *Ann Intern Med* 83:312, 1975.
121. Pichard, AD, Kay, R, et al. Large V waves in the pulmonary wedge pressure tracing in the absence of mitral regurgitation. *Am J Cardiol* 50:1044, 1982.
122. Aroesty, JM. Intra-Aortic Balloon Counterpulsation and Other Forms of Cardiopulmonary Support. In W Grossman and DS Baim (eds), *Cardiac Catheterization and Angiography* (4th ed). Philadelphia: Lea & Febiger, 1991. Pp 419–437.
123. Goodman, DJ, Rossen, RM, et al. Effects of nitroprusside on left ventricular dynamics in mitral regurgitation. *Circulation* 50:1025, 1974.
124. Chatterjee, K, Parmley, WW, et al. Beneficial effects of vasodilator agents in severe mitral regurgitation due to dysfunction of subvalvular apparatus. *Circulation* 48:684, 1973.
125. Hill, NS, Antman, EM, et al. Intravenous nitroglycerin: A review of pharmacology, indications, therapeutic effects and complications. *Chest* 79:69, 1981.
126. Keren, G, Bier, A, et al. Dynamics of mitral regurgitation during nitroglycerin therapy: A Doppler echocardiographic study. *Am Heart J* 112:517, 1986.
127. Keren, G, Bier, A, LeJemtel, TH. Improvement in forward cardiac output without a change in ejection fraction during nitroglycerin therapy in patients with functional mitral regurgitation. *Can J Cardiol* 2:206, 1986.
128. Keren, G, Katz, S, et al. Dynamic mitral regurgitation; an important determinant of the hemodynamic response to load alterations and inotropic therapy in severe heart failure. *Circulation* 80:306, 1989.
129. Bristow, MR, Ginsburg, R, et al. Decreased catecholamine sensitivity and β-adrenergic-receptor density in failing human hearts. *N Engl J Med* 307:205, 1982.
130. Lewis, KP. The use of amrinone in noncardiac surgery. *J Cardioth Anesth* 4 (Suppl 5):34, 1990.
131. Rackley, CE, Edwards, JE, et al. Aortic Valve Dis-

ease. In JW Hurst, RC Schlant, et al (eds), *The Heart* (7th ed). New York: McGraw-Hill, 1990. Pp 795–819.
132. Barlow, JB, Pocock, WA, et al. The significance of late systolic murmurs. *Am Heart J* 66:443, 1963.
133. Wann, LS, Gross, CM, et al. Diagnostic precision of echocardiography in mitral valve prolapse. *Am Heart J* 109:803, 1985.
134. Wann, LS, Grove, JR, et al. Prevalence of mitral prolapse by two dimensional echocardiography in healthy young women. *Br Heart J* 49:334, 1983.
135. Markiewicz, W, Stoner, J, et al. Mitral valve prolapse in one hundred presumably healthy young females. *Circulation* 53:464, 1976.
136. Procacci, PM, Savran, SV, et al. Prevalence of clinical mitral-valve prolapse in 1169 young women. *N Engl J Med* 294:1086, 1976.
137. Markiewicz, W, Stoner, J, et al. Mitral valve prolapse in one hundred presumably healthy females. *Circulation* 52 (Suppl II):77, 1975.
138. Kowalski, SE. Mitral valve prolapse. *Can Anaesth Soc J* 32:138, 1985.
139. Malcolm, AD. Mitral valve prolapse associated with other disorders. Causal coincidence, common link, or fundamental genetic disturbance? *Br Heart J* 53:353, 1985.
140. Crawford, MH. Mitral valve prolapse due to coronary artery disease. *Am J Med* 62:447, 1977.
141. Barlow, JB, Pocock, WA, Obel, IWP. Mitral valve prolapse: Primary, secondary, both or neither? *Am Heart J* 102:140, 1981.
142. Sakuma, T, Kakihana, M, et al. Mitral valve prolapse syndrome with coronary artery spasm: A possible cause of recurrent ventricular tachyarrhythmia. *Clin Cardiol* 8:306, 1985.
143. Gottdiener, JS, Sherber, HS, Harvey, WP. Midsystolic click and mitral valve prolapse following mitral commissurotomy. *Am J Med* 64:295, 1978.
144. Boudoulas, H, Kolibash, AJ, Jr, et al. Mitral valve prolapse and the mitral valve prolapse syndrome: A diagnostic classification and pathogenesis of symptoms. *Am Heart J* 118:796, 1989.
145. Gaffney, FA, Bastian, BC, et al. Abnormal cardiovascular regulation in the mitral valve prolapse syndrome. *Am J Cardiol* 52:316, 1983.
146. Davies, AO, Mares, A, et al. Mitral valve prolapse with symptoms of beta-adrenergic hypersensitivity. Beta-2 adrenergic receptor supercoupling with desensitization on isoproterenol exposure. *Am J Med* 82:193, 1987.
147. Shah, AA, Quinones, MA, et al. Pulsed Doppler echocardiographic detection of mitral regurgitation in mitral valve prolapse: Correlation with cardiac arrhythmias. *Cathet Cardiovasc Diagn* 8:437, 1982.
148. Devereux, RB, Perloff, JK, et al. Mitral valve prolapse. *Circulation* 54:3, 1976.
149. Davies, MJ, Moore, BP, Braimbridge, MV. The floppy mitral valve: Study of incidence, pathology, and complications in surgical, necropsy, and forensic material. *Br Heart J* 40:468, 1978.
150. Baker, PB, Bansal, G, et al. Floppy mitral valve chordae tendineae: Histopathologic alterations. *Hum Pathol* 19:507, 1988.
151. Symptomatology. In RM Jeresaty, *Mitral Valve Prolapse*. New York: Raven Press, 1979. Pp 38–44.
152. Crowe, RR. Mitral Valve Prolapse and Anxiety. In H Boudoulas and CF Wooley (eds), *Mitral Valve Prolapse and the Mitral Valve Prolapse Syndrome*. Mount Kisco, NY: Futura Publishing Co, 1988. Pp 511–523.
153. Gaffney, FA, Blomqvist, CG. Mitral Valve Prolapse and Autonomic Nervous System Dysfunction: A Pathophysiological Link. In H Boudoulas and CF Wooley (eds), *Mitral Valve Prolapse and the Mitral Valve Prolapse Syndrome*. Mount Kisco, NY: Futura Publishing Co., 1988. Pp 427–443.
154. Combs, RL, Shah, PM, et al. Effects of induced psychological stress on click and rhythm in mitral valve prolapse. *Am Heart J* 99:714, 1980.
155. Puddu, PE, Pasternac, A, et al. QT interval prolongation and increased plasma catecholamine levels in patients with mitral valve prolapse. *Am Heart J* 105:422, 1983.
156. Kligfield, P, Levy, D, et al. Arrhythmias and sudden death in mitral valve prolapse. *Am Heart J* 113:1298, 1987.
157. Boudoulas, H, Schaal, SF, et al. Mitral valve prolapse: Cardiac arrest with long term survival. *Int J Cardiol* 26:37, 1990.
158. Marks, AR, Choong, CY, et al. Identification of high-risk and low-risk subgroups of patients with mitral valve prolapse. *N Engl J Med* 320:1031, 1989.
159. Panidis, IP, McAllister, M, et al. Prevalence and severity of mitral regurgitation in the mitral valve prolapse syndrome: A Doppler echocardiographic study of 80 patients. *J Am Coll Cardiol* 7:975, 1986.
160. Gilbert, BW, Schatz, RA, et al. Mitral valve prolapse. Two dimensional echocardiographic and angiographic correlation. *Circulation* 54:716, 1976.
161. D'Cruz, IA, Shah, S, et al. Cross-sectional echocardiographic visualization of abnormal systolic motion of the left ventricle in mitral valve prolapse. *Cathet Cardiovasc Diagn* 7:35, 1981.
162. Cohen, MV, Shah, PK, Spindola-Franco, H. Angiographic-echocardiographic correlation in mitral valve prolapse. *Am Heart J* 97:43, 1979.

163. Cipriano, PR, Kline, SA, Baltaxe, HA. An angiographic assessment of left ventricular function in isolated mitral valvular prolapse. *Invest Radiol* 15:293, 1980.
164. Pasternak, RC, Thibault, GE, et al. Chest pain with angiographically insignificant coronary arterial obstruction. Clinical presentation and long-term follow-up. *Am J Med* 68:813, 1980.
165. Schwartz, DC, James, FW, Koplan, S. Exercise induced ST segment depression in children with mitral valve prolapse (abstract). *Circulation* 52:258, 1975.
166. Jeresaty, RM. Etiology of the mitral valve prolapse-click syndrome. *Am J Cardiol* 36:110, 1975.
167. Gottdiener, JS, Borer, JS, et al. Left ventricular function in mitral valve prolapse: Assessment with radionuclide cineangiography. *Am J Cardiol* 47:7, 1981.
168. Schaal, SF. Mitral Valve Prolapse: Cardiac Arrhythmias and Electrophysiological Correlates. In H Boudoulas and CF Wooley (eds), *Mitral Valve Prolapse and the Mitral Valve Prolapse Syndrome*. Mount Kisco, NY: Futura Publishing Co, 1988. Pp 567–590.
169. Boudoulas, H, Kligfield, P, Wooley, CF. Mitral Valve Prolapse: Sudden Death. In H Boudoulas and CF Wooley (eds), *Mitral Valve Prolapse and the Mitral Valve Prolapse Syndrome*. Mount Kisco, NY: Futura Publishing Co, 1988. Pp 591–605.
170. Chesler, E, King, RA, Edwards, JE. The myxomatous mitral valve and sudden death. *Circulation* 67:632, 1983.
171. Bharati, S, Granston, AS, et al. The conduction system in the mitral valve prolapse syndrome with sudden death. *Am Heart J* 101:667, 1981.
172. Mason, JW, Koch, FH, et al. Cardiac biopsy evidence for a cardiomyopathy associated with symptomatic mitral valve prolapse. *Am J Cardiol* 42:557, 1978.
173. Horhreiter, C, Niles, N, et al. Mitral regurgitation: Relationship of noninvasive right and left ventricular performance descriptors to clinical and hemodynamic findings and to prognosis in medically and surgically treated patients. *Circulation* 73:900, 1986.
174. Frishman, WH, Sonnenblick, EH. β-Adrenergic Blocking Drugs. In JW Hurst, RC Schlant (eds), *The Heart* (7th ed). New York: McGraw-Hill, 1990. Pp 1712–1731.
175. Winkle, RA, Lopes, MG. Propranolol for patients with mitral valve prolapse. *Am Heart J* 93:422, 1977.
176. Siskind, SJ (personal communication). Booth Memorial Medical Center, Flushing, NY.
177. Dajani, AS, Bisno, AL, et al. Prevention of bacterial endocarditis. Recommendations by the American Heart Association. *JAMA* 264:2919, 1990.
178. MacMahon, SW, Hickey, AJ, et al. Risk of infective endocarditis in mitral valve prolapse with and without precordial systolic murmurs. *Am J Cardiol* 59:105, 1987.
179. Drapkin, MS. Endocarditis after the use of an oral irrigation device. *Ann Intern Med* 87:455, 1977.
180. Corrigall, D, Bolen, J, et al. Mitral valve prolapse and infective endocarditis. *Am J Med* 63:215, 1977.
181. McKinsey, DS, Ratts, TE, Bisno, AL. Underlying cardiac lesions in adults with infective endocarditis: The changing spectrum. *Am J Med* 82:681, 1987.

8
Pericardial Disease

Kevin M. Glassman

Pericardial disease has been associated with a long list of medical and surgical illnesses. In general, the severity of this condition depends on whether the process of pericardial involvement has been acute or chronic, the underlying disorder that led to changes in the pericardium, and the amount of compensatory changes in cardiovascular function necessary to overcome any compressive or restrictive properties of the pericardium. Surgical intervention for a patient with symptomatic pericardial disease is a rare event in most centers. In busy trauma or cardiac centers, pericardial disease may be seen more often in the acute setting, usually with a brief period of serious myocardial compression. Once this compression is surgically relieved, the anesthetic management is usually simpler. However, in some instances the relief of acute tamponade can lead to disastrous complications, such as in the patient with a complicated dissection of the ascending aorta, in whom release of the tamponade can lead to acute rises in aortic root pressures, with resultant rupture of the aorta and death [1]. Anesthesiologists will more likely be called on to care for a patient with subclinical pericardial disease, manifested as a complication of another underlying illness. If the operative procedure is noncardiac, the anesthesiologist does not have the luxury of surgical relief of the cardiac compression at some point, and the intraoperative as well as postoperative management becomes very complex. Proper care of these patients requires a firm understanding of the physiologic alterations common to pericardial disease, as well as the effects that anesthetics will have on an already compromised heart.

PERICARDIAL TAMPONADE

Pericardial effusions are caused by both acute and chronic diseases that involve the pericardium. The most ominous effect of these accumulations of fluid, cardiac tamponade, occurs when the volume of effusion impedes myocardial filling to the point that the patient becomes symptomatic. Common signs and symptoms of cardiac tamponade include increased heart rate, light-headedness due to hypotension, syncope, ascites, weakness, cough, orthopnea, chest pain, and distended jugular veins. Most patients with pericardial tamponade are treated outside the operating room with medical management or needle aspiration using ultrasound guidance [2]. There has been a good deal of debate in the literature concerning the proper management of medical patients with symptomatic effusions requiring drainage of the pericardium. Some recommend needle aspiration unless the procedure will likely be repeated several times over the course of the patient's illness. Singh and Newmark [3], in

Table 8-1. Causes of cardiac tamponade

Malignant disease
Idiopathic pericarditis
Uremia
Acute myocardial infarction
Diagnostic procedures
Bacteria
Tuberculosis
Radiation
Myxedema
Dissecting aortic aneurysm
Postpericardiectomy syndrome
Systemic lupus erythematosus
Cardiomyopathy
Trauma

Source: Modified from BA Guberman, NO Fowler, PJ Engel, et al. Cardiac tamponade in medical patients. *Circulation* 64: 633–640, 1981.

a study of uremic patients, suggested pericardiocentesis only in dire emergencies. They recommended surgical correction of the effusion as first-line therapy.

Anesthesiologists will commonly encounter patients in the operating room who are being treated for complications of their primary illness, with pericardial effusions and tamponade as associated findings. The incidence of pericardial effusions in patients with cancer has been variously quoted as 2 to 21 percent as determined by autopsy. Metastasis to the pericardium occurs most frequently in lung and breast carcinoma, followed by lymphoma, leukemia, and melanoma, in order of decreasing frequency [4–6]. In one series, over 90 percent of patients had either lung or breast primaries [7]. In an autopsy study by Thurber and colleagues [5], 189 patients were diagnosed with metastatic malignancy of the pericardium. Of these, 29 percent had clinically significant involvement during life, and the cause of death was judged to be a direct result of the pericardial metastasis in 36 percent. Considering the number of cancer patients taken to the operating room for corrective or palliative procedures, the likelihood of the anesthesiologist encountering a patient with pericardial effusion or tamponade, or both, in this population of patients is rather high. Cardiac tamponade can occur in various other conditions, with acute tamponade present in 3 to 6 percent of patients after open heart operations [8]. Approximately 10 percent of patients with chronic renal failure who are receiving hemodialysis will develop tamponade, and 15 to 55 percent manifest uremic pericarditis [3]. Other likely causes of pericardial tamponade in medical patients are presented in Table 8-1.

In the trauma patient, the possibility of encountering pericardial tamponade should be kept in mind, even if this is not the patient's primary reason for coming to the operating room. In a patient with direct chest injuries, the suspicion is always high. In a patient with blunt trauma or other indirect injuries, the anesthesiologist should consider the possibility of undetected tamponade on initial emergency room evaluation.

Physical Findings and Diagnostic Evaluation

The classic description of a triad of findings in the patient with pericardial tamponade was by Beck in 1935 [9]. Decreased arterial pressure, increased venous pressure, and a small quiet heart are usual (Table 8-2). However, many medical patients with chronic effusions leading to tamponade lack one or more of these signs. An enlarged "bottle-shape" cardiac silhouette on chest x-ray is common once at least 250 ml fluid or blood is present. Pulsus paradoxus is also quite common, though not universal or specific for tamponade. A paradoxical pulse is defined as at least a 10 mm Hg decrease in arterial systolic pressure during inspiration [10]. A proposed mechanism of pulsus paradoxus is augmented right heart filling during inspiration, which creates an increase in pericardial pressure. This rise in pericardial pressure causes further compression of the

Table 8-2. Clinical signs of cardiac tamponade

Pulsus paradoxus
Distant heart sounds
Arterial hypotension
Tachycardia
Elevated central venous pressure
Electrical alternans
Decreased ECG voltage
Nonspecific ST-T wave changes

left ventricle, leading to a decrease in cardiac output and blood pressure [10]. An inspiratory increase in the jugular venous pressure (Kussmaul's sign) is usually associated with constrictive pericarditis, but rarely occurs in uncomplicated cardiac tamponade.

Electrocardiographic findings of tamponade consist of nonspecific ST and T-wave changes, ischemia, decreased electrical voltage, and electrical alternans [4, 11]. Though these ECG changes are seen commonly, many patients lack one or more of these findings. Decreased electrical voltage is due to a short-circuiting effect of the pericardial fluid on the heart's electrical impulses as detected by the ECG. Electrical alternans, due to changes in the heart's position resulting from rotational pendular movements, occurs in 10 to 15 percent of patients [12]. Since the heart is suspended in a relatively large volume of fluid, it tends to move more freely than normal, and rocks back and forth between systole and diastole. When the heart swings anteriorly, it is closer to the chest wall, and a taller R wave results with every other beat. As it recoils to its normal position, the R wave decreases in amplitude as the heart moves away from the chest wall [11]. The rotational motion of the heart is usually confined by the mediastinal structures and the pressure of the lungs. Heart rate, volume of fluid, and viscosity of the pericardial fluid are interrelated in the production of electrical alternans.

Echocardiography has been described as the most reliable indicator of pericardial tamponade, able to detect as little as 15 ml fluid [13]. Exaggerated motion of the heart within the pericardial sac is described [14], as well as the presence of a sonolucent space between the pericardial and epicardial echoes (Fig. 8-1). If the pericardium is filled with clotted blood rather than fluid, echocardiography may be unable to make the diagnosis because of similar densities of clotted blood and muscle.

Anatomy and Pathophysiology

The pericardium consists of a visceral pericardium covering the surface of the heart and a parietal pericardium, which together enclose the pericar-

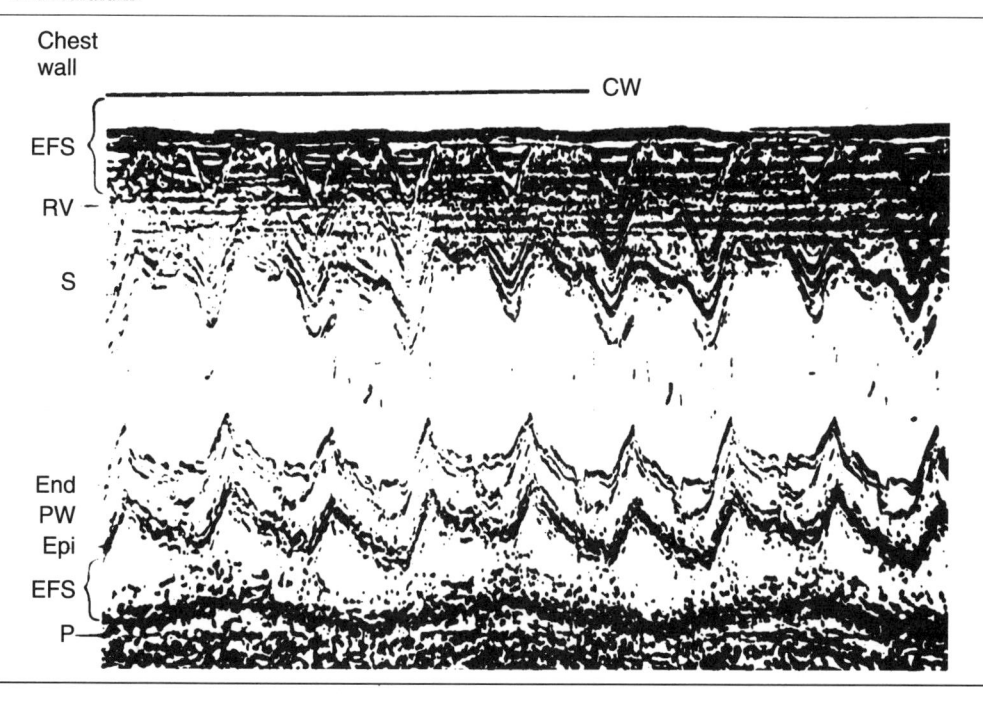

Fig. 8-1. M-mode echocardiogram of a patient with a pericardial effusion. Note the effusion (EFS) between the epicardium (Epi) and the pericardium (P). RV = right ventricle; PW = posterior wall; S = septum; End = endocardium.

dial space. The pericardial cavity normally contains 25 to 50 ml clear fluid, which is an ultrafiltrate of plasma. This fluid is normally drained through an interconnecting plexus of epicardial and endocardial channels that eventually drain into a large lymph node near the aortic root. The majority of this fluid, as well as lymphatic circulation of the heart, drains into the mediastinal lymph nodes.

The pericardium functions to protect the heart from acute dilatation, and isolates it from other structures in the mediastinum, preventing adhesions and infection while maintaining the heart in optimal position and shape. With the pericardium intact, interaction between the right and left ventricles is enhanced. As the left ventricle dilates, intrapericardial pressure increases, inhibiting the filling of the right ventricle. This limited filling of the right ventricle prevents overload of the pulmonary circulation, and thus helps to prevent pulmonary edema. While there is controversy in the literature concerning the functional roles of the pericardium, it is clear that this structure is not essential for life. The pericardium is often removed or left open after cardiac surgery, with few untoward effects on the patient. Tamponade occurs when fluid accumulates in the pericardial sac and prevents proper filling of the heart. As fluid accumulates, pressure rises within the sac, forcing the ventricular chamber size to decrease. This external pressure interferes with diastolic filling of the ventricle and cardiac output falls. The sympathetic nervous system initially compensates for the fall in stroke volume and cardiac output by increasing heart rate and systemic vascular resistance. As the pressure and volume within the pericardium increase, sympathetic compensatory mechanisms are unable to maintain normal cardiac output, stroke volume continues to decline, and systolic arterial pressure falls.

As ventricular diastolic pressure increases, coronary perfusion pressure steadily declines, ultimately leading to myocardial ischemia. Arrhythmias are frequent, due to a mismatch of myocardial oxygen supply and demand. Increased heart rate and contractility needed to overcome tamponade require an increase in oxygen demand. However, rising ventricular end diastolic pressures, wall tension, and a shorter diastolic filling period, plus hypotension, all lead to significant declines in myocardial oxygen delivery.

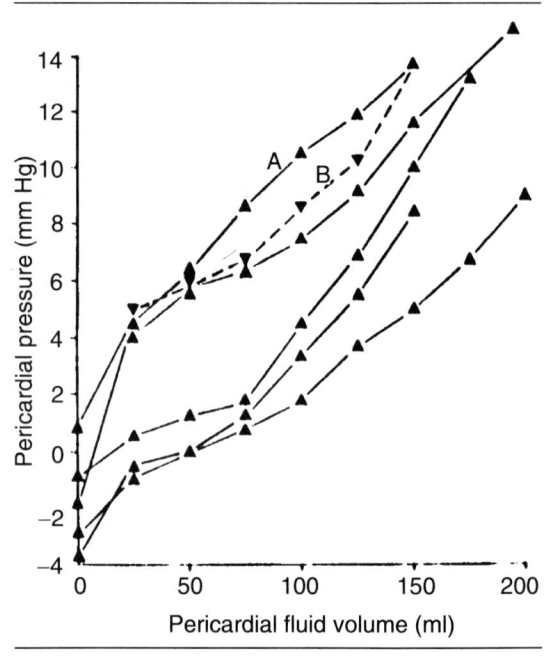

Fig. 8-2. Pericardial pressure-volume relationship in the baboon. Note the rapid rise in pressures at higher volumes. (A) and (B) denote the same animal, with addition and removal of saline from the pericardium, respectively. (Reprinted with permission from CT Moller, CG Schoonbee, and C Rosendorff, Haemodynamics of cardiac tamponade during various modes of ventilation. Br J Anaesth 51:409–414, 1979.)

The parietal pericardium is a stiff collagenous membrane that resists acute expansion. If pericardial fluid accumulates rapidly, as in trauma or iatrogenic causes such as central venous catheter placement, the fibrous pericardium is incapable of acute expansion and tamponade occurs at relatively small volumes. If fluid accumulates more gradually, with time the fibrous pericardium can stretch and accommodate larger volumes. At some point, a critical volume is reached beyond which additional fluid leads to rapid decompensation and tamponade. Rapid accumulation of as little as 200 ml pericardial fluid may precipitate tamponade, as opposed to a capacity of greater than 2 liters given several weeks to develop [15]. However, when the volume in a chronically dilated pericardium is at its critical point, the addition of small amounts of fluid will cause rapid tamponade (Fig. 8-2).

The increased pericardial pressure is transmitted to all four chambers of the heart, resulting in a classic equalization of several diastolic pressures. As measured by pulmonary artery catheter, the right atrial, right ventricular end diastolic, central venous, and pulmonary artery diastolic pressures are nearly equal to intrapericardial pressure, which may be elevated as high as 20 mm Hg or more [16].

Pulsus paradoxus is an exaggerated decrease in systolic blood pressure during inspiration in the presence of an elevated intrapericardial pressure. Normally, there is a 5 to 10 mm Hg decrease in arterial systolic pressure with inspiration, but in the case of a paradoxical pulse the pressure may drop as much as 20 mm Hg or more. It has been described in a varying number of patients, and is by no means specific or pathognomonic for tamponade, as it has been reported in patients with severe chronic obstructive pulmonary disease or asthma without tamponade. A significant effusion may exist without pulsus paradoxus, and it may also be difficult to elicit in the face of hypotension, arrhythmias, and respiratory distress. This decline is due to an imbalance during inspiration between an increase in pulmonary venous capacitance and a smaller augmentation in venous return to the right side of the heart. This relative imbalance leads to a decrease in left-sided filling and output on the next cycle and a decrease in arterial systolic pressure. There is also a shift in the intraventricular septum during increased right ventricular filling with inspiration, which further decreases left ventricular filling [17].

When the pericardium is filled with fluid, the increase in right ventricular volume with inspiration causes an increase in right ventricular pressure that is transmitted to the pericardium. The resultant increase in pericardial pressure further compresses the left ventricle, preventing filling and a decline in arterial systolic pressure (Fig. 8-3).

Effects of Ventilation

Induction of general anesthesia in the face of pericardial tamponade has resulted in severe hypotension, ischemia, and cardiac arrest, in part due to positive-pressure ventilation [18, 19]. It has been recommended that if general anesthesia is

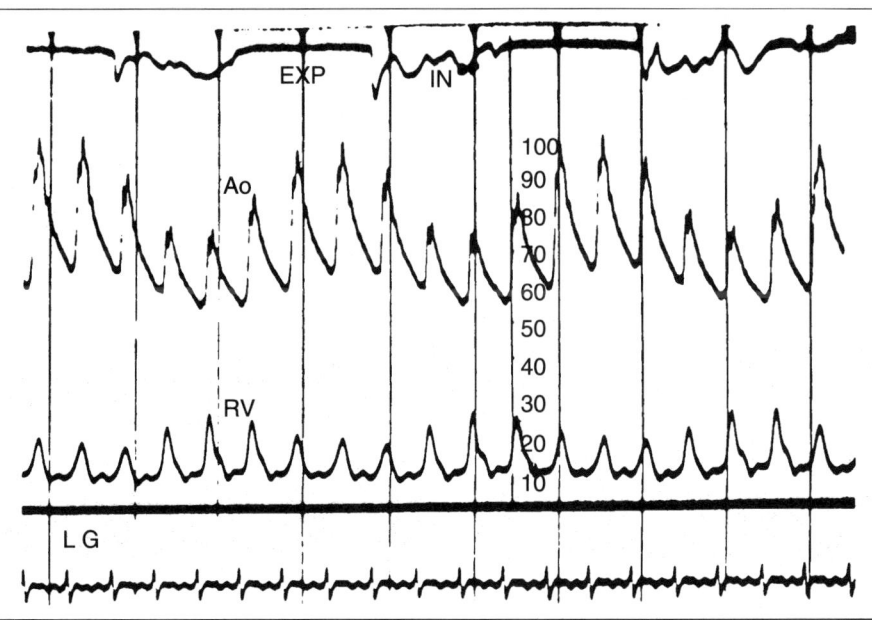

Fig. 8-3. Arterial pressure tracing in a patient with pericardial tamponade, demonstrating pulsus paradoxus. Note the more than 10 mm Hg decline in aortic pressure (Ao) during inspiration (INSP). (Reprinted with permission from R Shabetai et al. The hemodynamics of cardiac tamponade and constrictive pericarditis. *Am J Cardiol* 26:480, 1970.)

required for a patient with a pericardial effusion or tamponade, an anesthetic using spontaneous respirations should be employed, because positive-pressure ventilation may diminish cardiac output [20].

Intermittent positive-pressure ventilation produces a significant decrease in both transmural right ventricular end diastolic pressure and cardiac output over and above that produced by cardiac tamponade with the patient breathing spontaneously. If positive end expiratory pressure is added to this, a further reduction in cardiac output can be expected [20]. The mechanism for this decrease in cardiac output is a decrease in right heart venous return with positive pressure. Any drop in right-sided output is reflected as a decrease in left-sided return and subsequent decrease in cardiac output. This mechanism is consistent with studies linking left ventricular stroke volume to right ventricular stroke volume one or two beats earlier [21]. The addition of positive end expiratory pressure will further decrease right-sided venous return and the transmural right ventricular end diastolic pressure [21, 22] (Fig. 8-4). The use of high-frequency jet ventilation has been shown to preserve cardiac output by lowering peak airway and intrapericardial pressures relative to conventional mechanical ventilation [23].

Hemodynamics of Fluid Status

One of the hallmarks of pericardial tamponade is an elevated central venous pressure (CVP). This increase is required to overcome the pressure being exerted on the right atrium and right ventricle by the fluid-filled pericardium. As long as the CVP is above the pericardial pressure, right ventricular output and filling will be well maintained. Once the central venous pressure falls, the right ventricular end diastolic volume and pressure fall and cardiac output decreases. As the intrapericardial pressure increases, compensatory changes such as tachycardia and vasoconstriction are less likely to maintain blood flow and arterial pressure. As a compensatory mechanism, in the face of arterial hypotension, renal retention of salt and water occurs, which leads to an increase in CVP and maintenance of cardiac output. Any decrease in CVP related to perioperative fluid or blood loss can lead to severe hypotension and ischemia. The goal of

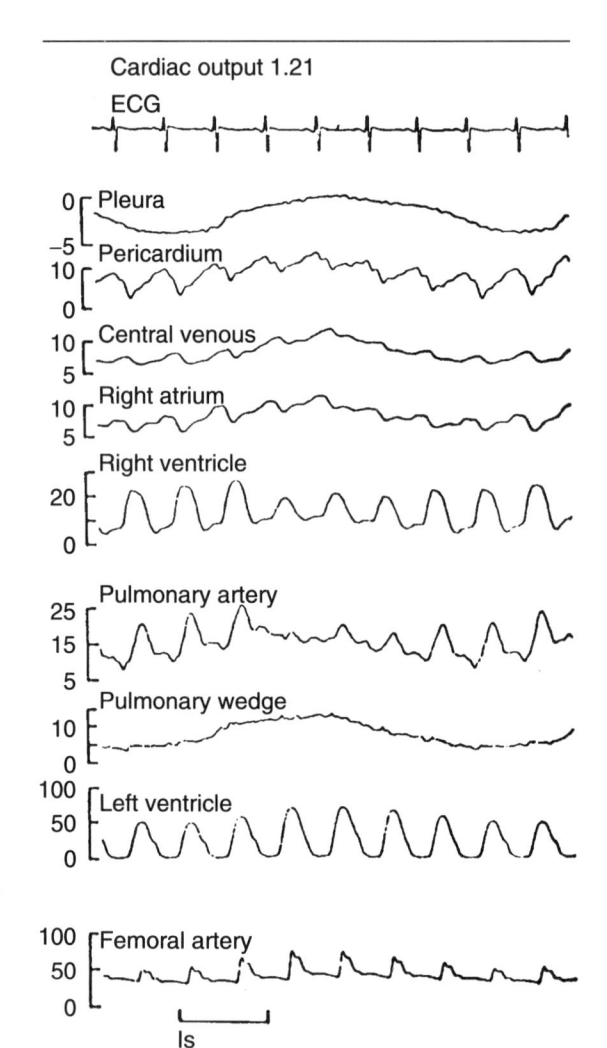

Fig. 8-4. Cardiac output, ECG, and pressure tracings in the baboon with saline-induced cardiac tamponade and intermittent positive-pressure ventilation. Note the simultaneous rise in pleural and pericardial pressures, while right ventricular pressure declines. Several beats later, arterial pressure falls. The same animal with spontaneous respirations has a cardiac output of 1.66 liters per minute. (Reprinted with permission from CT Moller, CG Schoonbee, and C Rosendorff, Haemodynamics of cardiac tamponade during various modes of ventilation. Br J Anaesth 51:409–414, 1979.)

the anesthesiologist should be to maintain the CVP at levels optimum for the calculated Starling curve of the individual patient. Ideally, this curve should be plotted preoperatively based on the measurements of cardiac output versus CVP and pulmonary capillary wedge pressure (PCWP). If the patient is dehydrated or has suffered acute blood loss preoperatively, elevated CVP, pulsus paradoxus, and jugular venous distention may be masked until the blood volume is restored [24].

Pressure-volume Curves

The normal pressure in the pericardial space is essentially the same as that in the pleural space, with a mean pressure near zero. With the addition of fluid to the pericardial space, pressure rises, quite slowly at first if the pericardium is relaxed, then steeply when the pericardium becomes tense. When the volume of fluid increases rapidly, the stiff pericardium does not stretch easily, and tamponade can result rapidly with as little as 200 ml fluid. In contrast, if the volume of fluid rises slowly, the pericardium can expand gradually, and contain as much as 2 liters of fluid before hemodynamic compromise occurs. Thereafter, pressure again rises rapidly. Hypervolemia increases the resting pericardial pressure and raises the slope of the pericardial pressure-volume curve. The undesirable effect of hypervolemia may be offset by an increase in the cardiac output and venous return to the right ventricle. Hypovolemia does not change the level of the resting pericardial pressure, but lowers the slope of the pressure-volume curve measured during tamponade [25] (Fig. 8-5).

The rise in pericardial pressure can be seen indirectly by a careful examination of the central venous or right atrial pressure tracing. Since the main effect of an elevated pericardial pressure is to resist filling of the ventricle, a change is seen in the normal pressure tracing. Systemic venous return is compromised during diastole, resulting in a loss of the usual y descent of this pressure curve. The atrium essentially fills only during systole, when the ventricular volume is decreasing and the pericardial pressure exerts less of an inhibitory force on the atrium. A prominent x descent and loss of the y descent on the central venous tracing are characteristic of tamponade.

The x descent occurs during ventricular systole

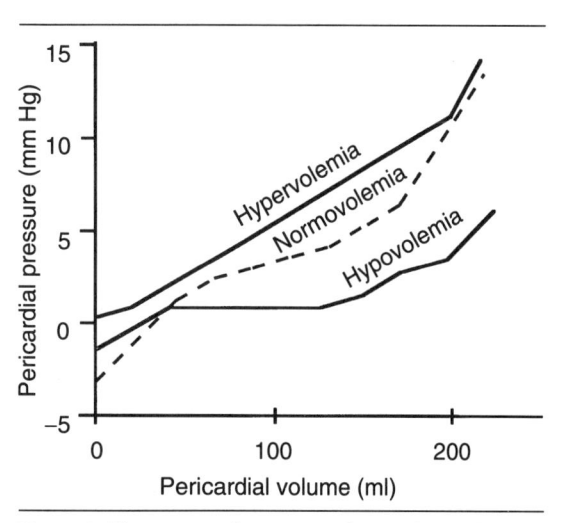

Fig. 8-5. Illustration of pressure-volume relationship within the pericardial sac dependent on the overall volume status of the patient. Note that the hypovolemic patient will have a considerably lower pericardial pressure given the same volume of pericardial fluid as the hypervolemic patient.

and is a result of downward displacement of the base of the heart and tricuspid valve as well as continued atrial relaxation. The y descent usually occurs after opening of the tricuspid valve and during rapid inflow of blood from the right atrium into the ventricle [26] (Fig. 8-6).

Removal of as little as 50 ml fluid from the pericardium once tamponade has resulted can dramatically improve the clinical condition of the patient, and may be lifesaving [25].

Monitoring

Due to the potentially life-threatening complications of cardiac tamponade and effusion, extensive perioperative monitoring is essential. The patient should be connected to standard monitoring, such as blood pressure cuff, pulse oximeter, end-tidal carbon dioxide, and temperature. An ECG is also standard, but can be optimized by a modified V_5 lead to monitor for left ventricular ischemia. An arterial line should be used to monitor beat-to-beat pressure, and to watch for changes in magnitude of pulsus paradoxus, which, if present, would indicate possible worsening tamponade. Patients may require inotropic support, which also necessitates

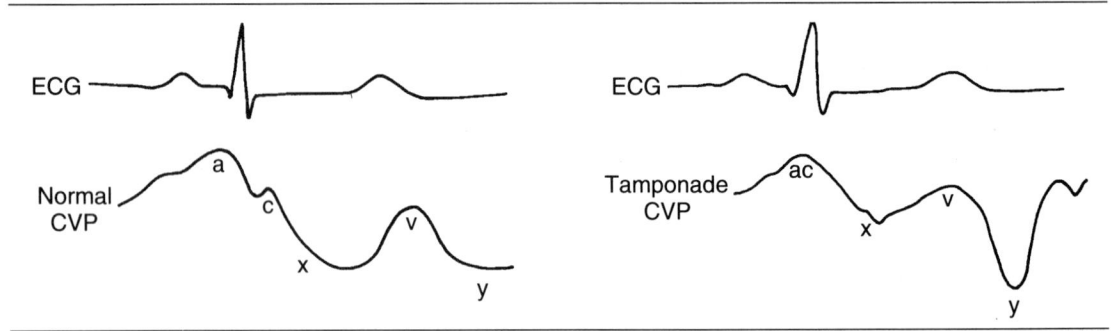

Fig. 8-6. Schematic of a normal central venous pressure tracing and a typical tracing seen in the patient with pericardial tamponade. Note that the x descent is a result of atrial relaxation as well as downward displacement of the base of the heart and tricuspid valve during ventricular systole, and is accentuated in tamponade. The normal y descent occurs after opening of the tricuspid valve as blood flows rapidly into the ventricle from the atrium. This portion of the tracing is often attenuated during pericardial tamponade.

continuous arterial pressure monitoring. Arterial blood gases should be drawn preoperatively as a baseline, then periodically during the procedure. Urine output should be monitored closely as another sign of fluid status.

While a central venous catheter may be sufficient for some patients a pulmonary artery catheter is more appropriate. It will enable the anesthesiologist to produce a Starling curve for the patient, as well as to closely monitor the effects of anesthetics on the cardiac output and filling pressures. These monitors will allow for a safer induction period, as well as help in the possible diagnosis of acute hemodynamic decompensation, causes of which may include additional myocardial depression from anesthetics and decreased filling pressures due to anesthetic agents or regional anesthesia, positive-pressure ventilation, or preexisting cardiac disease [18, 27]. Obviously, immediate surgical therapy for life-threatening cardiac tamponade should not be delayed for the purpose of placing invasive monitors, but when time allows, these monitors will enable the anesthesiologist to administer anesthesia in a much safer manner.

Optimizing the Patient's Condition Preoperatively

In significant pericardial effusions and tamponade, it is important to optimize fluid status and maintain the CVP at higher than normal levels. The elevated CVP helps to counteract the restrictive forces of the pericardial fluid that prevent chamber filling. Maintenance of filling pressures as high as 25 to 30 mm Hg or more may be necessary [16].

Debate continues as to the appropriate supportive therapy for these patients, with many authors suggesting vigorous fluid expansion and the use of vasodilators such as nitroprusside. Volume expansion can be accomplished with the use of crystalloids, blood, or colloid. Others have shown that the hemodynamic benefits of volume expansion and nitroprusside infusion are limited in patients with acute tamponade [28]. This therapy seems more helpful in slower-developing cardiac decompensation, with surgical drainage or pericardiocentesis more effective in the acute setting.

Administration of catecholamines (dobutamine, isoproterenol) may help maintain arterial pressure, coronary perfusion, and cardiac output, but some evidence suggests that they may be of limited value in acute tamponade [29]. Arrhythmias are common in these patients, and even minimal amounts of hypoxia or hypercarbia should be avoided. Preoperative sedation should be minimized or withheld, as it may lead to respiratory depression, hypercarbia, and hypoxia.

Isoproterenol and dobutamine, which increase myocardial contractility without increasing systemic vascular resistance, will augment cardiac output. Norepinephrine and other alpha agonists are contraindicated because they primarily increase systemic vascular resistance, leading to a decrease in cardiac output in tamponade.

Metabolic acidosis frequently develops secondary to an increase in systemic vascular resistance and decreased cardiac output, and this acidosis further worsens the cardiac output. Treatment with 0.5 to 1.0 mEq/kg sodium bicarbonate can correct this acidosis, and will counteract its negative effect on cardiac output [30]. Digitalis is not of proven value for treatment of low cardiac output associated with cardiac tamponade; this may be due to the large increase in systemic vascular resistance that may accompany administration of this drug.

Management of Anesthesia

Induction of general anesthesia has resulted in rapid hemodynamic deterioration in the patient with pericardial effusion and tamponade, at times leading to cardiac arrest [31]. These patients respond poorly to resuscitative efforts unless the effusion is drained surgically. It has been suggested that the optimal anesthetic management of tamponade includes subxiphoid drainage of the tamponade under local anesthesia before induction of general anesthesia. This approach is still debated, with others recommending general anesthesia before the release of tamponade in an attempt to provide a paralyzed, cooperative patient for surgery. The management of acute tamponade in the setting of trauma is challenging for the anesthesiologist and surgeon. Despite sedation and local infiltration of the chest, these patients can become confused, and violent, and move about on the operating room table. This can lead to lacerations of the myocardium, coronary arteries, or pneumothorax, even with direct surgical drainage. Because of these problems, many surgeons prefer general rather than local anesthesia before drainage of the tamponade.

As noted earlier, if general anesthesia is required, spontaneous respirations should be preserved, since positive pressure ventilation can diminish cardiac output. Once the tamponade has been decompressed by pericardiotomy or pericardiocentesis, general anesthesia can be administered more easily. It should be noted that removal of the pericardial fluid should be accomplished slowly. Pulmonary edema has been precipitated by the rapid drainage of large pericardial effusions, which abruptly relieves right heart compression, leading to a sudden increase in venous return. This can cause left ventricular overload while the systemic vascular resistance is still elevated, and can result in pulmonary edema [32, 33]. In addition, pericardiocentesis has also been associated with lacerations of the myocardium and coronary arteries, puncture of the ventricle, and pneumothorax.

If relief of increased pericardial pressure is not possible before induction of anesthesia, the goal is maintenance of cardiac output. Reductions in contractility, heart rate, and venous return to the right heart should be avoided. Induction and maintenance of anesthesia are often with ketamine or benzodiazepines plus nitrous oxide. Pancuronium is a useful muscle relaxant if skeletal paralysis is required, due to the tachycardia it can produce.

Ketamine is very useful for induction and maintenance of anesthesia due to its circulatory effects. It increases heart rate, contractility, and systemic vascular resistance. It is prudent to keep in mind that patients with tamponade and long-standing hemodynamic deterioration may be under the effects of maximal endogenous catecholamine stimulation before induction of anesthesia, and even ketamine may result in hypotension, and myocardial depression [27]. All inhalational and most intravenous anesthetics decrease myocardial contractility and cause peripheral vasodilation [34, 35].

Induction of anesthesia with benzodiazepines, followed by maintenance of anesthesia with nitrous oxide and fentanyl plus pancuronium, has also been used successfully in patients with tamponade [36].

The use of catecholamines to maintain cardiac output and systemic vascular resistance has been advocated by many. However, the use of isoproterenol has been shown to increase epicardial blood flow more than endocardial flow, which may be less helpful in the face of ischemia [16]. In dogs, catecholamines have been shown to increase blood flow only to the myocardium, not to the brain or kidneys, despite a doubling of cardiac output [29]. The use of nitroprusside is controversial, but its presumed benefit in increasing cardiac output secondary to a decline in systemic vascular resistance can be offset by a decrease in venous return unless the patient is well hydrated [37]. Primary arteriolar vasodilators such as hydralazine have been shown to be more effective in increasing cardiac output [16].

Since patients with pericardial effusions and tamponade have relatively fixed stroke volumes, they rely more on heart rate for cardiac output, and bradycardia should be avoided because of its likely decrease in cardiac output. Atropine has been used to counteract the depressor vagal reflex described in both early and late tamponade [38, 39].

In the special case of acute cardiac tamponade complicating dissection of the ascending thoracic aorta, a different approach to anesthetic management is suggested. The release of tamponade may lead to a sudden rise in systolic blood pressure and cardiac output, which may cause an already compromised aorta to rupture. Norman and Mycyk [1] successfully managed this type of patient with femoral-femoral bypass, vasodilation, and β-blockade. Management as previously described led to aortic rupture and exsanguination of another patient with similar disease.

Use of Inhalational Agents

The patient with pericardial tamponade is utilizing all the endogenous resources available to maintain cardiac output and forward blood flow, and thus should be treated as a patient with severe impairment of left ventricular function. As all of the currently used inhalational agents lead to some degree of myocardial depression, their use should be discouraged intraoperatively. These agents are poorly tolerated by these patients and may result in greater than anticipated decreases in blood pressure. Of the three most widely used agents, isoflurane would be the more appropriate choice, due to its greater peripheral vasodilation.

Nitrous oxide has been used successfully by many, combined with narcotics and muscle relaxants. High-dose fentanyl (50–100 μg/kg) has been recommended for patients who cannot tolerate even minimal myocardial depression [40]. The drawback of this technique is that the patient usually remains intubated postoperatively. More traditional doses of opioids must be combined with other drugs, such as nitrous oxide, to assure complete amnesia. Although nitrous oxide has been combined with opioids successfully in critically ill patients, there have been reports of significant circulatory changes, including reductions in blood pressure and cardiac output [41]. The mechanism of these changes is suggested by increases in pulmonary artery occlusion pressures when nitrous oxide is used [42].

Patients with pericardial effusions from metastatic cancer have often been treated aggressively with chemotherapeutic agents that may be cardiotoxic. These agents may lead to an underlying cardiomyopathy in addition to a compressed ventricle from tamponade. Inhalational agents should be avoided in these patients.

Use of Noninhalational General Anesthesia

Agents that decrease venous return to the heart, depress cardiac output, significantly reduce systemic vascular resistance, or create extremes in heart rate should be avoided. Keeping these fundamentals in mind, agents such as thiopental or other barbiturates are poor choices for induction of general anesthesia. Etomidate has been described as a reliable induction agent by some, but its use is not widespread due to other side effects, such as adrenal suppression even after single doses. Propofol may have fewer circulatory changes associated with its use than barbiturates, but has also been described as leading to significant hypotension on induction in critically ill patients, and should be avoided.

Benzodiazepines can be used for induction of anesthesia and cause little circulatory change or decrease in cardiac output when used alone. Their combination with fentanyl, however, can produce reductions in blood pressure and cardiac output [36, 43]. The use of benzodiazepines as preoperative medication should be limited because of possible respiratory depression. This will lead to hypoxia and hypercarbia, which will worsen any preexisting ischemia.

As discussed earlier, ketamine is a useful induction agent for these patients, with a good margin of safety. It maintains heart rate, myocardial contractility, and systemic vascular resistance, but will also lead to an increase in myocardial oxygen demand.

High-dose fentanyl will maintain hemodynamic stability during induction, but will likely result in a prolonged intubation postoperatively. Shorter-acting narcotics such as alfentanil (Alfenta) may be a more logical choice if hemodynamic stability and an extubated patient at the end of surgery are desired. Induction doses of 30 to 50 µg/kg will be required, and a continuous infusion of 1 to 2 µg/kg/min can be maintained intraoperatively.

Pancuronium is a widely used muscle relaxant for these patients due to its preservation of increased heart rate. It is especially useful in combination with opioids to prevent bradycardia. Atracurium, vecuronium, and metocurine have also been used as relaxants with good success.

Use of Regional Anesthesia

Patients with cardiac effusion and tamponade may be candidates for regional anesthesia, provided a technique is employed that allows adequate analgesia without interference in respiratory and circulatory function. Hyperbaric spinal anesthesia is not a recommended option for these patients due to the abrupt decline in venous return and hypotension that may develop. Hypobaric spinal anesthesia can be considered, for example, in the case of orthopedic surgery of the lower extremities, due to its less profound decrease in sympathetic tone and venous return. Adequate preoperative volume loading is essential, as well as aggressive hemodynamic monitoring. Continuous spinal anesthesia with fractionated dosing is an alternative approach, although this technique has recently come under scrutiny due to several reported cases of cauda equina syndrome following its use [44].

Epidural anesthesia should be considered where applicable, due to the slower hemodynamic shifts and easily titrated dosing to achieve adequate anesthesia. Again, proper fluid loading is essential. Extra care must be taken to ensure that inadvertent administration of local anesthetic into the cerebrospinal fluid or blood is avoided during fractionated dosing.

If the patient is scheduled to have a high abdominal procedure, regional anesthesia should be avoided due to the likely compromise of respiratory function associated with high thoracic levels of anesthesia.

Other regional techniques, such as ankle blocks, wrist blocks, axillary blocks, and Bier's blocks, can be used for procedures of the extremities. Interscalene and supraclavicular blocks should be avoided due to their associated complications, which may lead to rapid intubation and hemodynamic instability.

Example of Emergency Operation

A 60-year-old man with metastatic lung carcinoma and pericardial effusion is brought to the operating room for emergency exploratory laparotomy for possible bowel ischemia. He has a blood pressure of 100/60, pulse of 96, and respiratory rate of 20.

Initially, this patient should have invasive monitors placed for intraoperative management. These should include an arterial line, central venous catheter or pulmonary artery catheter, and two large-bore intravenous lines. He should receive supplemental oxygen during transport to the operating room. No preoperative medication should be administered.

Initial measurements of CVP, PCWP, pulmonary artery pressure, and arterial pressure, as well as cardiac output and pulsus paradoxus, should be recorded. Boluses of 500 ml crystalloid should be administered if initial cardiac output is low, and additional outputs recorded until optimum filling pressures and cardiac output are reached.

Rapid-sequence induction with alfentanil, ketamine, and succinylcholine is one possible method of maintaining hemodynamic stability while protecting this patient from aspiration. Inotropes, such as dobutamine, isoproterenol, and dopamine, should be available. Maintenance of anesthesia can be provided by continuous infusion of alfentanil, nitrous oxide, and oxygen with controlled ventilation until the patient recovers from muscle paralysis. At this point, spontaneous respiration can resume unless the surgical team requires continuous paralysis. If paralysis is needed, pancuronium is the relaxant of choice, especially with the combined use of alfentanil.

Filling pressures should be maintained at levels to provide maximum cardiac output, with consideration given to the large third-space fluid sequestration common during these procedures. Hematocrit should be checked at regular intervals to assure that excessive crystalloid is not administered in place of needed colloid. It should be recalled that these patients are prone to ischemia secondary to the changes in coronary blood flow and wall tension that accompany pericardial effusion and tamponade. Hemodilution and anemia will only aggravate ischemia.

Any change in hemodynamic stability should initially be corrected with crystalloid or colloid, followed by the application of inotropic support. Bicarbonate therapy is important for the prompt correction of acidosis, which can interfere with the effectiveness of inotropic agents as well as myocardial contractility.

Postoperative Management
Depending on the hemodynamic stability of the patient intraoperatively, extubation can be considered immediately postoperatively if the surgical procedure was not extensive. Otherwise, a more prolonged intubation with stabilization of fluid shifts postoperatively can be considered, with slow weaning and frequent blood gas analysis until extubation is complete. High-frequency jet ventilation should be used if available for postoperative ventilatory support to promote more stable hemodynamics and cardiac output.

Central venous pressures as well as pulmonary artery wedge pressure should be maintained above normal to overcome compressive forces of the effusion.

ACUTE AND CHRONIC PERICARDITIS

When comparing the physiologic effects of pericarditis with tamponade, it is important to emphasize their similarities and differences. Some differences between chronic pericarditis and cardiac tamponade will lead to changes in management. In chronic pericarditis the pericardial space is frequently obliterated and scarred, and the pericardium is adherent to the epicardium. This creates an impedance to filling of the ventricle, as in tamponade, but also causes an impairment in myocardial contractility, not usually seen with tamponade. The combination of impaired filling and contractility can decrease cardiac performance more than in tamponade alone [45].

In constrictive pericarditis, pulsus paradoxus usually occurs in only 30 percent of patients, whereas it is much more common in tamponade. Atrial fibrillation is seen very often in pericarditis, whereas sinus rhythm is one of the hallmarks of tamponade [25]. A common feature of both disorders is the impedance of diastolic filling and expansion of both ventricles, and near equalization of atrial, ventricular diastolic, and pulmonary artery diastolic pressures.

Constrictive pericarditis was at one time a rather common pathologic finding in poorly treated infections such as tuberculosis or endocarditis. With the widespread use of antibiotics over the past several decades, this cause has diminished and today pericarditis is more commonly a complication of myocardial infarction, viral infection, metastatic tumors, renal failure, cardiac trauma, systemic lupus erythematosus, collagen-vascular diseases, and rheumatoid arthritis (Table 8-3). As a result, many of these patients, who may at some point require surgery for their underlying illness, will have involvement of the pericardium complicating their operative course.

Fifteen to twenty percent of patients who expe-

Table 8-3. Common causes of pericarditis

Infectious
    Tuberculosis
    Bacterial, i.e., endocarditis
    Viral, i.e., Coxsackie B, influenza, ECHO
    Meningococcal disease
    Gonococcal disease
    Fungal, i.e., histoplasmosis, blastomycosis, toxoplasmosis
Idiopathic
Acute myocardial infarction
Postmyocardial infarction syndrome (Dressler's syndrome)
Postcardiotomy syndrome
Connective tissue/systemic diseases
    Rheumatoid arthritis
    Rheumatic fever
    Scleroderma
    Systemic lupus erythematosus
    Takayasu's arteritis
    Sarcoidosis
    Multiple myeloma
    Amyloid disease
Radiation
Chronic renal failure
Neoplasms
    Metastatic
    Lymphoma
    Leukemia
Drugs, i.e., hydralazine, procainamide, penicillin

rience a myocardial infarction will likely develop pericarditis, usually within the first week after infarction [46]. In contrast, Dressler [47] described a syndrome of postmyocardial infarction pericarditis, which usually develops 2 to 3 months after the initial infarct. Some investigators have suggested an etiology of pericarditis in Dressler's syndrome and in the postcardiotomy syndrome to be related to an immune complex response. Serum antibodies directed at the myocardium in both these disorders have been described [26]. Postcardiotomy syndrome is an acute nonspecific pericarditis that occurs after cardiac surgery or cardiac trauma, usually within 10 days to 2 months [26, 48, 49]. When the pericardium is closed following cardiac surgery, with placement of intrapericardial and mediastinal tubes for drainage, a decreased incidence of postcardiotomy syndrome has been demonstrated [50]. Pericarditis has been described as a complication of chronic renal failure in 40 to 50 percent of these patients [51, 52].

Pathophysiology

Acute pericarditis is an inflammatory process of the pericardium that involves the accumulation of fibrin on the pericardial surface and usually an associated serous effusion. If the initial inflammatory process is untreated, it may lead to chronic constrictive pericarditis. A more prolonged course of pericarditis, or recurrent acute events, may also lead to chronic changes in the pericardium, with related scarring and constriction. As noted earlier, chronic constrictive pericarditis resembles tamponade in that both processes restrict ventricular diastolic filling and reduce stroke volume. All four chambers of the heart are usually equally involved in the inflammatory process, and decreased filling can be seen in each. As with tamponade, ventricular diastolic pressures, pulmonary artery diastolic pressure, right atrial pressure, and PCWP are near equal. In chronic pericarditis, the myocardium cannot contract freely because of scar formation and thickening of the pericardium. The compliance of the "lumped" system comprising the ventricle and the pericardium is decreased, leading to impairment of ventricular filling and reduction in stroke volume and cardiac output [24].

Diagnosis

Typically, a patient with acute pericarditis will complain of symptoms similar to those of a patient with ischemic heart disease. There is an acute onset of severe chest pain, usually located midsternum, sometimes extending to the back and left shoulder. In some cases the pain may radiate to the abdomen, causing confusion with other possible surgical diagnoses. Shortness of breath due to chest pain is common, as well as a low-grade fever. The feature that most easily differentiates acute pericarditis from myocardial ischemia is that the degree of pain is significantly diminished if the patient sits up. In addition, the pain is usually continuous rather than intermittent, as frequently seen in ischemic chest pain. A friction rub, best heard at the left sternal border, is one of the classic findings in acute pericarditis. It has been described as leathery in quality, and increases in intensity on exhalation with the patient sitting upright. Sinus tachycardia and other rhythm disturbances, such as atrial flutter or fibrillation, have been described in these patients with varying frequencies.

Most patients with acute pericarditis do not manifest elevations in their serum creatinine kinase levels, which is another useful method of differentiating these findings from those of myocardial ischemia. Early ECG changes seen in pericarditis include concave ST segment elevations in the precordial leads, T-wave inversions, and atrial rhythm disturbances. As the process evolves into a chronic constrictive pericarditis, the electrocardiogram may show low-voltage QRS complexes, notched P waves that are broadened (P mitrale), and persistence of inverted T waves.

Chest radiography may reveal normal to small heart size with pericardial calcifications, or a slightly enlarged heart size due to a pericardial effusion, plus a left pleural effusion. Pulsus paradoxus is present in only about one third of patients with constrictive pericarditis, as opposed to tamponade [25].

Although constrictive pericarditis involves both the right and left heart, the more pronounced clinical manifestations are usually a result of right ventricular failure. These include venous congestion, which eventually leads to hepatosplenomegaly, ascites, exaggerated distention of the neck veins during inspiration (Kussmaul's sign), and peripheral edema. These findings may be seen in patients with moderately severe or end-stage disease [17].

Echocardiography may be a useful tool in the diagnosis of chronic pericarditis, although it is more helpful in cases of tamponade. Findings include a thickened anterior and posterior pericardium, and a small echo-free space separating the pericardium from the epicardial surface.

Anesthetic Management

In general, the treatment of acute pericarditis consists of identifying the underlying cause, if possible, and providing appropriate therapy. This may include antibiotics, nonsteroidal antiinflammatory drugs, analgesics, and bed rest. If the acute phase of pericarditis is associated with an effusion or tamponade, management is the same as that of tamponade of any other etiology (such as trauma). Unless tamponade is present, acute pericarditis in and of itself should not pose any special concerns to the anesthesiologist and should not place the patient in an especially high risk for surgery, with the possible exception of an increased incidence of atrial and ventricular arrhythmias. Left stellate ganglion block has been employed, albeit infrequently, for relief of continuous pain from pericarditis.

The patient with chronic constrictive pericarditis will likely develop many more problems intraoperatively, as compared to the patient with uncomplicated acute pericarditis. Because the pericardium is thickened and scarred, filling of the ventricles is restricted, cardiac output is reduced, and a clinical picture similar to that of tamponade emerges. Patients with early constrictive pericarditis may improve with aggressive medical therapy, but many do not and progress to more advanced stages of disease. If symptoms persist despite medical therapy, or the patient shows signs of hemodynamic compromise, surgery and pericardiectomy are usually indicated. Patients with unrelenting precordial chest pain may also be considered candidates for surgery [53, 54].

Patients who undergo pericardiectomy for constrictive pericarditis do not usually show any rapid, dramatic hemodynamic improvement, as do patients with tamponade. In fact, some investigators have found no measurable improvement in cardiac output, CVP, or mean arterial pressure after removal of the diseased pericardium at the conclusion of surgery [55]. Central venous pressure and cardiac output may remain similar to preoperative values for more than 48 hours after surgery. By 2 to 5 days postoperatively, however, CVPs usually decline, and by 4 weeks most values return to normal [56]. Walsh and associates [57] have suggested that the reason for this sluggish improvement is partially the failure to remove the sclerotic epicardium as well as the parietal pericardium. Removal of the epicardium is, however, associated with multiple complications, including damage to the myocardium and coronary vessels.

Removal of an adherent and scarred pericardium is technically difficult for most surgeons, and usually requires extensive manipulation of the heart. These maneuvers can exacerbate hypotension as the heart is manually compressed, and may lead to arrhythmias, or acute hemorrhage if the ventricle or atria are lacerated. Pericardiectomy is usually performed with the cardiopulmonary bypass unit (CPB) readily available should inadvertent tearing of the thin right ventricular wall or atria occur during dissection. The routine use of CPB has been advocated by some surgeons because of the hemodynamic stability it affords and easier operating conditions for a more extensive removal of the pericardium [58, 59]. The routine use of CPB, however, is associated with full heparinization and increased blood loss from raw cardiac surfaces, necessitating massive blood transfusions. Median sternotomy allows for wide exposure of the heart and easy cannulation for CPB, but a left thoracotomy incision has also been used, with good exposure and the advantage of not requiring elevation of the heart during dissection.

The extent to which the pericardium needs to be resected to relieve constriction remains controversial [60, 61]. Some believe that removal of pericardium over the ventricles is adequate, while others argue that complete pericardiectomy is necessary. The latter approach will likely lead to more complications, as dissection over the atria is more delicate and will likely lead to more arrhythmias.

The principles of anesthetic management previously discussed for patients with cardiac tamponade are similar for the patient with constrictive pericarditis. The similarities in their physiologic derangements require much the same emphasis on perioperative anesthetic care. Invasive hemodynamic monitoring for the patient with pericarditis requires an arterial line. Placement of a right radial artery catheter is preferred, in the event a left thoracotomy incision for pericardiectomy is used. Additionally, a pulmonary artery catheter is recommended for pericardiectomy, but also for the patient scheduled for noncardiac surgery, due to the fluctuations in cardiac output and increased filling pressures common with pericarditis.

The anesthetic management of the patient with pericarditis centers around avoidance of bradycardia or extreme tachycardia, because cardiac output is often rate dependent due to limited ventricular diastolic filling. Avoidance of drugs or techniques that greatly decrease venous return or directly depress the myocardium is recommended, and isoproterenol or other inotropes can often be used to increase heart rate and improve cardiac output [18]. As with tamponade, combinations of opioids, ketamine, benzodiazepines, and nitrous oxide have been most successful for perioperative management. Muscle relaxants, such as pancuronium, metocurine, vecuronium, and atracurium, have been used with equal success. The use of pancuronium in combination with opioids to offset potential bradycardia is a wise choice unless the patient is uremic, in which case vecuronium or atracurium may be a better alternative.

During pericardiectomy, cardiac arrhythmias are frequent, and a defibrillator and antiarrhythmic drugs such as lidocaine and procainamide should be readily available. At least two large-bore peripheral intravenous lines should be started preoperatively to provide access for rapid fluid administration in the event of massive blood loss during pericardiectomy. These points require less emphasis if the patient is having noncardiac surgery, but an understanding of the problems that may arise and adequate preparation can reduce risk to the patient intraoperatively.

If the patient continues to show signs of low coronary perfusion pressures and cardiac output, the use of inotropic agents and the intraaortic balloon pump should be a part of the postoperative management [59].

Although the long-term survival of patients with pericardial disease depends on their underlying disease, short-term outcome can be improved with diligent monitoring and careful anesthetic management. The care of these patients is a challenge to even the most skilled clinician, and a well-planned anesthetic will generally lead to a rewarding outcome.

REFERENCES

1. Norman, PH, Mycyk, T. Dissection of ascending thoracic aorta complicated by cardiac tamponade. *Can J Anaesth* 36:470–472, 1989.
2. Williams, C, Soutter, L. Pericardial tamponade. *Arch Intern Med* 94:571–584, 1954.
3. Singh, S, Newmark, K. Pericardiectomy in uremia. *JAMA* 228:1132–1135, 1974.
4. Theologides, A. Neoplastic cardiac tamponade. *Semin Oncol* 5:181–192, 1978.
5. Thurber, D, Edwards, J, Anchor, R. Secondary malignant tumors of the pericardium. *Circulation* 26:228–241, 1962.
6. Cohen, G, Peery, T, Evons, J. Neoplastic invasion of the heart and pericardium. *Ann Intern Med* 42:1238–1245, 1955.
7. Osuch, J, Khandekar, J. Emergency subxiphoid pericardial decompression for malignant pericardial effusion. *Am Surg* 51:298–300, 1985.
8. Weeks, KR, Chatterjee, K, Block, S, et al. Bedside hemodynamic monitoring: Its value in the diagnosis of tamponade complicating cardiac surgery. *J Thorac Cardiovasc Surg* 71:250–252, 1976.
9. Beck, CS. Two cardiac compression triads. *JAMA* 104:714–716, 1935.
10. Guberman, BA, Fowler, NO, Engel, PJ, et al. Cardiac tamponade in medical patients. *Circulation* 64:633–640, 1981.
11. Fowler, NO. The electrocardiogram in pericarditis. *Cardiovasc Clin* 5:255–267, 1973.
12. Surawicz, B, Lasseter, KC. Electrocardiogram in pericarditis. *Am J Cardiol* 26:471–474, 1970.
13. Horowitz, MS, Schultz, CS, et al. Sensitivity and specificity of echocardiographic diagnosis of pericardial effusion. *Circulation* 50:239–247, 1974.
14. Settle, HP, Adolph, RJ, Fowler, NO, et al. Echocardiographic study of cardiac tamponade. *Circulation* 56:951–959, 1977.
15. White, JB, Macklin, S, et al. Cardiac tamponade: A review of diagnosis and anaesthetic and surgical management illustrated by three case reports. *Ann R Coll Surg Engl* 70:386–391, 1988.

16. Lake, CL. Anesthesia and pericardial disease. *Anesth Analg* 62:431–443, 1983.
17. Fowler, NO. Diseases of the pericardium. *Curr Probl Cardiol* 2:6–38, 1978.
18. Kaplan, JA, Bland, JW, Jr, Dunbar, RW. The perioperative management of pericardial tamponade. *South Med J* 69:417–419, 1976.
19. Cyna, AM, Rodgers, RC, Meterlane, H. Hypotension due to unexpected cardiac tamponade. *Anaesthesia* 45:140–142, 1990.
20. Moller, CT, Schoonbee, CO, Rosendorff, C. Haemodynamics of cardiac tamponade during various modes of ventilation. *Br J Surg* 51:409–414, 1979.
21. Guntheroth, WG, Morgan, BC, Mullins, GL. Effects of respiration on venous return and stroke volume in cardiac tamponade. *Circ Res* 20:381–390, 1967.
22. Quist, J, et al. Hemodynamic responses to mechanical respiration with PEEP: The effect of hypervolemia. *Anesthesiology* 42:45, 1975.
23. Goto, K, Goto, H, Benson, KT, et al. Efficacy of high-frequency jet ventilation in cardiac tamponade. *Anesth Analg* 70:375–381, 1990.
24. Agner, RC, Gallis, HA. Pericarditis: Differential diagnostic considerations. *Arch Intern Med* 139:401–412, 1979.
25. Shabetai, R, Fowler, NO, Guntheroth, WG. The hemodynamics of cardiac tamponade and constrictive pericarditis. *Am J Cardiol* 26:480–489, 1970.
26. Legler, DC. Uncommon Diseases and Cardiac Anesthesia. In JA Kaplan (ed), *Cardiac Anesthesia* (2nd ed). Philadelphia: Saunders, 1987. Pp 785–831.
27. Stanley, TH, Weidauer, HE. Anesthesia for the patient with cardiac tamponade. *Anesth Analg* 52:110–114, 1973.
28. Kerber, RE, Gascho, JA, et al. Hemodynamic effects of volume expansion and nitroprusside compared with pericardiocentesis in patients with acute cardiac tamponade. *N Engl J Med* 307:929–931, 1982.
29. Martins, JB, Manuel, WJ, Marcus, ML, et al. Comparative effects of catecholamines in cardiac tamponade: Experimental and clinical studies. *Am J Cardiol* 46:59–66, 1980.
30. Stoelting, RK. Diseases of the Pericardium. In RK Stoelting and SF Dierdorf (eds), *Anesthesia and Coexisting Diseases* (2nd ed). New York: Churchill Livingstone, 1988. Pp 161–168.
31. Cassell, P, Cullum, P. The management of cardiac tamponade: Drainage of pericardial effusions. *Br J Surg* 54:620–626, 1967.
32. Vandyke, WH, Jr, Cure, J, Chakko, CS, et al. Pulmonary edema after pericardiocentesis for cardiac tamponade. *N Engl J Med* 309:595, 1983.
33. Shenoy, MM, Dhar, S, Gittin, R, et al. Pulmonary edema following pericardiotomy for cardiac tamponade. *Chest* 86:647–648, 1984.
34. Brown, BR, Crout, JR. A comparative study of the effects of five general anesthetics on myocardial contractibility. *Anesthesiology* 34:236–245, 1971.
35. Eger, EI, II, Smith, NT, Cullen, DJ, et al. A comparison of the cardiovascular effects of halothane, fluroxene, ether, and cyclopropane in man. *Anesthesiology* 34:25–41, 1971.
36. Konchigeri, HN, Levitsky, S. Anesthetic considerations for pericardiectomy in uremic pericardial effusion. *Anesth Analg* 55:378–382, 1976.
37. Fowler, NO, Gabel, M, Holmes, JC. Hemodynamic effects of nitroprusside and hydralazine in experimental cardiac tamponade. *Circulation* 57:563–567, 1978.
38. Freidman, HS, Lajam, F, Zaman, Q, et al. Effect of autonomic blockade on the hemodynamic findings in acute cardiac tamponade. *Am J Physiol* 232:5–11, 1977.
39. Freidman, HS, Lajam, F, Gomes, JA, et al. Demonstration of the depressor reflex in acute cardiac tamponade. *J Thorac Cardiovasc Surg* 73:278–286, 1977.
40. Lunn, JK, Stanley, TH, Eisele, J, et al. High dose fentanyl anesthesia for coronary artery surgery: Plasma fentanyl concentration and influences of nitrous oxide on cardiovascular responses. *Anesth Analg* 58:390–395, 1979.
41. Stoelting, RK, Gibbs, PS. Hemodynamic effects of morphine and morphine-nitrous oxide in valvular heart disease and coronary artery disease. *Anesthesiology* 38:45–52, 1973.
42. Lappas, DG, Buckley, MJ, Laver, MB, et al. Left ventricular performance and pulmonary circulation following addition of nitrous oxide to morphine during coronary-artery surgery. *Anesthesiology* 43:61–69, 1975.
43. Tomicheck, RC, Rosow, CE, Philbin, DM, et al. Diazepam-fentanyl interaction—hemodynamic and hormonal effects in coronary artery surgery. *Anesth Analg* 62:881–884, 1983.
44. Rigler, ML, Drasner, K, Krejcietc, TC, et al. Cauda equina syndrome after continuous spinal anesthesia. *Anesth Analg* 72:275–281, 1991.
45. Harvey, RM, Ferrer, MI, Cathcart, RT, et al. Mechanical and myocardial factors in chronic constrictive pericarditis. *Circulation* 8:695–707, 1953.
46. Kirsh, MM, McIntosh, K, Kahn, DR, et al. Postpericardiotomy syndrome. *Ann Thorac Surg* 9:158–179, 1970.

47. Dressler, W. The post–myocardial-infarction syndrome; a report of forty-four cases. *Arch Intern Med* 103:28–42, 1959.
48. Brown, DF, Older, T. Pericardial constriction as a late complication of coronary bypass surgery. *J Thorac Cardiovasc Surg* 74:61–64, 1977.
49. Cohen, MV, Greenberg, MA. Constrictive pericarditis: Early and late complications of cardiac surgery. *Am J Cardiol* 43:657–661, 1979.
50. Spencer, FC, Zeff, R, Williams, CD, et al. Influence of primary closure of the pericardium after open-heart surgery on the frequency of tamponade, postcardiotomy syndrome, and pulmonary complications. *J Thorac Cardiovasc Surg* 70:119–125, 1975.
51. Bailey, GL, et al. Uremic pericarditis: Clinical features and management. *Circulation* 38:582–591, 1968.
52. Wacker, W, Merrill, JP. Uremic pericarditis in acute and chronic renal failure. *JAMA* 156:764–765, 1954.
53. Kluge, T, Hall, TV. Surgery in acute and chronic pericarditis. *Scand J Thorac Cardiovasc Surg* 10:21–30, 1976.
54. Wychulis, AR, Connally, DC, McGoon, DC. Surgical treatment of pericarditis. *J Thorac Cardiovasc Surg* 62:608–617, 1971.
55. Coleman, AJ, Mayes, DG, Wheatley, DJ, et al. Immediate effects of pericardiectomy. *J Thorac Cardiovasc Surg* 66:803–806, 1977.
56. Harrison, EC, Crawford, DW, Lou, FYK. Sequential left ventricular function studies before and after pericardiectomy for constrictive pericarditis. *Am J Cardiol* 26:319–323, 1970.
57. Walsh, TJ, Baughman, KL, Gardner, TJ, Bulkley, BH. Constrictive epicarditis as a cause of delayed or absent response to pericardiectomy. *J Thorac Cardiovasc Surg* 83:126–132, 1982.
58. Copeland, JG, Stinson, EB, Griepp, RB, et al. Surgical treatment of chronic pericarditis using cardiopulmonary bypass. *J Thorac Cardiovasc Surg* 69:236–238, 1975.
59. McCaughan, BC, Schaff, HV, Piehler, JM, et al. Early and late results of pericardiectomy for constrictive pericarditis. *J Thorac Cardiovasc Surg* 89:340–348, 1985.
60. Kilman, JW, Bush, CA, Wooley, CF, et al. The changing spectrum of pericardiectomy for chronic pericarditis: Occult constrictive pericarditis. *J Thorac Cardiovasc Surg* 74:668–673, 1977.
61. Das, PB, Gupta, RP, Jairaj, PS, et al. Constrictive pericarditis and its surgical management. *Int Surg* 60:210–214, 1975.

9
Cardiomyopathies

PIERRE A. CASTHELY
SOOM YUNG LEE
CLAUDIA A. KOMER

Cardiomyopathies are diseases of heart muscle with multifactorial etiology associated with signs and symptoms of congestive heart failure. They are divided into three categories: dilated or congested cardiomyopathy, hypertrophic cardiomyopathy, and restrictive cardiomyopathy (Table 9-1). The mechanism of the heart failure is different in each group (Table 9-2; Fig. 9-1).

CONGESTIVE CARDIOMYOPATHY

The most common etiology of congestive cardiomyopathy is "idiopathic." Other etiologies include myocarditis due to nutritional deficit, alcohol abuse, infections, neuromuscular disease, and intoxication (heavy metals, doxorubicin). Ischemic cardiomyopathy is very common and is the main topic of this discussion. It is an anatomic condition resulting from the imbalance between the oxygen supply and the demand of the heart.

Ischemic Cardiomyopathy

Pathogenesis of Cardiomyopathy
Quantitative studies have indicated that involvement of 40 percent or more of the left ventricle in humans leads to severe myocardial dysfunction that may result in sudden cardiac death or acute congestive heart failure [1, 2]. Pump function is reduced in direct proportion to the amount of myocardium that is lost, that is, the ejection fraction falls as a function of infarct size [3–7].

Infarct size is an important determinant of prognosis, and a threshold of infarct dimension seems to predict impairment of ventricular dynamics [8]. On such a basis, a number of agents have been used to decrease the extent of myocardial necrosis [9, 10]. Despite normal intraventricular pressure, myocardial infarction and subsequent events create an overload via the Laplace relation because compensatory dilatation increases the ventricular radius and, thus, wall tension. Therapeutic interventions such as lowering the preload and afterload may reduce the extent of wall stress and its negative consequences and thereby improve ventricular performance.

Several studies have demonstrated that after large left ventricular infarcts, there is a relatively rapid development of right ventricular hypertrophy [11]. The precise mechanism by which a left ventricular myocardial infarction leads to right ventricular hypertrophy is currently unknown. Three possibilities have been considered: (1) an increase in right ventricular systolic pressure due to left-sided pump failure [12]; (2) pulmonary hypertension as a primary stimulus suggested by medial

Table 9-1. Classification of the common cardiomyopathies by etiology

Cause	Congestive (dilated)	Restrictive	Hypertrophic

Idiopathic	Idiopathic
	Postpartum
	Endocardial fibroelastosis
	    (dilated type)
		Endocardial fibroelastosis (restrictive type)
		Endomyocardial fibrosis
		    Davies' disease
		    Loeffler's disease
			Obstructive
			Nonobstructive

Ischemic	Coronary artery disease		
Toxic	Ethanol Heavy metal (i.e., cobalt) Doxorubicin		

Inflammatory	Infective
	    Viral
	    Diphtheria
	    Chagas' disease
	Noninfective
	    Rheumatic myocarditis
	    Systemic lupus erythematosus
	    Sarcoidosis
	    Polyarteritis
		Scleroderma
		Amyloid
		Neoplasm	

Metabolic	Thiamine deficiency Acromegaly Thalassemia	Hemochromatosis Glycogen storage disease	
Neuromuscular	Friedreich's ataxia Muscular dystrophy		

Source: Modified from MR Goldman and CA Boucher, Value of radionuclide imaging techniques in assessing cardiomyopathy. *Am J Cardiol* 46:1232–1236, 1980.

Table 9-2. Mechanisms of the cardiomyopathies

Classification	LVDV	LVEF	Mechanism of heart failure
Dilated (congestive)	↑↑	<0.40	Systolic impairment
Nondilated (restrictive)	↓, NL, ↑	0.30–0.70	Compliance abnormality
Hypertrophic	↓, NL, ↑	0.45–0.95	Compliance abnormality

LVDV = left ventricular diastolic volume; LVEF = left ventricular ejection fraction; ↑ = slightly increased; ↑↑ = greatly increased; NL = normal.

hypertrophy of the muscular branches of the pulmonary artery in infarcted subjects [13]; and (3) the right ventricle may constitute a functional unit with the infarcted left ventricle, contributing to the emptying of the left ventricular chamber during systole [13]. These events, either independently or combined, all lead to a greater pressure load on the right ventricle, resulting in concentric hypertrophy [14], before congestive heart failure develops.

Capillary Changes. Three fundamental structural properties of the capillary network are relevant to tissue oxygenation and are significant in the compensatory adaptation of the myocardium after infarction: capillary luminal volume density, capillary luminal surface density, and average diffusion distance from the capillary wall to the surrounding myocytes. These capillary parameters are functionally related to the volume of capillary blood available for gas exchange within the tissue, the capillary area available for oxygen transport from the blood to the tissue, and the diffusion path length to the sites of oxygen use and adenosine triphosphate (ATP) synthesis, respectively.

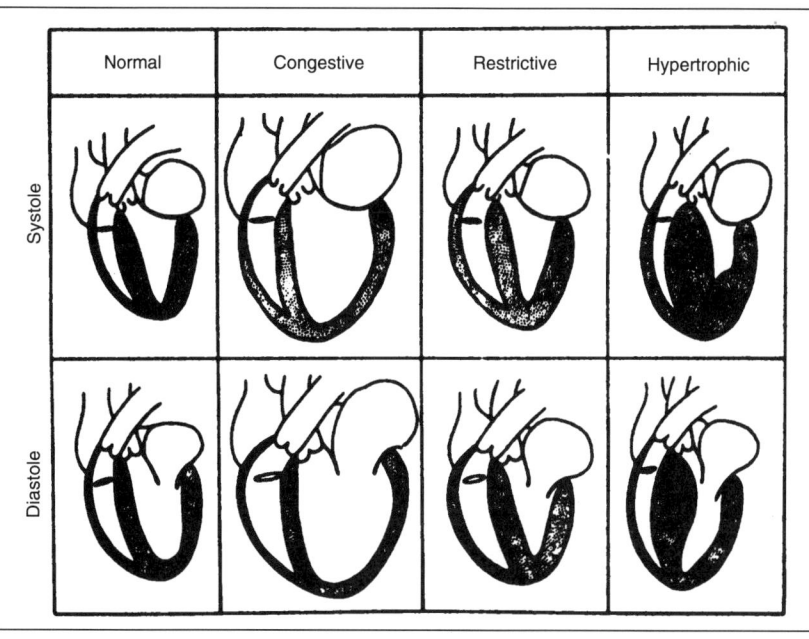

Fig. 9-1. Mechanism of heart failure in cardiomyopathy. (Reprinted with permission from MR Goldman and CA Boucher, The value of radionuclide imaging techniques in assessing cardiomyopathy. *Am J Cardiol* 46:1232, 1980).

Alterations of the capillary microcirculation within the surviving myocardium could be the mechanisms generating a sustained imbalance between oxygen supply and demand that in turn may lead to local ischemic and tissue damage. Myocyte necrosis, reactive hypertrophy of the remaining cells, replacement fibrosis, and increased collagen deposition in the interstitial space may all occur, providing the structural template of the postinfarction cardiomyopathic heart, which is characterized by thinning of the wall [15, 16], chamber dilatation, increased wall tension, and abnormal ventricular stiffness [17–20].

A deficit in the capillary network exists after infarction and the magnitude of this deficit increases with infarct size and proximity to the scarred region of the injured ventricle. This response of the coronary vasculature can be considered one of the major factors in the development of the cardiomyopathy that occurs in humans following myocardial infarction and in its progression into irreversible congestive heart failure and death.

Myocardial Changes. In patients in whom large portions of the left ventricle have been damaged after myocardial infarction, chronically increased work of the otherwise normal myocardium leads to progressive deterioration of the overloaded myocardial cells. However, the mechanisms by which sustained overloading causes the hypertrophied myocardial cells to deteriorate, die, and become replaced by fibrous tissue are not well understood. This process, which represents an unwelcome consequence of the compensation provided by the increased mass of overloaded myocardium, can be viewed as a "cardiomyopathy of overload" that probably plays an important role in determining the poor prognosis in the patient with congestive heart failure [21].

Although the causes of deterioration of the failing heart remain poorly understood, at least two pathogenic mechanisms appear likely to play a role in this important process: chronic energy starvation and complex changes in the composition of the hypertrophied heart.

ENERGY STARVATION IN THE FAILING HEART. At least three mechanisms could lead to a state of energy starvation in the cells of the chronically overloaded heart. Chronic overloading causes each myocardial cell to sustain an increased level of work output because the adult heart has little or no capacity for cell division. Hypertrophy, by increasing the size of the myocardial cells and thereby augmenting the number of sarcomeres that share the overload, would, reduce the load on each sarcomere. However, the compensation brought about by the increased muscle mass may not perfectly match the increased load; as a result, the rate of energy expenditure by each sarcomere of the hypertrophied heart would remain chronically elevated.

Secondly, there is a relative deficiency in the systems that provide high-energy phosphate compounds to meet the increased work of the overloaded heart in patients with congestive heart failure. This is due to the fact that in established myocardial hypertrophy, the fraction of cell volume occupied by myofibril is increased relative to mitochondrial mass [22, 23].

Thirdly, changes in the architecture of the hypertrophied heart could also exacerbate a state of energy starvation in the hypertrophied, failing heart. These changes, which include increased intercapillary distance and a decreased number of transverse capillary profiles per square millimeter [24], would increase the diffusion distance for substrates, notably oxygen, which are essential for energy production by the hypertrophied heart.

CHANGES IN THE COMPOSITION OF THE HYPERTROPHIED HEART. In the heart's response to chronic overload, the altered expression of the genes that encode key myocardial proteins leads to the preferential synthesis of protein isoforms that determine a reduced rate of energy expenditure, and an overall change in composition that leads to the reappearance of proteins that had normally appeared earlier in fetal life [21]. The extent to which the expression of altered genes produces changes in the hypertrophied myocardium contributes to the progressive degeneration of the overloaded heart and may, in fact, represent the most important question for future research into the causes of the downhill course in these patients.

Pathophysiology. Dilated cardiomyopathy is characterized by a profound reduction in the left ventricular ejection fraction (LVEF). In cardiac impairment, due to systolic dysfunction, heart failure does not occur until the LVEF is less than 0.40 [25, 26]. The right ventricle may also dilate and its ejection fraction may be reduced. As myocardial contractility progressively declines, there is an increase in the left ventricular end diastolic volume and left atrial pressure aimed at maintaining the stroke volume (Starling's mechanism). The heart then dilates, the left atrial pressure increases, and heart failure ensues. Biventricular failure occurs in some patients. Mitral regurgitation is present in as many as two thirds of patients with dilated cardiomyopathy, but it is usually mild or moderate [27]. Left ventricular dilatation and a greatly reduced LVEF are more constant features of dilated cardiomyopathy than decreased cardiac output or elevated left atrial pressure [28].

β-Adrenergic Receptors in the Failing Heart
β-Adrenergic receptors are the most powerful means of quickly increasing the contractile state of both nonfailing and failing ventricular myocardium. In heart failure, both $β_1$- and $β_2$-adrenergic receptors and the inhibitory G protein (G_i) undergo regulatory changes that render the receptor–G protein–adenylate cyclase (RGC) complex less capable of mediating inotropic support. These changes consist of profound down-regulation in the $β_1$ receptor, mild uncoupling of the $β_2$ receptor, and mild up-regulation of the $G_{1α}$ subunit (Table 9-3). Although these changes may serve a protective function from the standpoint of minimizing exposure to cardiotoxic stimuli, they also compromise the ability of the failing heart to respond to the increased demand of stress or exercise.

When β-receptor subtypes were measured in the nonfailing and failing human heart [29, 30], an interesting and unexpected finding emerged. The percentage of $β_1$ receptors in failing human hearts

Table 9-3. Summary of receptor pathway abnormalities in the failing human heart

Constituent	Abnormality
$β_1$ receptor	Down-regulated
$β_2$ receptor	Uncoupled
$G_{1α}$	Up-regulated

$G_{1α}$ = alpha G inhibitory protein.

Table 9-4. Evidence that increased cardiac norepinephrine levels cause β_1-receptor down-regulation in the failing human heart

Coronary sinus and interstitial levels of norepinephrine are increased.
β_1-Receptor down-regulation may be correlated with increased coronary sinus norepinephrine level.
In model heart-cell systems, norepinephrine produces a prompt down-regulation in β_1- or β_2-like receptors.
The lower norepinephrine affinity receptors α_2 and β_2 do not down-regulate.
Selective β_1-receptor blockade may restore β_1-receptor density to normal.

---

was decreased relative to the nonfailing heart, with an average value of 63 percent compared to 80 percent, respectively [29]. This decrease in the percentage of β_1 receptors was due to a marked decrease in β_1-receptor density, which was lowered to 60 percent of control values. Because β_2-receptor density remained unchanged in the failing heart (see below), the selective loss in β_1 receptors led to a change in $\beta_1:\beta_2$ subtype ratio from approximately 80:20 in the nonfailing heart to 60:40 in the failing heart [8]. β_1-Adrenergic receptor density is markedly decreased in membranes that are derived from failing hearts with idiopathic dilated cardiomyopathy, as is subtype selective stimulation of adenylate cyclase and muscle contraction [29, 31]. That down-regulation of beta receptors may be due to increased cardiac norepinephrine levels (Table 9-4).

Effect of β-Adrenergic Agonist in the Failing Heart

Alteration of β-adrenergic responsiveness has been observed with both short-term [32, 33] and long-term [34] therapy with beta agonist. The degree of desensitization produced by individual beta agonist appears to be highly variable. For example, a decrease in the therapeutic response to dopamine can be observed after a 48-hour continuous infusion, whereas no change in efficacy is observed with a 48-hour infusion of dobutamine [32, 33]. However, tolerance to dobutamine administration does develop after longer periods of time [33]. Different beta agonists may also produce different degrees of β-adrenergic receptor down-regulation. Thus, the development of desensitization of the β-adrenergic agonist is variable and is probably dependent on multiple factors, including the individual beta agonist administered, the method of its administration, the baseline state of the β-adrenergic receptor–adenylate cyclase complex, and the effect of agonist administration on myocardial exposure to endogenous catecholamines [34].

Clinical Presentation

Symptoms of left or biventricular failure include dyspnea at rest or on exertion, extreme fatigability, and poor exercise tolerance. Chest pain may also occur and is more common in patients with ischemic cardiomyopathy. Episodes of pulmonary edema frequently aggravate the clinical picture and often require mechanical ventilation of the patient. Common signs include jugular venous distention, peripheral edema, ascites, hepatomegaly, S_3 gallop, and the murmur of mitral insufficiency.

Anesthetic Considerations

The role of the anesthesiologist is to provide anesthesia while maintaining stable cardiovascular parameters in these patients. The anesthetic technique should provide minimal depression in cardiac contractility while maintaining the preload and afterload. The anesthesiologist should also be prepared to assist the failing heart pharmacologically (amrinone, dobutamine, dopamine, epinephrine) and mechanically (intraaortic balloon counterpulsation). The induction of anesthesia is especially critical. A combination of positive pressure ventilation, airway obstruction, and blunting of sympathetic response can precipitate cardiovascular collapse in an already weak and hypokinetic heart. Respiratory and metabolic acidosis are poorly tolerated in the patient with end-state cardiac failure.

Of great concern to the anesthesiologist is the effect of the myopathy on the adrenergic system (down-regulation beta receptors). As was mentioned previously, the patient with end-stage cardiomyopathy has several hemodynamic abnormalities. Three basic abnormalities are seen in the patient with end-stage heart failure: impairment of

Fig. 9-2. Pressure-volume loop from a normal heart (*left*) and a heart with dilated cardiomyopathy (*right*). The stroke volume in the heart with cardiomyopathy is decreased when its systolic pressure is mildly elevated. LV = left ventricular.

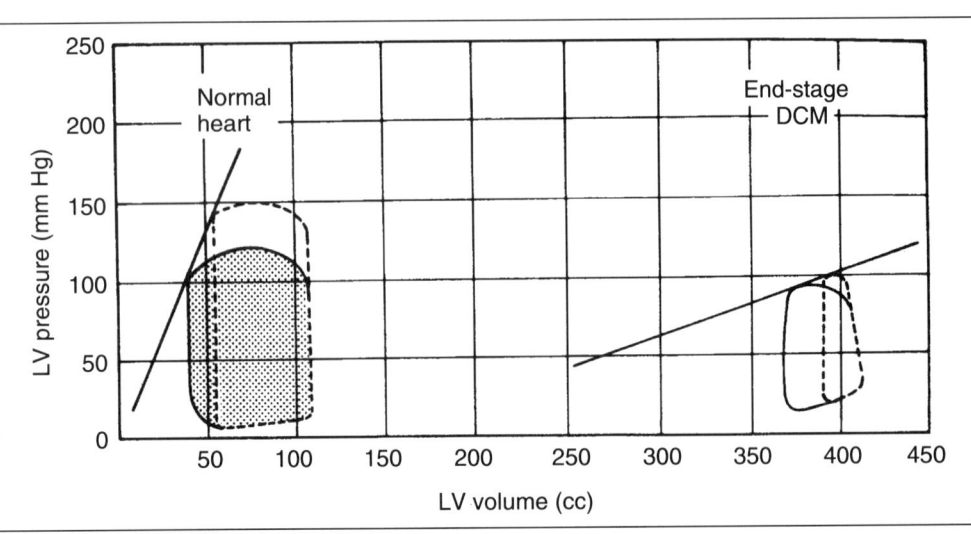

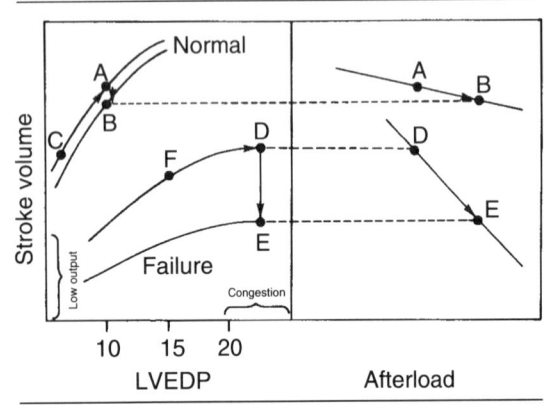

Fig. 9-3. Frank-Starling curves of a normal heart and a cardiomyopathic heart. Increase in afterload produces a small decrease in output in the normal heart (A → B) and a considerable decrease in output in the failing heart (D → E). LVEDP = left ventricular end diastolic pressure.

myocardial contractility, dependence on preload, and high sensitivity to afterload. Figure 9-2 shows the pressure-volume loops from a normal heart and a heart with end-stage cardiac failure. There is a marked decrease in stroke volume in the myopathic heart when its peak systolic pressure is mildly elevated. Wall tension increases due to ventricular dilatation and systolic function is markedly impaired. There are increases in end systolic and end diastolic volume.

Afterload Sensitivity. Ventricular wall stress is determined by the intraventricular pressure, intraventricular volume, and ventricular wall thickness. In the normal heart, wall stress declines immediately after ventricular ejection begins because the volume and radius of the ventricle decrease with ejection while its wall thickens with contraction [35, 36]. When the dilated myopathic ventricle contracts against an identical aortic pressure, wall force and stress rise much higher and peak later in systole because of the relatively small change in ventricular volume and negligible increase in wall thickness (Fig. 9-3).

Any maneuver that increases systemic vascular resistance without a concomitant increase in myocardial contractility will jeopardize the patient's well-being by affecting cardiac output and stroke volume.

Preload Dependence. The effect of preload on the heart is completely different in the failing heart than in the normal heart. In the normal heart, a small increase in end diastolic volume produces a large increase in stroke volume. In the failing heart, the sarcomere length is increased to maximum because of chronic dilatation of the heart. This heart has its preload reserve completely exhausted and an increase in preload produces no increase in stroke volume [36–39].

In the patient with dilated cardiomyopathy, the cardiac output is insensitive to increases in preload. Because these patients have fixed output, a small decrease in stroke volume can result in circulatory collapse (see Fig. 9-3). Preload should be kept constant, and any maneuver that affects venous return to the heart, such as positive end-expiratory pressure or use of vasodilators (sodium nitroprusside, nitroglycerin), should be avoided. Because the upper limit of stroke volume is fixed, cardiac output in these patients is rate dependent. Almost all are mildly to moderately tachycardic at rest. It is therefore important to avoid bradycardia in these patients at any cost.

Down-Regulation of Beta Receptors. As was previously mentioned, the down-regulation of beta receptors presents several problems for the anesthesiologist. There is a decrease in effectiveness of the usual inotropic agents on the heart because they act by stimulation of the β-adrenergic receptors. If cardiac function deteriorates following induction of anesthesia, a higher than usual dose of inotropes should be used. Another alternative is to use inotropes that bypass the beta receptor (calcium or amrinone) [40, 41]. Intraoperative administration of a beta agonist may also exacerbate the receptor deficit by converting the remaining functional receptors to the low-affinity, uncoupled state [42, 43].

Myocardial norepinephrine stores are decreased in advanced heart failure [44] and circulating norepinephrine levels are elevated [44, 45]. The norepinephrine re-uptake mechanisms of adrenergic nerve terminals in the failing myocardium are impaired [46], and coronary sinus blood levels of norepinephrine are not only elevated but exceed arterial blood levels [47]. Therefore, the failing heart is chronically exposed to very high levels of catecholamines.

Monitoring. Intraoperative monitoring of the patient with cardiomyopathy is similar to that used during major cardiac operations. Monitoring minimally consists of the following: (1) five-lead electrocardiogram, (2) pulse oximeter, (3) arterial catheter for measurement of blood pressure, (4) urinary catheter, (5) pulmonary artery catheter, and (6) capnography.

If the patient has severe right ventricular dysfunction, the use of a thermal dilution right ventricular ejection fraction catheter should also be considered [48, 49]. This modified catheter is equipped with a fast-response thermistor that measures beat-to-beat variations in the temperature of blood in the pulmonary artery and a ventricular electrode for measurement of the intracardiac electrogram. This device makes it easy to manage the patient with pulmonary hypertension and right ventricular strain because right ventricular end diastolic volume, end systolic volume, stroke volume, and ejection fraction can be calculated.

Anesthetic Management. The single most important consideration for induction of anesthesia in the patient with cardiomyopathy is that it be undertaken slowly [50]. Narcotics such as fentanyl and sufentanil are the agents most often used [51, 52]. They are usually administered in small boluses or by continuous infusion and titrated against various stimuli, such as oral airway insertion, Foley catheter insertion, and endotracheal intubation [51]. The synthetic narcotics are usually preceded by the administration of benzodiazepines such as midazolam, diazepam, or lorazepam. The use of benzodiazepines is not without complications. It may produce hypotension and decreased peripheral vascular resistance and add to myocardial depression when used in conjunction with high-dose narcotics [53]. Because of its cardiovascular effects, sodium thiopental and propofol are very seldom used in these patients. Muscle paralysis can be accomplished with any one of a number of muscle relaxants, including vecuronium, pancuronium, pipicuronium, atracurium, and doxacurium. Two common side effects during induction of anesthesia are bradycardia and hypoventilation. Bradycardia may be due to vagal stimulation or the synthetic narcotics (fentanyl and/or sufentanil). It can have deleterious effects because cardiac output in these patients is rate dependent. This can be attenuated by the administration of pancuronium as a muscle relaxant [54], using its vagolytic properties. Muscle rigidity may be induced by the administration of the narcotics and may result in inadequate ventilation, respiratory and metabolic acidosis, and elevated central venous pressure. These effects are very detrimental to the patient with severe right ventricular dysfunction, and can easily be prevented by the early administration of muscle relaxants.

There may be a delay in the onset of action of the drugs given, because of the low cardiac output and slow circulation time [50, 55], making the induction of anesthesia slower than usual. Furthermore, the volume of distribution of many of the drugs is decreased due to the action of diuretics. This thereby may elevate the blood and brain anesthetic concentration, exaggerating the initial drug effect [50, 56].

The potent inhalation drugs are very seldom used as primary-maintenance anesthetics in this patient population [54]. Halothane and enflurane are potent myocardial depressants that will worsen the severely impaired myocardial contractility seen in patients with cardiomyopathy [57, 58]. Isoflurane is a potent vasodilator and may produce severe hypotension in a patient who is sensitive to afterload changes. The use of nitrous oxide warrants caution and is still controversial. There are conflicting data regarding this drug's myocardial depressant and/or direct pulmonary vasoconstrictive properties [59, 60]. It seems prudent to avoid it in all patients with severe right ventricular dysfunction.

When anesthesia was maintained with the potent synthetic narcotics such as fentanyl and sufentanil, the hemodynamic responses to laryngoscopy, intubation, and surgical incision were greatly attenuated [61–65], and minimal myocardial depression was produced by those agents [61, 62, 66, 67]. Most of these patients have hepatomegaly and hepatic dysfunction due to severe heart failure. Therefore, the metabolism of some drugs may be delayed, and some patients may require prolonged mechanical ventilation if high doses of narcotics are used.

Intraoperatively, the hemodynamic parameters are very unpredictable due to the fact that patients with end-stage cardiac failure lack sufficient contractile reserve to generate a hypertensive response to noxious stimuli that activate the sympathetic nervous system [68]. Instead, these patients show progressive decreases in ejection fraction and stroke volume and increases in left ventricular end diastolic volume [68, 69]. The inotropes commonly used are dobutamine, dopamine, amrinone, epinephrine, and isoproterenol. Amrinone, a phosphodiesterase inhibitor, is especially important in patients who failed to respond to β-adrenergic drugs because of the down-regulation of beta receptors. It can be used alone or combined with other inotropic agents [70].

When planning the emergency anesthetic management of a patient with fixed cardiac output and end-stage cardiac failure, one should consider the risks for aspiration and hemodynamic changes due to the anesthetic agents used during the induction of anesthesia.

Many centers use the classic rapid-sequence induction technique with preoxygenation and cricoid pressure [50, 54]. Short-acting induction agents such as etomidate, midazolam, or ketamine can be used. Ketamine appears to be an ideal induction agent for the patient with end-stage cardiac failure because of its sympathomimetic effects. However, it should be remembered that these patients have a down-regulation of beta receptors that may make them less responsive to catecholamines, and ketamine can then produce severe hemodynamic depression due to direct myocardial depression [71]. Sufentanil has also been used for the rapid-sequence induction of anesthesia. Its use has been shown to preserve the hemodynamic profile, especially in the patient without impairment of ventricular function [61, 62].

RESTRICTIVE CARDIOMYOPATHIES

Restrictive cardiomyopathies are the least common of the cardiomyopathies in the Western countries. They are characterized by a primary abnormality of diastolic ventricular function with normal systolic function and internal ventricular dimensions. With increased interest in ventricular diastolic function and with the advanced diagnostic techniques, there have been concomitant increases in both awareness and understanding of restrictive cardiomyopathies.

Classification

Restrictive (nondilated) cardiomyopathy is most often classified by its functional impairment and loss of ventricular compliance [72]. While specific entities, such as amyloidosis [73], sarcoidosis [74], hemochromatosis [75], radiation, and diabetes [76], demonstrate the properties of restrictive diastolic impairments, they are not classified as a restrictive cardiomyopathy by the strict definition. The distinction between primary and secondary (specific heart disease) restrictive cardiomyopathy is not absolute. While amyloidosis confined to the heart is classified as a cardiomyopathy with restrictive features, generalized amyloidosis with cardiac involvement is classified as a specific heart disease. The following discussion is applicable to all disease states that exhibit restrictive pathophysiology. Specific disease states are also briefly discussed.

Etiology

Restrictive cardiomyopathy may be the result of multiple factors and causes [77]. The primary pathogenic mechanisms currently under investigation include hereditary, metabolic, hormonal, toxic, infectious, autoimmune, hypoxic, free radical, and altered vascular reactivity mechanisms [78–82].

Myocardial diastolic dysfunction may be idiopathic (enzymatic/metabolic disturbances), infiltrative (myocardial interstitium), or within myocardial cells (storage diseases). Endomyocardial fibrosis or hypereosinophilic syndrome typifies diastolic dysfunction that results from endomyocardial disease, although carcinoid, metastatic malignancies, radiation, and anthracycline toxicity may be associated with endomyocardial restriction (see Table 9-1).

There is mounting evidence that endomyocardial fibrosis, the most common form of restrictive cardiomyopathy in tropical countries, and Loeffler's hypereosinophilic syndrome, a more aggressive and progressive disorder in temperate areas, are due to the same disease process. Activated eosinophils, which mediate both entities, bind to immunogammaglobulin G and have increased peroxidases that have direct toxic effects on myocytes [83]. In Western countries, the most common causes of restrictive cardiomyopathy are idiopathic myocardial fibrosis and amyloidosis.

Pathophysiology

The pathophysiology of restrictive cardiomyopathy is one of impaired diastolic function. Ventricular distensibility decreases secondary to morphologic changes in the endocardium or the myocardium, or both, with normal or near normal systolic function, and, thus, is given the descriptive diagnoses of "nondilated, nonhypertrophic cardiomyopathy" or "congestive heart failure with normal systolic function."

Ventricular diastole (relaxation and filling) is not a passive event in which the blood fills by expansion of a compliant ventricle, but an active, complex process that requires energy (ATP) to restore ionic gradients across the sarcolemma. At physiologic heart rates, 80 percent of ventricular filling occurs during the rapid filling phase. The next phase, diastasis, normally accounts for less than 5 percent of filling. Finally, atrial systole contributes about 15 percent of normal ventricular filling.

In describing diastolic stress-strain relationships, myocardial stiffness is the change in stiffness of a muscle unit, while chamber stiffness refers to changes in muscle mass. Therefore, in restrictive cardiomyopathy both chamber stiffness and myocardial stiffness are increased, while ventricular hypertrophy is characterized by chamber stiffness without myocardial stiffness.

In restrictive cardiomyopathy, ventricular filling is completed in early diastole. Right and left ventricular end diastolic pressures increase, with minimal changes in end diastolic or systolic dimensions, resulting in a steep slope of the diastolic pressure-volume curve. Significant left ventricular hypertrophy or dilatation (left ventricular end diastolic volume > 100 ml/m^2) excludes the diagnosis of restrictive cardiomyopathy. The ventricular pressure tracing shows prominent A and V waves and an early diastolic dip followed by an elevated plateau (square root sign). Increased jugular venous pressure with prominence of the y descent is the characteristic clinical and hemodynamic hallmark of restrictive cardiomyopathy (Fig. 9-4). A hemodynamic profile of restrictive cardiomyopathy is described in Table 9-5.

The pathophysiology and hemodynamic presentation of restrictive cardiomyopathy and constrictive pericarditis are exceedingly similar

200   The Adult Patient

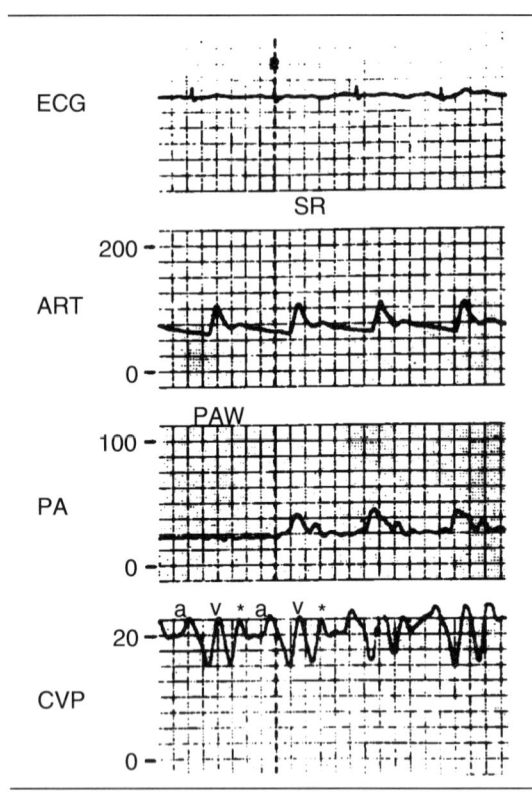

Fig. 9-4. Equalization of elevated diastolic filling pressures characteristic of restrictive cardiomyopathy. Note the prominence of A and V waves and y descent followed by an elevated plateau (square root sign). (Reprinted with permission from JB Mark: Central venous pressure monitoring: Clinical insights beyond the numbers. *J Cardiothorac Vasc Anesth* 5:163, 1991.)

(Table 9-6). Differentiation between the two by differences in filling pressures accentuated by exercise, volume loading, or induced premature ventricular beats have been proposed [84]. In fact, the differential diagnosis between constrictive pericarditis and restrictive cardiomyopathy is difficult and not always possible short of a histologic examination.

Gross pathologic examination of the end-stage restrictive cardiomyopathy reveals a normal-sized heart. The ventricular cavities may be obliterated by varying degrees of patchy fibrosis of the endocardium or myocardium, or both, depending on the primary process. The papillary muscle, atrioventricular valves, and conduction system may be involved. Endomyocardial biopsies play an important role in the diagnosis and classification of restrictive cardiomyopathy. The histopathologic features largely depend on the specific diseases and the stage of the disease. In advanced cases, histologic findings may be nonspecific and the absence of histologic abnormalities does not exclude the diagnosis of restrictive cardiomyopathy.

Clinical Manifestation

Due to their similar pathophysiology and hemodynamic profile, the clinical manifestation of restrictive cardiomyopathy is similar to that of constrictive pericarditis. The presentation and clinical course of restrictive cardiomyopathy are variable and dependent on the etiology of the restrictive pathophysiology [81, 85]. The criteria for clinical diagnosis of restrictive cardiomyopathy include heart failure resulting from a stiff left ventricle, normal left ventricular size and systolic function, and absence of left ventricular hypertrophy. Typical presentation consists of fatigue and exertional dyspnea, as there is inability to increase cardiac output by increasing heart rate without decreasing already compromised diastolic filling. Dyspnea and chest pain are not unusual. With endomyocardial fibrosis, atrioventricular regurgitation and mural thrombosis are common. Sometimes, right-sided signs and symptoms consisting of jugular venous distention with a prominent y descent, hepatomegaly, peripheral edema, ascites, and anasarca may dominate. The physical examination usually reveals tachycardia, narrow pulse pressure, and a protodiastolic gallop.

The chest x-ray will show cardiomegaly (biatrial) and pulmonary congestion with or without pleural effusions. The electrocardiogram often reveals arrhythmias, conduction defects (especially

Table 9-5. Hemodynamic profile of restrictive cardiomyopathy

Increased pulmonary wedge and right arterial pressures with "m" or "w" configuration

Ventricular pressure pulse, early diastolic dip and plateau, diminished compliance

Normal left ventricular end diastolic volume

Pulsus paradoxus in some instances

Preserved systolic function (ejection fraction = 0.52–0.76)

Kussmaul's sign may be present

Table 9-6. Findings in constrictive pericarditis and restrictive cardiomyopathy

Finding	Constrictive pericarditis	Restrictive cardiomyopathy
S_3 gallop	Absent	May be present
Pericardial knock	May be present	Absent
Palpable systolic apical impulse	Absent	May be present
Pericardial calcification	Present 50% of time	Absent
Pulsus paradoxus	May be present	May be present
Equal RV and LV diastolic pressure	May be present	May be present
Rate of LV filling	80% at 50% diastole	40% at 50% diastole
PEP/LVET	Avg. 0.31	Avg. 0.48 (congestive failure)
CT scan	Thickened pericardium	Normal pericardium

RV = right ventricle; LV = left ventricle; PEP = preejection period; LVET = left ventricular ejection time; CT = computed tomography.
Source: From NO Fowler, The Pericardium in Health and Disease. Mount Kisco, NY: Futura, 1985. Pp 301–329.

with amyloidosis and sarcoidosis), and nonspecific ST-T wave changes. Echocardiographic evaluation with Doppler analysis has been very important in evaluating systolic and diastolic function [86]. Radionuclide angiographic [87] and Doppler [88] assessment of diastolic filling have been utilized to differentiate between restrictive cardiomyopathy and constrictive pericarditis.

Cardiac catheterization in restrictive cardiomyopathy typically shows elevated biventricular diastolic pressures, the left ventricular end diastolic pressure usually exceeding the right by greater than 5 mm Hg. Central venous pressure is elevated to 15 to 20 mm Hg and pulmonary artery systolic pressure often exceeds 45 mm Hg [89]. Cardiac output is often severely reduced, while left ventricular systolic pressure and ejection fraction are maintained. Computed tomography [84] and nuclear magnetic resonance have provided further advances in the characterization of restrictive cardiomyopathy, as well as its differentiation from constrictive pericarditis.

Transvenous endomyocardial biopsy is mandatory for patients in whom the diagnosis of restrictive cardiomyopathy is considered. Although not specific, biopsy may reveal other causes of restrictive physiology that may benefit from accurate diagnosis and therapy, such as hemochromatosis.

Therapy for idiopathic restrictive cardiomyopathy is generally nonspecific and supportive. Diuretics and vasodilators are often used for congestive heart failure. However, caution needs to be exercised, as these agents may decrease already compromised ventricular filling. As the systolic function is normal, inotropic agents have little benefit. Antiarrhythmics and digitalis preparations are prescribed for arrhythmias and rapid ventricular response to atrial fibrillation. Pacemaker insertion may be indicated for severe conduction defects. As there is no effective therapy, death is usually due to arrhythmias and congestive heart failure.

Several specific diseases with restrictive cardiomyopathy physiology may respond to specific therapies. Phlebotomies [90] and iron chelation [91] therapy reduce myocyte iron deposition in hemochromatosis. Therapy with prednisone or hydroxyurea, or both, has been recommended for the hypereosinophilic syndrome. Sarcoidosis is treated with steroids. Endocardectomy and atrioventricular valve replacement have been performed with success for endomyocardial fibrosis [92]. Calcium channel blockers, which are known to improve diastolic function, have not been studied in the treatment of restrictive cardiomyopathy.

Anesthetic Management

Patients with restrictive cardiomyopathy may present for noncardiac surgery. Given the variety of diseases and wide spectrum of diastolic impairment, it is important to evaluate each patient individually. The anesthetic management of restrictive cardiomyopathy is similar to the management of cardiac tamponade. As cardiac output is maintained by increased filling pressures and tachycardia, the anesthetic plan should avoid drugs or maneuvers that decrease venous return, heart rate, or contractility. Severe tachycardia will shorten diastole and further reduce ventricular filling.

In addition to routine monitoring, invasive monitoring should be considered, depending on the patient's general status and the nature of the surgical procedure. Direct arterial pressure monitoring will provide beat-to-beat information on blood pressure and arterial wave form. Central venous pressures should be monitored to assess the trends in ventricular filling. A pulmonary artery catheter also allows for measurements of cardiac output, derived hemodynamic variables, and mixed venous oxygen saturation. Due to decreased ventricular compliance, elevated central venous pressures overestimate ventricular preload. Therefore, the changes in pressures and cardiac output are more important than absolute numbers. Transesophageal two-dimensional Doppler echocardiography provides assessment of ventricular filling and diastolic function.

Because patients with restrictive cardiomyopathy may have compromised hemodynamic reserve, induction of anesthesia must be performed carefully. Intravenous anesthetics such as opioids, ketamine, and etomidate that cause minimal myocardial and hemodynamic depression are preferred. Vasodilation and the subsequent decrease in ventricular filling may be encountered with propofol, benzodiazepines, curare, and atracurium. The myocardial depressant effects of inhalational anesthetic agents limit their use as a primary anesthetic agent. However, low-dose isoflurane may be utilized as a part of balanced anesthesia. Regional anesthetic techniques are beneficial in the avoidance of myocardial depressants and the decrease in venous return seen with institution of positive pressure ventilation. However, preload needs to be maintained when regional anesthesia is chosen and invasive hemodynamic monitoring is indicated.

HYPERTROPHIC CARDIOMYOPATHY

Hypertrophic cardiomyopathy (HCM) is a primary idiopathic disorder of the myocardium characterized by either symmetric or asymmetric ventricular hypertrophy. It appears to be transmitted genetically as an autosomal dominant trait with incomplete penetrance. Evidence of this disease is present in 25 percent of first-degree relatives of patients with HCM.

Brock [94] and Teare [95] brought attention to this disease entity in the late 1950s, describing nine subjects, all of whom at postmortem examination were reported to have ventricular septal hypertrophy. Subsequent to this original description, autopsy and echocardiographic studies demonstrated a much wider spectrum of ventricular involvement with remarkable variability in the site of the hypertrophic process [94, 95].

Asymmetric septal hypertrophy (ASH) occurs in over 90 percent of cases, and often exists with hypertrophy of the left ventricular free and posterior wall. Symmetric hypertrophy involving the septum and free wall has also been reported. Another distinctive feature of many patients with HCM is a dynamic pressure gradient in the subaortic region that may result in outflow tract obstruction and associated mitral regurgitation [96].

Tremendous technological advances have improved our understanding of the natural history, pathophysiology of characteristic systolic and diastolic abnormalities, clinical manifestations, and approach to treatment. However, the etiology of HCM remains unknown. Neither the cause of ASH, the predominant gross anatomic disorder, nor the cause of myocardial fiber disarray, the predominant histopathologic abnormality, has been established. This section focuses on the pathophysiologic mechanisms associated with HCM, the efficacy of pharmacologic and surgical therapy, and their implications on anesthetic management.

Pathophysiology

Gross Morphology
The characteristic morphologic feature of HCM is a thickened nondilated ventricle that exists in the absence of coexisting cardiac or systemic disease capable of producing such hypertrophy. The increase in ventricular mass is due almost entirely to an increase in the thickness of the ventricular wall, with the left ventricle usually being more involved in the hypertrophic process than the right [97] (see

Fig. 9-1). The atria are frequently hypertrophied and dilated as well [98].

The pattern of hypertrophy is particularly distinctive and frequently associated with disproportionate involvement of the interventricular septum. Hypertrophy commonly involves both the septum and anterolateral free wall [99].

Hypertrophic cardiomyopathy may be obstructive or nonobstructive in nature. In patients with subaortic obstruction, frequently referred to as idiopathic hypertrophic subaortic stenosis (IHSS), the basal septum is markedly thickened at the level of the mitral valve, and the cross-sectional area of the outflow tract at end diastole is decreased. In the nonobstructive form of HCM, the ventricular septum at the level of the mitral valve is less thickened, with a more distal distribution of septal hypertrophy and thus a larger outflow tract [100].

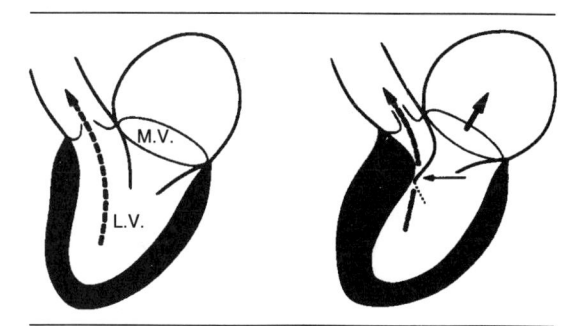

Fig. 9-5. Mechanism of outflow tract obstruction in the patient with hypertrophic cardiomyopathy. LV = left ventricle; MV = mitral valve. (Reprinted with permission from ED Wigle, Z Sasson, MA Henderson, et al, Hypertrophic cardiomyopathy: The importance of the site and extent of hypertrophy. A review. *Prog Cardiovasc Dis* 28:1, 1985.)

Histopathology

In his initial morphologic description, Teare [95] described HCM as characterized by short, plump, hypertrophied myocardial fibers, interspersed with loose, intercellular connective tissue that at times appeared to undergo a transformation to dense fibrosis. Foci of disorganized myocardial cells are located among areas of hypertrophied but otherwise normal muscle cells. This cellular disorganization and fibrosis are often extensive and may contribute to impaired systolic and diastolic function, or serve as a nidus for ventricular arrhythmias.

Small, abnormal, intramural coronary arteries are found in 80 percent of patients with HCM. The walls of these vessels are thickened, and lumens frequently appear narrowed. These abnormal intramural coronary arteries are commonly found in the intraventricular septum or adjacent to areas of extensive fibrosis, and may in fact be responsible for the development of myocardial ischemia [101].

Outflow Tract Obstruction

The presence of a dynamic pressure gradient in HCM has been a subject of considerable controversy over the past 30 years. This pressure gradient, which is associated with outflow tract obstruction, was initially thought to be due to a muscular sphincteric action in the subaortic area. Subsequent studies have demonstrated that with early rapid ejection, a Venturi effect occurs that draws the anterior leaflet of the mitral valve toward the bulging interventricular septum [97, 100, 102]. A pressure gradient is then generated between the left ventricular cavity and aortic outflow tract (Fig. 9-5).

The magnitude of the obstructive gradient is determined by the time of onset in systole of mitral leaflet–septal contact. Therefore, early and prolonged mitral leaflet–septal contact is associated with a high pressure gradient [103, 104], marked prolongation of left ventricular ejection time, and thus a greater percentage of stroke volume being ejected against obstruction [105]. Some degree of mitral regurgitation is a constant finding in patients with gradients and appears to correlate with the magnitude of outflow tract gradient [106, 107]. Small gradients arise from delayed and brief systolic anterior motion (SAM) septal contact. If mitral leaflet–septal contact occurs after 55 percent of the systolic ejection period, no pressure gradient develops [104]. Other factors that exacerbate SAM-septal contact include increased contractility and decreased preload and afterload.

Diastolic Dysfunction

Derangements in diastolic function are present in all patients with HCM, and probably contribute to the frequent symptoms of angina and dyspnea. Diastolic dysfunction results from both altered passive elastic properties that lead to reduced ventricular compliance and from impairment of active ventricular relaxation [108].

Reduced left ventricular compliance arises from a markedly thickened ventricular muscle mass. This is worsened by the characteristic myocardial scarring and fibrosis that occur. Impaired relaxation has also been demonstrated; however, the precise mechanism is unclear. It has been suggested that the inactivation process by which calcium ions are sequestered in the sarcoplasmic reticulum is impaired in hypertrophic conditions, leading to intracellular calcium overload and impaired relaxation [109]. In addition a disturbed end systolic pressure-volume relationship, altered afterload, impaired coronary blood flow, and regional wall stress may further contribute to this problem. Regardless, impaired relaxation leads to prolongation of isovolumetric relaxation time, reduction in the peak velocity of left ventricular filling, and, ultimately, elevated left ventricular filling pressures [108, 110, 111].

Reduced ventricular compliance and impaired relaxation imply that these patients are dependent on a large intravascular volume and that the maintenance of sinus rhythm is essential for adequate diastolic filling. The atrial contribution to ventricular filling is extremely important in HCM, and may approach 75 percent of total stroke volume.

Systolic Function

Left ventricular systolic performance in the majority of patients with HCM is normal or even supernormal, with ejection fractions of 80 percent or more being common [112]. This represents the influence of reduced afterload rather than augmented contractility. The increased ventricular mass decreases systolic wall stress (decreasing afterload), thus allowing for enhanced ejection [113].

In a small subset of patients with HCM, there is progressive myocardial scarring and wall thinning, left ventricular cavity dilatation, and reduced systolic performance. Such patients are usually severely symptomatic, and management is considerably different from that of the typical patient with hyperdynamic systolic function.

Myocardial Ischemia

Even in the absence of coronary artery disease, it is well documented that myocardial ischemia occurs in patients with HCM. Multiple factors are involved. First, hypertrophy itself occurs with inadequate expansion of the vascular compartment, rendering the tissue particularly vulnerable to acute decreases in myocardial blood flow. Various studies have demonstrated reduced coronary vasodilator reserve, such that increases in myocardial demands are not balanced by appropriate increases in coronary flow. The presence of abnormally narrowed intramural coronary arteries further diminishes coronary reserve [114, 115].

Left ventricular diastolic dysfunction is associated with an increased left ventricular diastolic pressure that may have a compressive effect on the intramyocardial vessels, especially limiting subendocardial blood flow. In addition, even under basal conditions the thickened myocardium is associated with markedly increased oxygen requirements. With the added demand resulting from outflow obstruction, myocardial oxygen requirements may not be met.

Once ischemia occurs, it may be self-perpetuating, resulting in further impairment of diastolic function, greater increase in end diastolic pressure, and ultimately compromised myocardial blood flow (Fig. 9-6).

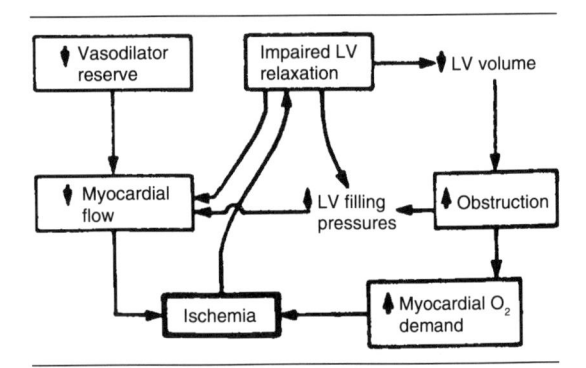

Fig. 9-6. Mechanisms of ischemia in hypertrophic cardiomyopathy.

Clinical Manifestations

Natural History

The natural history of HCM is varied. Most patients remain stable or have a slow progression

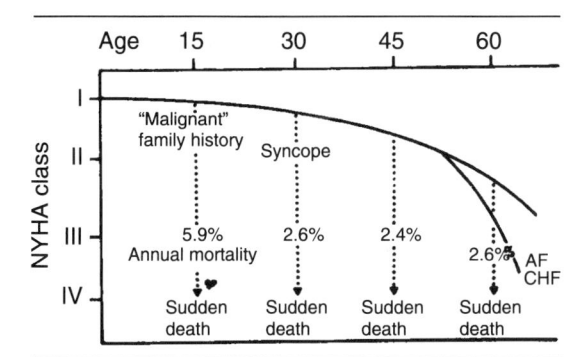

Fig. 9-7. The natural history of hypertrophic cardiomyopathy. NYHA = New York Heart Association; AF = atrial fibrillation; CHF = congestive heart failure. (Reprinted with permission from W McKenna. The Natural History of Hypertrophic Cardiomyopathy. In JA Shaver (ed), *Cardiomyopathies: Clinical Presentation, Differential Diagnosis and Management*. Philadelphia: Davis, 1987. P 138.)

of symptoms. The principal determinant of many manifestations of the disease is the extent of the hypertrophic process, although the degree of left ventricular hypertrophy does not necessarily correlate with prognosis. Regardless of clinical course, the annual mortality of patients with HCM is reported to be about 4 percent, with a high incidence of sudden death [74] (Fig. 9-7).

Data by Fighali and associates [116] suggest that radionuclide ejection fraction and peak ejection rate fall gradually in association with a small increase in left ventricular end systolic and end diastolic volume. Clinically significant impairment of systolic function develops in about 10 percent of patients; however, the progression to a dilated, poorly contracting left ventricle is rare. Most patients with HCM and progressive wall thinning become severely symptomatic before the left ventricle has the morphologic manifestations of a dilated ventricle [117].

Children with HCM have a similar course; however, in one of the largest series, 30 percent of children died suddenly during an average follow-up period of 9 years. Overall, children with HCM appear to have an annual mortality of about 6 percent [118]. In fact, unsuspected HCM is the most common abnormality found at autopsy of young athletes who die suddenly [119].

Identification of patients at risk for sudden death continues to be a challenging problem. Known risk factors include young age at diagnosis, family history of HCM, sudden death, and the occurrence of asymptomatic ventricular tachycardia on ambulatory Holter monitoring [120]. The mechanism of sudden death has not been proved; however, malignant arrhythmias have been implicated.

Symptoms

Symptoms in patients with HCM are caused by the complex interaction of various pathophysiologic mechanisms, and therefore correlation between a particular symptom and a single pathophysiologic mechanism does not always exist. Patients with mild and localized hypertrophy may have severe symptoms, whereas those with marked hypertrophy may have no symptoms. Similarly, patients with outflow tract obstruction may have comparable symptoms to those without obstruction.

Clinical symptoms of HCM include dyspnea, angina, syncope, and palpitations. Dyspnea, the most common, occurs in 75 percent of symptomatic patients and appears related to elevated left ventricular end diastolic pressures (LVEDP) that are secondary to left ventricular hypertrophy and reduced ventricular compliance [121]. Angina occurs in about 66 percent of symptomatic patients, reflecting increased left ventricular mass, abnormal ventricular relaxation prolonging systolic wall tension, and a decreased diastolic interval, thus reducing the time available for coronary flow; this is in addition to the many other factors that contribute to myocardial ischemia, including the imbalance in myocardial supply-demand, discussed previously. Importantly, coronary artery disease (CAD) occurs in 20 percent of adults with HCM and therefore must not be overlooked when such patients are evaluated [122]. Likewise, HCM should always be ruled out in the adult suspected of having CAD who is found to have normal coronaries on angiography.

Syncope is a symptom that occurs more frequently in patients with left ventricular outflow gradients, although there is little correlation with the magnitude of the gradient. Syncope is usually effort related, reflecting the inability to increase cardiac output with exertion. This is due to either outflow obstruction or impaired diastolic filling.

It may also be secondary to cardiac arrhythmias. In one study, 90 percent of patients complaining of syncope demonstrated recurrent atrial and ventricular arrhythmias during ambulatory ECG monitoring.

Palpitations are common and usually secondary to arrhythmias. Canedo and associates [122] reported a 70 percent incidence of supraventricular arrhythmias and an 82 percent incidence of premature ventricular complexes. Most patients had more than one type of arrhythmia, including 39 percent who had potentially life-threatening rhythm disturbances. McKenna and colleagues [123, 124] reported asymptomatic episodes of nonsustained ventricular tachycardia in 25 percent of patients with HCM, detected during ambulatory ECG monitoring. Although these episodes appear benign and are not associated with any ST-T segment change, two centers have reported nonsustained ventricular tachycardia to be associated with increased annual mortality [120, 125].

Atrial fibrillation is more common in the older patient and often is a poor prognostic sign. Atrial fibrillation may occur in patients with severe hypertrophy, resting left ventricular outflow gradients, and increased left atrial size. The onset of atrial fibrillation usually leads to a striking increase in symptoms, and prompt cardioversion is usually indicated.

Diagnostic Evaluation

Chest Roentgenogram. Findings on the standard chest roentgenogram are nonspecific. Cardiac size may vary from normal to markedly enlarged with little correlation between heart size and functional status of the patient, or severity of outflow tract pressure gradient. In fact, marked left ventricular hypertrophy with cavity dilatation may be present and yet cardiomegaly not observed on chest x-ray. Left atrial enlargement is frequently seen when mitral regurgitation is present.

Electrocardiogram. The ECG is clearly abnormal in the vast majority of patients with HCM. Electrocardiographic evidence of left ventricular hypertrophy is present in more than 50 percent of patients and seemingly correlates with the degree of hypertrophy as determined by two-dimensional echocardiography. ECG evidence of left ventricular hypertrophy is seen in more than 70 percent of patients with resting obstruction. Left axis deviation and left atrial enlargement may also be seen, the latter being related to coexistent mitral regurgitation [98].

ST segment T-wave anomalies are common and may closely resemble the ECG found in ischemic heart disease. A pseudoinfarction pattern with abnormal Q waves is relatively frequent, particularly involving the inferior and lateral leads.

Conduction abnormalities, specifically a shortened PR interval with normal QRS, occurs in about 5 to 10 percent of patients. These patients may be at increased risk of supraventricular tachyarrhythmias on the basis of preexcitation [126]. Ventricular arrhythmias have been demonstrated in about 75 percent of patients undergoing ambulatory ECG monitoring. Supraventricular tachycardia is present in up to 50 percent of patients studied [125, 126].

Echocardiography. Echocardiography has become the noninvasive standard for the evaluation of HCM. The echocardiogram is able to identify, as well as quantify, both morphologic and functional features of the left ventricle.

The cardinal feature of HCM on echocardiography is left ventricular hypertrophy, with great variability in the distribution of involvement. A thickened septum that is at least 1.3 to 1.5 times the thickness of the posterior wall when measured in diastole just before atrial systole has been the classic criterion for the diagnosis of ASH [98]. Typically, in HCM the septum is greater than 15 mm thick (normally < 11 mm). In addition, a small left ventricular outflow tract and systolic anterior motion of the mitral valve may be seen. Abnormalities of diastolic function are also present.

Angiography. In patients over 45 years of age with symptoms of ischemic pain, despite diagnosis of HCM on echocardiogram, it is necessary to perform angiography. Left ventriculography will demonstrate the hypertrophied ventricle with a small cavity in which movement of the anterior mitral valve leaflet encroaches on the outflow tract during systole. Any associated mitral regurgitation can be quantified. In addition, the coronary anatomy can be evaluated.

Medical Therapy

β-Adrenergic Blocking Agents

β-Adrenergic blockers have long been the mainstay of medical management and have been shown to provide symptomatic relief in up to two thirds of patients. This therapeutic effect appears to mediate by reduction in heart rate, inotropic state, and inhibition of sympathetic stimulation of the heart during physical or emotional stress [127].

β-Blockers may be effective in reducing the pressure gradient, particularly when associated with exertion. They have been shown to reduce myocardial oxygen demand by virtue of their negative chronotropic action, reducing myocardial ischemia. β-Blockers do not, however, appear to have clinically important effects on ventricular relaxation and filling [128]. They may play a role in the prevention of tachyarrhythmias. However, controlled studies to assess the impact of therapy on prognosis have not been performed.

Calcium Channel Blocking Agents

The greatest clinical experience has been with verapamil. Verapamil reduces symptoms and increases exercise tolerance in the majority of patients during short-term therapy, and sustained clinical improvement has been reported in over 50 percent of patients during long-term therapy [129].

Numerous studies have reported improved left ventricular diastolic function from both intravenous and oral verapamil administration, as well as reduced outflow tract obstruction. Verapamil improves diastolic filling by improved relaxation rather than by changes in compliance [130]. Propranolol has been shown to have no such effect.

The majority of patients receive only mild symptomatic improvement at lower doses and achieve more acceptable reduction of symptoms at higher doses. However, verapamil at high doses may be associated with adverse cardiac reactions, including sinus bradycardia and atrioventricular block, or hypotension. In patients with outflow obstruction and elevated pulmonary capillary wedge pressure (PCWP), high-dose verapamil therapy may precipitate acute pulmonary edema [131].

Other calcium channel blockers, including nifedipine, have been studied, but much less extensively than verapamil. Nifedipine does improve left ventricular relaxation and filling characteristics; however, it may potentially exacerbate outflow obstruction on the basis of reduced peripheral resistance [132].

Clinical trials with diltiazem have not been reported.

Disopyramide

Disopyramide has been used in patients with obstructive HCM primarily because of its negative inotropic action, which results in decreased myocardial contractility and decrease in obstructive pressure gradient. In addition, disopyramide, a potent antiarrhythmic, is beneficial in the treatment of ventricular arrhythmias, which commonly occur. The clinical experience with disopyramide to date is limited to those patients with resting obstruction.

Amiodarone

Symptomatic therapy with β- or calcium channel blocking agents does not reduce the incidence of ventricular arrhythmias. Amiodarone has been used in the treatment of ventricular tachyarrhythmias in HCM, and more recent data suggest that it may prevent sudden death. McKenna and associates [133] reported no deaths in 21 patients with HCM and ventricular tachycardia who received amiodarone for at least 3 years.

Surgical Therapy

Surgical therapy is aimed at abolishing the obstructive pressure gradient across the left ventricular outflow tract and may be indicated in patients who are unresponsive to medical management. The most common surgical procedure is ventriculomyectomy, in which a portion of the hypertrophied basal septum is excised, thereby widening the outflow tract. The efficacy of ventriculomyectomy in reducing or abolishing the subaortic pressure gradient in the immediate, short-, and long-term follow-up has been excellent. Left ventricular systolic performance is usually unaffected and remains hyperdynamic, while left ventricular diastolic function is often improved.

Anesthetic Considerations

Anesthetic management should be directed toward measures that are known to decrease subaortic obstruction, namely maintaining adequate intravascular volume, normalizing systemic vascular resistance (SVR), and avoiding any increase in myocardial contractility.

Any maneuvers that augment contractility, such as increased sympathetic stimulation from noxious stimuli, light anesthesia, and drugs such as epinephrine and digitalis, will further worsen obstruction. Decreased intravascular volume secondary to hypovolemia or injudicious use of venodilators will clearly enhance obstruction. Acute reductions in SVR from the vasodilating effects of anesthetic agents or use of vasodilating agents such as sodium nitroprusside will further worsen this subaortic gradient.

Premedication should be heavy, with the goal of decreasing apprehension and blunting activation of the sympathetic nervous system. Premedication with atropine may theoretically result in an increased heart rate, which in these patients could potentially shorten ventricular filling of the noncompliant ventricle. In addition, tachycardia will increase myocardial oxygen demands, and may initiate a vicious cycle of ischemia. Chronic β-blocker, calcium channel blocker, or antiarrhythmic therapy should be continued until the morning of surgery and promptly reinstituted in the postoperative period.

General anesthesia is more commonly used than regional techniques, specifically due to the risks of peripheral vasodilatation. The inhalational anesthetics are particularly beneficial for their dose-dependent myocardial depressant effects. Halothane is most commonly used, but carries some risk regarding the potentiation of arrhythmias, particularly junctional rhythms. Enflurane and isoflurane are associated with a more profound decrease in SVR. Induction agents, including benzodiazepines, barbiturates, and etomidate, can also be safely used. Ketamine has the potential of increasing myocardial contractility and is best avoided. The sole use of narcotics is probably not recommended, as they are unable to effectively depress the myocardium, and may be associated with a reduction in SVR.

Nondepolarizing muscle relaxation is acceptable, but the use of pancuronium may be associated with an increase in heart rate and contractility. Also d-tubocurare and atracurium may be associated with histamine release and a reduction in SVR that is undesirable.

Intraoperative monitoring should include an ECG system with the capability of monitoring V_5 and each of the six limb leads. Inspection of lead II is particularly valuable in the detection of arrhythmias. Direct arterial monitoring is advantageous in the rapid detection of arrhythmias that may cause hemodynamic compromise. In addition, changes in the shape of the arterial wave form may suggest outflow obstruction.

Central venous pressure (CVP) monitoring is limited by the marked differences between right and left ventricular compliance, and most probably will not offer valuable data to guide perioperative management. However, such access is helpful for the administration of vasoactive agents should they be necessary.

Pulmonary artery pressure monitoring can be helpful in assessing filling pressures and monitoring cardiac output, and allows for mixed venous sampling. Due to altered left ventricular compliance and the increased contribution of atrial contraction to final end diastolic pressure, the pulmonary capillary wedge pressure will underestimate LVEDP. It will, however, reflect LVEDP more accurately than the CVP would. Optimum filling pressures should be assessed using ventricular function curves; an A-V sequential paceport pulmonary artery catheter (PAC) may be particularly helpful, allowing overdrive pacing in the event of junctional arrhythmias, while maintaining the atrial kick [134].

Intraoperative arrhythmias should be treated aggressively. Junctional rhythms should be treated by assessing their cause. The concentration of inhalational agent used should be reduced and atropine given. Supraventricular or junctional tachycardia can be treated with small doses of propranolol. Verapamil also can be used; however, it has the potential of causing vasodilation, which will ultimately worsen outflow tract obstruction. If these rhythms are associated with hemodynamic compromise, cardioversion should be promptly performed.

In the absence of arrhythmia, intraoperative hypotension should be treated by increasing intravascular volume. Further support of perfusion pressure can be provided with phenylephrine. The use of calcium, inotropes, or beta agonist is contraindicated in HCM.

The intraoperative availability of two-dimensional transesophageal echocardiography may negate the need for intraoperative PAC placement. It allows online assessment of ventricular function and chamber dimensions, and an assessment of outflow obstruction.

REFERENCES

1. Page, DI, Caulfield, JB, Kastor, JA, et al. Myocardial changes associated with cardiogenic shock. *N Engl J Med* 285:133, 1971.
2. Caulfield, JB, Leinbach, R, Gold, H. The relationship of myocardial infarct size and prognosis. *Circulation* 53 (Suppl): 141, 1976.
3. Field, BJ, Russell, RO, Jr, Dowling, JT, et al. Regional left ventricular performance in the year following myocardial infarction. *Circulation* 46:679, 1972.
4. Gould, KL, Lipscomb, K, Hamilton, GW, et al. Left ventricular hypertrophy in coronary artery disease. A cardiomyopathy syndrome following myocardial infarction. *Am J Med* 55:595, 1973.
5. Moraski, RE, Russell, RO, Jr, Smith, M, et al. Left ventricular function in patients with and without myocardial infarction and one, two, or three vessel coronary artery disease. *Am J Cardiol* 35:1, 1975.
6. Cosby, RS, Giddings, JA, See, JR, et al. Late complications of myocardial infarction. *Adv Cardiol* 23:73, 1978.
7. Taylor, GJ, Humphries, JO, Mellits, ED, et al. Predictors of clinical course, coronary anatomy and left ventricular function after recovery from acute myocardial infarction. *Circulation* 62:960, 1980.
8. Sobel, BE. Infarct size, prognosis, and causal contiguity. *Circulation* 53 (Suppl 1): 146, 1976.
9. Hills, LD, Braunwald, E. Myocardial ischemia. *N Engl J Med* 296:1034, 1977.
10. Kloner, RA, Braunwald, E. Observations on experimental myocardial ischemia. *Cardiovasc Res* 14:371, 1980.
11. Anversa, P, Loud, AV, Levicky, V, et al. Left ventricular failure induced by myocardial infarction. I. Myocyte hypertrophy. *Am J Physiol* 248:H876, 1985.
12. Pfeffer, MA, Pfeffer, JM, Fishbein, MC, et al. Myocardial infarct size and ventricular function in rats. *Circ Res* 44:503, 1979.
13. Turek, Z, Grantner, M, Kubat, K, et al. Arterial blood gases, muscle fiber diameter and intercapillary distance in cardiac hypertrophy of rats with an old myocardial infarction. *Pflugers Arch* 376:209, 1978.
14. Anversa, P, Begni, C, McDonald, SL, et al. Morphometry of right ventricular hypertrophy induced by myocardial infarction in the rat. *Am J Pathol* 116:504, 1984.
15. Pfeffer, JM, Pfeffer, MA, Braunwald, E. Influence of chronic captopril therapy on the infarcted left ventricle of the rat. *Circ Res* 53:84, 1985.
16. Pfeffer, MA, Pfeffer, JM, Steinberg, C, et al. Survival after an experimental myocardial infarction: Beneficial effects of long-term therapy with captopril. *Circulation* 72:406, 1985.
17. Braunwald, E. Heart failure: Pathophysiology and treatment. *Am Heart J* 102:466, 1981.
18. Diamond, G, Forrester, JS. Effect of coronary artery disease and acute myocardial infarction on left ventricular compliance in man. *Circulation* 45:11, 1972.
19. Parmley, WW, Chuck, L, Chatterjee, K, et al. Acute changes in the diastolic pressure volume relationship of the left ventricle. *Eur J Cardiol* 4 (Suppl.): 105, 1976.
20. Johnson, RA, Palacios, I. Dilated cardiomyopathies of the adult. *N Engl J Med* 307:1051; 307:1119, 1982.
21. Katz, AM. Cardiomyopathy of overload. A major determinant of prognosis in congestive heart failure. *N Engl J Med* 322:100, 1990.
22. Anversa, P, Olivetti, G, Mellssari, M, Loud, AV. Stereological measurement of cellular and subcellular hypertrophy and hyperplasia in the papillary muscle of adult rat. *J Mol Cell Cardiol* 12:781, 1980.
23. Rabinowitz, M. Protein synthesis and turnover in normal and hypertrophied heart. *Am J Cardiol* 31:202, 1973.
24. Roberts, JT, Weam, JT. Quantitative changes in the capillary-muscle relationship in human hearts during normal growth and hypertrophy. *Am Heart J* 21:617, 1941.
25. Johnson, RA. Heart Failure. In RA Johnson, E Haber, WG Austen (eds), *The Practice of Cardiology*. Boston: Little, Brown, 1980. Pp 31–95.
26. Alexander, J, Dainiak, N, Berger, HJ, et al. Serial assessment of doxorubicin cardiotoxicity with quantitative radionuclide angiocardiography. *N Engl J Med* 300:378, 1979.
27. Field, BJ, Baxley, WA, Russell, RO, Jr, et al. Left ventricular function hypertrophy in cardiomyopathy with depressed ejection fraction. *Circulation* 47:1022, 1973.
28. Engler, R, Ray, R, Higgins, CB, et al. Clinical assessment and follow-up of functional capacity in patients with chronic congestive cardiomyopathies. *Am J Cardiol* 49:1832, 1982.
29. Bristow, MR, Ginsburg, R, Umans, V, et al. β_1-β_2-

adrenergic-receptor subpopulations in nonfailing and failing humans' ventricular myocardium: Coupling of both receptor subtypes to muscle contraction and selective β_1-receptor down-regulation in heart failure. *Circ Res* 297:309, 1986.
30. Brodde, OE, Schuler, S, Kretsch, R, et al. Regional distribution of β-adrenoceptors in the human heart: Coexistence of function β_1- and β_2-adrenoceptors in both atria and ventricles in severe congestive cardiomyopathy. *J Cardiovasc Pharmacol* 8:1235, 1986.
31. Bristow, MR, Hersberger, RE, Port, JD, et al. β_1 and β_2 adrenergic receptor mediated adenylate cyclase stimulation in nonfailing and failing human ventricular myocardium. *Mol Pharmacol* 35:295, 1989.
32. Leier, CV, Heban, PT, Huss, P, et al. Comparative systemic and regional hemodynamic effects of dopamine and dobutamine in patients with cardiomyopathic heart failure. *Circulation* 58:466, 1978.
33. Unverferth, DV, Blanford, M, Kates, RE, et al. Tolerance to dobutamine after a 72 hour continuous infusion. *Am J Med* 69:262, 1980.
34. Colucci, WS, Alexander, RW, Williams, GH, et al. Decreased lymphocyte beta-adrenergic-receptor density in patients with heart failure and tolerance to the beta-adrenergic agonist pirbuterol. *N Engl J Med* 305:185, 1981.
35. Gaasch, WH, Zile, MR. Evaluation of myocardial function in cardiomyopathic states. *Prog Cardiovasc Dis* 27:115, 1984.
36. Weber, KT, Janicki, JS. The heart as a muscle-pump system and the concept of heart failure. *Am Heart J* 98:371, 1979.
37. Parmley, WW. Pathophysiology of congestive heart failure. *Am J Cardiol* 56:7A, 1985.
38. Ross, J, Sonnenblick, EH, Taylor, RR, et al. Diastolic geometry and sarcomere lengths in the chronically dilated canine left ventricle. *Circ Res* 28:49, 1971.
39. Rackley, CE, Dalldorf, FG, Hood, WP, et al. Sarcomere length and left ventricular function in chronic heart disease. *Am J Med Sci* 259:90, 1970.
40. Ginsburg, R, Esserman, LJ, Bristow, MR. Myocardial performance and extracellular ionized calcium in a severely failing human heart. *Ann Intern Med* 98:603, 1983.
41. Colucci, WS, Wright, RF, Braunwald, E. New positive inotropic agents in the treatment of congestive heart failure. Mechanisms of action and recent clinical developments. *N Engl J Med* 314:290, 1986.
42. Ruffolo, RR, Kopia, GA. Importance of receptor regulation in the pathophysiology and therapy of congestive heart failure. *Am J Med* 80 (Suppl 2B):67, 1986.
43. Lefkowitz, RJ, Caron, MG, Stiles, GL. Mechanisms of membrane-receptor regulation. Biochemical, physiological, and clinical insights derived from studies of the adrenergic receptors. *N Engl J Med* 310:1570, 1984.
44. Chidsey, CA, Braunwald, E, Morrow, AG. Catecholamine excretion and cardiac stores of norepinephrine in congestive heart failure. *Am J Med* 39:442, 1965.
45. Cohn, JN, Levine, TB, Olivare, MT, et al. Plasma norepinephrine as a guide to prognosis in patients with chronic congestive heart failure. *N Engl J Med* 311:819, 1984.
46. Petch, MC, Naylor, WG. Uptake of catecholamines by human heart muscle in vitro. *Br Heart J* 41:336, 1979.
47. Swedberg, K, Chatterjee, K, Roizen, M, et al. Myocardial norepinephrine release in congestive heart failure (abstract). *Circulation* 66 (Suppl II): 23, 1982.
48. Kay, HR, Afshari, M, Barash, PG, et al. Measurement of ejection fraction by thermal dilution techniques. *J Surg Res* 34:337, 1983.
49. Hines, R, Barash, PG. Intraoperative right ventricular dysfunction detected with a right ventricular ejection fraction catheter. *J Clin Monit* 2:206, 1986.
50. Ream, AK, Fowles, RE, Jamieson, S. Cardiac Transplantation. In JA Kaplan (ed), *Cardiac Anesthesia*. Orlando: Grune & Stratton, 1987. Pp 111–135.
51. Gallo, JA, Jr, Corc, RC. Anesthesia for Cardiac Transplantation. In BR Brown (ed), *Anesthesia and Transplantation Surgery*. Philadelphia: Davis, 1987. Pp 91–107.
52. Berberich, JJ, Fabian, JJ. A retrospective analysis of fentanyl and sufentanil for cardiac transplantation. *J Cardiothorac Anesth* 1:200, 1987.
53. Tomicheck, RC, Rosow, CE, Philbin, DM, et al. Diazepam-fentanyl interaction—hemodynamic and hormonal effects in coronary artery surgery. *Anesth Analg* 62:881, 1983.
54. Hensley, FA, Jr, Martin, DE, Larach, DR, et al. Anesthetic management for cardiac transplantation in North America—1986 survey. *J Cardiothorac Anesth* 1:429, 1987.
55. Reitz, BA, Fowles, RE, Ream, AK. Cardiac Transplantation. In AK Ream and RP Fogdall (eds). *Acute Cardiovascular Management*. Philadelphia: Lippincott, 1982. Pp 549–567.
56. Benowitz, NL, Meister, W. Pharmacokinetics in patients with cardiac failure. *Clin Pharmacokinet* 1:389, 1976.
57. Shimosato, S, Yasuda, I, Kemmotsu, O, et al. Effect of halothane on altered contractility of isolated heart muscle obtained from data with experimen-

58. Kemmotsu, O, Hashimoto, Y, Shimosato, S. The effects of fluroxene and enflurane on contractile performance of isolated papillary muscles from failing heart. Anesthesiology 40:252, 1974.
59. Lappas, DG, Buckley, MJ, Laver, MB, et al. Left ventricular performance and pulmonary circulation following addition of nitrous oxide to morphine during coronary artery surgery. Anesthesiology 43:61, 1975.
60. Schulte-Sasse, U, Hess, W, Tarnow, J. Pulmonary vascular responses to nitrous oxide in patients with normal and high pulmonary vascular resistance. Anesthesiology 57:9, 1982.
61. Murkin, JM, Moldenhauer, CC, Hug, CC. High-dose fentanyl for rapid induction of anaesthesia in patients with coronary artery disease. Can Anaesth Soc J 32:320, 1985.
62. Reeder, DA, Newsome, LR, Moldenhauer, CC, et al. Hemodynamic or hormonal effects of rapid-sequence induction sufentanil. Society of Cardiovascular Anesthesia Ninth Annual Meeting, Scientific Abstract, 1987. P 88.
63. Barash, PG, Kopriva, CJ, Giles, R, et al. Global ventricular function and intubation: Radionuclear profiles. Anesthesiology 53:S109, 1980.
64. Demas, K, Wyner, J, Mihm, JG, et al. Anesthesis for heart transplantation. A retrospective study and review. Br J Anaesth 58:1357, 1986.
65. Barash, PG, Tarabadkar, S, Giles, R, et al. Preservation of global left ventricular function during intubation in patients with ischemic heart disease. Anesthesiology 55:A6, 1981.
66. Reve, JG. Anesthesia and cardiac transplantation. In TH Stanley and WC Petty (Eds), Anaesthesia and the Cardiovascular System. Boston: Martinus Nighott, 1984. Pp 217–224.
67. Strauer, BE. Contractile responses to morphine, piritramide, meperidine, and fentanyl: A comparative study of effects on the isolated ventricular myocardium. Anesthesiology 37:304, 1972.
68. Wynands, JE, Wong, P, Whalley, DG, et al. Oxygen fentanyl anesthesia in patients with poor ventricular function. Anesth Analg 62:476, 1983.
69. Tarabadkar, S, Kopriva, CJ, Sreenivasan, N, et al. Hemodynamic impact of induction in patients with decreased cardiac reserve. Anesthesiology 53:S43, 1980.
70. Gage, J, Rutman, H, Lucido, D, et al. Additive effects of dobutamine and amrinone on myocardial contractility and ventricular performance in patients with severe heart failure. Circulation 74:367, 1986.
71. White, PF, Way, WL, Trevor, AJ. Ketamine—its pharmacology and therapeutic uses. Anesthesiology 56:119, 1982.
72. Report of the WHO/ISFC task force on definition and classification of cardiomyopathies. Br Heart J 44:672, 1980.
73. Crockett, LK, Thompson, M, Dekker, A. A review of cardiac amyloidosis: Report of a case presenting as constrictive pericarditis. Am J Med Sci 264:149, 1972.
74. Wynne, J, Braunwald, E. The Cardiomyopathies and Myocarditides in Heart Disease. In E Braunwald (ed), Heart Disease: A Textbook of Cardiovascular Medicine (2nd ed). Philadelphia: Saunders, 1984. Pp 1410–1469.
75. Cutler, DJ, Isner, JM, Bracey, AW, et al. Hemochromatosis heart disease: An unemphasized cause of reversible restrictive cardiomyopathy. Am J Med 69:923, 1980.
76. Bouchard, A, Sanz, N, Botvinick, EH, et al. Noninvasive assessment of cardiomyopathy in normotensive diabetic patients between 20 and 50 years old. Am J Med 87:160, 1989.
77. Benotti, JR, Grossman, W. Restrictive cardiomyopathy. Ann Rev Med 35:113, 1984.
78. Aroney, C, Bett, N, Radford, D. Familial restrictive cardiomyopathy. Aust NZ J Med 18:877, 1988.
79. Fitzpatrick, AP, Shapiro, LM, Rickard, AF, et al. Familial restrictive cardiomyopathy with atrioventricular block and skeletal myopathy. Br Heart J 63:114, 1990.
80. Siegel, RJ, Shah, PK, Fishbein, MC. Idiopathic restrictive cardiomyopathy. Circulation 70:165, 1984.
81. Benotti, JR, Grossman, W, Cohn, PF. Clinical profile of restrictive cardiomyopathy. Circulation 61:1206, 1980.
82. Navarro-Lopez, F, Llorian, A, Ferrer-Roca, O, et al. Restrictive cardiomyopathy in pseudoxanthoma elasticum. Chest 78:113, 1980.
83. Spry, CJF, Tai, PC, Davies, J. The cardiotoxicity of eosinophils. Postgrad Med J 59:147, 1983.
84. Hosenpud, RJ, Nies, NR. Clinical, hemodynamic and endomyocardial biopsy findings in idiopathic restrictive cardiomyopathy. West J Med 144:303, 1986.
85. Hirota, Y, Shimizu, G, Kita, Y, et al. Spectrum of restrictive cardiomyopathy: Report of the national survey in Japan. Am Heart J 120:188, 1990.
86. Janos, GG, Arjunan, K, Meyer, RA, et al. Differentiation of constrictive pericarditis and restrictive cardiomyopathy using digitalized echocardiography. J Am Coll Cardiol 1:541, 1983.
87. Aroney, CN, Ruddy, TD, Dighero, H, et al. Differentiation of restrictive cardiomyopathy from pericar-

dial constriction: Assessment of diastolic function by radionucleotide angiography. *J Am Coll Cardiol* 13:1007, 1989.
88. Appleton, CP, Hatle, LK, Popp, RL, et al. Demonstration of restriction ventricular physiology by Doppler echocardiography. *J Am Coll Cardiol* 11:757, 1988.
89. Shabeti, R. Profiles in Constrictive Pericarditis, Cardiac Tamponade and Restrictive Cardiomyopathy. In W Grossman (ed), *Cardiac Catheterization and Angiography*. Philadelphia: Lea & Febiger, 1974. P 304.
90. Dbestani, A, Child, JS, Henze, E, et al. Primary hemochromatosis: Anatomic and physiologic characteristics of the cardiac ventricles and their response to phlebotomy. *Am J Cardiol* 54:153, 1984.
91. Ley, TJ, Griffith, D, Niehuis, AW. Transfusion hemosiderosis and chelation therapy. *Clin Hematol* 11:437, 1982.
92. Davies, J, Sapsford, R, Brookes, I, et al. Successful treatment of two patients with eosinophilic endomyocardial disease. *Br Heart J* 46:73, 1981.
93. Clark, CE, Heary, WL, Epstein, SE. Familial prevalence and genetic transmission of idiopathic hypertrophic subaortic stenosis. *N Engl J Med* 289:709, 1973.
94. Brock, R. Functional obstruction of the left ventricle (acquired aortic subvalvular stenosis). *Guy's Hosp Rep* 106:221, 1957.
95. Teare, D. Asymmetrical hypertrophy of the heart in young adults. *Br Heart J* 20:1, 1958.
96. Roberts, WC, Ferrans, VJ. Pathologic anatomy of the cardiomyopathies. Idiopathic dilated and hypertrophic types, infiltrative types and endomyocardial disease with and without eosinophilia. *Hum Pathol* 6:287, 1975.
97. Wigle, ED, Sasson, Z, Henderson, MA, et al. Hypertrophic cardiomyopathy. The importance of the site and the extent of the hypertrophy. A review. *Prog Cardiovasc Dis* 28:1, 1985.
98. Nishimura, RA, Giuliana, ER, Brandenburg, RO. Hypertrophic cardiomyopathy. *Cardiovasc Rev Rep* 4:931, 1983.
99. Maron, BJ, Gottdiener, JS, Epstein, SE. Patterns and significance of distribution of left ventricular hypertrophy in hypertrophic cardiomyopathy: A wide angle two dimensional echocardiographic study of 125 patients. *Am J Cardiol* 48:418, 1981.
100. Spirito, P, Maron, BJ. Significance of left ventricular outflow tract cross sectional area in hypertrophic cardiomyopathy: A two-dimensional echocardiographic assessment. *Circulation* 67:1100, 1983.
101. Maron, BJ, Wolfson, JK, Epstein, SE, et al. Intramural ("small vessel") coronary artery disease in hypertrophic cardiomyopathy. *J Am Coll Cardiol* 8:545, 1986.
102. Spirito, P, Maron BJ. Patterns of systolic anterior motion of the mitral valve in hypertrophic cardiomyopathy: Assessment by two dimensional echocardiography. *Am J Cardiol* 54:1039, 1984.
103. Pollick, G, Morgan, CD, Gilbert, BW, et al. Muscular subaortic stenosis: The temporal relationship between systolic anterior motion of the anterior mitral leaflets and the pressure gradient. *Circulation* 66:1089, 1982.
104. Pollick, C, Rakowski, H, Wigle, ED. Muscular subaortic stenosis: The quantitative relationship between systolic anterior motion and the pressure gradient. *Circulation* 69:43, 1984.
105. Maron, BJ, Gottdiener, JS, Arce, J, et al. Dynamic subaortic obstruction in hypertrophic cardiomyopathy: Analysis by pulsed Doppler echocardiography. *J Am Coll Cardiol* 6:1, 1985.
106. Kinoshita, N, Nimura Y, Okamoto, M, et al. Mitral regurgitation in hypertrophic cardiomyopathy: Non-invasive study by two-dimensional Doppler echocardiography. *Br Heart J* 49:574, 1983.
107. Wigle, ED, Adelman, AG, Auger, P, et al. Mitral regurgitation in muscular subaortic stenosis. *Am J Cardiol* 24:698, 1969.
108. Gaasch, WH, Levine, HJ, Quinones, MA, et al. Left ventricular compliance: Mechanisms and clinical implications. *Am J Cardiol* 38:645, 1976.
109. Morgan, MP, Morgan, KG. Intracellular calcium levels during contraction and relaxation of mammalian cardiac and vascular smooth muscle as detected with Aequorin. *Am J Med* 77:33, 1984.
110. Sanderson, JE, Gibson, DG, Brown, DJ, Goodwin, JF. Left ventricular filling in hypertrophic cardiomyopathy: An angiographic study. *Br Heart J* 36:661, 1977.
111. Hanrath, P, Mathey, DG, Siegert, R, et al. Left ventricular relaxation and filling patterns in different forms of left ventricular hypertrophy: An echocardiographic study. *Am J Cardiol* 45:15, 1980.
112. Murgo, JP, Alter, BR, Dorethy, JF, et al. Dynamics of left ventricular ejection in obstructive and non-obstructive hypertrophic cardiomyopathy. *J Clin Invest* 66:1369, 1980.
113. Pouleur, H, Rousseau, MF, van Eyll, C, et al. Force-velocity-length relations in hypertrophy and cardiomyopathy: Evidence of normal or depressed myocardial contractility. *Am J Cardiol* 52:813, 1983.
114. Cannon, RO, Rosing, DR, Maron, BJ, et al. Myocardial ischemia in patients with hypertrophic car-

diomyopathy: Contribution of inadequate vasodilator reserve and elevated left ventricular filling pressures. *Circulation* 71:234, 1985.
115. Pasternac, A, Noble, J, Streulens, Y, et al. Pathophysiology of chest pain in patients with cardiomyopathies and normal coronary arteries. *Circulation* 65:778, 1982.
116. Fighali, S, Krajcer, Z, Edelman, S, et al. Progression of hypertrophic cardiomyopathy into a hypokinetic left ventricle. Higher incidence in patients with mid-ventricular obstruction. *J Am Coll Cardiol* 2:288, 1987.
117. tenCate, FJ, Roelandt, J. Progression to left ventricular dilatation in patients with hypertrophic obstructive cardiomyopathy. *Am Heart J* 97:762, 1979.
118. McKenna, W, Deanfield, J, Farugui, A, et al. Prognosis in hypertrophied cardiomyopathy. Role of age and clinical, electrocardiographic and hemodynamic features. *Am J Cardiol* 47:532, 1981.
119. Maron, BJ, Roberts, WC, McAllister, HA, et al. Sudden death in young athletes. *Circulation* 62:218, 1980.
120. Maron, BJ, Savage, DD, Wolfson, JR, et al. Prognostic significance of 24 hour ambulatory electrocardiographic monitoring in patients with hypertrophic cardiomyopathy. A prospective study. *Am J Cardiol* 48:252, 1981.
121. Marcus, GB, Popp, RL, Stinson, EB. Coronary artery disease with idiopathic hypertrophic subaortic stenosis. *Lancet* 1:901, 1974.
122. Canedo, MI, Frank, MJ, Abdulla, AM. Rhythm disturbances in hypertrophic cardiomyopathy. Prevalence, relation to symptoms and management. *Am J Cardiol* 45:848, 1980.
123. McKenna, WJ, Chetty, S, Oakley, CM, et al. Arrhythmia in hypertrophic cardiomyopathy. Exercise and 48-hour ambulatory electrocardiographic assessment with and without beta-adrenergic blocking therapy. *Am J Cardiol* 45:1, 1980.
124. McKenna, WJ, England, D, Doi, YL, et al. Arrhythmia in hypertrophic cardiomyopathy, I. Influence on prognosis. *Br Heart J* 46:168, 1981.
125. Maron, BM, Wolfson, JR, Ciro, E, et al. Relation of electrocardiographic abnormalities and patterns of left ventricular hypertrophy identified by two-dimensional echocardiography in patients with hypertrophic cardiomyopathy. *Am J Cardiol* 51:189, 1983.
126. Krikler, DM, Davies, MJ, Rowland, E, et al. Sudden death in hypertrophic cardiomyopathy. Associated accessory atrioventricular pathways. *Br Med J* 43:245, 1980.
127. Thompson, DS, Nagvi, N, Juul, SM, et al. Effects of propranolol on myocardial oxygen consumption. Substrate extraction and hemodynamics in hypertrophic cardiomyopathy. *Br Heart J* 44:488, 1980.
128. Speiser, KW, Krayenbuehl, HP. Reappraisal of the effect of acute beta blockade on left ventricular filling dynamics in hypertrophic obstructive cardiomyopathy. *Eur Heart J* 2:21, 1981.
129. Rosing, DR, Condit, JR, Maron, BJ, et al. Verapamil therapy. A new approach to the pharmacologic treatment of hypertrophic cardiomyopathy. III. Effects on long term administration. *Am J Cardiol* 48:545, 1981.
130. Hess, OM, Grimm, J, Krayenbuehl, HP. Diastolic function in hypertrophic cardiomyopathy. Effects of propranolol and verapamil on diastolic stiffness. *Eur Heart J* 4 (suppl F): 47, 1983.
131. Epstein, SE, Rosing, DR. Verapamil: Its potential for causing serious complications in patients with hypertrophic cardiomyopathy. *Circulation* 64:437, 1981.
132. Betocchi, S, Cannon, RO, 3rd, Watson, RM, et al. Effects of sublingual nifedipine on hemodynamics and systolic and diastolic function in patients with hypertrophic cardiomyopathy. *Circulation* 72:1001, 1985.
133. McKenna, WJ, Oakley, CM, Krinkler, DM, et al. Improved survival with amiodarone in patients with hypertrophic cardiomyopathy. *Am J Cardiol* 54:802, 1984.
134. Jackson, JM, Thomas, S. Valvular Heart Disease. In JA Kaplan (ed), *Cardiac Anesthesia*, Vol 2. Orlando, FL: Grune & Stratton, 1987. Pp 602–609.

10
Arrhythmias and Conduction Abnormalities

PIERRE A. CASTHELY
MARK J. BADACH

Cardiac arrhythmias are very common in the surgical patient and are usually of little consequence. However, they remain the leading cause of morbidity and mortality in patients with heart disease [1–3]. With the recent advancements in electrophysiologic techniques, we see an ever increasing population of patients with chronic arrhythmias or varying degrees of heart block presenting both electively and emergently for noncardiac surgery. Further complicating the issues are the various antiarrhythmic drugs, or combinations thereof, that the patient might be receiving either chronically or acutely. The anesthetic management of these patients is challenging and demands a thorough understanding of the mechanisms of both normal and abnormal electrophysiology and conduction in the heart, as well as the mechanisms of actions of the various antiarrhythmic agents.

The myocardium is, like any other muscle, made of actin, myosin, and nerve. The electrical impulse that initiates myocardial excitation and contraction coupling normally originates at regular cyclic intervals in the sinoatrial (SA) node. This impulse is conducted rapidly through the atria and enters the atrioventricular (AV) node. Conduction through the AV node requires 0.2 seconds, which allows completion of both atrial excitation and contraction before ventricular excitation. At its inferior margin, the AV node forms the AV bundle of His, which divides into the left and right bundle branches and terminates in the branches known as Purkinje fibers. Ventricular systole is coupled to this electrical activation through altered membrane permeability in contracting cells. This allows intracellular sarcoplasmic and extracellular calcium to enter the cells. Intracellular calcium then binds the inhibitory protein troponin, which allows the interaction of actin with myosin and stimulates the myosin–adenosine triphosphatase (ATPase) hydrolysis. This transformation of chemical energy to mechanical energy causes contraction to occur.

In contracting myocardial cells, the action potential (AP) is conventionally subdivided into five phases. Phase 0 is rapid depolarization and is due to a change in the permeability of the cell membrane to sodium and calcium. It is initiated when an external stimulus reduces the resting membrane potential from approximately −90 mV to a level called the threshold potential, normally about −60 mV. The AP is propagated by the flow of current into adjacent nondepolarized areas of the membrane, which lowers the local adjacent potential to threshold. The rapid entry of sodium into the cell makes the inside of the cell positive relative to the exterior. Repolarization occurs during phases 1, 2, and 3, and begins with closing of the sodium channel. This results in a brief decrease in

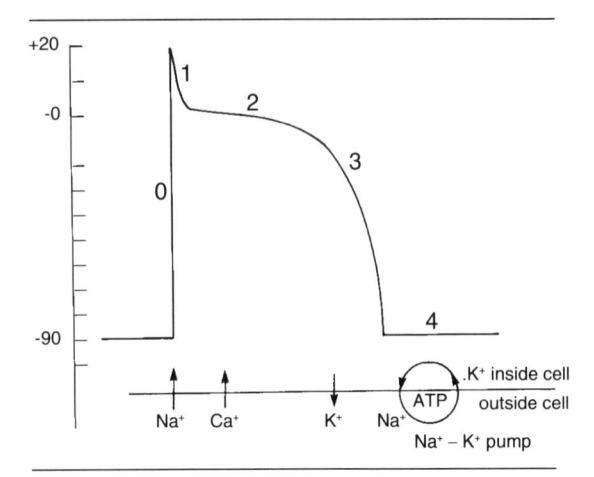

Fig. 10-1. Action potential of a typical myocardial cell.

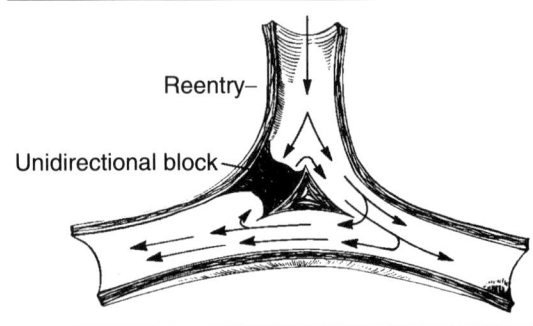

Fig. 10-2. Reentry and reflection. These mechanisms can occur when an area of unidirectional conduction block is coupled with depressed conduction.

membrane potential toward 0 mV (phase 1). During phase 2, or the plateau phase, calcium entry continues, and the cell remains depolarized and isoelectric. During phase 3, there is increased potassium permeability, resulting in potassium efflux as the membrane potential returns to its resting level of −90 mV. Before returning to −90 mV (at approximately the level of the threshold potential during phase 3), the cell can again be depolarized, but no propagated action potential will occur; this is the effective refractory period (ERP). At the end of phase 3, repolarization is complete. During phase 4, the normal ionic gradients are reestablished by the sodium-potassium pump (Fig. 10-1).

MECHANISMS OF ARRHYTHMIAS

Two major mechanisms have been proposed: abnormalities of impulse generation (automaticity) and abnormalities of impulse conduction. A combination of both has also been reported.

Impulse Generation

Arrhythmias caused by impulse generation are due to increased spontaneous phase 4 depolarization. Cells that undergo spontaneous phase 4 depolarization include: the sinus node, distal portions of the AV node, bundle of His, bundle branch His-Purkinje fibers, and specialized atrial fibers. These are, by definition, automatic and capable of impulse generation. Normal atrial or ventricular cells are incapable of impulse generation.

Impaired Conduction (Reentry)

Arrhythmias caused by conduction disturbances primarily involve the reentry mechanism. These may occur in zones of myocardial infarction, the His-Purkinje system, or the AV node. Several factors are required, as shown in Fig. 10-2, such as unidirectional block of impulse conduction in areas of injury and slow conduction via an alternate pathway. That conduction in the alternate pathway is usually slow enough to find the limb with unidirectional block repolarized and able to conduct the impulse retrograde and through the antegrade limb before an impulse from the pacemaker site. This may explain supraventricular tachyarrhythmias (atrial fibrillation and flutter), ventricular tachycardia, and premature ventricular contractions (PVCs).

CLASSIFICATION OF ANTIARRHYTHMIC AGENTS

The Vaughn-Williams classification is the one most widely used. With the introduction of the new antiarrhythmic agents, some modifications have been added (Table 10-1). There are four groups

Table 10-1. Classification of antiarrhythmic agents

Class	Effect	Drugs
IA	Local anesthetic	Quinidine, disopyramide, procainamide
IB	Local anesthetic	Lidocaine, phenytoin, tocainide, mexiletine
IC	Local anesthetic	Flecainide, encainide, lorcainide
II	β-Adrenergic blockade	Propranolol, timolol, acebutolol, esmolol
III	Prolong action potential duration and effective refractory period	Bretylium, amiodarone, N-acetylprocainamide
IV	Calcium channel blockade	Verapamil, diltiazem, lidoflazine

Table 10-2. Modified class I based on cellular electrophysiologic and clinical profiles

Class	Action	Rate of onset of block
IA	Depress phase 0 Slow conduction Prolong repolarization	Intermediate
IB	Little effect on phase 0 in normal tissue Depress phase 0 in abnormal fibers Shorten repolarization	Very fast
IC	Markedly depress phase 0 Profound slowing of conduction Slight effect on repolarization	Very slow

of antiarrhythmic agents. Group I has local anesthetic effects. Based on cellular electrophysiologic and clinical profiles, it is subdivided into three subgroups. Group IA includes quinidine, disopyramide, and procainamide. These all depress phase 0, slow conduction, and prolong repolarization. Group IB includes lidocaine, phenytoin, tocainide, and mexiletine. These shorten repolarization, increase fibrillation threshold, depress phase 0 in abnormal fibers, and have no effect on phase 0 in normal tissues. Group IC includes flecainide, encainide, and lorcainide. These markedly depress phase 0 and slow conduction, with minimal effect on repolarization. Group IB has the fastest rate of onset, followed by group IA, then group IC (Table 10-2). Group II has β-adrenergic blockade properties. Drugs in this group include propranolol, timolol, acebutolol, and esmolol. Group III prolongs action potential duration (APD) and ERP. Drugs in this group include bretylium and amiodarone. Group IV has calcium channel blockade properties, and agents include diltiazem, verapamil, and lidoflazine.

Human cardiac tissue is more specialized than is often appreciated. Consequently, antiarrhythmic agents are selective with regard to their site of action. For example, the effects of mexiletine are confined predominantly to the ventricular myocardium and the His-Purkinje system (Fig. 10-3), although modest activity on accessory pathway tissue has been reported. In contrast, encainide and flecainide affect almost all cardiac tissue, including the atrial myocardium, ventricular myocardium, AV node, and accessory pathways.

Quinidine

Quinidine is effective for both supraventricular and ventricular arrhythmias. It successfully converts atrial flutter or atrial fibrillation to sinus rhythm in about 10 to 20 percent of patients, with better success rates if the arrhythmia is of more recent onset and when the atrium is not enlarged. However, quinidine may accelerate the ventricular rate in atrial fibrillation or flutter, and should be preceded by AV nodal suppression with propranolol, digitalis, or verapamil. Quinidine, like other class IA agents, can be used for suppression of atrial and

Class IB drugs
Mexiletine

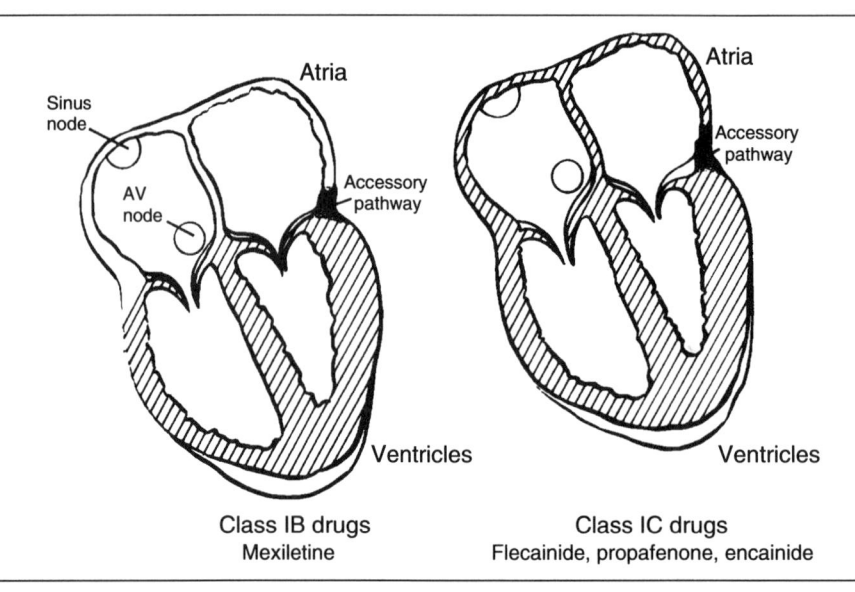

Class IC drugs
Flecainide, propafenone, encainide

Fig. 10-3. Examples of the sites of action of some antiarrhythmic drugs.

ventricular premature depolarization and sustained tachyarrhythmias.

Quinidine depresses phase 0 by blocking fast sodium channels in atrial and ventricular muscle and Purkinje fibers. Action potential amplitude and V_{max} of phase 0 are reduced more during ischemia and in partially depolarized fibers. The open channel has a high affinity for quinidine, resulting in more pronounced effects at higher rates [4, 5].

Like other class IA agents, quinidine also prolongs depolarization, resulting in prolongation of APD and ERP. By increasing the refractoriness of accessory pathways, quinidine can be used effectively to treat or prevent ventricular tachyarrhythmias in the Wolff-Parkinson-White syndrome.

α-Adrenergic blocking effects may cause significant hypotension, and this may be especially prominent in patients receiving concomitant vasodilators. This hypotensive effect is the principal limitation to intravenous administration. Myocardial contractility is maintained unless large doses are administered intravenously, in which case myocardial depression may contribute to hypotension. Oral administration is preferred, with virtually 100 percent absorption and peak serum levels in 2 hours.

Adverse side effects include a well-described interaction with digoxin [6]. Clinical digitalis toxicity occurs in 20 to 40 percent of patients receiving both agents [7]. Serum digoxin levels increase about twofold with therapeutic doses of quinidine. Individual dosing varies widely, and digitalis toxicity may occur when quinidine dosage is increased [8, 9].

Quinidine may produce syncope in 0.5 to 10.0 percent of patients during the first days of treatment. This is likely the result of a nonsustained polymorphic ventricular tachycardia of a specific variety, called "torsades de pointes" [9, 10] (Fig. 10-4).

Central nervous system (CNS) toxicity can manifest as tinnitus, hearing or visual disturbances, confusion, delirium, or psychosis. Electrocardiographic features of quinidine toxicity include conduction disturbances of varying degrees and even asystole. Prolongation of the QRS complex and QT interval, and SA node or AV node slowing, are also signs of toxicity.

Allergic thrombocytopenia is caused by antibodies to quinidine–platelet complexes; it may cause bleeding in patients receiving oral anticoagulants. Other allergic reactions include rash, fever, hemolytic anemia, and anaphylaxis.

Quinidine is primarily hydroxylated by the liver

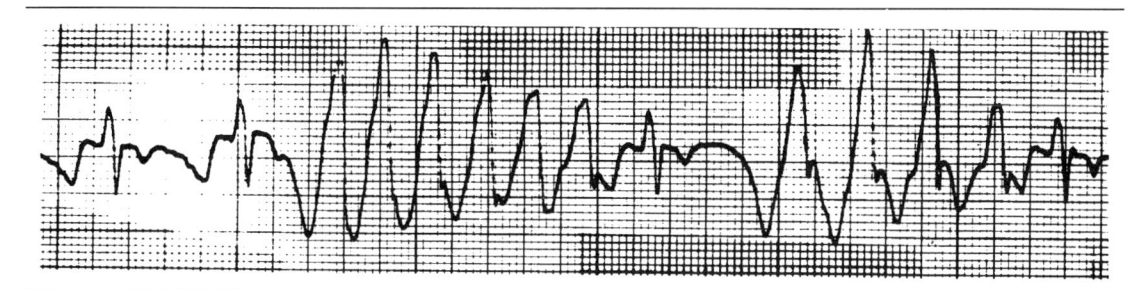

Fig. 10-4. Two brief episodes of torsades de pointes with spontaneous conversion to sinus rhythm. This nonsustained polymorphic ventricular tachycardia is a side effect of all group IA antiarrhythmic agents.

and is excreted in the urine. Drugs that induce hepatic enzymes may shorten the duration of action of quinidine.

Procainamide

Like quinidine, procainamide is effective for supraventricular and ventricular arrhythmias. Although these two drugs have similar electrophysiologic actions, either one may effectively suppress a supraventricular or ventricular arrhythmia that is refractory to the other drug. Administered intravenously, procainamide is an effective emergency treatment for ventricular arrhythmias that are unresponsive to lidocaine. Intramyocardial distribution of procainamide during ischemia is believed to be an important component of its therapeutic effect, and in a canine infarction model, higher concentrations of procainamide were present in ischemic areas [11].

Procainamide has electrophysiologic properties similar to those of quinidine, with fast channel sodium block causing a decreased V_{max} and amplitude of phase 0. An increased refractoriness and the effective refractory period to action potential duration ratio (ERP:APD) also occur. However, indirect anticholinergic effects may decrease AV nodal refractoriness (decreased ERP:APD). Both quinidine and procainamide decrease the frequency of ventricular tachycardia or fibrillation from R or T phenomenon [12]. Also, as with quinidine, indirect anticholinergic side effects may contribute to an increased ventricular response to atrial fibrillation or flutter, unless AV nodal conduction is suppressed. In high doses, procainamide may depress myocardial contractility. It may also produce peripheral vasodilatation via a mild ganglionic blocking action that impairs cardiovascular reflexes and warrants cautious administration to patients on a vasodilator.

Procainamide is metabolized by the liver and is excreted by the kidney. The metabolite, N-acetylprocainamide (NAPA) is an active compound and may also contribute to toxicity at apparently therapeutic procainamide levels in patients who have renal insufficiency.

A high incidence of adverse side effects limits chronic therapy, with 40 percent of patients requiring discontinuation within the first 6 months [13]. In almost all patients receiving chronic treatment, antinuclear antibodies develop, but this alone is not sufficient to discontinue therapy. In approximately 15 percent, signs or symptoms of a systemic lupus erythematosus (SLE)–like syndrome developed, and these patients were at risk for pleural effusions or possible lethal tamponade [14]. Symptoms usually disappear with discontinuation of the drug. The aromatic amino group on procainamide appears important for the induction of this SLE syndrome, because acetylating this amino group to form NAPA removes the SLE-inducing effect [15].

Blood counts should be performed at regular intervals because of possible agranulocytosis [16]. Ventricular tachyarrhythmias similar to those produced by quinidine can occur. Procainamide, unlike quinidine, will not elevate plasma digoxin levels. An interaction with cimetidine results in elevated plasma levels as a result of the decreased tubular secretion of procainamide [17].

Disopyramide

Disopyramide is approved in the United States only for oral administration. Like quinidine, it is effective for both supraventricular and ventricular arrhythmias, but it is more commonly utilized for the treatment of ventricular arrhythmias.

Disopyramide reduces the V_{max} of phase 0, prolongs the ERP and APD, and increases refractoriness via increasing the ERP:APD ratio. Disopyramide lengthens the conduction time in normal and depolarized Purkinje fibers and, like procainamide, reduces the disparity in APD between normal and infarcted cardiac tissue [18–20]. Disopyramide can increase SA node discharge rate and AV node conduction when these nodes are under cholinergic influences due to its vagolytic effects.

Intravenous disopyramide can cause profound hemodynamic deterioration from its negative inotropic effects and reflex increase in systemic vascular resistance (SVR) [21]. In patients with normal myocardial function, cardiac output (CO) usually decreases 10 to 15 percent. Half of the patients with a history of congestive heart failure (CHF) may have a recurrence of symptoms [21]. Therefore, disopyramide is contraindicated in patients with poor ventricular function and signs of pulmonary edema and CHF.

Most commonly, disopyramide produces dose-related anticholinergic side effects and should be avoided in patients with obstructive uropathy or closed-angle glaucoma. Anticholinergic symptoms may be minimized by concomitant administration of anticholinesterase agents [22].

Lidocaine

Lidocaine is useful for the acute treatment of ventricular arrhythmias of almost all types except those precipitated by an abnormally long QT interval. Lidocaine is also indicated for the treatment of PVCs that occur more frequently than five per minute, are closely coupled to the T wave, are multiform, or are grouped together [23]. The use of lidocaine for prophylaxis against ventricular arrhythmias in patients with acute myocardial infarction (MI) is controversial. Several studies have shown a decreased incidence of post-MI arrhythmias, whereas other investigators have not.

Lidocaine exerts its antiarrhythmic effect by decreasing the slope of phase 4 diastolic depolarization in Purkinje fibers. Lidocaine has no electrophysiologic effect on or above the AV node. Conduction velocity is not affected by lidocaine in normal tissue, but is significantly decreased in ischemic tissue [24]. The effects of lidocaine on APD and ERP vary by location. In ventricular muscle and Purkinje fibers, lidocaine significantly reduces the APD and ERP by blockage of the fast (tetrodotoxin-sensitive) sodium channels and consequently decreases entry of sodium into the cell (see Fig. 10-1). It has been suggested that intracellular calcium is also reduced because of the sodium-calcium exchange mechanism [25]. It has little, if any, effect on atrial fibers or accessory pathways and, unless preexisting SA node disease is present, lidocaine will not affect SA node activity. Due to the absence of supraventricular activity, lidocaine is only indicated in ventricular ectopy.

Adverse hemodynamic changes are rare unless left ventricular function is severely impaired. The most commonly reported adverse effects of lidocaine are dose-related manifestations of CNS toxicity, including dizziness, paresthesia, confusion, delirium, stupor, comas, and seizures. Therapeutic plasma concentration ranges from 1.5 to 5.0 μg/ml. Lidocaine undergoes extensive first-pass metabolism in the liver. The rate of clearance is extremely sensitive to altered hepatic blood flow. Clearance is markedly decreased in patients with liver disease or CHF, and in the elderly.

Phenytoin

Phenytoin's value as an antiarrhythmic agent is limited to atrial and ventricular arrhythmias caused by digitalis toxicity. Phenytoin is effective in abolishing the delayed afterpotentials responsible for automatic arrhythmias induced by digitalis preparations [26–28]. It is not effective in treating ventricular arrhythmias in patients with ischemic heart disease.

Intravenous phenytoin produces decreased left ventricular contractility and a corresponding increase in left ventricular end diastolic pressure (LVEDP) [29]. These potentially adverse acute hemodynamic effects are related to the rate of administration. Rates over 50 mg per minute are reported to result in cardiovascular collapse [29]. To achieve therapeutic plasma concentrations rapidly, 100 mg phenytoin should be given intravenously every 5 minutes.

Phenytoin toxicity most commonly causes CNS signs (nystagmus, nausea, vertigo, ataxia, and cerebellar dysfunction), and sometimes hypotension and respiratory arrest [30]. Other side effects (with chronic use) include gingival hyperplasia, megaloblastic anemia, hirsutism, hyperglycemia, and hypoglycemia. Thrombophlebitis, due to acidity of the parenteral preparation, may occur and can be minimized via administration into a central intravenous line. Chronic administration is not routinely utilized for control of arrhythmias.

Amiodarone

Amiodarone has been used to suppress a wide spectrum of supraventricular and ventricular tachyarrhythmias [31–35], and its efficacy exceeds or equals that of all other antiarrhythmic agents. However, because of its extremely long and variable half-life (13–103 days) and multiple adverse side effects, the use of amiodarone is very limited. Amiodarone should be among the last antiarrhythmic agents to be tried and is approved only for hemodynamically unstable ventricular arrhythmias (ventricular fibrillation or ventricular tachycardia) that are refractory to other agents or when these agents were not tolerated.

Like other class III agents, amiodarone blocks potassium channels and therefore prolongs repolarization during phase 3 of the action potential. Amiodarone, administered in usual doses (2.5–10.0 mg/kg), decreases left ventricular contractility (dp/dt), heart rate, and SVR.

The metabolism of amiodarone is predominantly through the liver. The drug exhibits alpha- and beta-receptor antagonism. It is highly protein bound. The full effects of the drug necessitate several weeks of use because of the prolonged loading period needed to achieve tissue concentrations. After cessation of amiodarone therapy, antiarrhythmic action may persist from 30 to 45 days [32, 36].

Adverse effects occur in about 75 percent of patients treated orally with 400 mg per day and require discontinuation of treatment in 4 to 20 percent of patients [37, 38]. Of the noncardiac adverse reactions, diffuse pulmonary fibrosis is the most serious, with a reported mortality up to 10 percent. The initial pulmonary inflammation can occur within 2 weeks, with a mean onset of 8 months [39], and usually is seen within the first 30 months of treatment. The mechanism is unclear but may relate to a hypersensitivity reaction or widespread phospholipidosis [40]. Chest roentgenograms every 3 months are recommended. Clinically, this pulmonary inflammatory complication may mimic deteriorating heart disease or pneumonia. Signs of dyspnea, nonproductive cough, fever, and pulmonary infiltrates on a chest x-ray are suggestive. Amiodarone must be discontinued if such changes develop.

Other noted side effects include dermal and corneal accumulation, resulting in a photosensitive dermatitis (20%) and corneal microdeposits (98%), respectively. Thyroid toxicity with either hyperthyroidism with elevated T_3 (1–2%) or hypothyroidism (1–5%) may occur. Other side effects include nausea, anorexia, tremor, ataxia, neuropathy, headaches, and hepatotoxicity.

Amiodarone binds cytochrome P450 hepatic enzymes and thus alters the metabolism of several drugs. There are increased plasma concentrations of antiarrhythmic drugs of groups IA, IB, IC, II, and III. Warfarin, digoxin, β-blockers, and calcium channel blockers also require reduced dosages and must be given cautiously [32]. Torsades de pointes, heart block, and atropine-resistant bradycardia have been reported when amiodarone is used in combination with class I antiarrhythmic agents [41].

Bretylium

Bretylium has been effective in treating patients with drug-resistant tachyarrhythmias [42–44]. It is recommended only for parenteral use in critically ill patients with life-threatening ventricular tachyarrhythmias that have not responded to other agents. Like lidocaine, it is also useful in treating out-of-hospital ventricular fibrillation [43–46].

Bretylium's mode of action is believed to be triphasic. After initially releasing norepinephrine, it prevents norepinephrine release from sympathetic nerve terminals. Initial catecholamine release may worsen some arrhythmias, such as those caused by digitalis excess or MI. The subsequent chemical sympathectomy results in prolongation of APD and ERP of atrial and ventricular muscle and Purkinje fibers. Bretylium significantly increases the ventricular fibrillation threshold [39]. Reduced disparity between APD and ERP in regions of normal and infarcted myocardium [47, 48], as well as its sympatholytic action, may account for some of its antifibrillatory effects.

During chronic bretylium maintenance, the sensitivity of β-adrenergic receptors to circulating catecholamines is increased. There are no vagal effects and no alteration in the sensitivity of cholinergic receptors.

Bretylium is not a myocardial depressant and initially may cause transient hypertension and an increase in heart rate. Significant hypotension may follow by blocking the efferent limb of the baroreceptor reflex; the vasoconstrictive reflexes are diminished, and orthostatic hypotension is common, although the supine patient may also become hypotensive.

This potential hypotension is the most significant side effect, and vasodilators may enhance this effect. Orthostatic hypotension may persist for several days after drug discontinuation.

β-Blockers

Only propranolol, metoprolol, acebutolol, esmolol, and timolol are approved for treating arrhythmias. At β-blocking concentration, propranolol slows spontaneous automaticity in the sinus node and Purkinje fibers that are being stimulated by adrenergic tone, but lacks this effect in the absence of adrenergic tone. Propranolol slows the sinus discharge rate in humans by 10 to 20 percent, while severe bradycardia can result if the heart is particularly dependent on sympathetic tone or if sinus node dysfunction is present. In high doses, β-blockers depress the fast sodium current and have quinidine-like actions, commonly referred to as "membrane-stabilizing" properties. However, this effect most likely plays only a minor antiarrhythmic role. In therapeutic concentrations, β-blockers do not alter resting membrane potentials, action potential, or refractoriness of atrial, Purkinje, or ventricular cells, when these tissues are not being perfused with catecholamines. However, in the presence of catecholamines, propranolol slows depolarization and can prolong the action potential in Purkinje fibers. It reduces the amplitude of digitalis-induced delayed afterpotentials and suppresses triggered activity in the Purkinje fibers [49].

The PR interval and AV nodal conduction time lengthen, but conduction in the normal His-Purkinje system remains unchanged even after high doses of propranolol. β-Blockers do not affect conduction in ventricular muscles, as evidenced by their lack of effect on the QRS complex, and they also insignificantly prolong the right ventricular effective refractory period.

β-Blockers depress cardiac contractility and may precipitate or worsen heart failure. By blocking beta receptors, an unopposed peripheral vasoconstriction may produce hypertension.

Other untoward effects include excessive slowing of heart rate and bronchospasm. Esmolol, the newest agent in this class, has recently been approved for use. Unlike propranolol, esmolol is $β_1$-selective. Another advantage is its rapid onset of action, which can also be terminated within minutes. It is metabolized by red blood cell esterases and is relatively safe in patients with both renal and hepatic failure. With a half-life of 9 minutes, esmolol infusions are currently finding widespread intraoperative use. Brief intraoperative suppression of the sympathetic response to a stimulus such as laryngoscopy or surgical incision is another area in which this agent is finding application.

Verapamil

The levorotatory stereoisomer of verapamil blocks the slow inward current carried by calcium, resulting in a reduced plateau height (phase 2) and duration of the Purkinje fiber action potential [50]. There is no effect on velocity, amplitude of sodium influx (phase 0), or resting membrane voltages in atrial and ventricular muscle, and no effect on the His-Purkinje system. Verapamil is the treatment of choice for several reentry-dependent supraventricular tachyarrhythmias. It terminates 60 to 80 percent of episodes of paroxysmal supraventricular tachycardia within several minutes [51–53].

Verapamil decreases the ventricular response (via the AV node) in the presence of atrial fibrillation or atrial flutter, particularly if the atrial flutter or fibrillation is of recent onset. Quinidine appears to be more effective than verapamil in establishing and maintaining sinus rhythm in patients with chronic atrial fibrillation. Data from animal models suggest that verapamil may be useful in preventing ventricular arrhythmias due to acute myocardial ischemia. In atrial fibrillation with Wolff-Parkinson-White (WPW) syndrome, verapamil may accelerate the ventricular response (by blocking normal but not accessory pathways), and therefore is contraindicated [51–55]. Cardiovascular collapse may occur if intravenous verapamil is given to patients with ventricular tachycardia. Therefore, a general rule of thumb is not to give intravenous verapamil to any patients with wide QRS tachycardia.

Verapamil, by blocking slow calcium channels, lowers intracellular calcium. This results in marked vasodilatation of coronary and peripheral vascular beds. Despite a direct depressant effect on SA node depolarization, the sinus rate usually does not change significantly in vivo, because verapamil's peripheral vasodilatation causes reflex sympathetic stimulation that maintains heart rate.

In patients with good left ventricular function, combined therapy with propranolol and verapamil appears to be well tolerated [56]. However, hypotension, bradycardia, AV block, and asystole are more likely to occur when verapamil is given to patients who are already receiving β-blocking agents [57]. Isoproterenol may be effective for treating bradyarrhythmias and calcium for treating hemodynamic compromise caused by this combination.

Adenosine

Adenosine is an endogenous nucleoside that occurs in all cells of the body. It slows conduction time through the AV node, can interrupt the reentry pathways through the AV node, and restores normal sinus rhythm in patients with paroxysmal supraventricular tachycardia. It does not work in atrial flutter, atrial fibrillation, or ventricular tachycardia. It has a very short half-life (10 seconds). The initial dose is 6 mg intravenous bolus over 2 seconds, which can be repeated 2 minutes later. Doses greater than 12 mg are usually needed. At the time of conversion to normal sinus rhythm, a variety of new rhythms may appear on the electrocardiogram. They generally last only a few seconds. These rhythms include PVCs, atrial premature contractions, sinus bradycardia, sinus tachycardia, and varying degrees of AV nodal block.

Intravenous adenosine is absolutely contraindicated in second- or third-degree AV block or sick sinus syndrome if the patient does not have a pacemaker.

ARRHYTHMIAS

Most arrhythmias that occur during anesthesia are supraventricular. They include premature atrial contraction, bradyarrhythmias, and junctional rhythms. In a study done by Kuner [58] in 154 patients undergoing anesthesia, junctional rhythms were most commonly followed by a wandering atrial pacemaker. The causes of arrhythmias are multifactorial and include the trauma of surgery, endogenous and exogenous catecholamines, drugs, hypoxia, electrolyte and acid-base abnormalities, and the underlying cardiac disease.

Intraoperative Causes of Arrhythmias

Anesthetic Agents
Halogenated hydrocarbons such as halothane or enflurane have been shown to produce dysrhythmias, probably by a reentrant mechanism [59]. In addition, these agents, especially halothane, have been shown to sensitize the myocardium to both endogenous and exogenous catecholamines. Other anesthetics such as cocaine and ketamine, which block the re-uptake of norepinephrine, can facilitate the development of epinephrine-induced dysrhythmias [60].

Abnormal Arterial Blood Gases or Electrolytes
Alterations of blood gases or electrolytes may lead to dysrhythmias, either by producing reentrant mechanisms or by altering phase 4 depolarization of conduction fibers.

Endotracheal Intubation
This may be the most common cause of arrhythmias during surgery. These arrhythmias are occasionally associated with severe hypertension [61].

Table 10-3. Common arrhythmias in surgical patients

Bradyarrhythmias
Sinus tachycardia
Supraventricular dysrhythmias
Premature ventricular contractions
Ventricular tachycardia
Heart block

Reflexes
Vagal stimulation may produce sinus bradycardias and permit ventricular escape mechanisms to occur. In addition, specific reflexes such as the oculocardiac reflex can produce severe rhythm disturbances during surgery [62].

Central Nervous System Stimulation
Many ECG abnormalities have been reported with intracranial pathology, especially subarachnoid hemorrhage, including changes in QT intervals, development of Q waves, ST segment changes, and the occurrence of U waves [63]. The mechanism of these arrhythmias appears to be changes in the autonomic nervous system.

Location of Surgery
Dental surgery is often associated with arrhythmias, since profound stimulation of both the sympathetic and parasympathetic nervous systems often occurs [64]. Junctional rhythms commonly are seen and may be due to stimulation of the autonomic nervous system via the fifth cranial nerve.

Insertion of Catheters or Wires in the Heart
Arrhythmias may be induced by the placement of a pulmonary artery catheter, often leading to PVCs.

Predisposing factors include recent MI, severe myocardial ischemia, and poor ventricular function [65]. The most common arrhythmias are enumerated in Table 10-3.

Bradyarrhythmias

Many factors predispose to bradyarrhythmias during anesthesia. They are illustrated in Table 10-4. The combination of anesthetic agents, vagal responses, and hypothermia is well known to produce bradycardia. All inhalation anesthetics depress sinus node activity (see Chap. 2). They slow the response of the sinus node by altering the slope of phase 4 depolarization, resulting in bradycardia. There appears to be a relationship between the effects of anesthetic agents and calcium flux [66].

Bradycardia may be a manifestation of sick sinus syndrome. Sick sinus syndrome is due to the inability of the sinus node to initiate impulses or conduct them out of the sinus node to the atrium. Symptomatic patients with prolonged sinus arrest or extreme bradycardia may require insertion of a temporary pacemaker. This syndrome may be accentuated after a stellate ganglionic blockade [67].

Narcotics used during general anesthesia, such as morphine sulfate, fentanyl, and sufentanil, may produce bradycardia, as a result of the direct action on the sinus node [68] (see Chap. 3). Among the other drugs used during anesthesia, muscle relaxants such as succinylcholine, d-tubocurare, and anticholinesterase agents (neostigmine, physostigmine, and edrophonium) can cause bradyarrhythmias. Another cause of bradycardia is hypothermia. Sympathetic outflow may also be blocked by drugs such as propranolol or by a regional anesthetic

Table 10-4. Factors that cause sinus bradycardia under anesthesia

Intrinsic to the patient
   Sick sinus syndrome
   Increased intracranial pressure
   Nonanesthetic drug related (i.e., propranolol, digoxin)
Vagal responses
   Reflex stimulation of nasopharynx, lateral rectus, bronchus, peritoneum, oculocardiac, etc.
   Acetylcholine-related drugs such as muscle relaxants (succinylcholine), neostigmine
Direct anesthetic agent related
   Inhalational (halothane, enflurane, isoflurane)
   Narcotic (fentanyl, sufentanil, morphine)

technique (spinal or epidural anesthesia), again causing bradycardia. An early manifestation of hypoxia in children is usually bradycardia. In adults, it is frequently overshadowed by the tachycardia produced by the increase in sympathetic outflow that follows any hypoxic episode.

With normal sinus rhythm, the atrial contribution to CO is 15 percent. However, in a patient with severe ischemic heart disease, aortic stenosis, or severe hypertension, it may account for as much as 40 percent of CO [69, 70]. In these patients loss of the "atrial kick" caused by a junctional bradyarrhythmia may result in hemodynamic collapse. The indications for treatment of bradycardia, which depend on the clinical setting, include hypotension, CHF, and signs of decreased cardiac output. Most of the bradycardias respond to the administration of atropine, isoproterenol, or transvenous cardiac pacing.

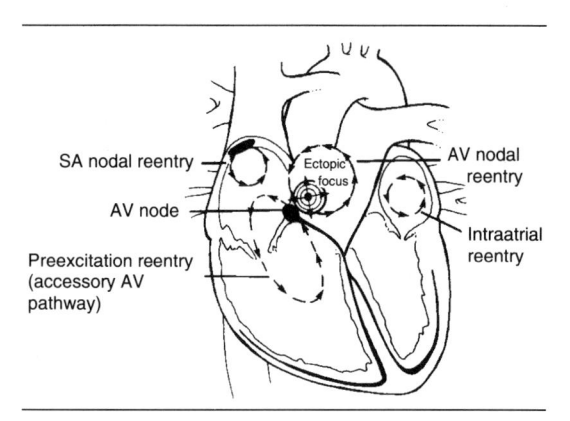

Fig. 10-5. Four anatomic reentry locations involved in paroxysmal supraventricular tachycardia. They include the SA and AV nodes, atrial muscle, and accessory AV pathways.

Sick Sinus Syndrome

Sick sinus syndrome is defined by severe sinus bradycardia and by sinus pause or arrest with escape. It frequently leads to atrial fibrillation. Most patients with sick sinus syndrome are elderly and have coronary artery disease. It can produce syncope and require permanent pacemaker implantation.

Sick sinus syndrome is an important condition for anesthesiologists to recognize. Elderly patients with sinus bradycardia or unexplained syncope, or both, must be fully evaluated before surgery is undertaken. If a sudden intraoperative long sinus pause or sinus arrest is noted, a pacemaker should be inserted. Advanced age, heart disease, and anesthetics may interact to produce this syndrome in the operating room.

Sinus Tachycardia

Sinus tachycardia is usually due to fever, hypoxia, hypovolemia, light anesthesia, and exogenous catecholamines. Sources of exogenously administered catecholamines include vasopressor infusions, use of local anesthetics with epinephrine, and topical cocaine with systemic absorption. It increases the oxygen demand of the heart and may precipitate myocardial ischemia. After the underlying cause is treated, small doses of propranolol or esmolol may be required to decrease the heart rate.

Supraventricular Tachycardia

Supraventricular tachycardia is commonly seen following surgery. A supraventricular arrhythmia with aberrant conduction may closely resemble ventricular tachycardia, and the nature of any tachycardia following surgery must be determined as soon as possible. Paroxysmal atrial tachycardia (PAT) is the common term for paroxysmal supraventricular tachycardias (PSVTs) originating in the atrium and AV junction (rate of 100–240 bpm). It is due to AV node reentry 58 percent of the time, atrial tachycardia 8 percent of the time, SA node reentry 4 percent of the time, and accessory AV connections 30 percent of the time (Fig. 10-5). When PAT converts to normal sinus rhythm, it does so suddenly. In nonhypotensive patients maneuvers to slow the ventricular rate can be tried. These include massage of the carotid sinus, application of pressure to the eyeball, and the Valsalva maneuver. If there is no response, these patients require prompt administration of β-blockers, calcium channel blockers, or adenosine. Edrophonium chloride (10 mg intravenously in adults) and digitalis may also slow the ventricular response to supraventricular tachycardia. Hypoten-

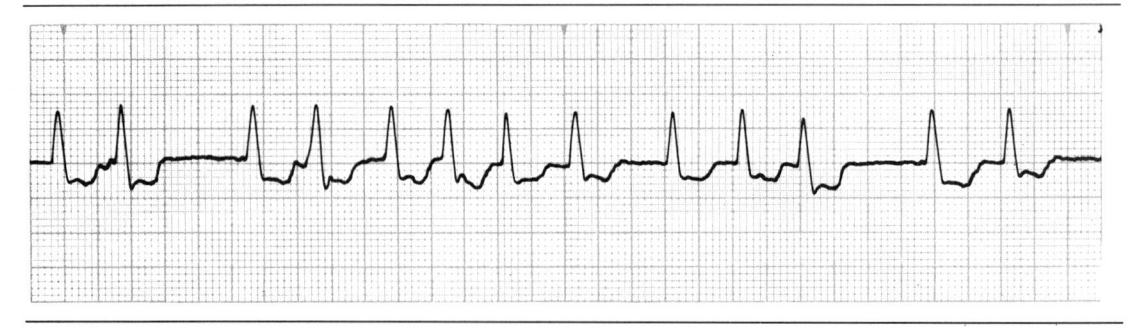

Fig. 10-6. Atrial fibrillation in a patient during general anesthesia.

sive patients should be treated by direct-current (DC) cardioversion.

Atrial Fibrillation

The occurrence of atrial fibrillation frequency results in decreased cardiac output and is detrimental to the surgical patient. When rapid atrial fibrillation is accompanied by hypotension, cardioversion is immediately indicated (Fig. 10-6). Premature ventricular contractions in the presence of atrial fibrillation should be a warning of possible digitalis toxicity.

β-Adrenergic blocking drugs are effective in the treatment of atrial fibrillation and supraventricular tachyarrhythmias (SVT). They prolong the conduction time through the AV node, thereby reducing the ventricular rate and improving ventricular function. The occurrence of SVT or atrial fibrillation in patients with underlying coronary artery disease may have serious consequences as a result of the rapid heart rate increasing the myocardial oxygen demand. Although β-blockers are beneficial in this setting, the relatively long duration of the older drugs limits their use during acute situations. However, esmolol may prove useful because of its unique pharmacokinetic profile. The efficacy and safety of esmolol in patients with SVT, atrial fibrillation, atrial flutter, and sinus tachycardia have been demonstrated in clinical studies. When the efficacy of esmolol was compared with that of intravenous verapamil in patients with either recent-onset or previous-onset atrial fibrillation or flutter [71] the mean reduction of heart rate with esmolol and verapamil was 24 and 31 percent, respectively. Hypotension occurred with equal frequency in both groups, but was more readily controllable in the patients treated with esmolol than in those treated with intermittent doses of verapamil (5–10 mg). Discontinuing or lowering the esmolol infusion caused the hypotension to resolve within 5 to 20 minutes.

Verapamil can also slow the ventricular response to atrial fibrillation and frequently converts paroxysmal supraventricular tachycardia or atrial flutter to a sinus rhythm. Intravenous bolus therapy of verapamil may result in hypotension that may be prevented by the slow administration of verapamil or by pretreatment with an intravenous dose of calcium. Calcium therapy reverses the hemodynamic effects of verapamil, but does not reverse the electrophysiologic effects. Frequently, a 30 percent reduction in the ventricular rate can be achieved with the initial dose of verapamil, but maximal clinical effects last only 30 to 45 minutes. To maintain this reduction of the heart rate, intravenous digoxin is necessary after rate reduction with verapamil. However, digoxin is not as effective as verapamil and may lack effectiveness in rate control during the stress of the perioperative period.

Since esmolol and verapamil have been shown to be equally effective in patients with atrial fibrillation or flutter, and because of the obvious advantage of the short duration of action of esmolol, it appears to be safer as the first-line drug. The other major advantage seems to be the higher conversion rate of atrial fibrillation to normal sinus rhythm during titration. In one study, 36 percent of the esmolol-treated patients were found to convert to normal sinus rhythm, versus only 12 percent with verapamil [71].

Digoxin has a slower onset of action than verapamil but is more useful for chronic treatment. One half of a digitalizing dose can be safely given over 5 minutes, with two additional doses of one quarter the digitalizing dose each administered over the next 2 to 3 hours. Additional doses can be based on the ventricular response.

Patients who are successfully electrically cardioverted usually have atrial fibrillation of less than one year's duration, a left atrial dimension of less than 45 mm by echocardiography, and no ventricular enlargement, and have had prior successful treatment of the precipitating factor. Anticoagulation should be considered before cardioversion in patients who remain in atrial fibrillation longer than 4 to 5 days and anticoagulation should be maintained for several weeks after establishment of sinus rhythm.

The anesthetic management of patients with atrial fibrillation begins with adequate digitalization preoperatively. This can be evaluated by noting the presence of a resting ventricular rate of 60 to 80 beats per minute that does not increase unduly with mild exercise. Preoperative correction of any diuretic-induced potassium deficit is important because hypokalemia potentiates digitalis toxicity. Patients with atrial fibrillation may have mitral valve disease associated with pulmonary hypertension. In those patients, the use of anesthetic agents that increase sympathetic stimulation, such as nitrous oxide or ketamine, may further increase pulmonary hypertension and should be avoided. Excess sympathetic activity can cause increased AV conduction of atrial impulses and a rapid ventricular rate.

Atrial Flutter

Atrial flutter is much less common than atrial fibrillation but shares the same predisposing factors. Atrial flutter is categorized into two types, I and II. In type I atrial flutter, there is a 2:1 AV block with a rate of 300 beats per minute and a ventricular rate of 150 beats per minute. The flutter waves are of a typical saw-tooth or biphasic appearance and are most commonly seen in leads II, III, aVF, and V_1 (Fig. 10-7). Type II atrial flutter exhibits a flat baseline, with positive flutter waves in the inferior leads and a rate usually greater than 350 beats per min-

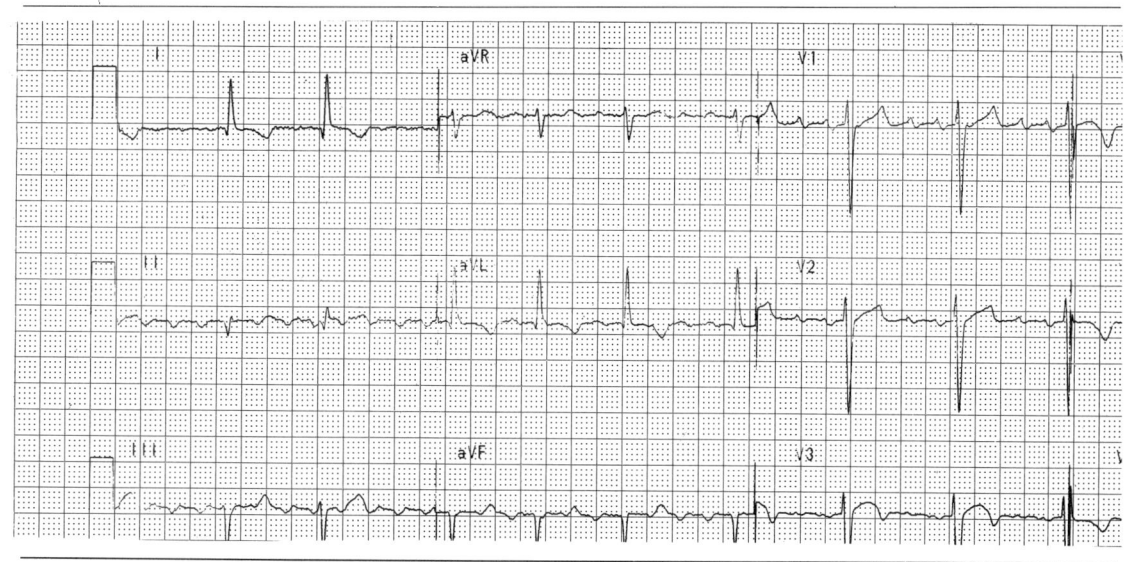

Fig. 10-7. Electrocardiogram showing atrial flutter with a variable block. Note the rapid atrial rate and saw-tooth appearance, usually obvious in V_1–V_2, II, III, and aVF. It is useful to remember that atrial flutter indicates structural heart disease, unlike atrial fibrillation, which could be present in normal hearts. Notice the ST-T changes indicating ischemia or injury.

ute. Atrial flutter is seen in patients with underlying heart disease such as rheumatic heart disease with enlarged atria; it is not commonly a manifestation of digitalis toxicity. The degree of block may vary and can change quite rapidly. One of the common problems associated with atrial flutter is that some drugs that are used for treatment of supraventricular dysrhythmias, such as quinidine, may be contraindicated early in the course of this condition. The reason is that the vagolytic action of these drugs will actually increase ventricular rate before converting the rhythm. This may lower CO unless the patient is treated with digitalis first. The treatment of choice for atrial flutter is cardioversion at low energy levels (10–25 joules) or rapid atrial pacing (overdrive suppression). As with PAT, atrial flutter can be successfully treated with verapamil, digoxin, or β-blockers.

Compared to fibrillation, atrial flutter is usually more difficult to treat. However, rapid atrial pacing in type I atrial flutter is effective, while type II atrial flutter frequently cannot be converted by rapid atrial pacing. Atrial pacing should proceed at a rate approximately 20 percent faster than the flutter rate. During rapid atrial pacing, a change in the morphology of the flutter pattern or a change in the ventricular response is a sign of overdrive suppression. In addition, a critical duration of rapid atrial pacing is required to convert atrial flutter. After interruption of atrial flutter, pacing should continue for approximately 30 seconds; pacing for shorter amounts of time may not be successful. Since atrial pacing thresholds are usually higher in atrial flutter and determination of capture is difficult, the maximum current (usually 20 amps on temporary pacemakers) is necessary for overdrive suppression. If suppression does not occur, it is usually because of inadequate rate, pacing duration, or current threshold.

Multifocal Atrial Tachycardia

Multifocal atrial tachycardia (MAT) is an arrhythmia that usually occurs in the seriously ill patient with chronic obstructive pulmonary disease (COPD). In most cases the ventricular rate is between 100 and 150 beats per minute. Aberrant ventricular conduction may also occur. Theophylline infusion is associated with this arrhythmia [72, 73]. Most of the patients go on to develop atrial flutter or fibrillation. Treating the underlying disease (COPD) is imperative. Correction and discontinuation of digoxin and theophylline will aid in the management of the arrhythmia. Recently, verapamil has been found to decrease the atrial and ventricular rates and to convert this arrhythmia to sinus rhythm in some patients [74].

Accelerated Junctional Rhythm

Accelerated junctional rhythm is an arrhythmia that is commonly seen during anesthesia with inhalational agents and a muscle relaxant such as pancuronium. It results from selective inhibition of sinus node automaticity by the inhalation anesthetic combined with an increase in atrioventricular junctional automaticity due to sympathetic stimulation [75]. It may respond to small doses of β-blockers. This arrhythmia may also be due to digitalis intoxication.

Wolff-Parkinson-White Syndrome

The WPW syndrome and its variants are grouped as the preexcitation syndrome, which consists of preexcitation via an accessory pathway. It is characterized by a short PR interval, bundle branch block, paroxysmal tachycardia, and the accessary bundle of Kent (Fig. 10-8). The initial slurring of the QRS complex is known as the "delta wave."

There are two other variants of this syndrome. The Lown-Ganong-Levine (LGL) syndrome is characterized by a short PR interval and normal QRS complex. Anatomically, the pathway of James bypasses the AV node and goes directly from the atrium to the bundle of His, producing the short PR interval but a normal QRS complex. The second variant is characterized by a normal PR interval and a delta wave and is associated with Mahaim fibers, arising just below the AV node and bypassing the Purkinje system (Fig. 10-8).

In 1975, Anderson and coworkers [76], representing the European study group for preexcitation, classified these syndromes into four basic anatomic subgroups: accessory atrioventricular connections, nodoventricular connections, fasciculoventricular connections, and AV nodal bypass tracts of three types: atrio-hisian bypass tract, intranodal bypass

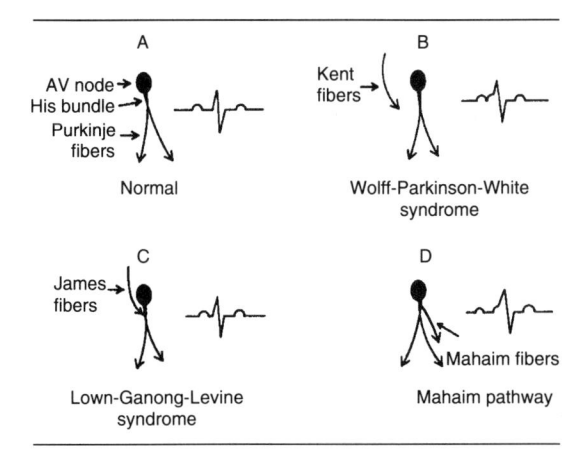

Fig. 10-8. Schematic diagram of the three most common anomalous conduction pathways associated with WPW syndrome.

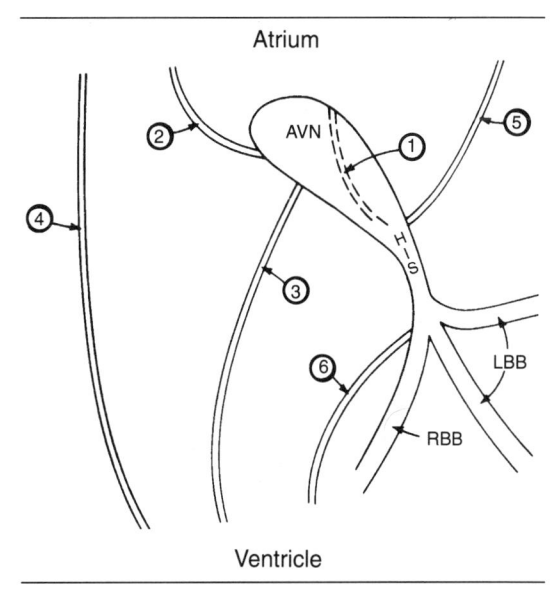

Fig. 10-9. Basic anatomic subgroups of accessory tracts in WPW syndrome. (1) Intranodal bypass tract; (2) posterior internodal tract; (3) nodoventricular bypass tract; (4) atrioventricular bypass tract; (5) atriohisian bypass tract; (6) fasciculoventricular bypass tract. AVN = atrioventricular node; RBB = right bundle branch; LBB = left bundle branch. (Reprinted with permission from ME Josephson, SF Seides, *Clinical Cardiac Electrophysiology*. Philadelphia: Lea & Febiger, 1979.)

tract, and posterior internodal tract. The relationships among these subgroups are demonstrated graphically in Fig. 10-9.

Arrhythmias, most commonly reentrant supraventricular, occur in 40 to 80 percent of patients with WPW syndrome [77]. The most common reentrant supraventricular tachycardia results from antegrade conduction across the normal conduction system, with retrograde conduction utilizing the accessory pathway [78, 79]. The reentrant loop may be established during ventricular stimulation if retrograde block occurs in the specialized conduction system, as is usually the case [80] (Figs. 10-10, 10-11).

Atrial fibrillation is also associated with the WPW syndrome, with a frequency ranging between 11.5 and 39.0 percent of cases [81–83]. The precise mechanism for this propensity to atrial fibrillation is unclear, but several possibilities have been suggested. The occurrence of supraventricular tachycardia at a higher than usual rate in patients with WPW syndrome may create electrical instability, which facilitates atrial fibrillation [84]. It may be a statistical occurrence whereby patients with atrial disease are prone to atrial premature depolarization (APD) and to atrial fibrillation, but the increased frequency of APDs may make these patients more likely to present with SVT and to thereby be recognized as having WPW syndrome. Other possibilities include the active role of the accessory pathway in promoting electrical instability by causing multiple atrial echoes via antegrade conduction, or a passive role in which the accessory pathway transmits the electronic effect of ventricular systole to the atrium, thereby promoting disparity of refractoriness and electrical instability. Because of the very fast conduction velocity and short refractory period of the accessory pathway, atrial fibrillation or atrial flutter may result in extremely fast ventricular rates (>300 bpm), which can lead to sudden death. These patients should have ablation of their bypass tracts. In patients with slower ventricular rates, whether the underlying rhythm is atrial flutter or PSVT, pharmacologic therapy is frequently sufficient.

If the QRS complex is wide, demonstrating preexcitation, intravenous procainamide or lidocaine is the drug of choice for the tachycardia [75, 85]. Intravenous verapamil and digoxin have been shown to increase the tachycardia rate in some pa-

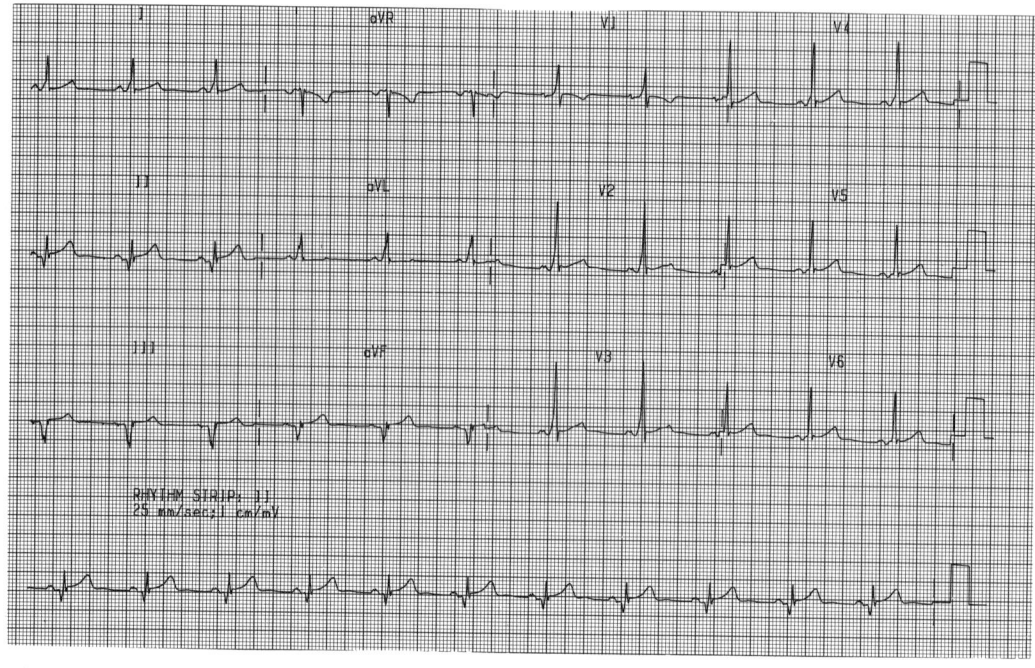

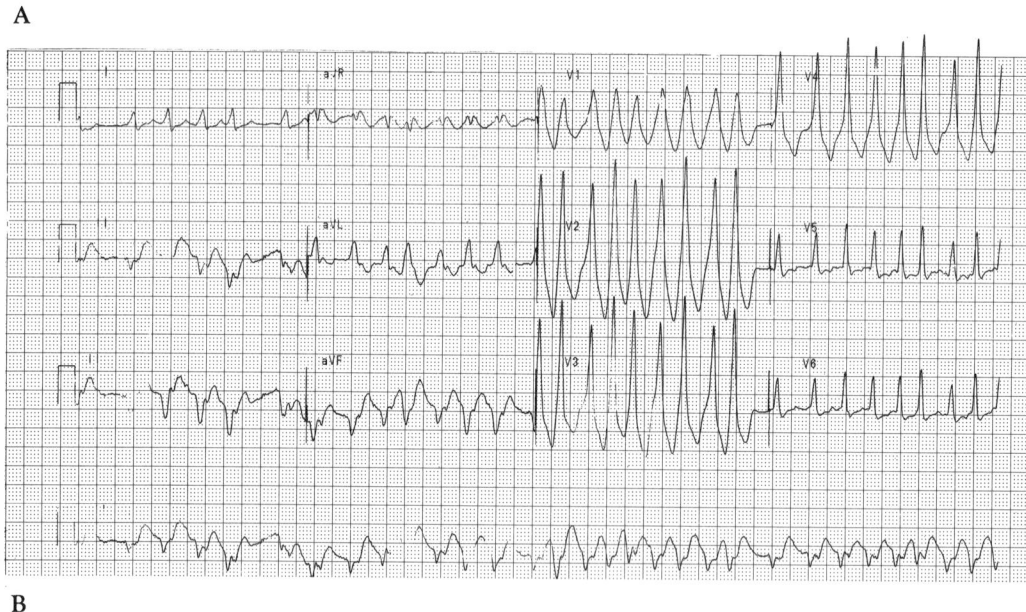

Fig. 10-10. A. Electrocardiogram from a patient with WPW syndrome during sinus rhythm. Note the short PR interval, wide QRS complex with the initial slurred delta wave indicating preexcitation of the ventricle via the bypass tract, and the Q waves in leads II, III, and aVF, which could be mistaken as inferior wall myocardial infarction (IWMI). B. Electrocardiogram of the same patient during atrial fibrillation indicating conduction antegradely over a bypass tract. Note the irregular rhythm (different RR intervals) with rapid ventricular response and the wide, bizarre, different QRS morphology.

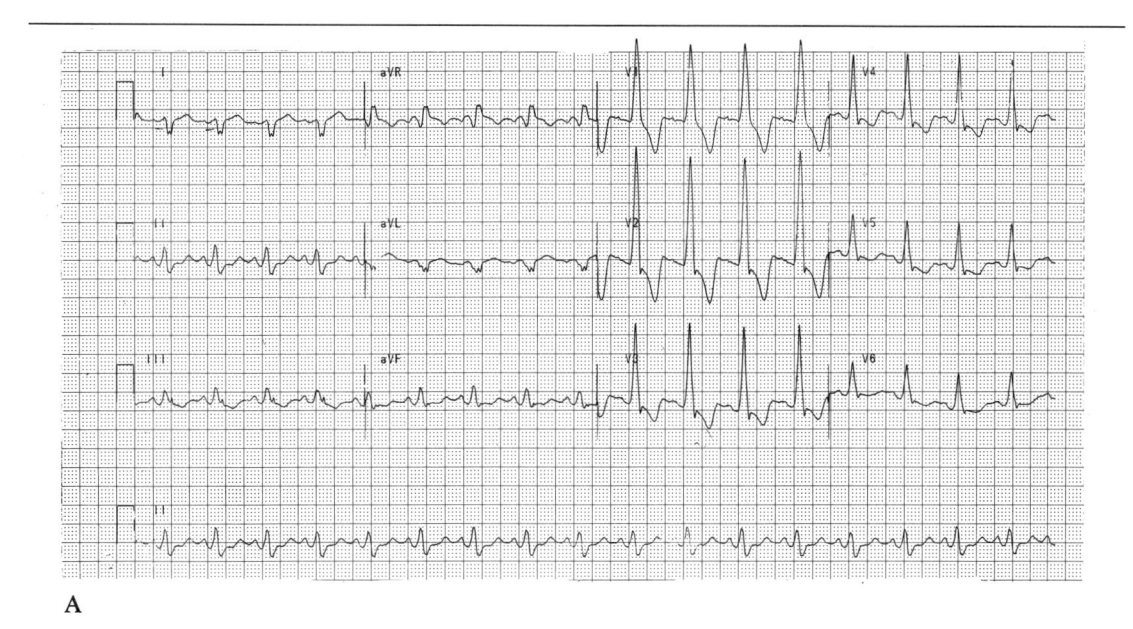

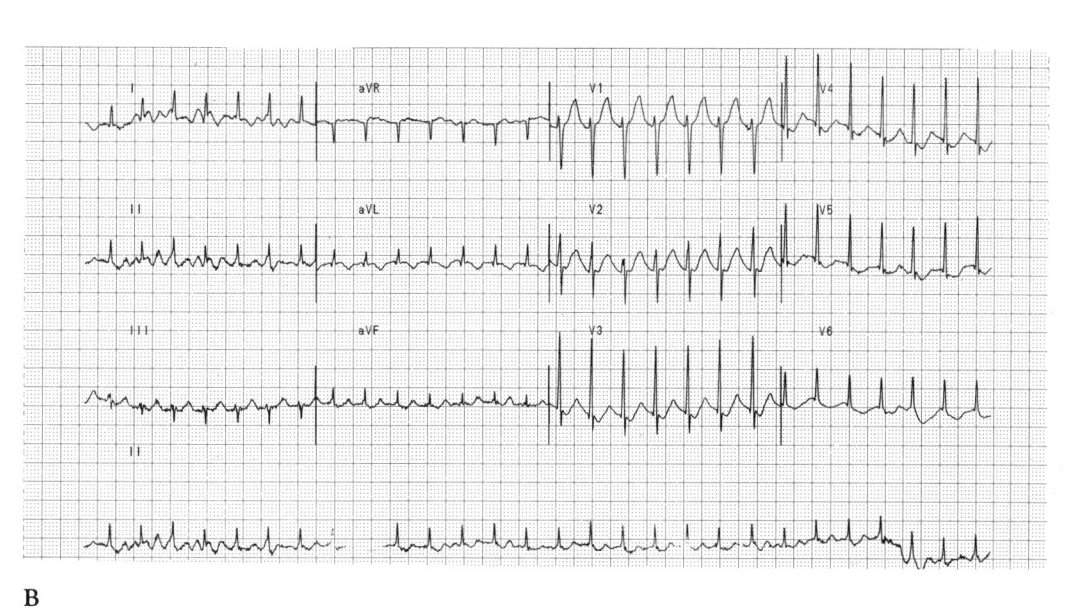

Fig. 10-11. A. Patient with WPW syndrome during sinus rhythm with delta waves in the precordial leads, making the recognition of short PR intervals difficult. Note the tall R in V$_1$ and wide QRS complex that could be mistaken for right bundle branch block (RBBB), however, there is no rSR′ or slurred S wave in V$_6$ that would be present in RBBB. B. Electrocardiogram of the same patient during SVT using the bypass tract retrogradely during atrioventricular reentry. Note that duration of the QRS is normalized to a narrow QRS tachycardia. Also note the regular rhythm.

Table 10-5. Recommendations for anesthetic management of the patient with WPW syndrome

Continue antiarrhythmic medication under surgery
Administer heavy preoperative sedation
Administer scopolamine instead of atropine because of its lesser cardiac vagolytic effects
Maintain adequate surgical analgesia to blunt the sympathetic stimulation to painful stimuli
Avoid muscle relaxants, such as pancuronium and gallamine, that produce tachycardia
Avoid reversal of muscle relaxants with atropine and neostigmine because it can accentuate the preexcitation pattern
Treat tachycardia with vagotonic maneuvers or β-blockers; if the tachycardia is associated with hypotension, give direct-current countershock

---

tients with wide QRS complexes and therefore are relatively contraindicated in WPW syndrome. However, after electrophysiologic study individual patients may demonstrate that verapamil or digoxin is suitable for their treatment. Chronic oral therapy includes the type IA antiarrhythmics or newer oral agents such as amiodarone and encainide. Encainide is a class IC [86, 87] antiarrhythmic agent that has been shown to be effective in treating supraventricular and ventricular tachycardia [88–90]. Its main advantage over other antiarrhythmic drugs is the lack of myocardial depressant effect in patients with abnormal left ventricular function [91]. Following administration of encainide, there is complete antegrade and retrograde block in up to 50 percent of patients with accessory pathways, a prolongation of the tachycardia cycle length, and prevention of a rapid ventricular response in patients with WPW syndrome who have atrial fibrillation and an accessory pathway with a short refractory period [92–94].

The treatment of a PSVT with a narrow QRS complex is the same as the treatment for most AV nodal reentry supraventricular tachycardias, that is, carotid sinus massage and/or verapamil, β-blockers, and so forth. When treating atrial fibrillation, quinidine and procainamide can be effective by suppressing antegrade conduction over the accessory pathway [95, 96]. Arrhythmias that are refractory to medical therapy are surgically treated by epicardial mapping and interruption of the accessory pathway (Table 10-5).

Premature Ventricular Contractions

Although PVCs are common in the surgical patient, they are important because they may serve as a warning of impending ventricular tachycardia and fibrillation. They must be treated aggressively [97, 98]. Indications for treatment include PVCs that occur six or more times per minute, those that are multifocal, and those that occur close to the preceding T wave.

Should the underlying cardiac rate be slow, overdrive pacing using atrial or ventricular wires may suppress the PVCs. The first step in treatment is the elimination of the underlying cause, such as arterial hypoxemia, myocardial ischemia, and other events associated with excessive sympathetic nervous system activity.

Lidocaine is the drug most commonly used to treat PVCs. A loading dose of 1 mg/kg intravenously is given, followed by maintenance doses of 1 to 4 mg per minute. Procainamide is often the second drug of choice when PVCs are refractory to lidocaine. An initial loading dose of 5 to 7 mg/kg slowly followed by a continuous infusion of 1 to 4 mg per minute is often sufficient.

Potassium may be very effective in suppressing PVCs, particularly in patients receiving digitalis therapy. Ideally, the serum potassium should be maintained between 4 and 5 mEq per liter throughout the perioperative period. Potassium will counteract the dysrhythmic effects of digitalis without suppressing its inotropic effects. However, potassium should not be used when prolonged atrioventricular conduction is observed, because it may cause complete heart block.

Bretylium tosylate is highly effective in reducing ventricular ectopy, and it may be particularly useful in cases in which such ectopy has been refractory to treatment with other drugs. Peripheral vasodilation and hypotension may be seen unless it is given slowly. The usual dosage is 7 mg/kg intravenously

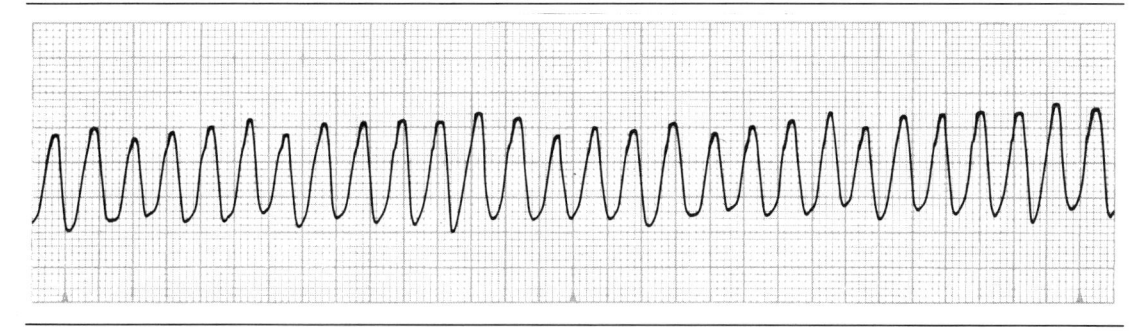

Fig. 10-12. Ventricular tachycardia following repair of thoracic aortic aneurysm.

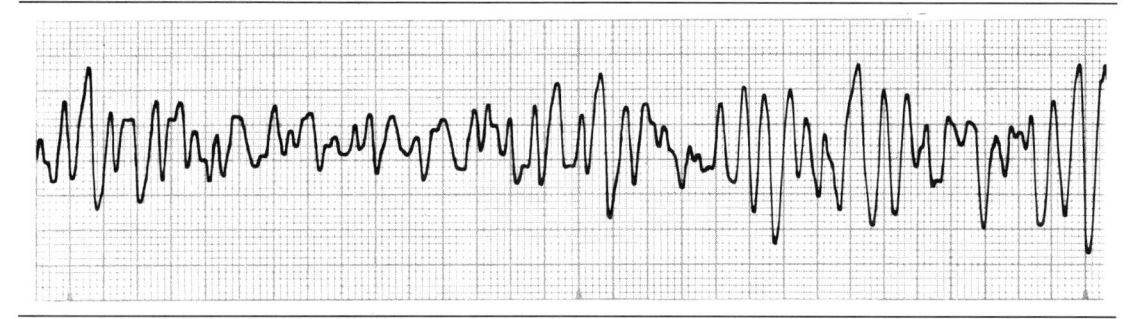

Fig. 10-13. Ventricular fibrillation in a patient previously treated for ventricular tachycardia.

followed by a continuous infusion of 1 to 4 mg per minute. Phenytoin sodium is particularly effective in suppressing the PVCs that are caused by digitalis toxicity.

Ventricular Tachycardia and Fibrillation

Ventricular tachycardia is usually defined as three or more consecutive PVCs [97] (Fig. 10-12). It may degenerate rapidly into ventricular fibrillation (Fig. 10-13). It should be considered life threatening and is usually seen in patients with coronary artery disease. The mechanism of ventricular tachycardia is either a focus with increased automaticity within the ventricle or an area where a reentry mechanism exists. Myocardial ischemia or infarction accounts for most cases of ventricular tachycardia and fibrillation in the perioperative period.

Ventricular tachycardia accompanied by hypotension is treated with cardioversion. Ventricular tachycardia without hypotension can be treated with lidocaine and, if that is unsuccessful, by cardioversion. Should lidocaine fail to control recurring ventricular tachycardia, procainamide and bretylium will generally be the drugs of choice. It should be noted, however, that procainamide and related drugs can cause prolongation of the QT interval and may precipitate ventricular tachycardia. Ventricular fibrillation is treated by cardioversion, followed by lidocaine, procainamide, or bretylium infusion.

ATRIOVENTRICULAR BLOCK

Atrioventricular block is an abnormality of impulse conduction between the atria and the ventricles.

The block can occur at several levels, either in the AV node, the His bundle, or the bundle branches. Blockade at any one of these locations may result in either partial or complete AV block.

First-Degree Atrioventricular Block

In first-degree AV block, conduction through the AV node is slow, resulting in a prolongation of the PR interval on the ECG. By itself it is not necessarily a dangerous phenomenon, implying a delay in conduction due to disease or drug effects on the AV node. In certain clinical situations it may allow a reentrant pathway to develop within the node, resulting in atrial arrhythmias. In addition, further deterioration in AV conduction can lead to a more severe degree of AV block.

Second-Degree Atrioventricular Block

Second-degree AV block is seen when some, but not all, atrial impulses conduct through the AV node to the ventricle [99]. There are two types, Mobitz type I and Mobitz type II. Mobitz type I (or Wenckebach) block is characterized by a PR interval that progressively prolongs for several beats, followed by a beat that is completely blocked. The site of this block is almost always within the AV node. In Mobitz type II block, there is no progressive prolongation of the PR interval. Every second, third, or fourth beat is not conducted. The site of Mobitz type II block is usually the His bundle or bundle branches. Mobitz type II is a serious form of AV conduction delay, and there is a significant risk of progression to complete heart block. If it is necessary to anesthetize a patient with Mobitz type II second-degree block, a pacemaker should be available in the operating room.

Third-Degree Atrioventricular Block

With third-degree, or complete, AV block, no atrial beats are conducted to the ventricle. The atria and ventricles beat independently. Ventricular activity is due to an escape rhythm in the conduction system distal to the AV node. All patients with Mobitz type II block and those with complete heart block are candidates for permanent pacemakers.

Bundle Branch Block

Bundle branch block can occur in any one of the three fascicles of the bundle of His: the right bundle, the anterosuperior fascicle of the left bundle, or the posteroinferior fascicle of the left bundle. A left bundle branch block is caused by a conduction block in both the left anterosuperior and left posteroinferior fascicles of the left bundle. The left bundle branch block is the most serious form of bundle branch block (Fig. 10-14). It is seen on the electrocardiogram as a wide-notched QRS (>120 msec) in leads I, aVL, and V_6. A left bundle branch block pattern is always associated with significant cardiac disease, whereas a right bundle branch block may or may not be of clinical significance. A right bundle branch block is seen on the electrocardiogram as a widened QRS with RR' in V_1 and V_2. Right bundle branch block is frequently associated with chronic lung disease and atrioseptal defects, or it may be insignificant (Fig. 10-15). Left anterior hemiblock is seen on the electrocardiogram as a left axis deviation with a small Q in lead I and an S in lead III. A left posterior hemiblock is seen on the electrocardiogram as a right axis deviation, an S in lead I and a small Q in lead III (Fig. 10-16). Bifascicular block occurs when right bundle block is present together with a block of one of the two left fascicles.

A theoretical concern in patients with bifascicular heart block is that such perioperative events as alterations in blood pressure, arterial oxygenation, or electrolyte concentrations might compromise conduction in the one remaining intact fascicle, leading to the acute onset of third-degree atrioventricular heart block. However, there is no evidence that surgery performed using general anesthesia or a regional technique predisposes to the development of third-degree block in patients with existing bifascicular block [100]. Therefore, placement of a prophylactic artificial cardiac pacemaker is not recommended before general or regional anesthesia in these patients. Conceivably, a temporary transvenous cardiac pacemaker should be placed before major surgical procedures when, additionally, the PR interval is prolonged on the preoperative electrocardiogram or there is a history of syncope, particularly in patients with block of the right bundle branch and the left posterior fascicle.

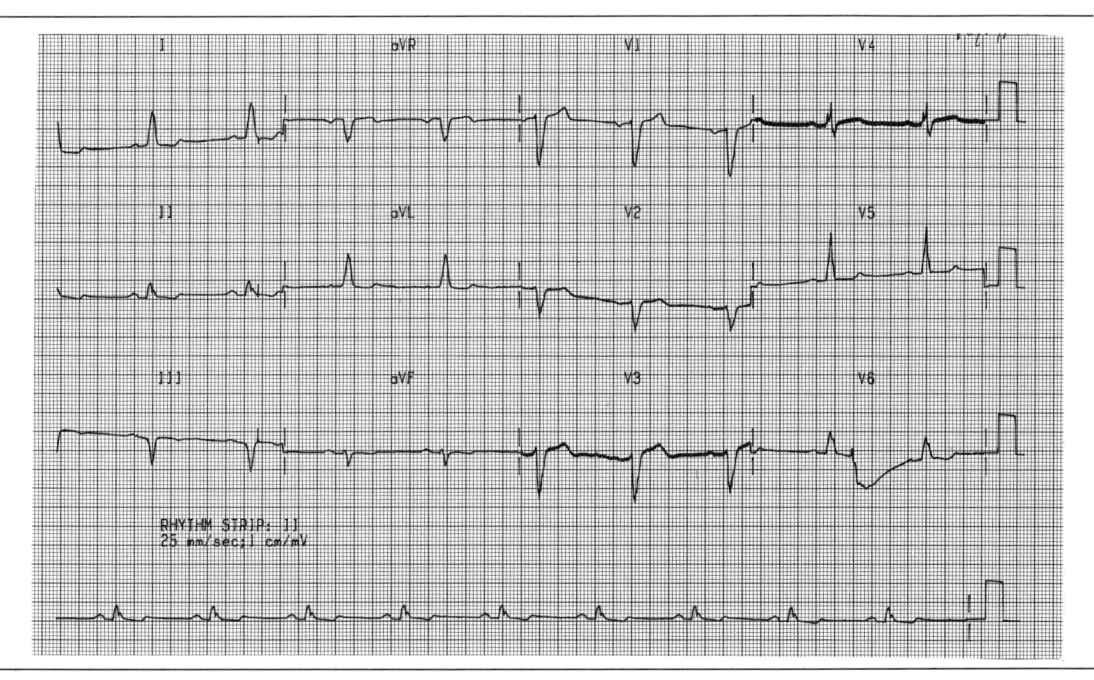

Fig. 10-14. Electrocardiogram showing left bundle branch block. Note the wide QRS complex of greater than 0.12 seconds, rS or QS in V_1, the wide "M-shaped" R wave in V_6, and the absence of normal q in leads I, aVL, and V_6.

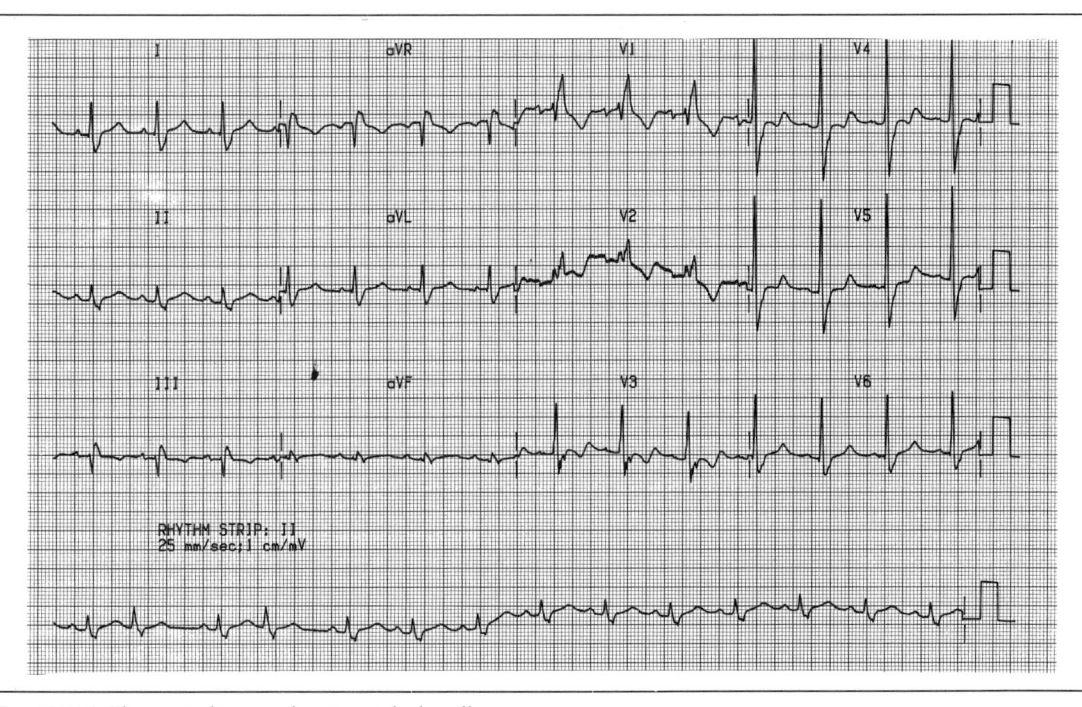

Fig. 10-15. Electrocardiogram showing right bundle branch block. Note that the broad QRS complex is greater than 0.12 seconds, with rSR′ in V_1–V_2 and a wide slurred S in V_6.

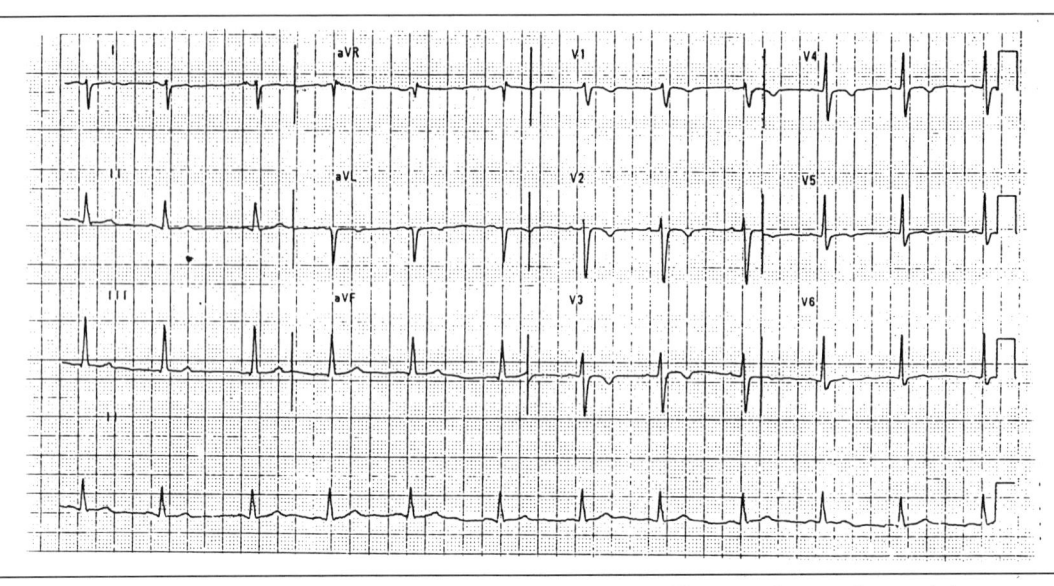

Fig. 10-16. Electrocardiogram showing left posterior hemiblock. Note the right axis deviation, the rS in lead I; and the qR in leads II, III, and aVF.

However, some symptomatic patients have undergone uneventful surgery without a prophylactic artificial pacemaker. A full discussion of the indications for temporary pacing (including passing a pulmonary artery catheter in a patient with preexisting block) is presented in Chap. 12.

ELECTROLYTE MANAGEMENT

The arrhythmogenic effects of hypokalemia and hypomagnesemia are also important. Magnesium is required as a cofactor for the Na^+-K^+ pump and the Ca-ATPase pump that maintains low intracellular calcium levels. Low serum magnesium levels reduce Na^+-K^+ pump activity, which increases Na^+-Ca^+ exchange; this in turn increases intracellular Ca^{++} and reduces intracellular K^+ concentrations. It is difficult to restore intracellular K^+ in the presence of low serum magnesium. Chronic magnesium depletion occurs in diuretic usage, aminoglycoside therapy, alcohol abuse, secondary aldosteronism, and malabsorption syndrome. Serum magnesium levels do not reflect intracellular magnesium levels, especially in chronic depletion. Reduced intracellular magnesium decreases calcium extrusion via Ca-ATPase pump, resulting in increased intracellular Ca^{++} currents, which are arrhythmogenic in triggered automaticity models. Clinically, magnesium is beneficial in digitalis toxic arrhythmias and in managing refractory ventricular arrhythmias, despite normal serum concentration.

Iseri and associates [101] recommend 2 gm $MgSO_4$ intravenously, given over 2 to 3 minutes, when ventricular arrhythmias are refractory to lidocaine and procainamide. A continuous infusion is begun with 10 gm given over 5 hours, and, especially if arrhythmias subside, a second 10 gm is given over 10 hours to restore intracellular magnesium levels; hypotension is a side effect that can be reversed easily with small doses of calcium. Serum K^+ and Mg^{++} should be closely monitored during magnesium and potassium therapy.

There are several concerns when patients with conduction abnormalities must undergo anesthesia and surgery. First, the arrhythmia may worsen intraoperatively. A second concern is the effectiveness of the antiarrhythmic agents that are available if severe hemodynamic instability occurs. A third concern is whether a transvenous pacemaker should be inserted before the induction of general anesthesia. Conduction disturbances high in the system such as the AV node generally are benign and so do not progress to severe conduction blockade. They respond very well to pharmacologic agents, and no hemodynamic instability occurs because of a fast escape pacemaker. However, disturbances lower in the system often result in hemodynamic instability and are more pathologic. They may require invasive treatment, such as insertion of temporary pacemakers or the use of a defibrillator.

The causes of arrhythmias during anesthesia are multifactorial and most of the time benign: general anesthesia, electrolyte abnormalities, acid-base imbalance, and hypoxia. Arrhythmias may also be attenuated or eliminated by general anesthesia. This could be due to relief of anxiety and loss of sympathetic stimulation, to an antidysrhythmic property of the anesthetic itself, or to the correction of acid-base and electrolyte imbalance. Prompt therapy and adequate monitoring will help decrease the morbidity and mortality associated with this frightening event during general anesthesia.

REFERENCES

1. Keefe, DL, Kates, RE, Harrison, DC. New antiarrhythmic drugs: Their place in therapy. *Drugs* 22: 363–400, 1981.
2. Podrid, PJ. Aggravation of ventricular arrhythmia: A drug-induced complication. *Drugs* 29 (Suppl 4): 33–44, 1984.
3. Willius, FA, Keyes, TE. A remarkable early reference to the use of inchona in cardiac arrhythmia. *Proc Staff Meet Mayo Clin* 17:294–296, 1942.
4. Mason, JW, Hondeghem, LM. Quinidine. *Ann NY Acad Sci* 432:162, 1984.
5. Weld, FM, Coromilas, J, Rothman, JN, Bigger, JN, Jr. Mechanisms of quinidine-induced depression of maximum up-stroke velocity in bovine cardiac Purkinje fibers. *Circ Res* 50: 369, 1982.
6. Leakey, EB, Jr, Reiffel, JA, Drusin, RE, et al. Interaction between quinidine and digoxin. *JAMA* 240: 533–534, 1978.
7. Smith, TW, Antman, EA, Friedman, PL, et al. Digitalis gylcosides: Mechanisms and manifestations of toxicity. *Prog Cardiovasc Dis* 26:412; 26:495; 27:21, 1984.
8. Selzer, A, Wray, HW. Quinidine syncope: Paroxysmal ventricular fibrillation occurring during treatment of chronic atrial arrhythmias. *Circulation* 30: 17, 1964.
9. Smith, WM, Gallagher, JJ. "Les torsades de pointes" and unusual ventricular arrhythmias. *Ann Intern Med* 93:578, 1980.
10. Roden, DM, Woosley, RL, Primm, K. Incidence and clinical features of the quinidine-associated long QT syndrome: Implications for patient care. *Am Heart J* 111:1088–1093, 1986.
11. Wenger, TL, Browning, DL, Masterton, E, et al. Procainamide delivers to ischemic canine myocardium following rapid intravenous administration. *Circ Res* 46:789–795, 1980.
12. Swartz, PJ. Idiopathic long QT syndrome progress and questions. *Am Heart J* 109:399, 1985.
13. Kosausky, BD, Taylor, J, Lorin, B, et al. Long-term use of procainamide following acute myocardial infarction. *Circulation* 47:1204–1210, 1973.
14. Anderson, RJ, Gentsin, E. Procainamide-induced pericardial effusion. *Am Heart J* 83:798–800, 1972.
15. Roden, DM, Reele, JB, Higgins, JB, et al. Antirrhythmic efficacy, pharmacokinetics, and safety of N-acetylprocainamide in human subjects: Comparison with procainamide. *Am J Cardiol* 46:463–468, 1980.
16. Ellrodt, AG, Murata, GH, Ridinger, MS, et al. Severe neutropenia associated with sustained release in procainamide. *Ann Intern Med* 100:197–201, 1984.
17. Polish, LB, Branch, RA, Fitzgerald, GA. Digitoxin-quinidine interaction: Potentiation during administration of cimetidine. *South Med J* 74:633–634, 1981.
18. Vaughn-Williams, EM. Disopyramide. *Ann NY Acad Sci* 432:189, 1984.
19. Myerberg, RJ, Bassett, AL, Epstein, K, et al. Electrophysiologic effects of procainamide in acute and healed experimental ischemia injury of cat myocardium. *Circ Res* 50:386, 1982.
20. Sasyniuki, BI, Kirs, T. Cellular electrophysiologic changes induced by disopyramide phosphate in normal and infarcted hearts. *J Ont Med* 4:20, 1976.
21. Podrid, PG, Schoenenberger, A, Lown, B. Congestive heart failure caused by oral disopyramide. *N Engl J Med* 302:614, 1980.
22. Teichman, SL, Fisher, JD, Matso, J, et al. Disopyramine-pyridostigmine: Report of a beneficial drug interaction. *J Cardiovasc Pharmacol* 7:108, 1985.
23. White, RD. Cardiovascular Pharmacology: Part 1. In KM McIntyre, AJ Lerins (eds), *Textbook of Advanced Clinical Life Support*. Dallas: American Heart Association, 1983. Pp 104, 107.
24. Kupersmith, J, Antman, EM, Hoffman, BF. In vivo electrophysiologic effects of lidocaine in canine acute myocardial infarction. *Circ Res* 36:84–91, 1975.
25. Shen, SS, Lederer, WJ. Lidocaine negative inotropic and antiarrhythmic actions. Dependence of shortening of action potential duration and reduction of intracellular sodium activity. *Circ Res* 57: 587, 1985.
26. Ferrier, GR. Digitalis arrhythmias: Role of oscilla-

tory after potentials. *Prog Cardiovasc Dis* 19:459, 1977.
27. Rosen, MR, Danils, P, Jr, Alonso, MB et al. Effects of therapeutic concentration of diphenylhydantoin on transmembrane potentials of normal and depressed Purkinje fibers. *J Pharmacol Exp Ther* 197:594–604, 1976.
28. Peon, J, Ferrier, CG, Moe, GK. The relationship of excitability to conduction velocity in canine Purkinje tissue. *Circ Res* 43:125–135, 1978.
29. Konn, RD, Kennedy, JW, Blackman, JR. The hemodynamic effects of diphenylhydantoin. *Am Heart J* 73:500, 1967.
30. Unger, AH, Sklaroff, HJ. Fatalities following intravenous use of sodium diphenylhydantoin of cardiac arrhythmias. *JAMA* 200:335, 1967.
31. Quart, BD, Gallo, DG, Sami, MH, et al. Drug interaction studies and encainide use in renal and hepatic impairment. *Am J Cardiol* 58:87C–95C, 1986.
32. Zipes, DP, Prystowsky, EN, Heger, JJ. Amiodarone: Electrophysiologic actions, pharmacokinetics, and clinical effects. *J Am Coll Cardiol* 3:1059–1071, 1984.
33. Coumel, P, Lucet, V, Ngoc, DD. The use of amiodarone in children. *PACE* 6:930, 1983.
34. Haeds, AH, Chiale, PA, Bandiere, JD, et al. Comparative antiarrhythmic efficacy of verapamil, 17-monochloracetyl-cymaline, mexiletine, and amiodarone in patients with severe chagasic myocarditis: Relation with the underlying arrhythmogenic mechanisms. *J Am Coll Cardiol* 7:114, 1986.
35. McKenna, WJ, Harris, L, Rowland, E, et al. Amiodarone for long-term management of patients with hypertrophic cardiomyopathy. *Am J Cardiol* 54:802, 1984.
36. Podrid, PJ. The new antiarrhythmic drugs. *Resident Staff Physician* 31:23–33, 1985.
37. Raeder, EA, Podrid, PJ, Lown, B. Side effects and complications of amiodarone therapy. *Am Heart J* 109:975, 1985.
38. Greene, HL, Graham, EL, Werner, JA et al. Toxic and therapeutic effects of amiodarone in the treatment of cardiac arrhythmias. *J Am Coll Cardiol* 2:1114, 1983.
39. Sobel, SM, Rakita, L. Pneumonitis and pulmonary fibrosis associated with amiodarone treatment: A possible complication of a new antiarrhythmic drug. *Circulation* 65:819, 1982.
40. Mason, JW. Amiodarone. *N Engl J Med* 316:455, 1987.
41. Marcus, FI, Fontaine, GH, Frank, R, et al. Clinical pharmacology and therapeutic applications of the antiarrhythmic agent, amiodarone. *Am Heart J* 101:480–493, 1981.
42. Harrison, EE, Amey, BD. The use of bretylium in prehospital ventricular fibrillation. *Am J Emerg Med* 1:1, 1983.
43. Olson, DW, Thompson, BM, Darin, JC, et al. A randomized comparison study of bretylium tosylate and lidocaine in resuscitation of patients from out-of-hospital ventricular fibrillation in a paramedic system. *Ann Emerg Med* 13:807, 1984.
44. Kerber, RE, Pandian, NG, Jensen, SR, et al. Requirements for transthoracic defibrillation: Experimental studies. *J Am Coll Cardiol* 7:397, 1986.
45. Haynes, RE, Chinn, TL, Copass, MK, et al. Comparison of bretylium tosylate and lidocaine in management in out-of-hospital ventricular fibrillation: A randomized clinical trial. *Am J Cardiol* 48:353, 1981.
46. Euler, DE, Scanton, PJ. Mechanisms of the effect of bretylium on ventricular threshold in dogs. *Am J Cardiol* 55:1396, 1985.
47. Wenger, TK, Lederman, S, Starmer, CF, et al. A method of quantitating antifibrillatory effects of drugs after coronary reperfusion in dogs: Improve outcome with bretylium. *Circulation* 69:142, 1984.
48. Lucchesi, BR. Rationale of therapy in the patient with acute myocardial infarction and life-threatening arrhythmias. A focus on bretylium. *Am J Cardiol* 54:14A, 1984.
49. Hewett, KW, Rosen, MR. Alpha- and beta-adrenergic interactions with ouabain-induced delayed after depolarization. *J Pharmacol Exp Ther* 229:188, 1984.
50. Gilmorin, RF, Zipes, DP. Basic Electrophysiology of the Slow Inward Current. In EM Antman, PH Stone (eds), *Cardiac Arrhythmia*. Mt. Kisco, NY: Futura, 1983.
51. Rickenberger, RL, Prystowsky, EN, Heger, JJ, et al. Effects of intravenous and chronic oral verapamil administration in patients with supraventricular tachyarrhythmias. *Circulation* 62:996, 1980.
52. Sung, RJ, Elser, B, McAllister, RG, Jr. Intravenous verapamil for termination of reentrant supraventricular tachycardia. Intracardiac studies correlated with plasma verapamil concentration. *Ann Intern Med* 93:682, 1980.
53. Hamer, A, Peter, T, Platt, M, et al. Effects of verapamil on supraventricular tachycardia inpatients with overt and concealed Wolff-Parkinson-White syndrome. *Am Heart J* 101:600, 1981.
54. Gulamhusein, SK, Ko, P, Carruthers, SG, et al. Acceleration of the ventricular response during atrial fibrillation in the Wolff-Parkinson-White syndrome after verapamil. *Circulation* 65:348, 1982.
55. McGovern, B, Garan, H, Ruskin, JN. Precipitation of cardiac arrest by verapamil in patients with Wolff-

Parkinson-White syndrome. *Ann Intern Med* 104: 791, 1986.
56. Fileet, WF, Johnson, TA, Graebner, CA, et al. Effects of verapamil on ischemia-induced changes in extracellular K^+, pH, and local activation in the pig. *Circulation* 73:837, 1986.
57. Pacer, M, Mellen, J, Medina, N, et al. Hemodynamic consequences of combined beta-adrenergic and slow calcium channel blockade in man. *Circulation* 65: 660, 1982.
58. Kuner, J. Cardia arrhythmia during anesthesia. *Disease of the Chest* 52:580–587, 1967.
59. Atlee, JL, Rusy, BF. Ventricular conduction times and AV nodal conductivity during enflurane anesthesia in dogs. *Anesthesiology* 47:498, 1977.
60. Koehntop, DE, Liao, JC, Van Bergen, FH. Effects of pharmacologic alterations of adrenergic mechanisms by cocaine, tropolone, aminophylline, and ketamine on epinephrine-induced arrhythmias during halothane–nitrous oxide anesthesia. *Anesthesiology* 46:83, 1977.
61. Fox, EJ, Sklar, GS, Hill, CH, et al. Complications related to the pressor response to endotracheal intubation. *Anesthesiology* 47:524, 1977.
62. Katz, RL, Bigger, JT. Cardiac arrhythmias during anesthesia and operation. *Anesthesiology* 33:193, 1970.
63. Smith, M, Ray, CT. Cardiac arrhythmias, increased intracranial pressure, and the autonomic nervous system. *Chest* 61:125, 1972.
64. Alexander, JP. Dysrhythmia and oral surgery. *Br J Anaesth* 43:773, 1971.
65. Angelini, L, Feldman, MI, Lufschnowski, R, et al. Cardiac arrhythmias during and after heart surgery: Diagnosis and management. *Prog Cardiovasc Dis* 16:469, 1974.
66. Bosnijak, ZJ, Kampine, JP. Effects of halothane, enflurane, and isoflurane on the SA node. *Anesthesiology* 58:314–321, 1983.
67. Rogers, MC, Battit, G, McPeek, B, et al. Lateralization of sympathetic control of the human sinus node: ECG changes of stellate ganglion block. *Anesthesiology* 48:139–141, 1978.
68. Pratilia, MG, Pratilia, V. Anesthetic agents and cardiac electromechanical activity. *Anesthesiology* 49:338–360, 1978.
69. Haldemann, G, Schoer, H. Haemodynamic effects of transient atrioventricular dissociation in general anaesthesia. *Br J Anaesth* 44:159–162, 1972.
70. Boba, A. Significant effects on the blood pressure of an apparently trivial atrial dysrhythmia. *Anesthesiology* 48:282–283, 1978.
71. Michelson, EL, Porterfield, JK, Das, G, et al. A comparison of esmolol and verapamil in the treatment of atrial fibrillation/flutter. *J Am Coll Cardiol* 7:157A, 1986.
72. Marchlinski, FE, Miller, JM. Atrial arrhythmias exacerbated by theophylline: Response to verapamil and evidence for triggered activity in man. *Chest* 88:931–934, 1985.
73. Levine, JH, Michael, JR, Guarineri, T. Multifocal atrial tachycardia: A toxic effect of theophylline. *Lancet* Jan 5, 1985. Pp. 12–14.
74. Levine, JH, Michael, JR, Guarineri, T. Treatment of multifocal atrial tachycardia with verapamil. *Med Intell* 312:21–25, 1985.
75. Breslow, MJ, Evers, AS, Lebowitz, P. Successful treatment of accelerated junctional rhythm with propranolol: Possible role of sympathetic stimulation in the genesis of the rhythm disturbances. *Anesthesiology* 62:180–182, 1985.
76. Anderson, RH, Becker, AE, Brechenmacher, C, et al. Ventricular preexcitation—a proposed nomenclature for its substrates. *Eur J Cardiol* 3:7, 1975.
77. Chung, KY, Walsh, TJ, Massie, E. Wolff-Parkinson-White syndrome. *Am Heart J* 69:116, 1965.
78. Sears, GA, Manning, GW. Wolff-Parkinson-White pattern in routine electrocardiography. *Can Med Assoc J* 87:1213, 1962.
79. Newman, BJ, Donoso, E, Friedberg, CK. Arrhythmias in the Wolff-Parkinson-White syndrome. *Prog Cardiovasc Dis* 9:147, 1966.
80. Wellens, HJ, Durrer, D. Patterns of ventriculoatrial conduction in the Wolff-Parkinson-White syndrome. *Circulation* 49:22, 1974.
81. Gallagher, JJ, Gilbert, M, Svenson, RH, et al. Wolff-Parkinson-White syndrome: The problem, evaluation, and surgical correction. *Circulation* 51:767, 1975.
82. Dreifus, LS, Haiat, R, Watanabe, Y. Ventricular fibrillation: A possible mechanism of sudden death in patients with Wolff-Parkinson-White syndrome. *Circulation* 43:520, 1971.
83. Wellens, HJ, Durrer, D. Wolff-Parkinson-White syndrome and atrial fibrillation: Relation between refractory period of the accessory pathway and ventricular rate during atrial fibrillation. *Am J Cardiol* 34:777, 1974.
84. Josephson, ME, Kastor, JA, Kitchen, JG, III. Lidocaine in Wolff-Parkinson-White syndrome with atrial fibrillation. *Ann Intern Med* 84:44–45, 1976.
85. Fenster, PE, Comess, KA, Marsh, R, et al. Conversion of atrial fibrillation to sinus rhythm by acute intravenous procainamide infusion. *Am Heart J* 106:501–504, 1983.
86. Sami, M, Mason, JW, Peters, F, et al. Clinical electrophysiologic effects of encainide, a newly devel-

oped antiarrhythmic agent. *Am J Cardiol* 49: 1270–1278, 1982.
87. Bigger, JN, Jr, Leakez, EB. Quinidine and digoxin—an important interaction. *Drugs* 24:229, 1982.
88. Wehmeyer, AE, Thomas, RL. Encainide: A new antiarrhythmic agent. *Drug Intell Clin Pharmacol* 20: 9–13, 1986.
89. Mason, JW. Basic and clinical cardiac electrophysiology of encainide. *Am J Cardiol* 58:18C–24C, 1986.
90. Jackman, WM, Zipes, DP, Naccarelli, GV, et al. Electrophysiology of oral encainide. *Am J Cardiol* 49:1270–1278, 1982.
91. Sami, MH. Acute intravenous and long-term oral hemodynamic effects of encainide. *Am J Cardiol* 58: 25C–30C, 1986.
92. Pool, PE. Treatment of supraventricular arrhythmias with encainide. *Am J Cardiol* 58:55C–57C, 1986.
93. Markel, ML, Prystowsky, EN, Heger, JJ, et al. Encainide for treatment of supraventricular tachycardias associated with the Wolff-Parkinson-White syndrome. *Am J Cardiol* 58:41C–48C, 1986.
94. Prystowsky, EN, Klein, GJ, Rinkenberger, RL, et al. Clinical efficacy and electrophysiologic effects of encainide in patients with Wolff-Parkinson-White syndrome. *Circulation* 69:278–287, 1984.
95. Gallagher, JJ, Svenson, RH, Sealy, WC, et al. The Wolff-Parkinson-White syndrome and the preexcitation dysrhythmias. *Med Clin North Am* 60: 101–123, 1976.
96. Narula, OS. Symposium of cardiac arrhythmias. IV. Wolff-Parkinson-White syndrome. *Circulation* 47: 872–886, 1973.
97. Kastor, JA, Horowitz, LN, Harken, AH, et al. Clinical electrophysiology of ventricular tachycardia. *N Engl J Med* 304:1004–1020, 1981.
98. Lown, B, Wolf, M. Approaches to sudden death from coronary heart disease. *Circulation* 44:103–142, 1971.
99. Zipes, DP. Second-degree atrioventricular block. *Circulation* 60:465, 1979.
100. Rooney, S, Goldiner, PL, Muss, E. Relationship of right bundle block and marked left axis deviation to complete heart block during general anesthesia. *Anesthesiology* 44:64–66, 1976.
101. Iseri, LT, Chung, P, Tobis, J. Magnesium therapy for intractable ventricular tachyarrhythmia in normomagnemic patients. *West J Med* 138:823, 1983.

11
Thoracic Aortic Disease

Gerald A. Schiff

Diseases of the aorta have been known since the time of Galen, who wrote "when the arteries are enlarged, the disease is called an aneurysm" [1]. Little was known of the clinical manifestations of the disease until 1555, when Vesalius diagnosed a pulsating tumor near the vertebrae in a patient's back and called it "a dilatation of the aorta" [2]. In 1761, Morgagni [3] reported the first description of both the clinical and the pathologic findings of aortic dissection. In the second century, a Roman physician, Antyllus, described proximal and distal ligation of an aneurysm and an incision to remove its contents [4]. In 1864, Moore and Morchison [5] inserted lengths of silver wire in a thoracic aneurysm in order to induce clot formation and Corradi, in 1879, added to this method the passage of a galvanic current through the wire [4]. In 1940, Pearse [6] called attention to the irritating properties of cellophane as a means of gradual occlusion of large arteries. By 1948, surgical techniques had advanced to allow resection and end-to-end anastomosis of a coarctation of the aorta [7]. In 1951, Oudot [8] of France first used a homograft to replace a thrombosed aortic bifurcation, while in 1953, DeBakey and Cooley [9] described the successful resection of a thoracic aortic aneurysm and replacement with a homograft. The current surgical technique of leaving the aneurysmal sac intact and restoring flow with an indwelling permanent graft has been popularized by the group at Baylor University and at the Texas Heart Institute [10].

ANATOMY

The aorta consists of thoracic and abdominal portions (Fig. 11-1). The thoracic aorta is composed of three segments, the ascending aorta, the aortic arch, and the descending thoracic aorta. The ascending aorta originates at the base of the heart and extends 5 to 6 cm cephalad to join the arch. Normally, the ascending aorta lies just to the right of the midline, with its proximal portion within the pericardial cavity. Nearby structures include the pulmonary trunk anteriorly, and the left atrium, right pulmonary artery, and right main-stem bronchus posteriorly.

The arch of the aorta gives rise to all of the brachiocephalic vessels. It courses slightly leftward in front of the trachea and then proceeds dorsally and inferiorly above the left main-stem bronchus to the left of the trachea and the esophagus. Other closely related structures include the left phrenic and vagus nerves to the left of the arch, and, inferiorly, the bifurcation of the pulmonary trunk and most of the left lung. The left recurrent laryngeal nerve also loops underneath it.

The descending thoracic aorta is the continua-

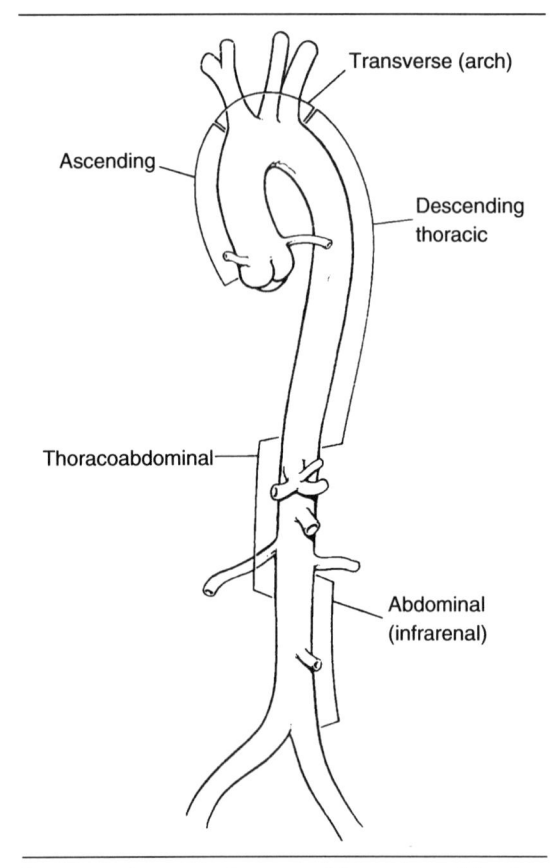

Fig. 11-1. Anatomic divisions of the aorta used for classification of aortic aneurysms according to location. (Reprinted with permission from DA Cooley, *Surgical Treatment of Aortic Aneurysms*. Philadelphia: Saunders, 1986. P 2.)

tion of the aorta beyond the arch. It lies in the posterior mediastinum to the left of the vertebral column, gradually courses in front of the vertebral column as it descends behind the esophagus, and passes through the diaphragm, usually at the level of the 12th thoracic vertebra.

A small but important segment called the aortic isthmus is the point at which the arch and descending thoracic aorta join. This is where coarctations of the aorta are usually located. It is also the point at which the mobile portion of the aorta becomes relatively fixed to the thorax by the pleural reflections, intercostal arteries, and left subclavian artery, thereby leaving this area especially vulnerable to traumatic injuries.

The abdominal aorta forms the continuation of the thoracic aorta, giving off the splanchnic vessels and ending in the aortic bifurcation at the level of the 4th lumbar vertebra.

Thoracic aortic disease can be divided into three major subgroups: aortic aneurysm, aortic rupture, and aortic dissection. These are discussed in the following sections. Aortic coarctation is discussed in Chap. 17.

THORACIC AORTIC ANEURYSM

There are many causes of thoracic aortic aneurysms. During the first part of the twentieth century, syphilis was by far the leading cause. In Boyd's review [11] of 4,000 aortic aneurysms, syphilis was implicated in 92 percent of patients. It typically would result in Luetic aortitis and an ascending aortic aneurysm. During the past 50 years, with the arrival of antibiotic therapy and the general decline of syphilis worldwide, atherosclerotic disease has appeared as the leading cause of thoracic aneurysms [12].

The location of these aneurysms has also changed. While only one quarter of all atherosclerotic aneurysms involve the thoracic aorta (most involve the abdominal aorta), the arch and descending thoracic aorta predominate. The shape has also changed. Syphilitic aneurysms tend to be saccular; atherosclerotic aneurysms are usually fusiform.

The atherosclerotic process leads to a weakening of the aortic wall, medial degeneration, and localized dilatation. Cholesterol deposits weaken the strength of the aortic wall and, especially in the presence of hypertension, contribute to the expansion of the aneurysm. The natural history of thoracic aortic aneurysms differs somewhat from that of abdominal aortic aneurysms in that spontaneous rupture is less common because a growing thoracic aneurysm usually causes earlier symptoms related to the compression of the surrounding structures. Pain is usually steady and occasionally pulsating, and may be extremely severe. The sternum and right thoracic cage may be eroded by large aneurysms of the ascending aorta, and the vertebral column and left ribs by descending thoracic aortic aneurysms. Wheezing, dyspnea, cough, hemoptysis, and recurrent pneumonia can result from compression of the tracheobronchial tree. Hoarseness may follow compression of the recurrent laryngeal nerve and dysphagia can arise from pressure against the esophagus.

The male-female ratio is 1.6:1.0 and the mean age at diagnosis is 69 [13]. Therefore, coexisting medical problems are very common, with preexisting hypertension occurring in 70 percent of patients, coronary artery disease in 44 percent, and chronic obstructive pulmonary disease in 34 percent. Thirty-four percent had had previous aneurysm surgery and 8 percent had undergone prior coronary artery bypass graft surgery.

TRAUMATIC RUPTURE OF THE AORTA

Aortic rupture usually results from an automobile accident. Death from exsanguination at the scene is the usual outcome. Most victims of aortic rupture are young men who are automobile drivers or passengers. Aortic rupture is twice as frequent in those ejected from a vehicle as in those not ejected. This injury can also occur in pedestrians struck by automobiles, motorcycle riders, and individuals who have fallen from great heights. In only 20 percent is the aortic rupture sufficiently contained to allow survival long enough to reach medical attention. The upper descending thoracic aorta just distal to the origin of the left subclavian artery is the most frequent site of rupture in patients who survive the trip to the hospital.

Most of the clinical features of aortic rupture are subtle and require a high index of suspicion from the emergency physician. Associated injuries can include extremity and/or pelvic fractures, rib and/or sternal fractures, central nervous system injuries, visceral ruptures, and body burns. The most common finding is hypertension in the upper extremities with widening of the pulse pressure. There is no evidence of an injured chest wall in approximately 50 percent of these patients. Once the diagnosis has been established, the most effective treatment is prompt surgical repair. Time is of the essence because of the constant risk of sudden rupture of the false aneurysm.

The general principles of emergency care of the seriously injured should be followed in all cases of suspected cardiovascular trauma. The airway is evaluated and secured by intubation, if necessary, in the emergency area. Oxygen is administered and ventilation is provided as required. As in most trauma patients, all precautions for emergency full-stomach rapid-sequence intubation should be taken. Multiple large-bore intravenous access routes should be established for fluid and blood resuscitation. A right radial arterial catheter should be placed for continuous blood pressure monitoring. Frequently, neurosurgical, general surgical, and orthopedic teams operate with the cardiothoracic team, and, therefore, the anesthesiologist must balance the individual needs of the various surgical teams [14], for example, the necessity to maintain hemodynamic stability with fluid and pharmacologic resuscitation in the face of possible increased intracranial pressure and cerebral ischemia.

THORACIC AORTIC DISSECTION

Acute aortic dissection is a relatively common life-threatening illness, with an incidence of approximately 20,000 new cases per year in the United States [15]. Aortic dissection originates from the sudden development of a tear in the aortic intima. This defect, when exposed to the force of arterial pressure, allows for disruption and destruction of the media and stripping of the intima from the adventitia along the aorta. It is uncertain whether the primary event in aortic dissection is rupture of the intima with secondary dissection into the media, or hemorrhage within diseased media followed by disruption of the adjacent intima and subsequent propagation of the dissection [16]. This process, termed *cystic medial necrosis*, most often is the result of chronic stress against the aortic wall, such as might occur with long-standing hypertension. Cystic medial necrosis also appears to be an intrinsic feature in the formation of aortic disease in patients with Marfan's syndrome [17] and Ehlers-Danlos syndrome [18]. Certain congenital cardiovascular abnormalities, especially coarctation of the aorta and bicuspid aortic valves, seem to predispose to aortic dissection [19]. An unexplained relationship exists between pregnancy and aortic dissection. About half of all dissections in women under the age of 40 occur during pregnancy, sometimes with extension to the coronary arteries [20].

Classifications

Many classifications have been described to categorize aortic dissections. DeBakey's classification describes three basic types in accordance with the origin and the extent of the dissection [21]. In type I, the dissection and the intimal tear start in the ascending aorta and extend distally for a variable distance, usually throughout the remaining aorta. Aortic valvular insufficiency is also frequently present.

Type II is characterized by a dissection that is limited to the ascending aorta. There is usually a transverse tear in the intima beginning just above the aortic valve, which terminates just proximal to the origin of the innominate artery. It is also often associated with aortic valvular insufficiency and is the type most likely to be found with Marfan's disease [22].

Type III is characterized by the fact that the dissecting process arises in the descending thoracic aorta, usually at or just distal to the origin of the left subclavian artery, and extends distally for a varying distance. Type III has been subdivided into IIIA and IIIB. Type IIIA is limited to the descending thoracic aorta while type IIIB extends into the abdominal aorta (Fig. 11-2).

Cooley [23] described a classification based on the site of origin of the dissection. Type A dissections have intimal tears occurring above the level of the coronary ostia. There may be extension of the dissection into the descending and abdominal aorta or beyond. Aortic valvular regurgitation frequently results and injuries to the coronary arteries may also occur. In type B dissections the site of origin is distal to the aortic arch and the dissection proceeds distally. In some instances, however, the dissection may also extend proximally into the ascending aorta (Fig. 11-3).

Still another classification, proposed by Daily and associates [24], is based on the approach to therapy. Type A includes all proximal dissections and those distal dissections that extend retrograde

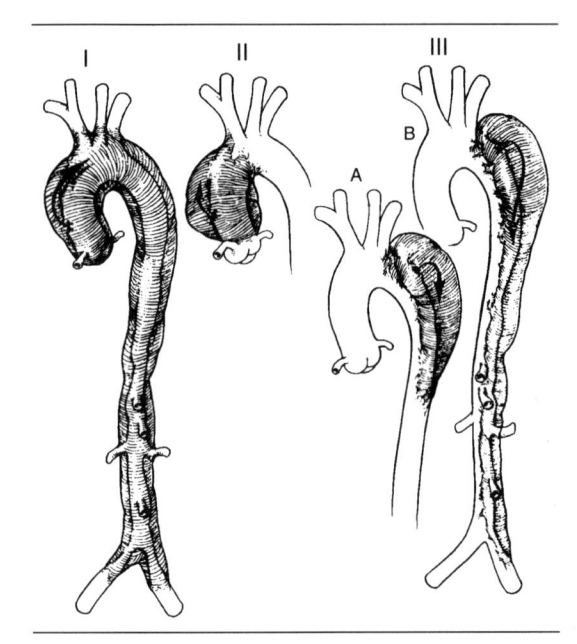

Fig. 11-2. DeBakey classification of dissecting aneurysms of the thoracic aorta. Type I: The dissection and the intimal tear arises in the ascending aorta and extends distally for a variable distance. Type II: The dissection is limited to the ascending aorta. Type III: The dissection arises in the descending thoracic aorta and extends distally for a variable distance. Type IIIA is limited to the descending thoracic aorta, and in type IIIB the dissection extends into the abdominal aorta. (Reprinted with permission from DA Cooley, *Surgical Treatment of Aortic Aneurysms*. Philadelphia: Saunders, 1986. P 44.)

to the arch and the ascending aorta. Type B refers to all other distal dissections without proximal extension.

Signs and Symptoms

By far the most common presenting symptom at aortic dissection is severe pain, which is found in over 90 percent of cases [25]. In fact, those patients without pain usually have suffered some disturbance of consciousness as a result of the dissection interfering with their cerebral blood flow. The pain, which is often described as having a "tearing" or "ripping" quality, is frequently most severe at its inception, contrasting with the pain of myocardial ischemia and infarction, which often increases in a

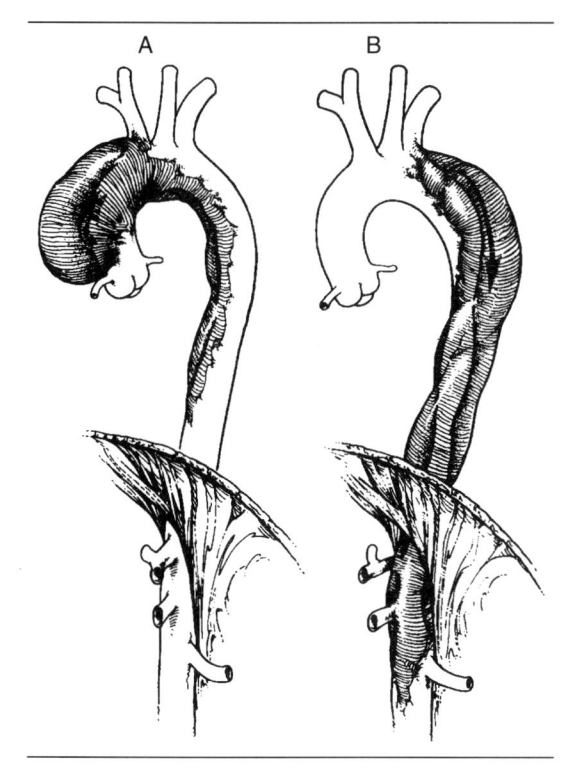

Fig. 11-3. Cooley classification of dissecting aneurysms, based on the site of origin. In type A aneurysms the intimal tear occurs transversely above the level of the coronary orifices. Type A cases may have extension of the dissection into the descending and abdominal aorta or beyond. In type B aneurysms the site of origin is distal to the aortic arch, and the dissection proceeds distally. In some instances, the dissection may extend proximally into the ascending aorta. Indications for surgical intervention vary between these two types of aneurysms, especially in acute cases. (Reprinted with permission from DA Cooley, *Surgical Treatment of Aortic Aneurysms*. Philadelphia: Saunders, 1986. P 45.)

crescendo pattern described as a squeezing or crushing pain. Vasovagal manifestations, such as diaphoresis, apprehension, nausea, vomiting, and lightheadedness, are common at the outset.

The location of the pain also helps in suggesting the diagnosis. Although pain may be felt simultaneously in the anterior and posterior chest with both proximal and distal dissection, the absence of posterior interscapular pain strongly mitigates against a distal dissection. Pain in the neck, throat, and arm is common in ascending aortic or arch dissections.

Other less common modes of presentation include congestive heart failure with or without associated chest pain, cerebrovascular accidents, syncope, paraplegia, and pulse loss with or without ischemic pain. Heart failure usually results from severe acute aortic regurgitation secondary to the dissection or from disruption of the origin of a coronary artery. Syncope without focal neurologic signs may signify rupture of the dissection into the pericardial cavity with cardiac tamponade [26].

Aortic regurgitation is an important feature of proximal dissection and occurs in over 50 percent of cases. There are three mechanisms of aortic regurgitation in proximal dissections: First, the dissection may dilate the aortic root, widening the annulus so that the aortic leaflets are unable to coapt in diastole; second, in an asymmetric dissection, pressure from the dissecting hematoma may depress one leaflet below the line of closure of the others; and third, the annular support of the leaflets or the leaflets themselves may be torn so as to render the valve incompetent.

Neurologic deficits associated with aortic dissection include cerebrovascular accidents, ischemic peripheral neuropathy, ischemic paraparesis, and disturbances of consciousness [27]. Each of these is more common with proximal dissection, but deficits in the lower extremities are equally frequent in proximal and distal dissection.

Other associated clinical manifestations include Horner's syndrome due to compression of the superior cervical sympathetic ganglion, vocal cord paralysis, and hoarseness from pressure against the left recurrent laryngeal nerve. Superior mediastinal syndrome with superior vena caval compression [28], tracheal or bronchial compression with bronchospasm [29], hemorrhage into the tracheobronchial tree with hemoptysis [30], hematemesis due to perforation into the esophagus [31], and heart block from retrograde burrowing of a dissection into the interatrial septum and then down into the atrioventricular (AV) node [32].

Pleural effusions result from rupture of the dissection into one of the pleural spaces. Additional complications may result from occlusion of important arteries by the dissection; mesenteric infarction, renal infarction, and myocardial infarction are among the most serious occlusive events (Table 11-1).

Table 11-1. Characteristics of type A and type B aortic dissections

Characteristic	Type A	Type B
Frequency	65–70%	30–35%
Average age	50–55 yr	60–70 yr
Associated hypertension	50%	80%
Arterial pressure on admission	50% normal or elevated 20% hypotensive	80% normal or elevated
Pain	Anterior, substernal	Posterior, midscapular
Associated atherosclerosis	+/−	++
Aortic regurgitation	50%	10%
Diastolic murmur	50%	10%
Pericardial effusion	++	++
Pleural effusion	+/−	++ (left pleura)
Syncope	++	Rare
Hemiparesis or hemiplegia	+	−
Paraparesis or paraplegia	+/−	+
Acute mortality	90–95%	40%
Renal-intestinal infarction	+	+
Myocardial infarction	+	Rare

− = absent; +/− = occasionally present; + = usually present; ++ = almost always present.
Source: Adapted with permission from MA Ergin, JD Galla, S Lansman, and RB Griepp, Acute dissections of the aorta: Current surgical treatment. Surg Clin North Am 65:721–741, 1985.

Diagnostic Techniques

Routine laboratory studies are not very helpful in making the diagnosis of aortic dissection. Anemia may develop from significant hemorrhage. A mild to moderate polymorphonuclear leukocytosis (10,000–14,000/mm^3) is common. Lactic acid dehydrogenase (LDH) and bilirubin levels are sometimes elevated because of hemolysis of blood sequestered within the false lumen. The electrocardiogram frequently shows left ventricular hypertrophy from preexistent hypertension and usually the absence of acute ischemic changes.

Diagnostic transthoracic ultrasound (M-mode) in combination with cross-sectional (two-dimensional) echocardiography is helpful in the detection of a proximal dissection by revealing a widened aortic root with delineation of the dissecting hematoma [33]. Computed tomographic (CT) scan with contrast injection is quite accurate in defining both ascending and descending thoracic aortic dissections, provided a false lumen is identified to distinguish the dissection from a fusiform aneurysm [34].

Chest roentgenography and aortic angiography provide the most substantive laboratory means of initial and definitive diagnosis, respectively. Chest roentgenography almost always reveals an abnormally widened aortic contour [35]. A localized bulge may overlay the site of the origin, and the aortic silhouette will be widened wherever the dissection extends.

The single most important study in the diagnosis of aortic dissection has been aortic angiography. A good study has three objectives: to establish a definitive diagnosis, to identify the site of origin of the dissection, and to delineate the extent of the dissection and the distal circulation to vital organs.

Transesophageal echocardiography (TEE) has recently appeared as the new gold standard in diagnosing aortic dissections [36]. Because of the close anatomic relationship between the esophagus and the thoracic aorta, TEE allows visualization of the entire thoracic aorta including the aortic arch. An intimal flap within the aorta separates the true and false lumens. In most cases the true lumen is compressed by the false lumen. They can be differentiated by: (1) the systolic enlargement of the true lumen on M-mode echocardiography, (2) the demonstration of systolic forward flow in the true lumen and delayed flow or no flow in the false lumen using pulse-wave Doppler echocardiography, and (3) the demonstration of entry jets during systole at the entry tear using color-flow Doppler.

TEE has an additional advantage in that in these critically ill patients, with a 2 percent mortality per hour [37] and associated poor hemodynamic status or diminished renal function, or both, the examination can be performed quietly and safely at the bedside, in the intensive care unit, or in the emergency department without radiologic dye. In fact, the accuracy of TEE has reached such a level that some surgeons are operating with only a TEE and without a preoperative aortogram [38] (Fig. 11-4).

Magnetic resonance imaging (MRI) is capable of noninvasively examining most thoracic aortic abnormalities with few limitations. Details of aortic dissection and aneurysm, including their size and extent and involvement of major arch and abdominal branch vessels, are often seen with MRI. The limitations of MRI stem from the long scan time and strong magnetic field used. The relatively long scan time implies a sensitivity to motion artifact, which makes MRI less applicable in uncooperative, unstable, or claustrophobic patients. Also, patients dependent on devices with ferromagnetic properties, such as pacemakers, pulmonary artery catheters, cerebral aneurysm clips, and ventilators, cannot be examined by MRI [39].

Initial Management

All patients, regardless of type of dissection, are started on aggressive medical therapy to control pain and to prevent rupture or extension of the aortic dissection as soon as the diagnosis is suspected [40]. The goals of medical therapy are to decrease the velocity of left ventricular contraction (dp/dt) [41] and to reduce the systolic blood pressure to the lowest acceptable level that will maintain adequate cardiac, cerebral, and renal perfusion. Patients are

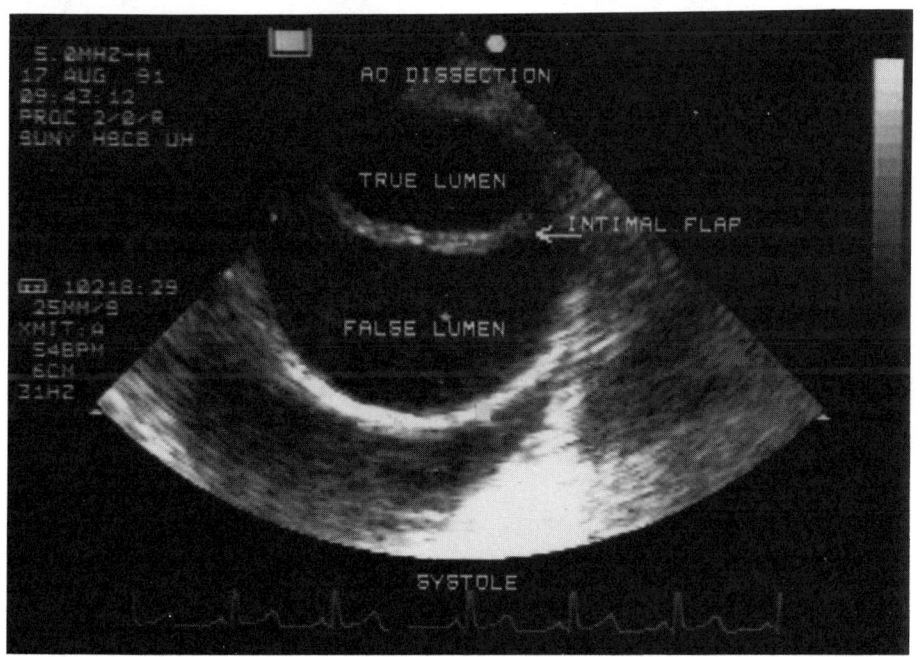

Fig. 11-4. A. Two-dimensional transesophageal echocardiographic image of an aortic dissection. The intimal flap is clearly visualized separating the true and false lumens within the aorta. Note the enlargement of the true lumen during systole. (*continued on next page*)

A

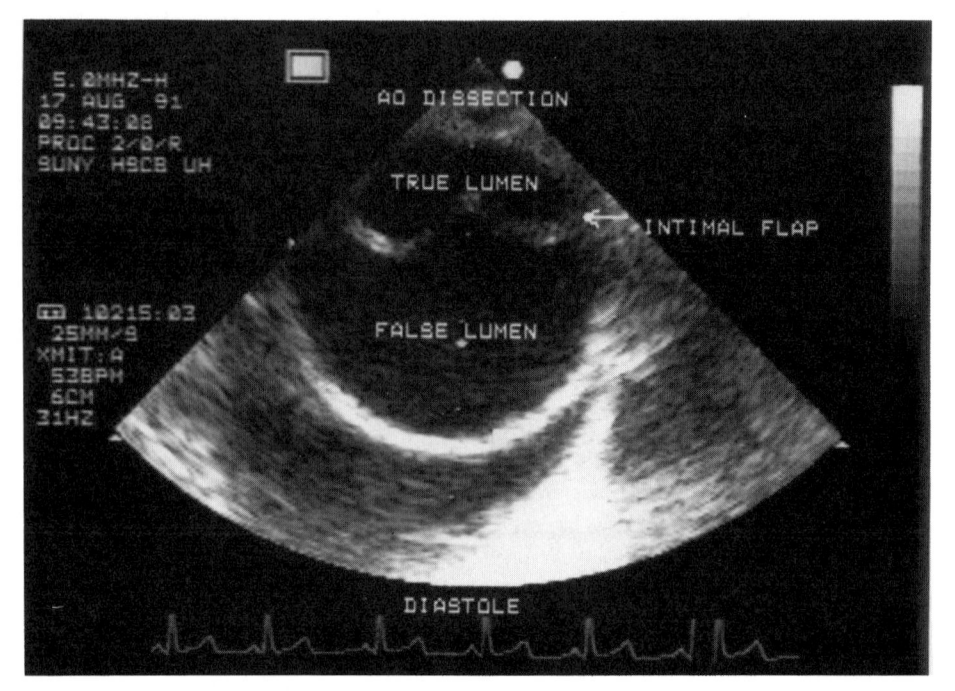

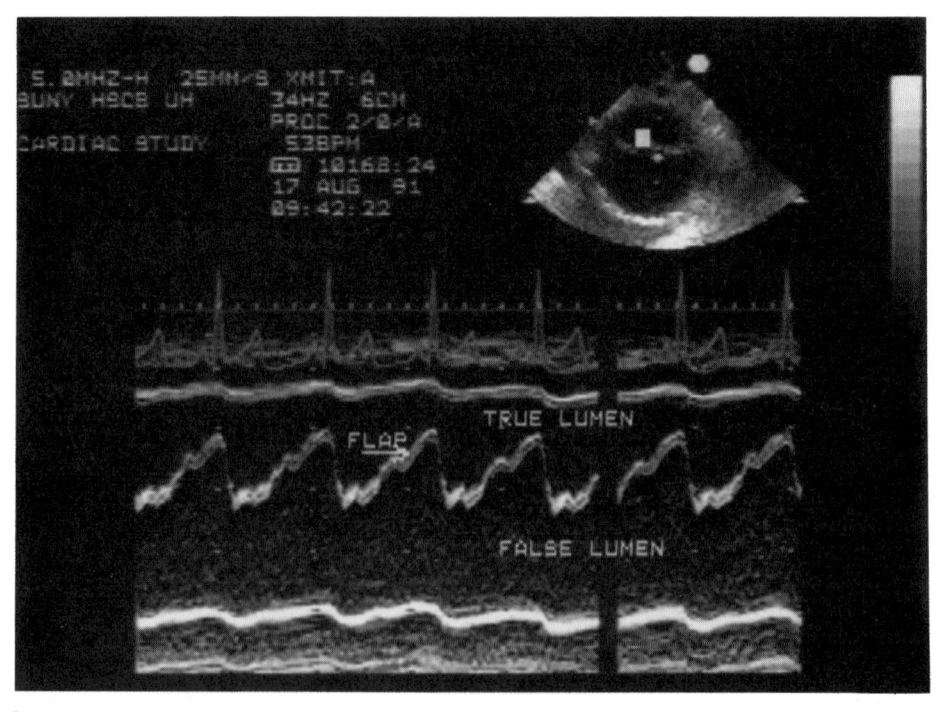

Fig. 11-4. (*continued*) B. The same patient during diastole. Note the decompression within the true lumen during diastole as the false lumen compresses the true lumen. C. M-mode image of thoracic aortic dissection. Note the systolic enlargement of the true lumen and the intimal flap separating the true lumen from the false lumen.

usually treated with intravenous morphine, to control pain caused by the dissection as well as to decrease anxiety levels and resultant catecholamine surges, which could cause an extension of the dissection. In addition, a combination of β-adrenergic blocking agents and vasodilators are used to control blood pressure. It is important to note that β-blockade should be established before the introduction of vasodilators; otherwise, any sudden drop in afterload would trigger an increase in left ventricular contractility and an increase in shearing force (dp/dt) to the aortic wall. β-Blockade can be induced with intravenous boluses of propranolol, 0.5 mg; labetalol, 5 to 10 mg; or esmolol, 0.5 to 1.0 mg/kg, followed by an intravenous infusion to reduce the heart rate to 60 to 70 beats per minute. In patients with asthma or severe chronic obstructive pulmonary disease, the β$_1$-selective esmolol or metoprolol, or verapamil, is preferred [42].

Vasodilator therapy is usually started with sodium nitroprusside titrated to reduce systolic blood pressure to 100 to 120 mm Hg, provided the patient continues to maintain an adequate urine output. Maintaining urine output will also help delay a build-up of cyanide through the excretion of the metabolite sodium thiocyanate [43].

A radial arterial catheter should be placed to accurately and continuously monitor arterial blood pressure and to obtain blood specimens for laboratory analysis. A left radial or femoral catheter should be placed in patients with a type A dissection as the innominate artery frequently is obstructed by the aortic crossclamp and/or may be involved in the aortic dissection. A right radial arterial line should be placed for all descending thoracic aortic aneurysm repairs as, similarly, the origin of the left subclavian artery may be occluded. A distal arterial line (femoral, dorsalis pedis, etc.) is usually placed in the operating room to measure perfusion pressures distal to the aortic crossclamp [44].

Continuous electrocardiographic monitoring should begin, with simultaneous lead II and V$_5$ capability to detect arrhythmias and myocardial ischemia. A central venous catheter is inserted to measure central venous pressure, as well as for the rapid administration of fluids and drugs. An internal jugular or median cephalic vein approach is frequently chosen, as the subclavian vein can be distorted or compressed by the enlarging aneurysm and accidental puncture of the aneurysm is possible. A pulmonary artery catheter should be inserted to measure hemodynamics and filling pressures, and as an aid in diagnosing pericardial tamponade in retrograde dissections. An indwelling bladder catheter should be inserted to measure hourly urine output, especially since descending thoracic aortic aneurysms have a tendency to extend to the abdominal aorta and disrupt renal artery perfusion. Proper judgment as to the appropriate balance between preoperative preparation and patient risk is extremely critical.

Upon the patient's arrival in the operating room, additional large-bore intravenous catheters for rapid fluid transfusion are placed. Pulse oximetry for continuous arterial oxygen saturation monitoring as well as end-tidal carbon dioxide analysis is also placed. Intraoperative TEE should be used to monitor cardiac function as well as to evaluate continuing aortic pathology. Core temperature monitoring to evaluate the effect of induced hypothermia should be used, and arterial blood gases, electrolytes, hematocrit, and coagulation studies should be rapidly available to the operating room team.

ANESTHETIC MANAGEMENT

Ascending Aortic Surgery

The induction of anesthesia should be tailored to the patient's pathology and condition. The scenario may range from a patient undergoing an elective repair of a dilated ascending aortic aneurysm without evidence of aortic valvular disease or dissection, to a patient rushed to the emergency room 30 minutes after eating a full dinner in cardiogenic shock from severe acute aortic valvular insufficiency secondary to a large proximal aortic dissection. In the acute setting the induction should be smooth and rapid but controlled with the aim to prevent tachycardia, increases in dp/dt, hypertension, and hypotension. Small to moderate doses of narcotics, benzodiazepines, ketamine, and thiopental, or some combination of these drugs, can be used, depending on the patient's hemodynamic and volume status. This should be followed by high-dose muscle relaxant, cricoid pressure, and rapid endotracheal intubation. For elective aneurysm repair higher induction doses of narcotics are used and a slower and more controlled increase in the depth of anesthesia is achieved. The addition of intravenous esmolol, sodium nitroprusside, lidocaine, further intravenous anesthetics, or the administration of potent inhalation agents can be used for more precise control of arterial blood pressure. The treatment of hypotension can include the infusion of fluids or the administration of a vasopressor such as phenylephrine. Multiple units of packed red blood cells should be available in the operating room, with fluid warmers, before the induction of anesthesia, as well as a Cell Saver to process and transfuse blood to the patient in the event of a sudden aortic rupture.

The femoral artery is cannulated for cardiopulmonary bypass and a single venous cannula is inserted into the right atrium for venous return to the bypass pump. If there is a significant risk of aortic rupture with sternotomy or if severe aortic insufficiency with pericardial tamponade is present, femoral arterial–femoral venous bypass can be instituted before sternotomy [45].

An isolated ascending aortic aneurysm can sometimes be resected and replaced with a single interpositional tubular graft [17]. Frequently, however, the coronary ostia or the aortic valve is involved, necessitating placement of an aortic valve conduit. Additionally, replacement of the proximal ascending aorta requires reestablishing coronary blood flow. The initial technique reported by Bentall and DeBono [46] in 1968 described replacing the aortic valve and proximal aorta with a valve conduit and reimplanting the coronary arteries directly into the conduit. More recently, Cabrol and associates [47] have introduced a technically easier procedure of connecting the right and left coronary ostia to a tubular graft and then creating a side-to-side anastomosis with the valve conduit to reestablish coronary blood flow. Additionally, intermittent coronary perfusion with cold cardioplegia can easily be given through the tubular graft for added myocardial protection (Fig. 11-5).

Surgery on the ascending thoracic aorta can involve long bypass times [48, 49] and, therefore, can

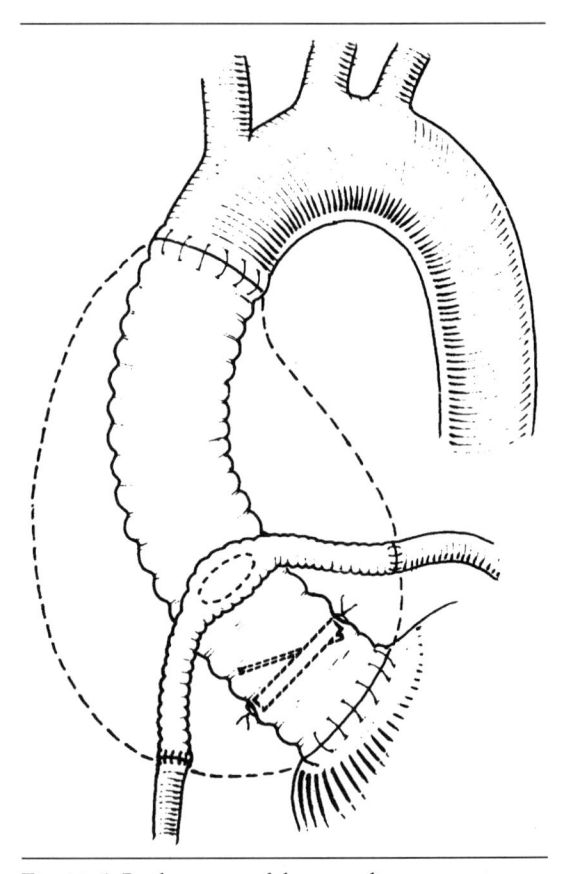

Fig. 11-5. Replacement of the ascending aorta using a tubular graft containing a prosthetic aortic valve and reimplantation of the coronary arteries by an intermediate tubular graft. (Reprinted with permission from C Cabrol et al, Long-term results with total replacement of the ascending aorta and reimplantation of the coronary arteries. *J Thorac Cardiovasc Surg* 91:17, 1986.)

be associated with pump-induced coagulation disorders, such as platelet dysfunction, dilution of clotting factors, or primary and secondary fibrinolysis. Complications in addition to hemorrhage include myocardial infarction, acute left ventricular failure requiring inotropic support, renal failure, and focal neurologic deficits [49].

Aortic Arch Repair

The basic principles of preoperative assessment and anesthetic induction for repair of the aortic arch are similar to those described for ascending aortic aneurysm repair. As the proximal ascending aorta will be crossclamped, total cardiopulmonary bypass is necessary to facilitate this procedure. The major difficulty encountered during aortic arch repair revolves around providing metabolic protection to the brain during the period that cerebral blood flow is interrupted (Fig. 11-6).

Profound hypothermia is a technique for cerebral protection that has long been used during surgical repair of congenital cardiac lesions in infancy [50, 51]. In 1975, Griepp and associates [52] introduced the concept of profound hypothermic circulatory arrest as a means of cerebral protection during the period that the brachiocephalic vessels must be opened when an arch aneurysm is being repaired. Ott, Frazier, and Cooley [53], in 1978, reported their results with profound hypothermic circulatory arrest and noted only one patient with postoperative cerebral deficits. In 1985, Casthely and colleagues [54] reported on a series of 17 patients in whom they had a successful result using deep hypothermia and circulatory arrest.

There is much controversy surrounding the methods of inducing hypothermia, as well as the question of what temperature is the effective endpoint. In 1971, Subramanian and associates [55] described the method of surface-induced deep hypothermia for cardiac surgery. Griepp [52, 54], in his initial descriptions, employed both surface and core cooling. Surface cooling was induced by placing the anesthetized patient on a cooling blanket set at 27°C. The entire body including the head and neck was packed with small plastic bags filled with ice chips. The genital organs, nose, eyes, ears, toes, and fingers were protected with gauze pads to avoid thermal injuries to these delicate areas. When the esophageal temperature reached 30°C, the ice was removed, the patient prepped and draped, and median sternotomy performed. The left femoral artery was cannulated for perfusion, the right atrium was cannulated for venous return, the patient was heparinized, and total cardiopulmonary bypass was commenced. The heart was arrested with cold cardioplegia in the usual manner. The patient's core continued to be cooled on cardiopulmonary bypass, while the surgical dissection continued until a rectal temperature of 12 to 14°C was achieved. At this point, after pharmacologic

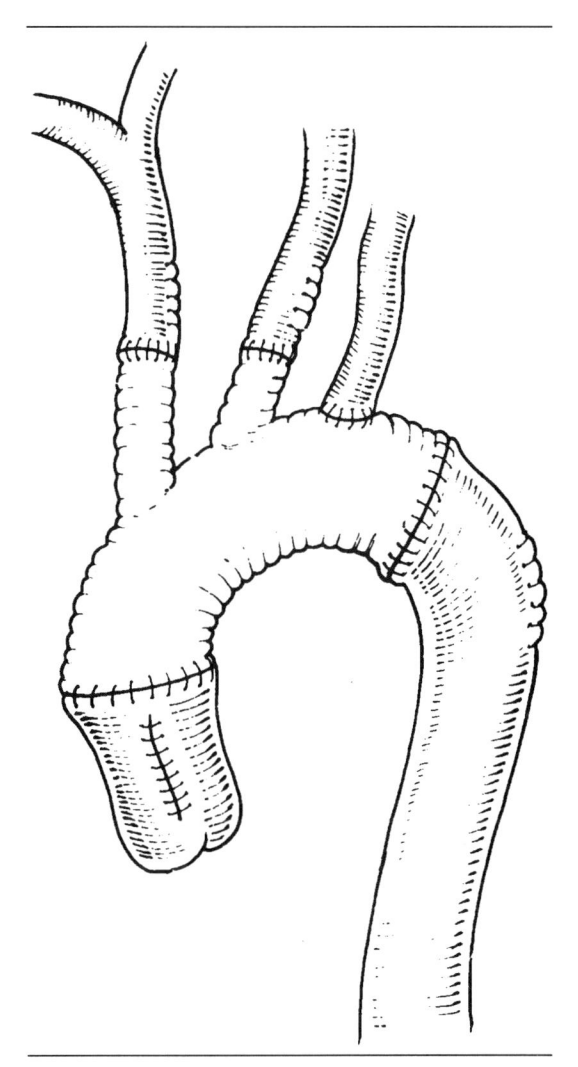

Fig. 11-6. Drawing illustrating complete replacement of the transverse aortic arch with a prosthetic graft. Note that the distal aortic anastomosis and all the brachiocephalic anastomoses must be performed with total circulatory arrest. (Reprinted by permission from ME DeBakey, Changing concepts in vascular surgery. *J Cardiovasc Surg* 27:367, 1986.)

intervention, the cardiopulmonary bypass pump was turned off, the arch vessels were individually clamped, and the aortic arch was opened. One of the complications initially associated with surface cooling was the difficulty in predicting the temperature at which a particular patient's heart would spontaneously fibrillate. Fibrillation at this time, with the chest closed, is especially dangerous due to the possibility of left ventricular distention. Additionally, defibrillation and resuscitation may be more difficult. Most centers now omit surface cooling.

Many authors have tried to identify the optimal temperature for cerebral protection. Ergin and Griepp [56] and O'Connor and associates [57] noted good cerebral protection for 60 minutes of circulatory arrest in dogs at 15°C and for periods of 15 to 59 minutes at temperatures ranging from 11 to 18°C in humans. Crawford and colleagues [58, 59], using only core cooling, found rectal temperatures of between 12 and 20°C to offer good cerebral protection for up to 75 minutes. They maintain the operating room at 15°C to prevent external rewarming by the environment. They believe that the optimal level of hypothermia safe for total circulatory arrest exists when the pupils are fully dilated and the electroencephalogram is isoelectric. This usually occurs at a rectal temperature of 22°C; however, considering the tendency toward upward drift, a lower temperature would be desirable at the onset of vessel occlusion.

The most important component of cerebral protection is hypothermia. However, other techniques are available to preserve cerebral function. Hemodilution, a common component of cardiopulmonary bypass technique, should be used for all circulatory arrest cases. Crystalloid, added to the priming solution of the bypass pump, lowers the hematocrit, thereby decreasing blood viscosity and improving the rheologic properties of blood [60, 61].

Various pharmacologic agents have been shown to be beneficial in reducing the incidence of neurologic injury in patients undergoing aortic arch repair. Thiopental, at a dose of 5 to 15 mg/kg bolus injection before total circulatory arrest, can reliably produce an isoelectric electroencephalogram and has been shown to offer some cerebral protection, particularly from particulate matter or air embolization, which can occur during aortic arch surgery [62]. Mannitol 0.5 gm/kg, given before cardiopulmonary bypass, may help to attenuate postischemic cerebral edema and has been shown to reduce infarct size in experimental models [63, 64]. The addition of furosemide may also attenuate increases in intracranial pressure [65]. These two drugs also have the advantage of helping to establish adequate urine output before and after circulatory arrest. A large dose of steroids (methylprednisolone; sodium succinate, 15 mg/kg; or dexamethasone, 0.5 mg/kg) is commonly given before total circulatory arrest; however, the experimental data to support this are inconclusive [54, 64, 66]. An additional dose of muscle relaxant should also be given before circulatory arrest since even at temperatures below 15°C, patients can make occasional gasping attempts at respiration and as the patient starts to rewarm, an unparalyzed muscle may start to shiver and cause an increase of oxygen consumption. Other drugs, such as phenytoin [67], the calcium channel blocker nimodipine [68], and possibly high-dose midazolam [69], have been reported to be potentially useful for cerebral protection.

Hyperglycemia should be avoided by minimizing the use of glucose-containing fluids during cardiopulmonary bypass. Neurologic outcome has been correlated negatively with increased levels of plasma glucose during cerebral ischemia. The mechanism of cerebral damage after glucose loading is believed to be an increased rate of anaerobic metabolism with greater lactate production, resulting in tissue damage during ischemia [66, 70]. Nitrous oxide should probably be avoided during circulatory arrest procedures, as well as in any other procedure that has a propensity for cerebral air embolization.

Before the crossclamps are removed from the cerebral vessels, the patient should be placed in a steep Trendelenburg position, the pump should be turned on slowly to fill the descending aorta and arch, and the clamps should be removed. The cerebral vessels can then gently be milked free of any isolated air pockets before complete cerebral blood flow is reestablished. Some recommend occluding carotid flow by manually pressing down on both carotid arteries during the first 30 seconds of reperfusion. The patient should be rewarmed to a rectal temperature of 36°C before cardiopulmonary bypass is terminated. One of the disadvantages of profound hypothermia is the long period of rewarming (78–139 minutes), which is often associated with excessive bleeding. One series described the use of 10 to 20 units of platelets, packed red blood cells, and fresh frozen plasma, which were given with protamine at the termination of cardiopulmonary bypass [58].

Shenaq and Crawford [71] believe that primary fibrinolysis is a major cause of deep hypothermic circulatory arrest–induced coagulopathy. They recommend combining protamine with ε-aminocaproic acid immediately upon the termination of cardiopulmonary bypass.

Descending Thoracic Aortic Surgery

The approach to a patient with a descending thoracic aortic aneurysm or a thoracoabdominal aortic aneurysm differs greatly from that of the previously described proximal lesions. While almost all patients with a type I or II aortic dissection are treated surgically, much controversy still exists regarding the appropriate management of type III lesions. Some authors recommend urgent surgical repair while others opt for initial medical therapy and then schedule elective surgical repair under optimal conditions [72–75]. The mortality for medically treated patients with type I or II dissections is 88 percent while the mortality for those treated surgically is only 23 percent. However, with type III injuries, the mortality is only 32 percent for medical therapy and 36 percent for surgical therapy [76]. In addition, while almost all proximal lesions are treated in the realm of cardiac surgery utilizing the cardiopulmonary bypass pump, distal lesions are frequently treated by vascular surgeons, without the assistance of cardiopulmonary bypass.

Intraoperative bleeding should be a major concern to the anesthesiologist when preparing for this operation. Since repair is frequently performed without the use of cardiopulmonary bypass, one must rely on peripheral sites for rapid fluid resuscitation. Saleh [77] reported that the average blood product usage at Baylor University included 10 units of packed red blood cells, 7.2 units of fresh frozen plasma, and 13 units of platelets. This author recommended four 14-gauge peripheral intravenous catheters, two in the upper extremities and two in the lower extremities, to rapidly replace volume; a single No. 8.5 French catheter was as effective as two 14-gauge peripheral lines. This was in addition to two arterial lines and a pulmonary artery catheter. Blood warmers should be used to maintain the patient's body temperature during the period of rapid transfusion, and a Cell Saver autotransfusion device can decrease the requirement for homologous blood product transfusion.

The induction of anesthesia is similar to that previously described for more proximal lesions. The aim should be to prevent tachycardia, hypertension, and hypotension. Most patients arrive in the operating room pretreated with β-blockers and vasodilators. In patients with acute dissection, the induction should be smooth and rapid but controlled. In these individuals, anesthesia should be induced intravenously, with small to moderate doses of narcotic, ketamine, benzodiazepine, or thiopental (or some combination of these drugs, depending on the starting blood pressure and the degree of hypovolemia present). This should be followed by profound muscle relaxation, cricoid pressure, and rapid endotracheal intubation. For elective aneurysm repair, higher doses of narcotics are used and a more controlled environment is achieved.

The descending thoracic aorta is more easily approached through a left thoracotomy incision than with a median sternotomy. Use of a double-lumen tube and one-lung anesthesia and ventilation is strongly advocated for these procedures, for many reasons. Firstly, as with other thoracic surgical procedures, surgical exposure of the left chest and the mediastinum is greatly assisted with collapse of the left lung. Secondly, the dilated dissected aorta can be adherent to many related structures and the delicate surgical dissection and mobilization of structures are easier with the left lung collapsed. Thirdly, surgical manipulation and retraction can result in bleeding into the lung parenchyma and with an unprotected dependent lung, this hemorrhage could spill over into the dependent right lung and could impair ventilation. This would be complicated further if the patient required heparinization. Therefore, one-lung ventilation offers many benefits to the patient.

It is imperative that the double-lumen tube be placed in the proper position to function properly. Before insertion both cuffs should be tested. The tracheal cuff, a low-pressure and high-volume balloon, can accommodate up to 20 cc air. The bronchial cuff, in proper position, should only require a maximum of 3 cc to fully occlude the bronchial lumen. Any additional volume could cause herniation of the cuff back toward the carina and result in obstruction of the contralateral lung. The tube is inserted with the bronchial tip curved concave facing anteriorly. Once the bronchial balloon passes the vocal cords, the stylet should be removed and the tube should be rotated 90 degrees. Left-sided tubes should be rotated to the left and right-sided tubes to the right. The tube should then be advanced until moderate resistance is felt. The tracheal cuff should be inflated to seal the trachea, and bilateral breath sounds should be confirmed. If breath sounds are only unilateral, a deep endobronchial intubation may have occurred and the tube should be withdrawn slightly [78]. Next, the bronchial cuff should be inflated and bilateral breath sounds should be checked again to ascertain that the bronchial cuff has not herniated to obstruct air flow to the other lung. Third, the individual lumens of the tube should be alternatively clamped and clear breath sounds should be present on the contralateral side, with absence of breath sounds on the ipsilateral side. It is very helpful to check the peak airway pressures while confirming proper tube placement to make sure that major increases in airway pressure are not occurring. Rupture of the bronchus is one of the more serious complications that can occur [79].

Currently, the optimal method for ascertaining tube placement is direct visualization of the carina with a fiberoptic bronchoscope. Smith and associates [80] demonstrated that when the double-lumen tube was thought to be in the correct position by auscultation and physical examination, fiberoptic bronchoscopy showed that 48 percent of tubes were, in fact, malpositioned. Pediatric fiberoptic bronchoscopes are available in 5.6-, 4.9-, and 3.6-mm external diameters. The 4.9-mm diameter bronchoscope can be passed through a 37 French and larger double-lumen tube. The 3.6-mm diameter bronchoscope can be passed through all standard double-lumen tubes. The larger-diameter bronchoscope will provide better optical detail of the respiratory tract. When the tube is properly positioned, the bronchial cuff should be visualized as being just distal to the carina in the appropriate mainstream bronchus.

The anesthesiologist should use an inspired oxygen concentration (FIO_2) of 1.0 during one-lung ventilation. This high FIO_2 helps to protect against hypoxemia. Normally, collapse of the nonventilated, nondependent lung results in hypoxic pulmonary vasoconstriction (HPV). This causes local increases in pulmonary vascular resistance (PVR) and diversion of blood flow to other better-oxygenated parts of the pulmonary bed (i.e., the dependent oxygenated and ventilated lung) [81]. Pulse oximetry must be used during one-lung ventilation (as with all anesthetics); however, in this case rapid assessment of oxygenation is extremely important and blood gas analysis may involve some delay [82]. It should be noted that the sensor should be placed on the right extremity or the head, lest the aortic crossclamp alter blood flow to the pulse oximeter sensor and erroneous readings be observed.

Many studies have shown that should the arterial oxygen saturation fall, the single most effective maneuver to increase PaO_2 during one-lung ventilation is the application of continuous positive airway pressure (CPAP) to the nondependent lung. This will increase perfusion to the ventilated lung and a low level of CPAP (5–10 cm H_2O) maintains the patency of the nondependent alveoli, allowing some apneic oxygenation to occur [83–85]. The application of high-level CPAP is not recommended as, at this pressure, the lung becomes overdistended and interferes with surgical exposure. CPAP can be applied to the nonventilated lung using a number of easy-to-construct apparatuses [86–89], the salient parts of which are an oxygen source, tubing to connect the oxygen source to the nonventilated lung, a pressure relief valve, and a pressure gauge (Fig. 11-7).

Positive end-expiratory pressure (PEEP) has been used on the dependent lung to increase PaO_2, with varying results [83, 84]. The beneficial effect of PEEP is an increased lung volume at end expiration (FRC), which improves the ventilation-perfusion (V/Q) relationship in the dependent lung. This increase in FRC prevents airway and alveolar closure at end expiration. However, PEEP has also been shown to cause compression of the small intraalveolar vessels and thereby to result in increased PVR. Since this increase is only limited to the dependent lung, blood flow can be diverted to the nondependent lung, increasing V/Q mismatch and further decreasing PaO_2.

Many of the anesthesiologist's concerns revolve around the effects of crossclamping the descending

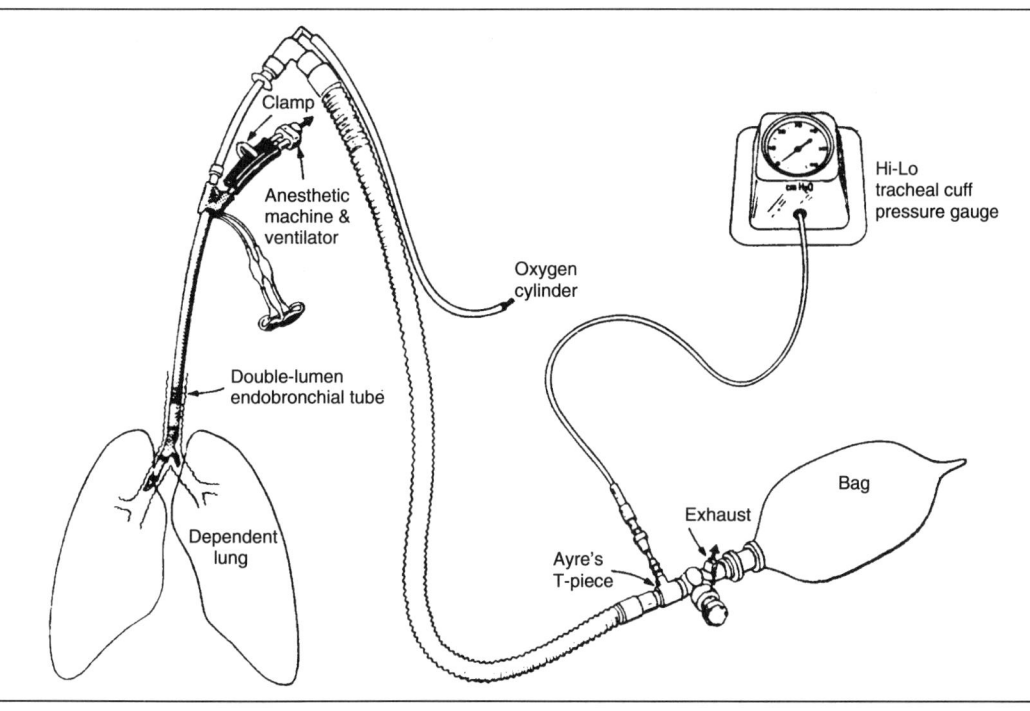

Fig. 11-7. A device for applying continuous positive airway pressure (CPAP) to the nonventilated lung during one-lung ventilation utilizing a pediatric system, an endotracheal cuff pressure gauge, and an exhaust valve. (Reprinted with permission from S Thiagarajah, C Job, and A Rao, A device for applying CPAP to the nonventilated upper lung during one-lung ventilation. *Anesthesiology* 60:254, 1984.)

thoracic aorta. When the aorta is crossclamped just distal to the origin of the left subclavian artery, there is a risk of paraplegia and paraparesis [90, 91]. Although the incidence is higher with distal descending aortic procedures, it can also occur following repair of coarctation, traumatic transections, and even resection of infrarenal aneurysms. The ischemic change is similar to that observed in the anterior spinal artery syndrome after occlusion of the arteria radicularis magna anterior (the artery of Adamkiewicz) [92]. This syndrome is characterized by loss of motor function and pinprick sensation, with preservation of vibratory and position sense [93].

One must understand the anatomy of the blood supply to the spinal cord to fully appreciate the relationship of spinal cord damage to aortic crossclamping. The blood supply of the spinal cord, first described in 1882 by Adamkiewicz [94], is provided by two posterior spinal arteries and one anterior spinal artery. In the adult, six to eight radicular arteries, branches of the intercostal arteries, supply the single anterior spinal artery, with between 10 and 23 arteries supplying the posterior spinal arteries. The anterior spinal artery is quite variable and may be well developed, being fed by few radicular branches, or it may be small and segmental and associated with a greater number of radicular arteries [95]. The anterior spinal artery supplies at least 75 percent of the cord, leaving only 25 percent or less to be supplied by the posterior spinal arteries. Superiorly, the anterior spinal artery is supported by collaterals, which derive from the circle of Willis, and inferiorly by radicular branches from the internal iliac arteries. Flow in these vessels is rarely affected by aortic crossclamping [96]. Collateral circulation through the anterior spinal artery at the lower thoracic and lumbar area is precarious, with the principal arterial supply to the anterior spinal artery in this region coming from the artery of Adamkiewicz [97] (Fig. 11-8).

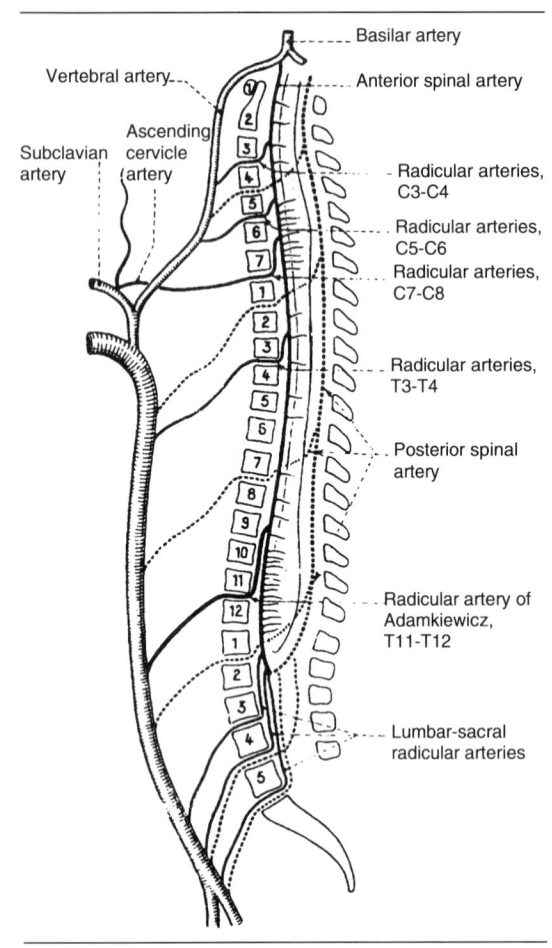

Fig. 11-8. Diagram of spinal cord blood supply. Note radicular arteries supplying both the anterior and posterior spinal arteries. Also note large distal radicular artery of Adamkiewicz joining the anterior spinal artery between T9 and T11. (Reprinted by permission from JE Connolly, Prevention of paraplegia secondary to operations on the aorta. *J Cardiovasc Surg* 27:410, 1986.)

Table 11-2. Origin of the artery of Adamkiewicz

Spinal segment	Percentage of patients in whom Adamkiewicz occurs
T5–T8	15
T9–T12	60
L1	14
L2	10
Below L3	<2

The artery of Adamkiewicz leaves the aorta as a single branch in over 60 percent of cases and is also quite variable in its origin (Table 11-2). This extreme variability in blood supply and the variability in continuity of the anterior spinal artery contribute to the unpredictability of cord preservation during thoracic aortic surgery [92].

High resistance is a characteristic of any blood supply based on small collateral vessels. Moreover, fluid pressure in the cerebrospinal fluid represents a second barrier to blood flow. Spinal cord ischemia occurs whenever the capillary perfusion pressure drops below the intraspinal pressure. Spinal cord perfusion pressure (SCPP) equals the mean arterial pressure (MAP) minus intraspinal pressure (ISP). Therefore, if the MAP supplying the artery of Adamkiewicz is decreased as a result of surgical transection of this artery or if the origin of the artery lies between the proximal and distal aortic crossclamps, the spinal cord will be ischemic. Similarly, ischemia may also occur as a result of an increase in intracranial or intraspinal pressure developing during the period of aortic crossclamping [98–100]. For these reasons, distal blood pressure high enough to overcome these resistances is necessary to ensure flow and maintain cord viability. Many authors have attempted to decrease intraspinal pressure as a method to improve neurologic outcome. In the 1960s, Blaisdell and Cooley [98] and Miyamoto and associates [101] reported that the drainage of cerebrospinal fluid before aortic crossclamping, in dogs, significantly decreased the incidence of paraplegia. Oka and Miyamoto [102] and McCullough and associates [103] confirmed the earlier data and stressed the importance of spinal cord perfusion pressure. They noted a 100 percent incidence of paraplegia in dogs, which did not have an adequate relative perfusion pressure and no paraplegia if the pressure gradient between the distal aorta and the cerebrospinal fluid was maintained at 15 mm Hg or greater. Wadouh and colleagues [92], using a porcine model, saw no improvement in neurologic outcome with cerebrospinal fluid drainage, in contrast to the previous reports.

The effect of sodium nitroprusside and aortic crossclamping on intraspinal pressure has generated much controversy. Crossclamping the descending thoracic aorta will cause an increase in arterial blood pressure above the crossclamp that is 30 to 48 percent over the preclamp values [104–109]. It will also cause a decrease in arterial blood pressure below the crossclamp of 78 to 89 percent. Simultaneous measurements show an increase in cerebrospinal fluid pressure. A possible mechanism of the rise in intraspinal pressure after crossclamping of the thoracic aorta is that as the proximal aortic pressure exceeds the limits of cerebral autoregulation, cerebral blood flow and cerebral blood volume increase, thereby causing an increase in intracranial pressure and in intraspinal pressure. The addition of sodium nitroprusside, as demonstrated by Nugent and colleagues [105] and Shine and Nugent [105a], will cause a further decrease in distal aortic pressures and a further increase in intraspinal pressure, placing spinal cord perfusion pressure in the ischemic range. It is recommended that pressures in the femoral artery and spinal cord be monitored during the crossclamp period, and if the perfusion pressure approaches ischemic levels, a shunting procedure should be performed.

Other methods have been tried to decrease the incidence of spinal cord ischemia. Blaisdell and Cooley [98] showed that removing cerebrospinal fluid reduces intraspinal pressure and decreases the incidence of paraplegia. This practice is still followed in some centers. One should note that the cerebrospinal fluid should not be drained during the period when cerebrospinal fluid pressure is high to protect against possible herniation; therefore, it should be removed before aortic crossclamping. Additionally, if paraplegia does occur after spinal fluid drainage, a subdural hematoma at the level of the drainage catheter must be ruled out despite the fact that spinal cord ischemia is more probable.

Mild hypothermia has been shown to be protective against spinal cord ischemia. Vacanti and Ames [106] showed in the rabbit model that a temperature reduction of 3°C during the period of circulatory impairment caused a doubling of the duration of ischemia that could be reversibly sustained. Pontius and associates [107] showed that the spinal cord can recover normal function after ischemia of 60 minutes' duration at a whole-body temperature of 30°C. Coles and colleagues [108], in a canine model, showed that hypothermic perfusion of the spinal cord itself could similarly offer protection during aortic crossclamping.

Drummond and associates [109], using a rabbit model, demonstrated that moderate elevation of the serum glucose before and during the period of spinal cord ischemia is associated with a markedly poorer neurologic outcome. This difference could not be explained by differences in osmolarity, cardiovascular function, or systemic acid-base parameters. It may be a result of increased lactate production during or after the period of ischemia similar to that seen with hyperglycemia in the face of cerebral ischemia [70]. For this reason, routine administration of dextrose-containing solutions is not recommended.

Laschinger and associates [110], using a dog model, demonstrated spinal cord protection by corticosteroids. Dogs pretreated with steroids had no neurologic injury, while dogs not pretreated had a 67 percent incidence of spastic paraplegia. This protective effect of steroids does not seem to be related to an effect on spinal cord perfusion pressure, but rather has a stabilizing effect on the cellular level.

Kirshner and associates [111], in a dog model, demonstrated that a combination of hypothermic crystalloid perfusate, barbiturates, and superoxide dismutase significantly decreased the neurologic deficits after 40 minutes of aortic occlusion. In 1991, Granke and colleagues [112] also demonstrated significantly decreased neurologic deficits in dogs pretreated with cerebrospinal fluid drainage and intravenous superoxide dismutase.

Crossclamping the descending thoracic aorta has major implications regarding myocardial function as well. It will consistently increase the mean arterial pressure above the crossclamp by approximately 30 to 48 percent [104, 105, 113–116]. Central venous pressure increases approximately 5 mm Hg and pulmonary capillary wedge pressure (PCWP) will also increase between 2 and 12 mm Hg. Cardiac index will decrease [117]. Transesophageal echocardiography is a useful adjunct to the standard thermodilution pulmonary artery catheter in monitoring the acute effects of aortic crossclamping on myocardial function [118]. Sodium nitroprusside or nitroglycerin has been used for acute management of left ventricular failure secondary to aortic crossclamping.

Another method involves mechanically shunting blood from an area proximal to the aortic crossclamp to the distal aorta. This has the additional benefit of shunting blood to the distal aorta, which will increase spinal cord perfusion pressure and protect against spinal cord ischemia (as long as the blood supply to the spinal cord does not originate between the proximal and distal crossclamps). Many techniques have been described with and without the use of an extracorporeal pump system.

The Gott shunt is a heparin-coated tubular shunt that is used in many centers [119]. The proximal end can be placed in either the ascending aorta, the transverse arch, the left subclavian artery (if the proximal crossclamp is certain to be placed distal to the origin of the subclavian artery), or the apex of the left ventricle. The distal end of the shunt can be inserted directly into the lower descending thoracic aorta, or into the left femoral artery, in which case the lower thoracic and abdominal aortas are perfused retrogradely [120]. Because the Gott shunt is heparin coated, systemic heparinization is not required and intrathoracic bleeding is minimized [121].

Right atrial-to-femoral artery bypass has also been described [122, 123]. May and associates [122] used nonthrombogenic, polyurethane polyvinylgraphite–coated tubing for perfusing the lower half of the body. A cannula is inserted into the right atrium through the femoral vein and returns the blood to the femoral artery with the help of a pump. This perfuses the lower half of the body with mixed venous blood while the patient is ventilated with 100 percent oxygen. The PaO_2 in the mixed venous blood ranged from 34 to 41 mm Hg; the authors reported no adverse effects when the lower part of the body was perfused with blood at a low PaO_2. Despite these findings, some centers will use a pump-oxygenator circuit. The anesthesiologist manipulates the cardiovascular system, with the aim of achieving a normal or slightly increased upper-body arterial pressure while avoiding a left atrial pressure above 18 mm Hg.

The most frequently used method today is the left atrial-to-femoral artery bypass [124]. The necessity for an oxygenator is avoided as oxygenated blood is removed from the left atrium and reperfused into the femoral artery. This simultaneously reduces preload, effectively unloading the left ventricle, as well as maintaining perfusion to the distal aorta and spinal cord. The method also eliminates the necessity to cannulate the femoral vein and avoids the risk of causing postoperative venous thrombosis. Left atrial pressure can be measured by a pressure line incorporated into the cannula and flow rates can be set at 1.5 liters per minute to maintain a left atrial pressure of approximately 5 to 8 mm Hg. Laschinger and associates [125] have also shown that adjusting the distal aortic blood pressure to a mean of 60 mm Hg or greater will help to avoid paraplegia (Fig. 11-9).

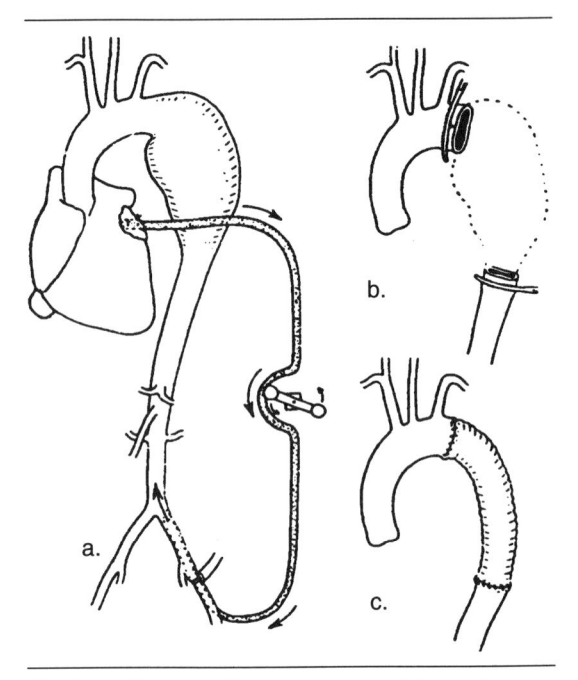

Fig. 11-9. Drawings illustrating repair of descending thoracic aortic aneurysm by excision and graft replacement utilizing left atrial to left femoral artery bypass pump. (Reprinted by permission from ME DeBakey, Changing concepts in vascular surgery. *J Cardiovasc Surg* 27:367, 1986.)

The technique of somatosensory evoked potentials (SSEP) has brought an added dimension to central nervous system monitoring [126]. Three types of evoked potentials are commonly used in the clinical setting. Visual and auditory evoked potentials are used during neurosurgical procedures to assess the function of their respective pathways

[127]. SSEPs, initially used during orthopedic surgery to monitor spinal cord integrity during procedures such as Harrington rod placement [128], appear to be helpful in monitoring for spinal cord ischemia during thoracic aortic crossclamping. SSEPs are generated by an electrical stimulus applied to nerves of the upper and lower extremities. These potentials are then transmitted along the dorsal ganglia, the posterior columns of the spinal cord, and the lemniscal pathways through the thalamus to the cerebral cortex. Evoked potentials can be monitored at many points along this pathway, for example, the posterior tibial nerve is stimulated and the response is recorded in the cerebral cortex. Cunningham and associates [129] and Laschinger and colleagues [125] have shown that this aspect of spinal cord function disappears 5 to 10 minutes after a crossclamp is applied to the thoracic or thoracoabdominal aorta. They have also demonstrated that distal aortic perfusion restores spinal cord blood flow, maintains SSEPs, and restores the function temporarily lost by a brief period of inadequate perfusion of the distal aorta.

Somatosensory evoked potential monitoring is not without its own shortcomings. First, one should note that normal SSEPs during crossclamping do not guarantee freedom from neurologic deficits. There are numerous case reports of paraplegia occurring postoperatively when SSEPs were normal during the entire intraoperative period [130–132]. It has been postulated that this occurs because while SSEP monitors the function of the dorsal columns of the spinal cord, ischemia and paraplegia from aortic crossclamping involves ischemia to the anterior motor cells. Second, it has been shown that inhalation anesthetics [133, 134], barbiturates [135], temperature [136], changes in hematocrit [137], blood pressure fluctuations [138], and arterial oxygen tension [139] can all interfere with SSEP wave forms and reliability. Third, the question arises as to what one should do after the disappearance of SSEP when the aorta has already been crossclamped and opened for repair. Cunningham and associates [129] reported the return of SSEPs after the reimplantation of three intercostal arteries. This may be a solution when the origin of the artery of Adamkiewicz lies between the crossclamps.

It is certainly clear from all previous studies that the single most reliable predictor of postoperative paraplegia is an extended ischemic period from a prolonged crossclamp time. Katz and associates [140] showed a dramatic increase in the probability of paraplegia after 30 minutes of crossclamping in patients who were not shunted to the distal aorta. Crawford and colleagues [141] found no difference in outcome between patient groups with the presence or absence of SSEP monitoring. Additionally, they reserved shunting procedures only for those patients with decreased preoperative ventricular function. They maintain that the major protection against paraplegia is a short crossclamp time. Shunting can extend the duration of crossclamping but the upper limits are unknown. Increasing distal aortic perfusion pressure, decreasing the intraspinal pressure, reimplanting the intercostal arteries, cooling the patient, and giving pharmacologic agents that may offer spinal cord protection are recommended, but still provide no guarantee.

Other postoperative complications add to the morbidity and mortality from this procedure. Pulmonary complications are more frequent in operations performed through a left thoracotomy approach than for operations performed through a median sternotomy [142]. Postoperative moderate or severe renal dysfunction requiring dialysis develops in about 25 percent of patients, with an increased incidence in patients more than 70 years old [143]. Preexistent renal dysfunction, evidence of diffuse atherosclerosis, the use of the pump bypass, and hemodynamic instability all significantly correlated with the development of postoperative renal failure [144]. Finally, postoperative hypotension should be avoided since late paraplegia can develop in patients who have marginally adequate collateral circulation and who have had the origin of the artery of Adamkiewicz resected.

The Patient with Thoracic Aortic Disease Presenting for Noncardiac Surgery

The consensus is that patients with type I or II dissections should be operated on emergently with the anesthetic management outlined earlier in this chapter. Occasionally, however, patients who have coexisting thoracic aortic disease require anesthesia for other procedures. These include the patient with a descending thoracic aneurysm on medical therapy who requires an orthopedic procedure on a lower extremity or the pregnant patient with an ascending aortic aneurysm who presents for labor and possible cesarean section.

Preoperative assessment should include some analysis of the patient's aortic pathology. Echocardiography is an accurate, noninvasive method of assessing aortic disease, and provides an objective indicator of the progression of the lesion by comparing the findings with earlier studies. When forming an anesthetic plan, one should remain cognizant of the patient's aortic pathology. Abrupt changes in hemodynamics are to be avoided, especially sudden bursts of tachycardia and rapid lowering of systemic vascular resistance, as this increases contractility and dp/dt against the aortic wall and can precipitate aortic rupture. Regional anesthesia is not contraindicated; however, the risks and benefits should be weighed for the individual patient. Care should be taken while raising the sensory level, with close attention to changing hemodynamics. Monitoring with an arterial line and a pulmonary artery catheter is recommended. In addition, two large, peripheral intravenous catheters should be placed and 8 units of packed red blood cells should be available. The induction of general anesthesia similarly should be controlled, with the avoidance of sudden tachycardia, hypotension, or hypertension. Appropriate pain management should be employed well into the postoperative period to assure a smooth emergence and recovery from surgery and anesthesia [145].

REFERENCES

1. Galen, J. *Observations on Aneurysm*. Translated by JE Erickson. London: Sydenham Society, 1944.
2. Osler, W. Aneurysm of the abdominal aorta. *Lancet* 2:1089, 1905.
3. Morgagni, GB. De Sedibus et causes morborum per anatomen indagitis. Veneties, 1761. In A Alexander (trans): *The Seats and Causes of Diseases Investigated by Anatomy*. London: Miller and Cedele, 1769.
4. Cooley, DA. *Surgical Treatment of Aortic Aneurysms*. Philadelphia: Saunders, 1986. Pp 1–7.
5. Moore, CH, Morchison, C. On a method of procuring consolidation of fibrin in certain incurable aneurysms. *Med-Chir Trans* 47:129, 1864.
6. Pearse, HE. Experimental studies on the gradual occlusion of large arteries. *Ann Surg* 112:923, 1940.
7. Shumacker, HB, Jr. Coarctation and aneurysm of the aorta: Report of a case treated by excision and end to end suture of the aorta. *Ann Surg* 127:655, 1948.
8. Oudot, J. La greffe vasculaire dans les thromboses du carrefour aortique. *Resse Med* 59:234, 1951.
9. DeBakey, ME, Cooley, DA. Successful resection of aneurysm of thoracic aorta and replacement by graft. *JAMA* 152:673, 1953.
10. DeBakey, ME, Cooley, DA, Crawford, ES, Morris, GC. Aneurysms of the thoracic aorta: Analysis of 179 cases treated by resection. *J Thorac Surg* 36:393, 1958.
11. Boyd, LJ. A study of four thousand reported cases of aneurysm of the thoracic aorta. *Am J Med Sci* 168:654, 1924.
12. Joyce, JW, Fairbairn, JF, II, Kincaid, OW, Juergons, JL. Aneurysms of the thoracic aorta, a clinical study with special reference to prognosis. *Circulation* 29:176, 1964.
13. Pressler, V, McNamara, JJ. Thoracic aortic aneurysm: Natural history and treatment. *J Thorac Cardiovasc Surg* 79:489, 1980.
14. Hilgenberg, AD, Moncure, AC. Cardiovascular Surgical Emergencies. In EW Wilkins (ed), *Emergency Medicine: Scientific Foundations and Current Practice* (3rd ed.) Baltimore: Williams & Wilkins, 1989.
15. Roberts, WC. Aortic dissection: Anatomy, consequences and causes. *Am Heart J* 101:195, 1981.
16. Wheat, MW, Jr. Pathogenesis of Aortic Dissection. In RM Doroghazi, EE Slater (eds), *Aortic Dissection*. New York: McGraw-Hill, 1983.
17. Symbas, PN, Baldwin, BJ, Silverman, ME. Marfan's syndrome: The aneurysms of the ascending aorta and aortic regurgitation: Surgical treatment and new histochemical observations. *Am J Cardiol* 25:483, 1970.
18. Antani, J, Srinivas, HV. Ehlers-Danlos syndrome and cardiovascular abnormalities. *Chest* 63:214, 1973.
19. Fukuda, T, Tadavarthy, SM, Edwards, JE. Dissecting aneurysm of aorta complicating aortic valvular stenosis. *Circulation* 53:169, 1976.
20. Kitchen, DH. Dissecting aneurysm of the aorta in pregnancy. *J Obstet Gynecol Br Commonwealth* 81:410, 1974.
21. DeBakey, ME, Henley, WS, Cooley, DA, et al: Surgical management of dissecting aneurysms of the aorta. *J Thorac Cardiovasc Surg* 49:130, 1965.

22. Crawford, ES. Marfan's syndrome: Broad spectral surgical treatment of cardiovascular manifestations. *Ann Surg* 198:487, 1983.
23. Cooley, DA. Surgical treatment of aortic aneurysms. Philadelphia: Saunders, 1986. Pp 43–46.
24. Daily, PO, Trueblood, HW, Stinson, EB, et al. Management of acute aortic dissection. *Ann Thorac Surg* 10:237, 1970.
25. Slater, EE. Aortic dissection: Presentation and diagnosis. In RM Doroghazi, EE Slater (eds), *Aortic Dissection*. New York: McGraw-Hill, 1983.
26. Slater, EE, DeCantis, RW. The clinical recognition of dissecting aortic aneurysm. *Am J Med* 60:625, 1976.
27. Weisman, AD, Adams, RD. Neurological complications of dissecting aortic aneurysms. *Brain* 67:69, 1944.
28. Riley, DJ, Liv, RT, Saxanoff, S. Aortic dissection: A rare cause of the superior vena cava syndrome. *J Med Soc NJ* 78:187, 1981.
29. Buja, ML, Ali, N, Roberts, WC. Stenosis of the right pulmonary artery: A complication of acute dissecting aneurysm of the ascending aorta. *Am Heart J* 83:89, 1972.
30. McCarthy, C, Dickson, CH, Besterman, EMM, et al. Aortic dissection with rupture through ductus arteriosus into pulmonary artery. *Br Heart J* 34:284, 1972.
31. Roth, JA, Parekh, MA. Dissecting aneurysms perforating the esophagus. *N Engl J Med* 299:776, 1978.
32. Thiene, G, Rossi, L, Becker, AE. The atrioventricular conduction system in dissecting aneurysms of the aorta. *Am Heart J* 98:447, 1979.
33. Victor, MF, Mintz, GS, Kotler, MN, et al. Two dimensional echocardiographic diagnosis of aortic dissection. *Am J Cardiol* 48:1155, 1981.
34. Heiberg, E, Wolverson, M, Sundaram, M, et al. CT findings in thoracic aortic dissection. *Am J Radiol* 136:13, 1981.
35. Earnest, F, Muhm, JR, Sheedy, PF. Roentgenographic findings in thoracic aortic dissection. *Mayo Clin Proc* 54:43, 1979.
36. Borner, N, Erbel, R, Braun, B, et al. Diagnosis of aortic dissection by transesophageal echocardiography. *Am J Cardiol* 54:1157, 1984.
37. Jamieson, WRE, Munro, AI, Miyagishima, RT, et al. Aortic dissection: Early diagnosis and surgical management are the keys to survival. *Can J Surg* 25:145, 1982.
38. Taams, MA, Gussenhoven, WJ, Schippers, LA, et al. The value of transesophageal echocardiography for diagnosis of thoracic aortic pathology. *Eur Heart J* 29:1308, 1988.
39. Fisher, MR. Application of MRI in Vascular Surgery. In JJ Bergan, JS Yao (eds), *Arterial Surgery—New Diagnostic and Operative Techniques*. Orlando, FL: Grune & Stratton, 1988.
40. De Sanctis, RW, Doroghazi, RM, Austen, WG, Buckley, MJ. Aortic dissection. *N Engl J Med* 317:1060, 1987.
41. Prokop, EK, Palmer, RF, Wheat, MW. Hydrodynamic forces in dissecting aneurysms: In-vitro studies in a Tygon model and in dog aortas. *Circ Res* 27:121, 1970.
42. Crawford, ES. The diagnosis and management of aortic dissection. *JAMA* 264:2537, 1990.
43. Wheat, MW, Jr. Intensive Drug Therapy. In RM Doroghazi, EE Slater (eds), *Aortic Dissection*. New York: McGraw-Hill, 1983. Pp 165–192.
44. Kopman, EA, Ferguson, TB. Intraoperative monitoring of femoral artery pressure during replacement of aneurysm of descending thoracic aorta. *Anesth Analg* 56:603, 1977.
45. Norman, PH, Mycyk, T. Dissection of ascending thoracic aorta complicated by cardiac tamponade. *Can J Anaesth* 36:470, 1989.
46. Bentall, M, DeBono, A. A technique for complete replacement of the ascending aorta. *Thorax* 23:338, 1968.
47. Cabrol, C, Pavie, A, Gandjbakhch, I, et al. Complete replacement of the ascending aorta with reimplantation of the coronary arteries. New Surgical approach. *J Thorac Cardiovasc Surg* 81:309, 1981.
48. Mayer, JE. Composite replacement of the aortic valve and ascending aorta. *J Thorac Cardiovasc Surg* 76:816, 1978.
49. Kouchoukos, NT. Replacement of the ascending aorta and aortic valve with a composite graft. Results in 86 patients. *Ann Surg* 192:403, 1980.
50. Muraoka, R, Shirotani, H. Open heart surgery in infants and small children utilizing profound hypothermia and limited cardiopulmonary bypass. *J Jap Surg Soc* 78:1009, 1977.
51. Rittenhouse, EA, Mohri, H, Dillard, DH, Merendino, KA. Deep hypothermia in cardiovascular surgery. *Ann Thorac Surg* 17:63, 1974.
52. Griepp, RB, Stinson, EB, Hollingsworth, JF, Buehler, D. Prosthetic replacement of the aortic arch. *J Thorac Cardiovasc Surg* 70:1051, 1975.
53. Ott, DA, Frazier, OH, Cooley, DA. Resection of the aortic arch using deep hypothermia and temporary circulatory arrest. *Circulation* 58 (Suppl):I–227, 1978.
54. Casthely, PA, Fyman, PN, Abrams, CM, et al. Anaesthesia for aortic arch aneurysm repair: Experience with 17 patients. *Can Anaesth Soc J* 32:73, 1985.

55. Subramanian, S, Wagner, H, Vlad, P, Lambert, E. Surface induced deep hypothermia in cardiac surgery. J Pediatr Surg 6:612, 1971.
56. Ergin, MA, Griepp, RB. Progress in treatment of aneurysms of the aortic arch. World J Surg 4:535, 1980.
57. O'Connor, JV, Wilding, T, Farmer, C. The protective effect of profound hypothermia on the canine central nervous system during one hour of circulatory arrest. Ann Thorac Surg 41:255, 1986.
58. Crawford, ES, Saleh, SA. Transverse aortic arch aneurysm: Improved results of treatment employing new modifications of aortic reconstruction and hypothermic cerebral circulatory arrest. Ann Surg 194:180, 1981.
59. Crawford, ES, Snyder, DM. Treatment of aneurysms of the aortic arch: A progress report. J Thorac Cardiovasc Surg 85:237, 1983.
60. Merrill, EW, Gilliland, ER, Cokelet, G, et al. Rheology of human blood, near and at zero flow: Effects of temperature and hematocrit level. Biophys J 3:199, 1963.
61. Gordon, RJ, Ravin, M, Daicoff, GR, Rawitscher, RE. Effects of hemodilution on hypotension during cardiopulmonary bypass. Anesth Analg 54:482, 1975.
62. Nussmeier, NA, Arlund, C, Slogoff, S. Neuropsychiatric complications after cardiopulmonary bypass: Cerebral protection by a barbiturate. Anesthesiology 64:165, 1986.
63. Yoshimoto, T, Sakamoto, T, Watanabe, T, et al. Experimental cerebral infarction: III. Protective effect of mannitol in thalamic infarction in dogs. Stroke 9:217, 1978.
64. Little, JR. Modification of acute focal ischemia by treatment with mannitol and high dose dexamethasone. J Neurosurg 49:517, 1978.
65. Cottrell, JE, Robustelli, A, Post, K, Turndorf, H. Furosemide and mannitol-induced changes in intracranial pressure and serum osmolality and electrolytes. Anesthesiology 47:28, 1977.
66. Todd, MM, Drummond, JC. Cerebral protection during cardiac surgery. In JA Kaplan (ed), Cardiac Anesthesia: Cardiovascular Pharmacology, Vol 2. New York: Grune & Stratton, 1983. P 551.
67. Artru, AA, Michenfelder, JD. Cerebral protective, metabolic, and vascular effects of phenytoin. Stroke 11:377, 1980.
68. Steen, PA, Gisvold, SE, Milde, JH, et al. Nimodopine improves outcome when given after complete cerebral ischemia in primates. Anesthesiology 62:406, 1985.
69. Nugent, M, Artru, AA, Michenfelder, JD. Cerebral metabolic, vascular, and protective effects of midazolam maleate: Comparison to diazepam. Anesthesiology 56:172, 1982.
70. Lanier, WL, Stangland, KJ, Scheithauer, BW, et al. The effects of dextrose infusion and head position on neurologic outcome after complete cerebral ischemia in primates: Examination of a model. Anesthesiology 66:39, 1987.
71. Shenaq, S, Crawford, ES. Personal communication to author, 1988.
72. Ergin, MA, Galla, JD, Lansman, S, Griepp, RB. Acute dissections of the aorta: Current surgical treatment. Surg Clin North Am 65:721, 1985.
73. Wolfe, WG, Moran, JF. The evolution of medical and surgical management of acute aortic dissection (editorial). Circulation 56:503, 1977.
74. Doroghazi, RM, Slater, EE, DeSanctis, RW, et al. Long term survival of patients with treated aortic dissection. J Am Coll Cardiol 3:1026, 1984.
75. Wheat, MW, Jr, Palmer, RF, Bartley, TD, Seelman, RC. Treatment of dissecting aneurysms of the aorta without surgery. J Thorac Cardiovasc Surg 50:364, 1965.
76. Applebaum, A, Karp, RB, Kirklin, JW. Ascending vs. descending aortic dissections. Ann Surg 183:296, 1976.
77. Saleh, SA. Anesthesia and monitoring for aortic aneurysm surgery. World J Surg 4:689, 1980.
78. Brodsky, JB, Shulman, MS, Mark, JBD. Malposition of left-sided double-lumen endobronchial tubes. Anesthesiology 62:667, 1985.
79. Burton, NA, Fall, SF, Lyons, T, Graeber, GM. Rupture of the left main-stem bronchus with a polyvinylchloride double-lumen tube. Chest 83:928, 1983.
80. Smith, G, Hirsch, N, Ehrenwirth, J. Sight and sound: Can double-lumen endotracheal tubes be placed accurately without fiberoptic bronchoscopy? Br J Anaesth 58:1317, 1987.
81. Benumoff, JL. One-lung ventilation and hypoxic pulmonary vasoconstriction: Implications for anesthetic management. Anesth Analg 64:821, 1985.
82. Brodsky, JB, Shulman, MS, Swan, M, Mark, JBD. Pulse oximetry during one-lung ventilation. Anesthesiology 63:212, 1985.
83. Capan, LM, Turndorf, H, Patel, K. et al. Optimization of arterial oxygenation during one-lung anesthesia. Anesth Analg 59:847, 1980.
84. Cohen, E, Eisenkraft, JB, Thys, DM, et al. Oxygenation and hemodynamic changes during one-lung ventilation. J Cardiothorac Anesth 2:34, 1988.
85. Alfery, D, Benumoff, JL, Trousdale, FR. Improving oxygenation during one-lung ventilation: The effects of PEEP and blood flow restoration to the non-ventilated lung. Anesthesiology 55:381, 1981.

86. Hannenberg, AA, Satwicz, PR, Dienes, RS, Jr, O'Brien, JC. A device for applying CPAP to the non-ventilated upper lung during one-lung ventilation II. *Anesthesiology* 60:254, 1984.
87. Thiagarajah, S, Job, C, Rao, A. A device for applying CPAP to the non-ventilated upper lung during one-lung ventilation. *Anesthesiology* 60:253, 1984.
88. Lyons, TE. A simplified method of CPAP delivery to the non-ventilated lung during unilateral pulmonary ventilation. *Anesthesiology* 61:217, 1984.
89. Arandia, HY, Patel, VU. PEEP and the Mapleson D circuit. *Anesthesiology* 62:846, 1985.
90. Adams, HD, Van Geertruyden, HH. Neurologic complications of aortic surgery. *Ann Surg* 144:574, 1956.
91. Costello, TG, Fisher, A. Neurological complications following aortic surgery: Case reports and review of the literature. *Anaesthesia* 38:230, 1983.
92. Wadouh, F, Lindemann, EM, Arndt, CF, et al. The arteria radicularis magna anterior as a decisive factor influencing spinal cord damage during aortic occlusion. *J Thorac Cardiovasc Surg* 88:1, 1984.
93. Foo, D, Rossier, AB. Anterior spinal artery syndrome and its natural history. *Paraplegia* 21:1, 1983.
94. Adamkiewicz, A. Die Blutgefasse des Menschlichen Ruckermarkesoberflache. Sitzungersberichte der Akademi der Wissenschaften in Wien. *Mathematische-naturwissenschaftliche klasse*. 85:101, 1882.
95. Connolly, JE. Prevention of paraplegia secondary to operations of the aorta. *J Cardiovasc Surg* 27:410, 1986.
96. Laschinger, JC, Izumoto, H, Kouchoukos, NT. Evolving concepts in prevention of spinal cord injury during operations of the descending thoracic and thoracoabdominal aorta. *Ann Thorac Surg* 44:666, 1987.
97. Hill, CS, Jr, Vasquez, JM. Massive infarction of spinal cord and vertebral bodies as a complication of dissecting aneurysm of the aorta. *Circulation* 25:997, 1962.
98. Blaisdell, FW, Cooley, DA. The mechanism of paraplegia after temporary thoracic aortic occlusion and its relationship to spinal fluid pressure. *Surgery* 51:351, 1962.
99. Berendes, JN, Bredee, JJ, Schipperheyn, JJ, Mashhour, YAS. Mechanisms of spinal cord injury after cross-clamping of the descending thoracic aorta. *Circulation* 66 (Suppl 1):I-112, 1982.
100. Crawford, ES, Rubio, PA. Reappraisal of adjuncts to avoid ischemia in the treatment of aneurysms of descending thoracic aorta. *J Thorac Cardiovasc Surg* 66:693, 1973.
101. Miyamoto, K, Keno, A, Wada, T, Kimoto, S. A new and simple method of preventing spinal cord damage following temporary occlusion of the thoracic aorta by draining the cerebrospinal fluid. *J Thorac Cardiovasc Surg* 16:188, 1960.
102. Oka, Y, Miyamoto, K. Prevention of spinal cord injury after cross-clamping of the thoracic aorta. *Jpn J Surg* 14:159, 1984.
103. McCullough, JL, Hollier, LH, Nugent, M. Paraplegia after thoracic aortic occlusion: Influence of cerebrospinal fluid drainage. Experimental and early clinical results. *J Vasc Surg* 7:153, 1988.
104. Molina, JE, Cogordan, J, Einzig, S, et al. Adequacy of ascending aorta–descending aorta shunt during cross-clamping of the thoracic aorta for prevention of spinal cord injury. *J Thorac Cardiovasc Surg* 90:126, 1985.
105. Nugent, M, Kaye, MP, McGoon, DC. Effects of nitroprusside on aortic and intraspinal pressures during thoracic aortic cross-clamping. *Anesthesiology* 61:A68, 1984.
105a. Shine, T, Nugent, M. Sodium nitroprusside decreases spinal cord perfusion pressure during descending thoracic aortic cross-clamping in the dog. *J Cardiothorac Anesth* 4:185, 1990.
106. Vacanti, FX, Ames, A. Mild hypothermia and Mg^{++} protect against irreversible damage during CNS ischemia. *Stroke* 15:695, 1984.
107. Pontius, RG, Brockman, HL, Hardy, EG, et al. The use of hypothermia in the prevention of paraplegia following temporary aortic occlusion: Experimental observations. *Surgery* 36:33, 1954.
108. Coles, JG, Wilson, GJ, Sima, AF, et al. Intraoperative management of thoracic aortic aneurysm: Experimental evaluation of perfusion cooling of the spinal cord. *J Thorac Cardiovasc Surg* 85:292, 1983.
109. Drummond, JC, Moore, SS, Zivin, JA, Shapiro, JM. The effect of hyperglycemia on neurologic outcome following spinal cord ischemia in the rabbit. *Anesth Analg* 66:S43, 1987.
110. Laschinger, JC, Cunningham, JN, Jr, Cooper, MM, et al. Prevention of ischemic spinal cord injury following aortic cross-clamping: Use of corticosteroids. *Ann Thorac Surg* 38:500, 1984.
111. Kirshner, DL, Kirshner, RL, Heggeness, LM, DeWeese, JA. Spinal cord ischemia: An evaluation of pharmacologic agents in minimizing paraplegia after aortic occlusion. *J Vasc Surg* 9:305, 1989.
112. Granke, K, Hollier, LH, Zdrahal, P, Moore, W. Longitudinal study of cerebral spinal fluid drainage in polyethylene glycol–conjugated superoxide dismutase in paraplegia associated with thoracic aortic cross-clamping. *J Vasc Surg* 13:615, 1991.
113. Roberts, AJ, Nora, JD, Hughes, WA, et al. Cardiac

and renal responses to cross-clamping of the descending thoracic aorta. *J Thorac Cardiovasc Surg* 86:732, 1983.
114. Symbas, PN, Pfaender, LM, Drucker, MH, et al. Cross-clamping of the descending aorta: Hemodynamic and neurohumoral effects. *J Thorac Cardiovasc Surg* 85:300, 1983.
115. Gelman, S, Reves, JG, Fowler, K, et al. Regional blood flow during cross-clamping of the thoracic aorta and infusion of sodium nitroprusside. *J Thorac Cardiovasc Surg* 85:287, 1983.
116. Kozody, R, Palahniuk, RJ, Wade, JG, et al. The effect of subarachnoid epinephrine and phenylephrine on spinal cord blood flow. *Can Anaesth Soc J* 31:503, 1984.
117. Kouchoukos, NT, Lell, WA, Karp, RB, Samuelson, PN. Hemodynamic effect of aortic clamping and decompression with a temporary shunt for resection of the descending thoracic aorta. *Surgery* 85:25, 1979.
118. Roizen, MF, Beaupre, PN, Alpert, RA, et al. Monitoring with two-dimensional transesophageal echocardiography. Comparison of myocardial function in patients undergoing supraceliac, suprarenal-infraceliac, or infrarenal aortic occlusion. *J Vasc Surg* 1:300, 1984.
119. Gott, VL. Heparinized shunts for thoracic vascular operation. *Ann Thorac Surg* 14:219, 1972.
120. Donahoo, JS, Brawley, RK, Gott, VL. The heparin coated vascular shunt for thoracic aortic and great vessel procedures: A ten-year experience. *Ann Thorac Surg* 23:507, 1977.
121. Akins, CW, Buckley, MJ, Daggett, W, et al. Acute traumatic disruption of the thoracic aorta: A ten-year experience. *Ann Thorac Surg* 31:305, 1981.
122. May, IA, Ecker, RR, Iverson, LIG. Heparinless femoral venoarterial bypass without an oxygenator for surgery on the descending thoracic aorta. *J Thorac Cardiovasc Surg* 73:387, 1977.
123. Cooley, DA, Belmonte, BA, DeBakey, ME, Latson, JR. Temporary extracorporeal circulation in the surgical treatment of cardiac and aortic disease: Report of 98 cases. *Ann Surg* 145:898, 1957.
124. DeBakey, ME. Changing concepts in vascular surgery. *J Cardiovasc Surg* 27:367, 1986.
125. Laschinger, JC, Cunningham, JN, Jr, Nathan, IM, et al. Experimental and clinical assessment of the adequacy of partial bypass in maintenance of spinal cord blood flow during operations on the thoracic aorta. *Ann Thorac Surg* 36:417, 1983.
126. Chiappa, KH, Ropper, AH. Evoked potentials in clinical medicine: II. *N Engl J Med* 306:1205, 1982.
127. Grundy, BL. Monitoring of sensory evoked potentials during neurosurgical operations: Methods and applications. *Neurosurgery* 11:556, 1982.
128. Engler, GL, Spielholz, NI, Bernhard, WN, et al. Somatosensory evoked potentials during Harrington instrumentations for scoliosis. *J Bone Joint Surg* 60:528, 1978.
129. Cunningham, JN, Jr, Laschinger, JC, Merkin, HA, et al. Measurement of spinal cord ischemia during operations upon the thoracic aorta: Initial clinical experience. *Ann Surg* 196:285, 1982.
130. Takaki, O, Okumura, F. Application and limitation of somatosensory evoked potential monitoring during thoracic aortic aneurysm surgery: A case report. *Anesthesiology* 63:700, 1985.
131. Ginsberg, HH, Shetter, AG, Randzens, PA. Postoperative paraplegia with preserved intraoperative somatosensory evoked potentials: Case report. *J Neurosurg* 63:296, 1985.
132. Zornow, MH, Drummond, JC. Intraoperative somatosensory evoked responses recorded during onset of the anterior spinal artery syndrome. *J Clin Monit* 5:243, 1989.
133. Clark, DL, Rosner, BS. Neurophysiologic effects of general anesthetics: I. The electroencephalogram and sensory evoked responses in man. *Anesthesiology* 38:564, 1973.
134. Rosner, BS, Clark, DL. Neurophysiologic effects of general anesthetics: II. *Anesthesiology* 39:59, 1973.
135. Drummond, JC, Todd, MM, U, HS. The effect of high dose thiopental on brain stem auditory and median nerve somatosensory evoked responses in humans. *Anesthesiology* 63:249, 1985.
136. Coles, JG, Lowry, NJ, Pearce, JM, et al. Cerebral monitoring of somatosensory evoked potentials during profoundly hypothermic circulatory arrest. *Circulation* 70 (Suppl):I-96, 1984.
137. Nagao, S, Roccaforte, P, Moody, RA. The effects of isovolemic hemodilution and reinfusion of packed erythrocytes on somatosensory and visual evoked potentials. *J Surg Res* 25:530, 1978.
138. Grundy, BL, Nash, CL, Jr, Brown, RH. Arterial pressure manipulation alters spinal cord function during correction of scoliosis. *Anesthesiology* 54:249, 1981.
139. Grundy, BL, Heros, RC, Tung, AS, Doyle, E. Intraoperative hypoxia detected by evoked potential monitoring. *Anesth Analg* 60:437, 1981.
140. Katz, NM, Blackstone, EH, Kirklin, JW, Karp, RB. Incremental risk factors for spinal cord injury following operation for acute traumatic aortic transection. *J Thorac Cardiovasc Surg* 81:669, 1981.
141. Crawford, ES, Crawford, JL, Safi, HJ, et al. Thora-

142. Miller, DC, Stinson, EB, Oyer, PE, et al. Operative treatment of aortic dissections: Experience with 125 patients over a sixteen-year period. *J Thorac Cardiovasc Surg* 78:365, 1979.
143. Livesay, JJ, Cooley, DA, Ventemiglia, RA, et al. Surgical experience in descending thoracic aneurysmectomy with and without adjuncts to avoid ischemia. *Ann Thorac Surg* 39:37, 1985.
144. Svenson, LG, Coselli, JS, Safi, HJ, et al. Appraisal of adjuncts to prevent acute renal failure after surgery on the thoracic or thoracoabdominal aorta. *J Vasc Surg* 10:230, 1989.
145. Mangano, DT. Anesthesia for the Pregnant Cardiac Patient. In SM Shnider, G Levinson (eds), *Anesthesia for Obstetrics* (2nd ed). Baltimore: Williams & Wilkins, 1987. P 370.

(coabdominal aortic aneurysms: Preoperative and intraoperative factors determining immediate and long term results of operations in 605 patients. *J Vasc Surg* 3:389, 1986.)

12
Patients with Pacemakers

DAVID AMAR
JAY N. GROSS

The progressive aging of the population has been associated with increasing numbers of patients with implanted pacemakers. Pacemaker technology is rapidly evolving, with increasingly complex devices designed to emulate normal cardiovascular electrophysiology and hemodynamics. Comprehension of basic pacemaker terminology and concepts and recognition of pacemaker malfunction in the perioperative period are essential skills for anesthesiologists. There is also a patient cohort who requires temporary pacing while undergoing surgery. This chapter reviews basic concepts of temporary pacing and management of patients with permanent pacemakers during the perioperative period.

TEMPORARY PACING

General Indications

There are three broad general indications for temporary pacing (Table 12-1). First, pacing is indicated in symptomatic patients whose symptoms (syncope or near-syncope) are related to sinus node dysfunction or second-degree atrioventricular (AV) block. These conduction abnormalities may be the result of acute myocardial damage, drug intoxication, electrolyte imbalance, or degenerative conduction disease. Second, pacing is indicated in asymptomatic patients at significant risk for development of symptoms or hemodynamic compromise from a bradyarrhythmia and this risk exceeds those associated with temporary pacing. This includes new-onset complete and Mobitz II second-degree heart block and the development of specific conduction abnormalities in the setting of acute myocardial infarction (see Table 12-1). Inferior myocardial infarction is frequently associated with transient sinus and AV nodal dysfunction and only occasionally results in permanent damage to the conduction system. When conduction abnormalities develop during anterior infarction, it is more indicative of damage to the His-Purkinje system, with a higher likelihood of unreliable escape rhythms and development of fixed complete heart block [1].

Third, pacing is indicated in patients with difficult to diagnose or uncontrolled tachycardias. Intracardiac electrograms may aid in differentiating between supraventricular and ventricular arrhythmias. Reentrant tachyarrhythmias, a frequent mechanism in both supraventricular and ventricular arrhythmias, may often be terminated with rapid pacing. Suppression of bradycardia-dependent tachydysrhythmias is occasionally possible with "overdrive" pacing at rates 10 to 25 percent higher than the spontaneous rate. Overdrive pacing is particularly effective in patients with drug-induced QT prolongation and "torsades de pointes" (see Chap. 10).

Table 12-1. Indications for temporary pacing

Symptomatic (e.g., syncope, etc.)
   Congenital or acquired complete heart block
   Type I (Wenckebach) second-degree heart block
   Type II second-degree heart block
   Bradydysrhythmia due to sinus node dysfunction (these may be due to chronic conduction disease, acute myocardial infarction, drug intoxication, or electrolyte imbalance)
   Atrial fibrillation with slow ventricular response
Asymptomatic
   New-onset acquired complete heart block
   Post–cardiac surgery complete heart block
   Type II second-degree heart block
   Acute myocardial infarction
      New-onset bifascicular block (LBBB, RBBB + LAHB, or RBBB + LPHB)
      New bundle branch block with transient complete AV block
      Type II second-degree AV block
      Complete heart block
      RBBB or LBBB and first-degree or type I second-degree AV block
      Alternating RBBB and LBBB
      RBBB with alternating LAHB and LPHB
      Preexisting RBBB and new LAHB and first-degree AV block
Tachycardia (prevention or treatment)
   Bradycardia-dependent arrhythmia
   Reentrant arrhythmias (overdrive pacing)

LBBB = left bundle branch block; RBBB = right bundle branch block; LAHB = left anterior hemiblock; LPHB = left posterior hemiblock.
Source: Adapted from DR Holmes, Temporary Cardiac Pacing. In S. Furman, DL Hayes, and DR Holmes (eds), *A Practice of Cardiac Pacing* (2nd ed). Mount Kisco, NY: Futura, 1989.

Perioperative Indications

Individuals with preexisting "stable" conduction abnormalities who are undergoing surgery represent a subset of patients at somewhat, but poorly quantified, increased risk for development of serious perioperative bradyarrhythmias. There are few specific data available to predict the actual risk to these patients and the advent of noninvasive transcutaneous pacemakers (NTP) has greatly changed the approach to their management. In patients with bifascicular block and mild or uncertain symptoms, temporary pacing should be available, but is not required before surgery [2]. The addition of a first-degree AV block (prolonged PR interval) to a bifascicular block, that is, trifascicular block, places patients at increased risk for development of complete heart block. In asymptomatic patients with trifascicular block, temporary pacing should be readily available before the induction of anesthesia. In symptomatic patients with trifascicular block, a permanent pacemaker is generally warranted and, therefore, temporary pacing should be initiated before surgery if there is insufficient time to insert a permanent pacemaker [3].

Patients with preexisting left bundle branch block who require pulmonary artery catheterization run the risk of irritation of the ventricular septum and induction of complete heart block during insertion of the catheter [4, 5]. Several options are available. The NTP is probably the ideal method for this situation. Its adhesive electrodes should be placed before central venous access is obtained [6], and it is useful to determine the pacing threshold prior to catheter insertion. This may be done by applying the posterior electrode first and then moving the anterior electrode to the position providing the lowest pacing threshold. Other options include the availability of a temporary transvenous pacemaker wire that can be quickly introduced once central access is achieved. A pacing pulmonary artery catheter (one that has pacing atrial and ventricular electrodes on its outer surface) can also be used; however, these catheters have fewer ports, are somewhat less compliant than the usual pulmonary artery catheters, and may be cumbersome to insert. Additionally, pacing capture is somewhat unpredictable since the pacing electrode is on the outer surface, and requires the pulmonary artery catheter to touch the ventricular wall and not to float within the ventricular cavity. Pacing catheters do have the advantage of being able to sequentially pace atrioventricularly, a feature that may be of great importance in patients who are reliant on their atrial kick, for example, those with aortic stenosis, left ventricular hypertrophy, mitral stenosis, or severe ischemic cardiomyopathy. In contrast, some pulmonary catheters have designated paceports, through which pacing wires can be introduced directly into the right ventricle or right atrium, or both. Pacing with these catheters is much more reliable because their wires exit the pulmonary artery catheter and touch the ventricular wall; thus, they would work even with a floating pulmonary artery catheter. Additionally, if the recently introduced AV paceport catheter is used, AV sequential pacing is possible.

Neither form of pacing by pulmonary artery catheter is a guaranteed protection against complete heart block, since the catheters need to be in place, that is, in the pulmonary artery, in order for their pacing functions to work. Frequently, when complete AV block is seen during the insertion of a pulmonary artery catheter, it occurs when the catheter enters the right ventricle and is not as yet in a position to pace. A previously advocated approach of temporary transvenous pacemaker insertion followed by fluoroscopy-guided insertion of a pulmonary artery catheter is now seldom done [7]. Thus, the NTP is the method most useful for these patients. Additionally, patients who require pulmonary artery catheterization and have a temporary or recently implanted permanent transvenous pacemaker (less than 4 weeks old) in place, should only be "instrumented" with the aid of fluoroscopy [8].

Methods

Noninvasive Transcutaneous Pacemakers (NTPs)

The use of the NTP has been shown to be safe and efficacious in clinical trials involving both adults and children [9]. It is currently recommended as a second-line therapy of symptomatic bradycardia after atropine [10] and may be beneficial when used early during cardiopulmonary resuscitation [11]. NTP has been used successfully in the perioperative period in patients undergoing noncardiac [12] as well as cardiac [13] surgical procedures. Other applications of the NTP include overdrive pacing of supraventricular and ventricular tachydysrhythmias [14, 15], temporary pacing in the cardiac catheterization laboratory [9, 16], and treatment of postcardioversion [17], hyperkalemia [18], and drug-associated [19] bradyarrhythmias.

The NTP can operate in the asynchronous, or VOO (Appendix A), or synchronous (ventricular inhibited pacing, or VVI) modes. Skeletal muscle is maximally activated by high-intensity stimuli of short duration (<1 msec). In contrast cardiac muscle activation is facilitated by longer-duration (40–50 msec) stimuli. Electrode placement for maximal efficacy and minimal skeletal muscle discomfort should have the anterior (negative) electrode placed to the left of the xiphoid process and inferior to the left nipple along the costal margin. The posterior (positive) electrode should be placed between the interior border of the left scapula and the thoracic spine.

A study of healthy human volunteers found no increase of myocardial enzymes after 30 minutes of transcutaneous pacing [20]. NTP's most limiting feature is the skeletal muscle discomfort it causes. Local skin irritation or erythema is also common. The risk of inducing ventricular tachycardia or fibrillation with NTP is quite rare and self-limited [9, 21]. Controversy regarding NTP electrophysiology exists. One report [22] described simultaneous atrial and ventricular activation while others [23, 24] reported ventricular activation with retrograde atrial conduction. Similarly uncertain is whether NTP causes paradoxical motion of the interventricular septum, which is typically seen during right ventricular pacing. Hemodynamically, the NTP has been shown to cause a rise in atrial, pulmonary artery, and mean aortic pressures in a study of 16 patients undergoing cardiac catheterization [16]. Another investigation [25] demonstrated a significant decrease in left ventricular systolic pressure during use of the NTP when compared to sinus rhythm or AV sequential pacing, but hemodynamics were similar to those of VVI pacing. Our preliminary experience with the NTP in patients undergoing elective thoracic surgery indicates that systolic arterial pressure is significantly decreased during use of the NTP. This is associated with paradoxical ventricular septal wall motion and simultaneous atrial and ventricular contractions, as seen by transesophageal echocardiography [26].

Of clinical importance is the significant discrepancy between the "set" pacing rate of the NTP and the actual resultant heart rate (Table 12-2). This is due to an additional 100-msec delay provided to facilitate sensing of intrinsic QRSs before initiation of pacing, and this idiosyncrasy is especially important when considering burst-pace termination of supraventricular or ventricular tachyarrhythmias.

The NTP has many applications in the perioperative period and thus is an important new tool for anesthesiologists. In addition to the use of the NTP in treating life-threatening bradycardia, this device

Table 12-2. Rate settings of the noninvasive transcutaneous pacemaker

Pacing rate setting (msec)*	Actual heart rate (msec)*
30	29
40	38
50	46
60	55
70	63
80	71
90	78
100	86
110	93
120	100
130	107

*Comparison of heart rate (HR) and pacing rate. This assumes that every paced beat is sensed.

Actual heart rate = $\dfrac{60{,}000 \text{ (msec)}}{\text{Pace rate (msec)} + 100 \text{ msec}}$

Example: Pace rate = 60 ppm

HR = $\dfrac{60{,}000 \text{ msec}}{1{,}000 \text{ msec} + 100 \text{ msec}}$ = 55 bpm

Source: Provided as a technical communication by Zoll Medical Co., Woburn, MA.

Table 12-3. Perioperative use of the NTP

Standby
Insertion or replacement of a permanent pacemaker
Possible intraoperative malfunction of a permanent pacemaker (electrocautery, battery depletion, lead dislodgment, myopotentials, shock wave lithotripsy, K^+ imbalance, myocardial infarction)
Central venous or pulmonary artery catheterization of a patient with preexisting left bundle branch block
For postcountershock pulseless rhythms
Patients with a bifascicular block
  Normal PR interval (symptomatic)
  Prolonged PR interval (asymptomatic)

Treatment
As outlined in the section on indications for temporary pacing

---

is readily available in the standby mode for many situations (Table 12-3) that previously were managed with temporary transvenous pacing.

Transesophageal Atrial Pacemakers

The use of transesophageal atrial pacing (TAP) has been shown to be safe and effective in the treatment of bradycardia in anesthetized adults and children [27–30]. More recently, atrial pacing thresholds were described in anesthetized patients with the use of a modified esophageal stethoscope [31].

TAP can be used to treat sinus bradycardia or an AV junctional rhythm amenable to atrial pacing. Patients with atrial fibrillation or high-degree AV block will not respond to TAP. In fact, sinus bradycardia or AV junctional bradycardia in the perioperative setting is generally transient and responsive to atropine, whereas most life-threatening bradycardias result from severe AV block that cannot be treated with this mode of pacing. Thus, its clinical utility in the perioperative period is fairly limited; when used appropriately, however, TAP can provide for superior hemodynamics via atrial pacing.

Transvenous Temporary Pacemakers

The lifesaving nature of temporary transvenous pacing (TTP) has been well established [32]. Most TTP systems sense and pace the right ventricle, but compromise atrioventricular synchrony (Fig. 12-1). VVI transvenous pacing is generally associated with a decrease in systolic blood pressure and cardiac output due to loss of atrioventricular synchrony and the atrial contribution to diastolic filling [33, 34]. The advent of AV sequential temporary pacing (DVI), and most recently temporary DDD pacing (in which both the atrium and ventricle may be sensed and paced), provides more physiologic pacing modes. As was mentioned earlier, temporary dual-chamber pacing may be particularly useful in patients with noncompliant ventricles (e.g., individuals with aortic stenosis, hypertrophic cardiomyopathy, myocardial ischemia, right ventricular infarction, etc.), where the atrial contribution to cardiac output may be as high as 40 percent [35]. Despite the limitations of ventricular pacing, it remains the mainstay of reliable temporary pacing, and is the standard method for emergent heart rate support.

Placement of Temporary Transvenous Pacemaker Catheters. Several types of pacing catheters and leads are available (Table 12-4), the majority of which are bipolar. The placement of rigid (Dacron

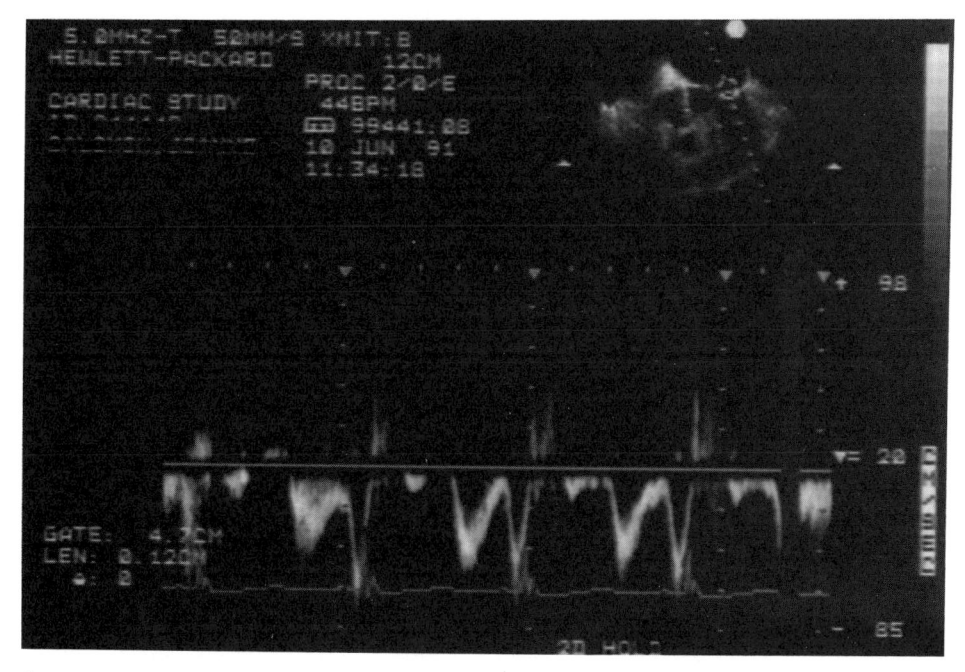

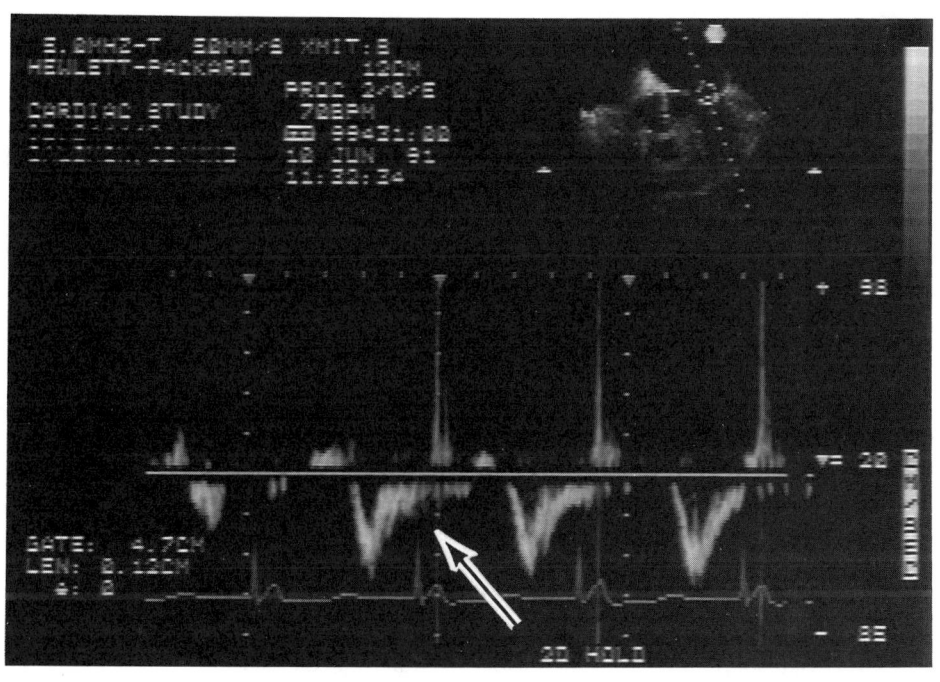

Fig. 12-1. A. Normal transmitral Doppler flow velocities seen by transesophageal echocardiography in a patient with sinus rhythm. Left ventricular filling consists of a rapid early (E) filling phase and a second atrial (A) contribution phase. B. Transmitral Doppler velocities in the same patient during transvenous VVI pacing. Note that the atrial contribution is lost (absence of the A wave).

Table 12-4. Temporary transvenous leads

Type		Fluoroscopy	Mode
Atrial	Atrial "J" lead	Required	AAI
Ventricular	Balloon-tipped lead (flexible)	Not required	VVI
	Flexible bipolar lead	Not required	
	Pacing pulmonary artery catheter	Not required	
	Paceport pulmonary artery catheter	Not required	
	Rigid (woven Dacron) bipolar	Required	
	Quadripolar (rigid)	Required	
Dual chamber	Separate atrial and ventricular leads	Required	DVI
	Multielectrode catheter for atrial and ventricular pacing	Required	
	Pacing pulmonary artery catheter	Not required	
	AV sequential paceport pulmonary artery catheter	Not required	

woven) catheters should be done under fluoroscopy because of the risk of cardiac perforation. These catheters, once properly positioned, tend to remain stable and provide more reliable pacing than flexible leads. The more flexible balloon-tipped pacemaker catheters are floated into the central circulation in the same manner as pulmonary artery catheters. Electrocardiographic-guidance is necessary to position the lead appropriately; fluoroscopy is helpful but rarely required. Preformed J-shaped atrial leads are available that permit atrial or dual-chamber temporary pacing. Alternatively, a multipolar catheter can be positioned into the right ventricle in a manner that allows the proximal electrodes to sense and/or pace the atrium.

Technique. The most common central venous access sites for placement of TTP are the subclavian and internal jugular veins. Other areas used include the femoral, external jugular, and brachial veins. The latter group allows avoidance of a number of potential complications related to subclavian or internal jugular access, but is generally less stable and may restrict patient mobility; furthermore, each of these "safer" approaches has its own specific limitations. A retrospective review found the antecubital vein route associated with the highest rate of arrhythmias, loss of ventricular capture, and right ventricular perforation [36]. Femoral insertion usually necessitates fluoroscopy and the site may be difficult to keep stable and sterile. Regardless of the site chosen for central venous access, meticulous aseptic technique should be followed.

Ventricular placement of a balloon flotation or soft nonballoon lead is recommended in urgent situations when fluoroscopy is unavailable. Before the lead is advanced, the distal electrode should be connected to the chest lead of a surface ECG cable in order to direct the lead to the desired location, which is suggested by the appearance of a distinct ventricular electrogram in association with a "current of injury" (i.e., local ST elevation). With continuous ECG monitoring the catheter is advanced until the tip is in the apex of the right ventricle as determined by the ECG (tracings shown in Fig. 12-2). The right ventricular apex is the most stable position and usually provides adequate pacing and sensing thresholds. Pacing thresholds should be less than 1 mA and the position of the pacemaker lead should be stable despite deep breathing or coughing.

Once initial placement is established by ECG or fluoroscopy, the distal (negative) and proximal (positive) pacing electrodes are connected to the pacemaker generator. With the pacemaker turned off, the output is set at 5.0 mA and the rate is set at 10 to 15 ppm (pulses per minute) above the intrinsic heart rate. The pacemaker is then turned on and 1:1 capture is verified on ECG. The output is gradually decreased until 1:1 capture is lost and stimulation threshold is defined as the output just above where capture was lost. The final setting of the output should be at 5 mA or two to three times the value of the stimulation threshold. In order to determine the sensitivity threshold, the R-wave sensitivity is set between 1.5 and 3.0 mV and the rate is set at 10 ppm below the intrinsic rate. If sensing is intact, the pacing output will be inhib-

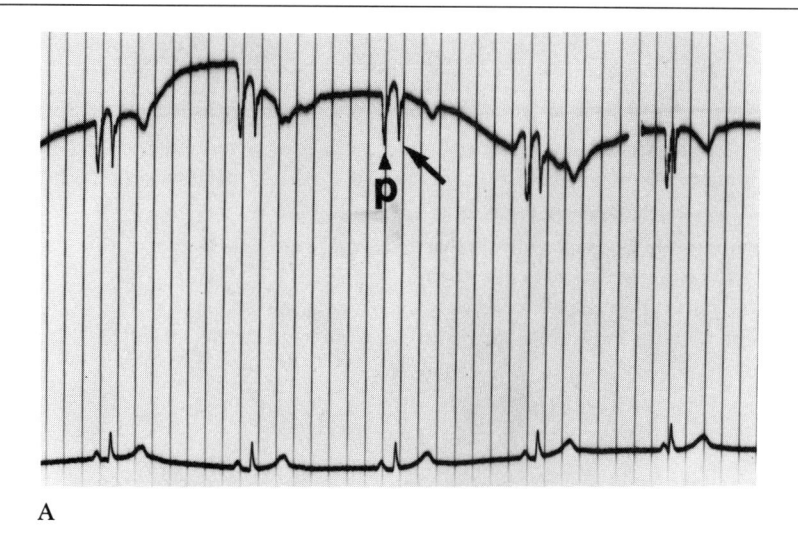

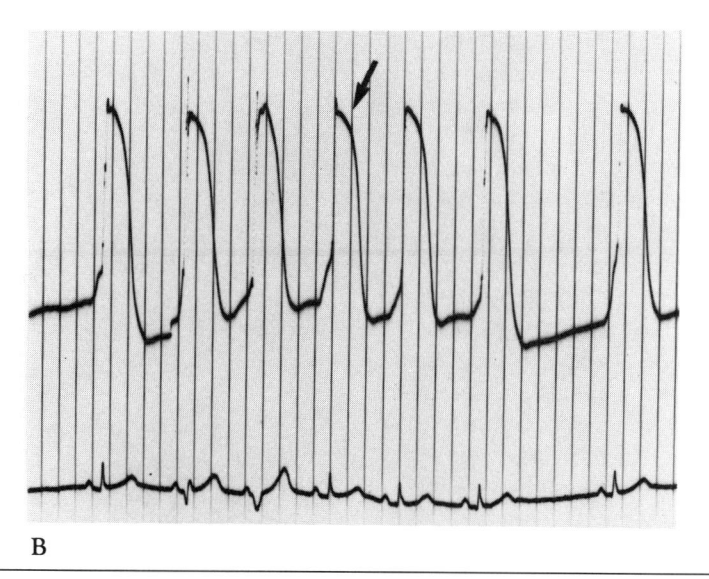

Fig. 12-2. Electrocardiogram-guided advancement of a temporary transvenous bipolar electrode. A. This electrogram represents the ECG tracing, with the pacing wire located in the right atrium. Note that the size and configuration of the P wave (p) resembles the intrinsic QRS complex (*arrow*). For comparison a simultaneous surface electrogram is provided. B. When the pacing electrode is in the right ventricle, the P waves disappear. Note that increasing pressure on the endocardium by the pacing electrode causes an increase in the electrogram amplitude and marked ST-segment elevation (*arrow*) or "current of injury." The second and third complexes are premature ventricular contractions.

ited and the sensing indicator will begin flashing in synchrony with the intrinsic R waves. At this point, the sensitivity dial should be turned counterclockwise (less sensitive) until the pacemaker begins to pace. The sensitivity control should be set at two to three times the sensitivity threshold. Routine setting of the temporary pacemaker to maximal sensitivity should be avoided, as it predisposes to "oversensing" noise, which may result in inappropriate and potentially dangerous episodes of nonpacing. Typical temporary pacemaker settings are shown in Table 12-5, and a troubleshooting guide during TTP is provided in Table 12-6.

DVI pacing pulmonary artery catheters are positioned in a routine manner by tracing identification of the pulmonary artery and wedge positions. Once the catheter is in position, temporary AV sequential pacing can be instituted and parameters similar to those in Table 12-5 can be set. Thermodilution cardiac outputs, as well as systemic and pulmonary arterial blood pressures, should be measured during AV sequential pacing. The desirable AV interval is the one at which the cardiac output is maximized while pulmonary artery pressure increases are minimized or even reduced. One example of customary measurements obtained during dual-chamber pulmonary artery catheter pacing is shown in Table 12-7. As was discussed earlier, many cardiologists with experience in using pacing pulmonary artery catheters find them more rigid and less reliable in assuring proper pacing than conventional temporary pacing lead systems and their use is less desirable when rapid emergent pacing is needed. In contrast, the paceport catheters discussed earlier have received high marks in two reports [37, 38].

Post-Pacemaker Insertion Care. All transvenous pacemaker catheters should be properly secured

Table 12-6. Troubleshooting guide during transvenous temporary pacing

Malfunction	Possible cause
Loss of pacemaker artifact	R-wave sensitivity too high Battery depletion Loose or broken wires Wire short circuit
Failure to capture without loss of pacemaker artifact	Lead malposition Battery depletion Poor electronic insulation Output setting too low Cardiac perforation
Rate malfunction	Faulty pacemaker generator
Loss of sensing	Lead malposition R-wave sensitivity too low Faulty pacemaker generator Electromagnetic interference
Oversensing	R-wave sensitivity too high Electromagnetic interference
Pacemaker-induced arrhythmias	Undersensing Electromagnetic interference
Chest wall or diaphragmatic stimulation	Output too high Cardiac perforation

Source: Adapted from Temporary Pacing Ready Reference Chart. Minneapolis: Medtronic, 1983.

Table 12-5. Temporary pacemaker settings (general guidelines)*

Ventricular demand (VVI)
Rate: 60–80 ppm, or 10 ppm above the patient's rate
Output: 3–5 mA
Sensitivity: 1.5 mV

AV sequential (DVI)
AV interval: 150 msec
Rate: 60–80 ppm, or 10 ppm above the patient's rate
Output: 3–5 mA (atrial and ventricular)
Ventricular sensitivity: 1.5 mV

*Appropriate variations are dependent on numerous patient characteristics and technical factors.

Table 12-7. Positioning of pacing pulmonary artery catheters: effect of the AV interval*

Pacing mode	Heart rate (bpm)	AV interval (msec)	Pulmonary artery pressure (mm Hg)	Cardiac output (liters/min)
VVI	70	—	54/24	3.2
DVI	70	175	43/24	3.0
DVI	70	250	33/18	4.2

*Example in one patient.

with nonabsorbable sutures to avoid dislodgment of the pacing lead. Antiseptic care and dressing should be applied. All electrical appliances in the room, such as an ECG monitor or the patient's bed, should be properly grounded so that microshock to the heart via the pacing wires is avoided. Even minimal current transmitted to the heart through the pacing leads may cause ventricular arrhythmias. Baseline chest x-ray and ECG (while pacing) are required to confirm location and function of the pacemaker system as well as to evaluate for complications (e.g., pneumothorax, etc.). ECG monitoring is required for patients who have transvenous temporary pacemakers to document the underlying rhythm and the need for pacing, and to detect intrinsic or pacing-induced arrhythmias. Pacing and sensing thresholds must be verified on a daily basis. A significant increase in the pacing threshold may be the first sign of lead dislodgment.

Meticulous nursing care is essential, with special attention to daily dressing changes of the puncture site. The external pacemaker generator should be pinned to the patient's gown or kept in a pouch hung about the patient's neck to prevent unnecessary traction on the pacing wires. In a patient who requires a transvenous pacemaker, and who is receiving systemic anticoagulation, extreme care should be exerted when central access is obtained. Once a temporary pacing lead is secured, anticoagulation, if indicated, should be employed with caution. Prophylactic administration of antibiotics before insertion of a transvenous pacemaker is generally not required.

Complications. The most frequent complication of temporary pacing is loss of capture due to lead dislodgment. Dislodgment should be suspected when marked increases in stimulation threshold occur and/or there is a deterioration in sensing function. Transient loss of capture may occur in an unstable lead when small variations in position occur. There are reports of patients with temporary pacemakers who were noted to have recurrent loss of capture concomitant with light positive pressure ventilation applied by face mask during induction, apparently secondary to the associated ventricular volume changes and interventricular septum shifts [39]. The incidence of right ventricular perforation is low, and is more commonly seen with a rigid pacing lead [36, 40]. Clinical signs of perforation include a postinsertion friction rub, loss of capture, diaphragmatic stimulation, a change in the QRS complex (from left bundle branch block to right bundle branch block) and, rarely, pericardial tamponade. A case of electrode tip–induced endocarditis, sepsis, and right ventricular perforation has been reported [41]. If perforation is suspected the lead should be withdrawn. Other complications include pneumothorax, hemothorax, arterial puncture, bacteremia, and local infection.

Epicardial Pacing

Permanent pacing via epicardial leads is almost exclusively reserved for patients undergoing concomitant cardiac surgery. Temporary epicardial pacing is frequently employed in patients undergoing cardiac surgery. Temporary wires are usually placed on the atrium and ventricle to allow for postoperative dual-chamber pacing. Following recovery from open heart surgery, these pacing wires may be associated with self-limited arrhythmias and, rarely, pericardial tamponade [42].

PERMANENT PACING

Implantation Indications

Guidelines for permanent pacemaker implantation have been established by the Joint American College of Cardiology/American Heart Association Task Force on Assessment of Cardiovascular Procedures and adapted by Medicare [43]. These guidelines encompass both indications for permanent pacing and recommendations for appropriate pacing mode selection.

Indications for implantation are categorized as: class I: chronic or recurrent conditions in which implantation is necessary and generally accepted; class II: conditions in which pacemakers are often used but opinions vary as to the need for a device; and class III: circumstances in which it is generally agreed that a pacemaker is not needed.

Sinoatrial dysfunction and AV conduction abnormalities are the principal indications for permanent pacemaker implantation. The association of symptomatic bradycardia, and its persistence or likelihood for recurrence, strengthens the indication for permanent pacing. Other influencing factors include underlying cardiac or cerebrovascular disease, the need for medication that may affect AV or sinoatrial function, and the patient's lifestyle (e.g., driving).

AV Block

Complete heart block (CHB) and symptomatic type II second-degree AV block are class I indications; asymptomatic type II second-degree AV block is considered class II. Asymptomatic type I second-degree AV block is usually categorized as class III, but the onset of symptoms or evidence of infra-hisian block indicates the need for implantation. Isolated first-degree AV block falls into class III.

Fascicular Block

Asymptomatic patients with bifascicular and trifascicular block should not receive prophylactic pacing. However, the presence of concomitant transient AV block or recurrent syncope without an alternative plausible explantation is an indication for permanent pacing.

Post-Myocardial Infarction

Temporary pacing indications for transient conduction abnormalities during myocardial infarction (MI) are different than permanent pacing indications in post-MI survivors. Persistent or transient high-grade second-degree AV block or CHB in association with bundle branch block (BBB) requires permanent pacing. Isolated second-degree AV block and first-degree AV block with BBB are class II. Transient AV block without an intraventricular conduction delay—typically in the setting of inferior wall MI—or with a left anterior hemiblock (LAHB), and isolated LAHB are in class III.

Sinus Node Dysfunction

Sinus node dysfunction (SND) or sick sinus syndrome (i.e., sinus bradycardia or arrest, sinoatrial block, paroxysmal supraventricular tachycardia, and/or bradycardic rhythms) requires the correlation of rhythm to symptoms before permanent pacing is considered. SND associated with documented symptoms, either spontaneous or related to required medications, is an indication for implantation. Asymptomatic bradycardia, whether spontaneous or in response to medication, falls into class III.

Hypersensitive Carotid Sinus Syndrome

This syndrome is an uncommon cause of syncope. Reproducible provocative testing with carotid sinus massage (CSM) or head tilt, which elicits a symptomatic asystolic period greater than 3 seconds due to sinus arrest or high-grade AV block, may confirm this diagnosis. Recurrent syncope, reproducible with CSM off medication, is a class I indication for a pacemaker, as is syncope due to bradycardia produced with head tilt. Recurrent syncope, with provoked asymptomatic asystole, is a class II indication. Asymptomatic or minimally symptomatic patients who demonstrate an asymptomatic response to CSM provocation are in class III.

Pacing Mode Indications

The rapid evolution of pacemaker technology and availability of single-chamber, dual-chamber, and rate-modulated units provide a wide range of options for device management of bradyarrhythmias. Optimal pacemaker selection requires careful analysis of the patient's overall clinical profile. Cardiac conduction disturbances, left ventricular function, associated coronary artery disease, comorbid states, medication, anticipated activity levels, implant and programming expertise, and cost factors must all be considered.

The most widely utilized single-chamber pacing modes include atrial inhibited pacing (AAI), rate-modulated AAI pacing (AAIR), VVI, and rate-modulated VVI pacing (VVIR). The pacemaker mode code is shown in Appendix A. Dual-chamber pacemakers provide for the potential of sensing and pacing both chambers while maintaining AV synchrony, that is, DDD pacing. Other dual-chamber modes include those that do not involve atrial pacing (VDD), those that provide for dual-chamber pacing without atrially tracked ventricular pacing (DDI), and rate-modulated DDD pacing (DDDR). Rate-modulated or adaptive-rate pacemakers use electronic "sensors" rather than atrial activity to modify the pacing rate. Clinically available sensors include those that monitor motion, temperature, oxygen saturation, impedance variations, and intracardiac potentials. The anesthetic considerations in patients with these implanted devices are discussed below.

Atrial inhibited pacing is most appropriate for patients with symptomatic sinus bradydysrhythmias and intact AV conduction. Patients with chronotropic insufficiency, that is, inadequate heart rate response to activity or stress, may be best managed with AAIR pacing.

Ventricular inhibited pacing is ideal for patients with persistent AV block and atrial dysrhythmias or in those in whom the maintenance of AV synchrony is believed to be less important. Patients with persistent atrial flutter/fibrillation, infirm or inactive patients, and those in whom follow-up study will be difficult are good candidates for this basic mode of pacing. VVIR pacing is recommended for subsets of patients who are active and would benefit from rate response during routine daily activities.

The presence of intact retrograde ventriculoatrial conduction, which may be determined at the time of pacemaker implant, is a relative contraindication to VVI pacing due to the risk of developing the "pacemaker syndrome" [40]. This syndrome refers to the constellation of signs and symptoms related to the adverse hemodynamic and electrophysiologic consequences of single-rate ventricular pacing. The symptoms may range from vague dizziness and palpitations to overt hypotension and low-output state. This syndrome is largely a result of loss of AV synchrony.

Dual-chamber pacing (i.e., DDD mode) is the mode of choice in patients with AV block, intact atrial function, and retrograde conduction or pacemaker syndrome. Patients with sinus node dysfunction and questionable AV conduction should be considered for DDD pacing. The DDDR mode is indicated in physically active patients with chronotropic incompetence.

Those patients with frequent supraventricular tachyarrhythmias (SVT) could be managed by the recently developed DDI (sensing/fixed rate pacing of both chambers) or DDIR (rate-modulated DDI pacing) modes. The VDD mode is regaining importance since the development of the "single-pass" lead (i.e., one lead achieves both atrial sensing and ventricular sensing/pacing), which allows AV synchrony and avoids implantation of an independent atrial lead.

Preoperative Evaluation

Investigation of the patient with a pacemaker should begin with a general evaluation of the patient. Patients who require pacemakers often have significant organic heart disease. As many as 50 percent of these patients have significant atherosclerotic heart disease, 20 percent may have hypertension, and 10 percent may have diabetes mellitus [44]. In addition, these patients may be receiving a variety of cardiac medications and thus require careful preoperative evaluation of their cardiopulmonary reserve. Attention should then be directed toward pacemaker-specific issues. Information regarding the initial indication for implantation and the patient's subsequent "pacemaker dependence" is important in determining the risk from transient pacer dysfunction during the perioperative period. Details about the implantation and follow-up study are quite helpful. Most patients receive identification cards specifying the type, model number, and manufacturer of their device and the date of its implantation. This information can be used to determine the status of the battery, the mode of pacing (i.e., VVI, DDD, etc.), and the various settings that were originally programmed at implant. Patients followed at pacemaker centers are evaluated by periodic clinical visits or via transtelephone monitoring, or both, and are least likely to suffer perioperative pacemaker malfunction due to unappreciated battery depletion or other pacing system failure. Medtronic Inc. (Minneapolis, MN) distributes pocket guides detailing the model numbers, manufacturers, basic pacing modes, and magnet/battery function of nearly all commercially available pacemakers. Individual anesthesiologists or anesthesia departments can easily obtain these handbooks and make them available for reference.

Further evaluation of the patient should include "routine" preoperative laboratory tests with special attention to potassium. Hypokalemia and hyperkalemia may render endocardial cells more refractory to pacing. In theory, hyperkalemia can promote pacing-induced ventricular arrhythmias but this is rarely seen. Peaked T waves may result from hyperkalemia and be falsely interpreted by the pacemaker as intrinsic ventricular complexes, leading to inappropriate inhibition of pacing. A patient in whom an MI has developed in the region of an implanted pacing lead may develop increased thresholds and loss of pacing, and will thus require a higher pacing output.

A preoperative ECG demonstrates the patient's rhythm and provides a crude assessment of the degree of dependence on the pacemaker. If the patient is unpaced, vagal maneuvers (carotid massage or Valsalva) may slow the intrinsic heart rate sufficiently to induce pacing, or magnet application to the pulse generator will transiently induce asynchronous pacing and allow determination of pacing capture. Capture is determined by noting consistent cardiac stimulation after a paced event (i.e., QRSs immediately follow ventricular pacing and P waves occur after atrial paced events). When pacing asynchronously, competition with intrinsic rhythms may occur; "noncapture" due to competition per se is physiologic and does not in any way indicate pacing malfunction. A preoperative chest x-ray is examined for the location and integrity of the pacing lead(s) (Fig. 12-3), and some pulse generators have a radiopaque symbol to aid in identification.

Should concerns remain following this initial assessment, a cardiology consultation is appropriate. A more thorough evaluation of the pacemaker involves use of a device-specific programmer to systematically analyze pacing and sensing threshold, refractory periods, and, where appropriate, many other parameters, including rate-modulation settings, AV delays, upper and lower rate limits, pacing and sensing polarities, and so forth. Reprogramming of the device can be performed at this time if so desired. Special concerns regarding specific procedures or use of electrocautery can be addressed (this issue is discussed in the following section). In pacer-dependent patients, the availability of a programmer and a cardiologist with specific understanding of pacing issues is highly desirable. If such expertise is not available, the manufacturer can be contracted to have a representative available in the operating room. A list of the leading pacemaker manufacturers is provided in Appendix B.

Effects of Diagnostic and Therapeutic Interventions on Permanent Pacemaker Function

Electrocautery

Electrocautery can potentially affect implanted pulse generators in one of several ways. Electrocautery units may generate electromagnetic fields as high as 60 V per meter. Pacemakers are designed to sense lower electromagnetic fields on the order of 0.1 V per meter. Inappropriate inhibition or triggering of pacer output during cautery commonly occurs as a result of sensing electromagnetic interference [45], and is most troublesome in pacemaker-dependent patients. Cautery may also induce transient asynchronous pacing due to reversion to the "noise mode," or reprogramming to the "back-up mode" [46], which necessitates resetting the device. When cautery must be used, problems can be minimized by limiting cautery to brief bursts and low energies, use of bipolar cautery systems, or positioning of the ground plate in a location remote from the pacing system, restricting use to areas at least 6 in. from the pulse generator, and when logistically and clinically appropriate, programming the device to an asynchronous pacing mode. Whenever feasible the electrical pathway between the cautery probe and ground plate should be perpendicular to the pacemaker lead system to further reduce exogenous currents in the pacing system. If polarity is a programmable option in a pulse generator, it should be set in the bipolar configuration to minimize the effects of outside electrical interference. Application of a magnet over a device during cautery is not recommended, as it enhances the chances of inappropriate device reprogramming in those pacemakers that require magnet application to access the programming circuit [47]. This problem will not occur in units that only use a radio frequency link for programming.

In addition to the self-limited problems just described, serious, albeit infrequent, untoward events may occur. Destruction of pacemaker circuitry with loss of pacemaker function [48], conduction of electrical impulses with resultant increases in pacing thresholds, myocardial thermal burns or initiation of ventricular fibrillation [49], and the induction of a "runaway pacemaker" [50] have all been reported. Thus, the benefits of electrocautery dur-

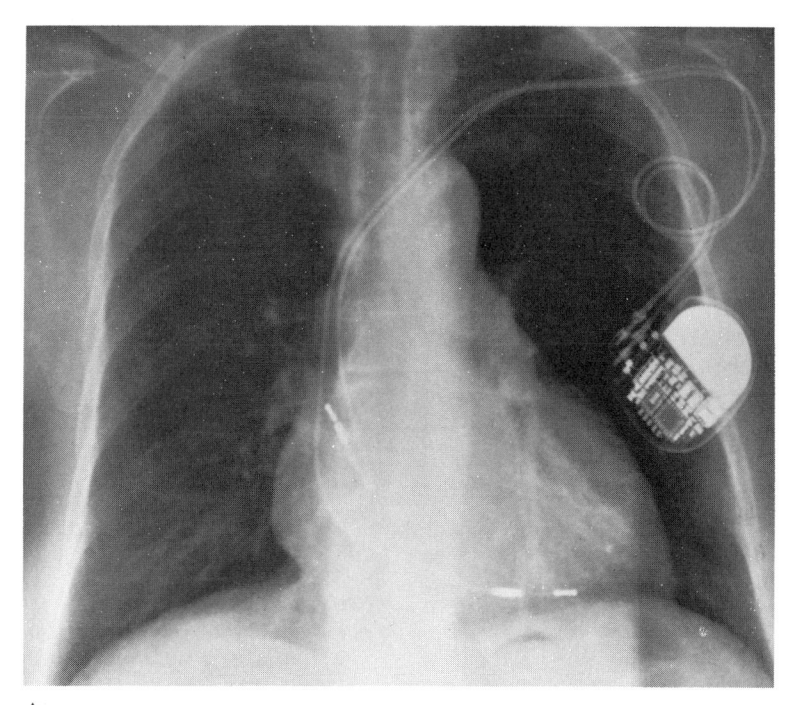

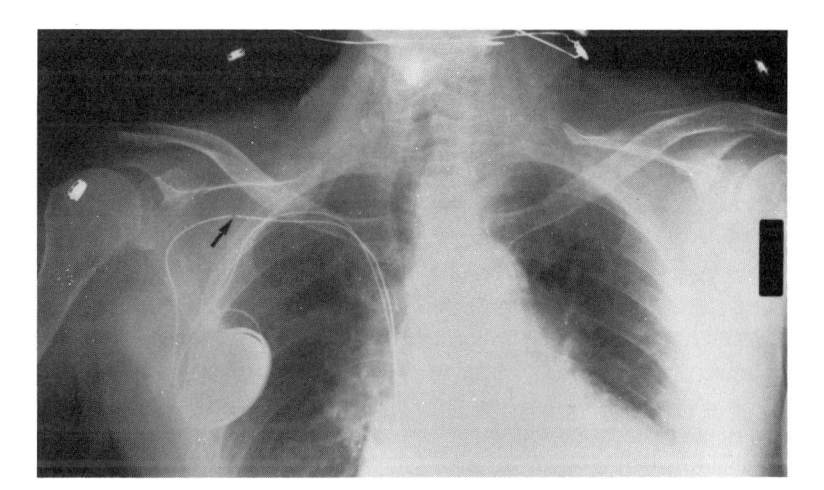

Fig. 12-3. A. The normal positions of the atrial and ventricular pacing electrodes. The atrial "J" lead is properly positioned in the right atrial appendage. The ventricular lead is located in the right ventricular apex. B. A fractured pacing electrode (*arrow*).

ing surgery must be weighed against potential complications in pacemaker patients and should account for the degree of pacemaker dependence, proximity of the operative field to the pulse generator, and type of cautery utilized. Careful pre- and postoperative assessment of pacemakers exposed to electrocautery is indicated.

Direct-Current Cardioversion

Despite the protective features incorporated in current-day pacemakers, external direct countershock can reprogram or destroy the circuitry of these devices [51, 52]. Defibrillation paddles should be kept as far away from the pulse generator and lead as possible. Anteroposterior positioning of the paddles is the configuration believed to carry the least risk. The lowest possible voltage should be used for defibrillation. Following defibrillation, the ECG should be observed, with simultaneous palpation of the carotid pulse. If defibrillation does not result in effective pulsatile flow, cardiopulmonary resuscitation (CPR) should be continued while alternatives are considered.

Lithotripsy

Lithotripsy is a new modality for the treatment of urinary tract calculi and gallstones. Calculi are disintegrated by shock waves generated by underwater high-voltage discharges that are synchronized to the patient's QRS. The presence of a permanent pacemaker was initially considered a contraindication to lithotripsy because of concern about potential pacer malfunction or destruction from barotrauma or electrical interference [53, 54]. Recent reports of in vitro and in vivo experience suggest that lithotripsy [55, 56] poses little to no risk of damaging pacemakers, and the transient sensing and output abnormalities that occur can be managed by the following guidelines: (1) The pacemaker device should be 6 in. or greater from the focal point of the lithotripsy; (2) rate-modulated devices, particularly those with piezoelectric crystals that sense vibration, should be programmed out of the activity mode; (3) DDD pacemakers should be programmed to VVI or VVD, or can be left in DDD in patients with intact native AV conduction; and (4) the ECG and lithotripsy should be synchronized to ensure delivery of the shock waves in the ventricular refractory period.

Magnetic Resonance Imaging

Magnetic resonance imaging (MRI) may deleteriously affect pacemakers because of the magnetic and radio frequency fields that are generated. These magnetic forces can physically rotate and move an implanted pacemaker device, and induce asynchronous pacing in most devices as a result of forced closure of the "reed switch." While MRI exposure does not appear to induce physical damage to pacemakers, it can cause transient periods of extremely rapid pacing rates in some devices (up to 3,000 bpm) [57]. MRI can seriously affect implantable cardioverter defibrillators (see below) by causing inappropriate charging of capacitors, device deactivation, or false arrhythmia detection [58]. MRI exposure must be considered contraindicated in most, if not all, patients with implanted pacemakers and cardioverter defibrillators.

Perioperative Management of Rate-Modulated Pacemakers

Currently, all Food and Drug Administration (FDA) approved rate-modulated pacemakers operate on the basis of one of three "sensor" parameters: vibratory sensation, change in blood temperature, or minute ventilation. Activity-sensing pacemakers detect body movement by a piezoelectric crystal built into the pacemaker unit. Physical activity may cause vibrations in the 5- to 40-Hz range that will in turn stimulate electrical impulses by the pacemaker. The device is programmed individually so that proportionate increases in activity produce a corresponding rise in the paced rate.

An anesthetic consideration of activity-sensing pacemakers is that vigorous position changes or surgical manipulations [59] will cause a transient increase in heart rate. Postoperative shivering, seizure activity, or electroconvulsive therapy may induce a tachycardia [60]. Fasciculations or myoclonus from intravenously injected anesthetics are of short duration and are unlikely to affect the paced heart rate.

Respiration-sensing pacemakers are programmed to increase heart rate in response to a matched increase in ventilation during exercise. These pacemakers detect changes in the electrical impedance of the thorax, which varies with changes in tidal volume and respiratory rate (minute ventilation) [61].

An anesthetic consideration of respiration-sensing pacemakers is that deliberate or inadvertent mechanical hyperventilation may lead to pacemaker-mediated tachycardia and hypotension [62]. Lack of understanding of the above mechanism can lead to inappropriate diagnosis of the tachycardia and to potentially harmful intervention.

Other sensing pacemakers increase heart rate in response to increase in blood temperature, QT interval, and myocardial contractility (right ventricular dp/dt), or decreased mixed venous oxygen saturation. With the exception of the temperature-sensing pacemakers, the others are not FDA approved.

Another anesthetic consideration is that perioperative change in body temperature, myocardial contractility, and mixed venous oxygen saturation may frequently occur during major surgery. Those changes may be extreme and of multifactorial etiology. Rapid fluid infusions, ventilation parameters, use of inotropes and vasodilators, myocardial ischemia, and sepsis can all affect the paced heart rate.

Rate modulation per se offers little in hemodynamic benefit during the immediate perioperative period, and maintaining patients in a rate-modulated mode may predispose them to inappropriate pacing rates. Thus, it is preferable to reprogram these devices to conventional, non–rate-modulated settings before surgery.

Implantable Cardioverter Defibrillators

Implantable cardioverter defibrillators (ICDs) are designed to detect and terminate malignant ventricular arrhythmias. First-generation systems required epicardial placement of patches and sensing leads, tunneling of the leads to a subcutaneous pocket in the abdomen, and attachment to a device that delivered a direct-current (DC) shock in response to rapid ventricular arrhythmias. Newer systems undergoing investigation have multiple additional capabilities, including antibradycardia and antitachycardia pacing, and are adaptable to nonthoracotomy transvenous lead systems.

Candidates for ICDs are patients who have inducible, sustained ventricular tachycardia or patients resuscitated following a cardiac arrest caused by a ventricular arrhythmia not associated with a myocardial infarction. Upon detection of rapid arrhythmias, a capacitor-charging cycle begins, followed by a defibrillation discharge. If ventricular tachycardia is detected, the discharge is synchronized with the R wave. If the arrhythmias persist, this sequence is repeated three times.

The previously discussed precautions and concerns relating to pacemakers apply to ICDs as well [63]. In addition, ICDs should generally be deactivated before operative procedures by an external programming device, as the "noisy" perioperative environment may lead to false detection of "arrhythmias" and result in delivery of inappropriate shocks or rapid ventricular pacing. These high-risk and "unprotected" patients require particularly careful monitoring of cardiac rhythm and electrolyte and metabolic status, and an external defibrillator should be easily accessible. X-rays that document the location of all the hardware implanted should be present in the operating room to help avoid inadvertent damage to the ICD system during the time of thoracic or abdominal surgery.

REFERENCES

1. Klein, RC, Vera, Z, Mason, DT. Intraventricular conduction defects in acute myocardial infarction: Incidence, prognosis, and therapy. *Am Heart J* 108: 1007, 1984.
2. Berg, GR, Kotler, MN. The significance of bilateral bundle branch block in the preoperative patient. *Chest* 59:62, 1971.
3. Horowitz, LN. Temporary Cardiac Pacing: Indications, Techniques and Management. In AH Hakki (ed), *Ideal Cardiac Pacing*. Philadelphia: Saunders, 1984. Pp 86–105.
4. Thompson, IR, Dalton, BC, Lappas, DG, et al. Right bundle-branch block and complete heart block caused by the Swan-Ganz catheter. *Anesthesiology* 51:359, 1979.
5. Sprung, CL, Pozen, RG, Rozanski, JJ, et al. Advanced ventricular arrhythmias during bedside pul-

monary artery catheterization. *Am J Med* 72:203, 1982.
6. Eissa, NT, Kvetan, V. Guide wire as a cause of complete heart block in patients with preexisting left bundle block. *Anesthesiology* 73:772, 1990.
7. Morris, D, Mulvihill, D, Lew, WYW. Risk of developing complete heart block during bedside pulmonary artery catheterization in patients with left bundle-branch block. *Arch Intern Med* 147:2005, 1987.
8. Zaidan, JR. Pacemakers. *Anesthesiology* 60:319, 1984.
9. Zoll, PM, Zoll, RH, Falk, RH, et al. External noninvasive temporary cardiac pacing: Clinical trials. *Circulation* 71:937, 1985.
10. Standards and guidelines for cardiopulmonary resuscitation (CPR) and emergency cardiac care (ECC). *JAMA* 255:2905, 1986.
11. Barthell, E, Toriano, P, Olson, D, et al. Prehospital external cardiac pacing: A prospective, controlled clinical trial. *Ann Emerg Med* 17:1221, 1988.
12. Berliner, D, Okun, M, Peters, RW, et al. Transcutaneous temporary pacing in the operating room. *JAMA* 254:84, 1985.
13. Kelly, JS, Royster, RL, Angert, KC, et al. Efficacy of noninvasive transcutaneous cardiac pacing in patients undergoing cardiac surgery. *Anesthesiology* 70:747, 1989.
14. Luck, JC, Davis, D. Termination of sustained tachycardia by external noninvasive pacing. *PACE* 10:1125, 1987.
15. Luck, JC, Grabb, BP, Artman, SE, et al. Termination of sustained ventricular tachycardia by noninvasive pacing. *Am J Cardiol* 61:574, 1988.
16. Feldman, MD, Zoll, PM, Aroesty, JM, et al. Hemodynamic response to noninvasive external cardiac pacing. *Am J Med* 84 (Pt 1):395, 1988.
17. Sharkey, SW, Chaffee, V, Kapsner, S. Prophylactic external pacing during cardioversion of atrial tachydysrhythmias. *Am J Cardiol* 55:1632, 1985.
18. Clinton, JE, Zoll, PM, Zoll, R, et al. Emergency noninvasive external cardiac pacing. *J Emerg Med* 2:155, 1985.
19. Kenyon, CJ, Aldinger, GE, Joshipuraj, P, et al. Successful resuscitation using external cardiac pacing in beta adrenergic antagonist-induced bradysystolic arrest. *Ann Emerg Med* 17:711, 1988.
20. Madsen, JK, Pedersen, F, Grande, P, et al. Normal myocardial enzymes and normal echocardiographic findings during noninvasive transcutaneous pacing. *PACE* 11:1188, 1988.
21. Voorhees, WD, II, Foster, KS, Geddes, LA, et al. Safety factor for precordial pacing: Minimum current thresholds for pacing and for ventricular fibrillation by vulnerable period stimulation. *PACE* 7:356, 1984.
22. Vargese, PJ, Bren, G, Ross, A. Electrophysiology of external pacing: A comparative study with endocardial pacing (abstract). *Circulation* 66 (Suppl II):II-349, 1982.
23. Falk, RH, Ngai, STA, Kumaki, DJ, et al. Cardiac activation during external cardiac pacing. *PACE* 10:503, 1987.
24. Prochaczek, F, Gaiecka, J, Machalski, M, et al. Diagnostic transcutaneous cardiac pacing examination of the ventriculo-atrial conduction (abstract). *PACE* 11 (Suppl):856, 1988.
25. Trigano, JA, Remond, JM, Mourot, F, et al. Left ventricular pressure during transcutaneous pacing (abstract). *PACE* 11:856, 1988.
26. Amar, D, Scher, C, Burt, M, et al. Noninvasive pacing in the lateral decubitus position and one-lung ventilation (abstract). *Anesth Analg* 74:S6, 1992.
27. Bachofen, JE, Schauble, JF, Rogers, MC. Transesophageal pacing for bradycardia. *Anesthesiology* 61:777, 1984.
28. Buchanan, D, Clements, F, Reves, JG, et al. Atrial esophageal pacing in patients undergoing coronary artery bypass grafting: Effects of previous cardiac operations and body surface area. *Anesthesiology* 69:595, 1988.
29. Greeley, WJ, Reves, JG. Transesophageal atrial pacing for the treatment of dysrhythmias in pediatric surgical patients. *Anesthesiology* 68:282, 1988.
30. Cung, DC, Townsend, GE, Kerr, CR. The optimum site and strength-duration relationship of transesophageal indirect atrial pacing. *Anesthesiology* 65:428, 1986.
31. Pattison, CZ, Atlee, JL, III, Mathews, EL, et al. Atrial pacing thresholds measured in anesthetized patients with the use of an esophageal stethoscope modified for pacing. *Anesthesiology* 74:854, 1991.
32. Furman, S, Robinson, G. The use of an intracardiac pacemaker in the correction of total heart block. *Surg Forum* 9:245, 1958.
33. Konstadt, SN, Reich, DL, Thys, DM, et al. Importance of atrial systole to ventricular filling predicted by transesophageal echocardiography. *Anesthesiology* 72:971, 1990.
34. Littleford, PO. Physiologic temporary pacing: Techniques and indications. *Clin Prog Pacing Electrophysiol* 2:236, 1984.
35. Benchimol, A, Ellis, JG, Dimond, EG. Hemodynamic consequences of atrial and ventricular pacing in patients with normal and abnormal hearts. *Am J Med* 39:911, 1965.

36. Hynes, JK, Holmes, DR, Jr, Harrison, CA. Five-year experience with temporary pacemaker therapy in the coronary care unit. *Mayo Clinic Proc* 58:122, 1983.
37. Trankina, MF, White, RD. Perioperative cardiac pacing using an atrioventricular pacing pulmonary artery catheter. *J Cardiothorac Anesth* 3:154, 1989.
38. Lumb, PD. Atrioventricular sequential pacing with transluminal atrial and ventricular pacing probes inserted via a pulmonary artery catheter: A preliminary comparison with epicardial wires. *J Clin Anesth* 1:292, 1989.
39. Thiagarajah, S, Azar, I, Agres, M, et al. Pacemaker malfunction associated with positive-pressure ventilation. *Anesthesiology* 58:565, 1983.
40. Hill, PE. Complication of permanent transvenous cardiac pacing: A 14-year review of all transvenous pacemakers inserted at one community hospital. *PACE* 10 (pt I):564, 1987.
41. Lyons, C. Sepsis and pacemaker malfunction. *Arch Intern Med* 142:540, 1982.
42. Hoidal, CR. Pericardial tamponade after removal of an epicardial pacemaker wire. *Crit Care Med* 14:305, 1986.
43. ACC/AHA Task Report. Guidelines for implantation of cardiac pacemakers and antiarrhythmic devices. *J Am Coll Cardiol* 8:1, 1991.
44. Furman, S. Cardiac pacing and pacemakers. I. Indications for pacing bradyarrhythmias. *Am Heart J* 93:523, 1977.
45. Furman, S, Parker, B. Electrosurgical device interference with implanted pacemakers. *JAMA* 239:1910, 1978.
46. Belott, PH, Sands, S, Warren, J. Resetting of DDO pacemakers due to EMI. *PACE* 7:169, 1984.
47. Damino, KB, Smith, TC. Electrocautery induced reprogramming of a pacemaker using a precordial magnet. *Anesth Analg* 62:609, 1983.
48. Gould, L, Chandrakandt, P, Betzu, R, et al. Pacemakers failure following electrocautery. *Clin Prog Pacing Electrophysiol* 4:53, 1986.
49. Orlando, JH, Jones, D. Cardiac pacemaker induced ventricular fibrillation during surgical diathermy. *Anaesth Intensive Care* 3:321, 1975.
50. Heller, LI. Surgical electrocautery and the runaway pacemaker syndrome. *PACE* 13:1084, 1990.
51. Das, G, Eaton, J. Pacemaker malfunction following transthoracic countershock. *PACE* 4:487, 1981.
52. Gould, L, Patel, S, Gomes, GL, et al. Pacemaker failure following external defibrillation. *PACE* 4:575, 1981.
53. Device disintegrates upper urinary stones. *FDA Drug Bull* 15:6, 1985.
54. Report of AUA Ad Hoc Committee to study the safety and clinical efficacy of current technology of percutaneous lithotripsy and non-invasive lithotripsy. Baltimore: American Urologic Assoc Inc, May, 1986.
55. Fetter, J, Patterson, D, Aram, G, et al. Effects of extracorporeal shock wave lithotripsy on single chamber rate response and dual chamber pacemakers. *PACE* 12:1494, 1989.
56. Cooper, D, Wilkoff, B, Masterson, M, et al. Effects of extracorporeal shock wave lithotripsy on cardiac pacemakers and safety in patients with implanted cardiac pacemakers. *PACE* 11:1607, 1988.
57. Hayes, DL. Practical Considerations. In S Furman, DL Hayes, OR Holmes (eds), *A Practice of Cardiac Pacing*. Mount Kisco, NY: Futura, 1989. Pp 606–607.
58. Bach, SM, Shapland, HE. Engineering Aspects of Implantable Defibrillators. In S Saksena, N Goldschlager (eds), *Electrical Therapy for Cardiac Arrhythmias*. Philadelphia: Saunders, 1990. P 337.
59. Andersen, C, Oxhoj, H, Arnsbo, P, et al. Pregnancy and cesarean section in a patient with a rate responsive pacemaker. *PACE* 12:386, 1989.
60. Andersen, C, Madsen, GM. Rate-responsive pacemakers and anaesthesia. *Anaesthesia* 45:472, 1990.
61. Mond, H, Strathmore, N, Kertes, P, et al. Rate responsive pacing using a minute ventilation sensor. *PACE* 11:1866, 1988.
62. Madsen, GM, Andersen, C. Pacemaker-induced tachycardia during general anaesthesia: A case report. *Br J Anaesth* 63:360, 1989.
63. Gaba, DM, Wyner, J, Fish, KJ. Anesthesia and the automatic implantable cardioverter/defibrillator. *Anesthesiology* 62:786, 1985.

Appendix A: The NASPE/BPEG (NBG) Pacemaker Code

Position and category

I Chamber(s) paced	II Chamber(s) sensed	III Response to sensing	IV Programmability, rate modulation	V Antitachyarrhythmia function(s)
O—None	O—None	O—None	O—None	O—None
A—Atrium	A—Atrium	T—Triggered	P—Simple	P—Pacing
V—Ventricle	V—Ventricle	I—Inhibited	M—Multiprogrammable	S—Shock
D—Dual (A & V)	D—Dual (A & V)	D—Dual (T & I)	C—Communicating (telemetry)	D—Dual (P & S)
			R—Rate modulation	

NASPE/BPEG = North American/British Pacing and Electrophysiology Group; A & V = atrial and ventricular; T & I = dual (atrial/ventricular) and inhibited; P & S = pacing and shock.

Appendix B: Pacemaker Manufacturers Index

Manufacturer	Telephone no.*
American Pacemaker Co.	(617) 890-5656
Biotronik	(800) 547-0934
	(503) 635-3594
Cardiac Control Systems	(904) 445-5450
Cardiac Pacemaker Inc.	(800) 328-9588
	(612) 631-3000
Cardio-Pace Medical	(612) 483-6787
Cordis Corp.	(800) 327-2490
	(305) 551-2000
Cook Pacemaker Co.	(800) 245-4715
	(412) 845-8621
Coratomic	(800) 245-6886
	(412) 349-1811
ELA Medical	(612) 935-2033
Intermedics Inc.	(800) 231-2330
	(713) 233-8611
Medtronic Inc.	(800) 328-2518
	(612) 547-4000
Pacesetter Systems Inc.	(800) 423-5611
(Siemens Pacesetter)	(818) 362-6822
Siemens Elema	(800) 423-5611
(Siemens Pacesetter)	(818) 362-6822
Teletronics	(800) 525-7042
	(303) 790-8000

*These are 24-hour emergency telephone numbers. When calling, request the clinical engineering division and have the pacemaker model number handy.

13
Postcardiac Surgical Patients

JOSEPH I. SIMPSON
ZVI ZISBROD

With the advent of recent technology, patients are now surviving cardiac surgery in much greater numbers than in years past. While elective noncardiac surgery would not be scheduled in the immediate or early postoperative cardiac surgical patient, occasionally some of these patients need to come to the operating room emergently for noncardiac surgery (Table 13-1). While perhaps the most common cause of emergency noncardiac surgery in the postoperative cardiac surgical patient is mediastinal bleeding and cardiac tamponade, other surgical emergencies do occur, principally abdominal or peripheral vascular, or both [1].

The hemodynamic and consequently anesthetic considerations in these patients may vary widely. On one end of the spectrum, these patients may be hemodynamically stable and "fixed" from a cardiac point of view, while on the other end of the spectrum, they may be in cardiogenic shock, requiring inotropic and perhaps even intraaortic balloon pump (IABP) support.

These patients may have a variety of pathophysiologic disorders that may complicate the anesthetic management of their emergent noncardiac surgery. These include hemodynamic and myocardial insufficiency [2, 3], respiratory problems [4], coagulation disorders [5], acute renal failure [6], arrhythmias, and acute neurologic deficits [7] (Table 13-2).

In the first part of this chapter, we discuss these common pathophysiologic problems and their impact on the anesthetic management of these patients. In the second part of this chapter, we discuss the most common surgical emergencies that will cause these patients to present to the operating room. Since mediastinal bleeding and tamponade are really within the purview of cardiac surgery, they are not discussed here.

POSTOPERATIVE PATHOPHYSIOLOGIC CONSEQUENCES OF CARDIAC SURGERY

Hemodynamic

Hypotension

Hemodynamic problems following cardiac surgery include hypotension, hypertension, and low-output syndrome (Table 13-3). The most common hemodynamic problem seen in this patient population is hypotension. Hypotension may be caused by a variety of etiologies, including vasodilatation, sepsis, hypovolemia, and, more ominously, ventricular failure.

Table 13-1. Noncardiac surgical emergencies following cardiac surgery

Femoral artery thrombectomy
Femoral artery reconstruction or aortofemoral bypass
Cholecystectomy
Resection of gangrenous bowel
Extremity amputation
Exploratory laparotomy for pancreatitis
Vagotomy and pyloroplasty
Antrectomy
Fasciotomy for compartment syndrome

Table 13-2. Common abnormalities following cardiac surgery

Arrhythmias
Conduction abnormalities
Cardiogenic shock
Low-output syndrome
Hypovolemia
Coagulopathy
Acute renal failure
Sepsis
Respiratory insufficiency
New neurologic injury

Table 13-3. Hemodynamic problems after cardiac surgery

Low-output syndrome
Biventricular failure
Vasodilatation
Hypotension
Hypertension
Arrhythmias

Vasodilatation

Vasodilatation can be seen in the early (drug induced, temperature equilibration) or late (sepsis) postoperative periods. Treatment will depend on the cause and may include the use of α-adrenergic agonists such as phenylephrine or norepinephrine (Levophed) infusions. Adding an inhalational anesthetic to a patient who is vasoconstrictor dependent may produce profound hypotension; a major regional anesthetic may have the same effect. Use of a narcotic-ketamine combination may prove the safest method, although narcotics can cause mild vasodilatation and ketamine may produce hypotension in the patient with catecholamine depletion (see Chap. 3).

Low-output Syndrome and Ventricular Dysfunction

Most cardiac surgical patients have some ventricular dysfunction postoperatively [2]. Causes for this are multifactorial and include acute myocardial infarction [8], poor myocardial protection during cardiopulmonary bypass, reperfusion injuries [9], and myocardial edema. Many patients will exhibit improvement in this ventricular dysfunction over the first few days following cardiac surgery.

Some patients will exhibit severe left ventricular dysfunction early, which may improve after 24 to 48 hours. This has been termed the *stunned myocardium* [10]. Causes may include reperfusion injury [9] worsened by calcium entry [11], prolonged ischemia [10], and inadequate myocardial protection during cardiopulmonary bypass.

Almost all of these patients with ventricular dysfunction will require inotropic support in the postoperative period, and thus when they present to the operating room for their emergency noncardiac surgery they may be on various beta agonist or alpha and beta agonist infusions (Table 13-4).

In some cases the ventricular dysfunction may be so severe that the patient may require an IAPB. The physiology of the IAPB is too involved to be discussed in this chapter. Briefly, the IAPB improves coronary blood flow, lowers left ventricular afterload, improves cardiac output, and decreases left ventricular stroke work and left ventricular wall stress [12] (Fig. 13-1; Table 13-5). The most frequent complication of IAPB is leg ischemia from obstruction to flow or clot formation, or both, in the femoral artery. Severe leg ischemia is frequently an indication for discontinuing IAPB and an emer-

Table 13-4. Inotropic infusions used to treat ventricular dysfunction after cardiac surgery

Epinephrine
Dopamine
Dobutamine
Amrinone
Norepinephrine
Isoproterenol

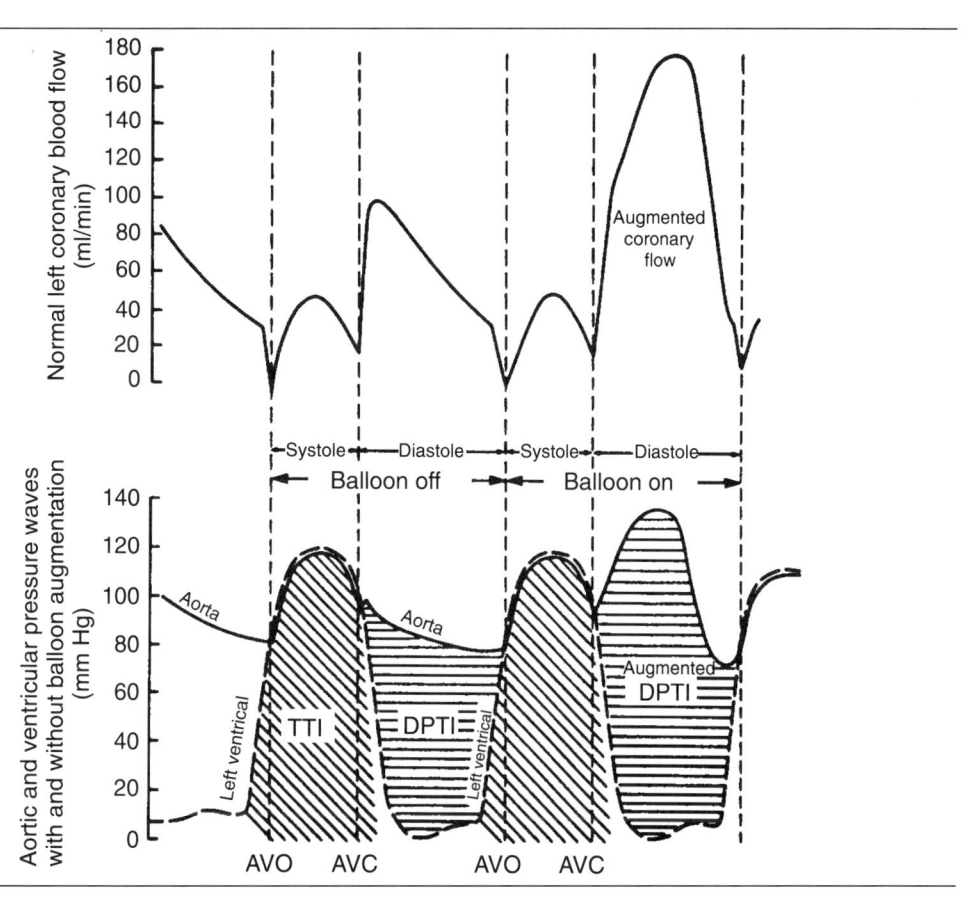

Fig. 13-1. *Top:* Blood flow in the left coronary artery with and without intraaortic balloon counterpulsation. Note that normal left coronary blood flow occurs mostly in diastole, and diastolic left coronary blood flow is greatly increased during balloon counterpulsation. *Bottom:* Simultaneous aortic and left ventricular pressure tracings. TTI is the area under the ventricular and aortic pressure curves during systole. DPTI is the area under the left ventricular and aortic pressure curves during diastole. With balloon inflation during diastole, both aortic diastolic pressure and coronary perfusion pressure are increased. DPTI is also increased, improving the myocardial oxygen supply-demand ratio, which is estimated by the DPTI:TTI ratio. AVO = aortic valve open; AVC = aortic valve closed. (Reprinted with permission from GA Maccioli, WJ Lucas, and EA Norfleet, The intra-aortic balloon pump: A review. *J Cardiothorac Anesth* 2:365–373, 1988.)

gency embolectomy or femoral artery reconstruction may be necessary. Other less common complications include thrombocytopenia, embolic events, aortic injury, and bowel ischemia [13] (Table 13-6).

The anesthetic management of these patients

Table 13-5. Physiologic effects of IAPB

Increased coronary blood flow
Decreased left ventricular afterload
Decreased left ventricular wall stress
Increased cardiac output
Increased renal blood flow

Table 13-6. Complications of intraaortic balloon counterpulsation

Ipsilateral leg ischemia
Femoral artery thrombosis
Thrombocytopenia
Aortic injury
Bowel ischemia
Thromboembolic events
Gas embolism

for emergency noncardiac surgery can be very difficult. They are unlikely to tolerate anesthetic drugs with negative inotropic qualities (barbiturates, propofol, inhalation anesthetics, nitrous oxide, etc.). Belo and Mazer [13] showed in the dog model that halothane and isoflurane will worsen the already depressed ventricular function of the stunned myocardium.

Anesthetics with minimal myocardial effects, such as fentanyl, sufentanil, and etomidate, may prove to be the drugs of choice. As discussed earlier (and in Chap. 3) while ketamine usually causes hemodynamic stimulation, it may produce severe myocardial depression in a patient with catecholamine depletion, and patients receiving inotropic infusions may be catecholamine depleted.

Hypertension

In the immediate postoperative period, cardiac surgical patients may exhibit severe hypertension [14]. Causes of this hypertension can be multifactorial and include inadequate anesthesia, sympathetic nervous system overdrive, activation of the renin-angiotensin system [15], and rebound effect of drugs chronically taken preoperatively (β-blockers clonidine, etc.).

These patients are frequently receiving high doses of vasodilators or α- and β-blockers, or both, to treat this hypertension (nitroglycerin, nitroprusside, esmolol, labetalol, etc.). Additionally, these patients are frequently heavily medicated and sedated. It is important to note that induction of anesthesia (for emergency noncardiac surgery) in such a patient may lead to a precipitous fall in blood pressure. Blood pressure should be invasively monitored and careful titration of anesthetic agents as well as vasodilators is required.

Respiratory Pathology

In most patients pulmonary function deteriorates early after cardiac surgery and slowly improves over the first few days, but some of the changes can last several weeks. Causes of this dysfunction include reduction of lung volume, median sternotomy, mucous plugging, atelectasis, pump lung, V/Q mismatch, and cardiogenic pulmonary edema.

All lung volumes, with the possible exception of the residual volume, are reduced after cardiac surgery [16]. Dead space ventilation is increased, and a restrictive pulmonary pattern may develop. Causes of these decreased lung volumes include pain, decreased chest wall compliance, and diaphragmatic dysfunction [17]. Cardiogenic pulmonary edema is another cause of pulmonary dysfunction after cardiac surgery and is usually treated with inotropes, vasodilators, and diuretics [18].

Postperfusion lung injury or "pump lung" is an increasingly rarer event following modern cardiopulmonary bypass [19]. Although the mechanism is not clear, causes may include microvascular and alveolar lung injury by microemboli with a subsequent inflammatory response. Mucous plugging, atelectasis, and pneumonia are occasionally seen after cardiac surgery, and patients sometimes require frequent bronchoscopies for removal of mucous plugs and reexpansion of collapsed areas of lung.

Many of these patients will require prolonged intubation and mechanical ventilation. They will arrive at the operating room intubated, possibly requiring positive end expiratory pressure, making transport from the intensive care unit to the OR difficult. Transport of these patients should always include portable pulse oximetry monitoring. Induction of anesthesia for emergency noncardiac surgery may further worsen their already compromised respiratory function. These patients will usually require a high concentration of inspired oxygen, which may preclude the use of anesthetic agents such as nitrous oxide.

Arrhythmias

Postcardiac surgical patients frequently have varying types of arrhythmias (Table 13-7). Anesthetic management of the patient with arrhythmias is

Table 13-7. Common arrhythmias following cardiac surgery

Ventricular tachycardia
Frequent premature ventricular contractions
Atrial fibrillation
Atrial flutter
Complete heart block
Supraventricular tachycardia

discussed in Chap. 10. Many of these patients will be on antiarrhythmic drug infusions when they arrive at the OR. Some of these drugs are myocardial depressants, and anesthetic agents added to them can precipitate hemodynamic collapse (see Chap. 10).

Coagulation

In the early postoperative period following cardiac surgery, severe coagulopathies can develop. Causes include thrombocytopenia, platelet dysfunction, primary fibrinolysis, heparin rebound, and, less commonly, factor deficiencies and disseminated intravascular coagulation (DIC).

Platelet counts frequently decrease 25 to 30 percent during cardiopulmonary bypass [20]. Causes for this decrease include dilution by the pump prime and platelet destruction by the pump rollers, pump suction, oxygenators, and filters. In addition to platelet loss, significant platelet dysfunction occurs following cardiopulmonary bypass, which may affect large platelets more than small ones [21].

Heparin rebound may occur in the early postoperative period. This is usually adequately treated with additional protamine. Primary fibrinolysis frequently occurs following cardiopulmonary bypass. It is thought to be caused by disruption of cell membranes on bypass, leading to the release of plasminogen activator substances [22]. Secondary fibrinolysis is usually part of a DIC picture, and only occurs with some other precipitating factor (sepsis, drug reaction, etc.). Primary fibrinolysis can be treated with ϵ-aminocaproic acid.

Clotting factor deficiencies also occur following cardiopulmonary bypass. However, most of these factors only decrease 30 to 40 percent, leaving enough (60–70%) functioning factors for adequate hemostasis in the majority of cases [23, 24]. Factors V and VIII seem to be especially vulnerable to the effects of cardiopulmonary bypass.

Patients with a coagulopathy who present to the OR for emergent noncardiac surgery carry a significant increased morbidity. Bleeding problems should be treated based on etiology. Platelets should be given if the platelet count is low or if the results of thromboelastography or sonoclot analysis indicate platelet dysfunction. Desmopressin acetate [25] may improve platelet dysfunction by causing release of factor VIIIC from endothelial tissue. Protamine can be used to treat heparin rebound, aminocaproic acid to treat primary fibrinolysis (but not secondary fibrinolysis), and fresh frozen plasma to treat factor deficiencies.

Renal Failure

Acute renal failure can occur following cardiac surgery. The incidence ranges from 2 to 30 percent [26, 27]. Mortality from acute renal failure in this setting approaches 60 percent. Predisposing factors include preoperative renal insufficiency, cardiogenic shock, intraaortic balloon counterpulsation, diabetes, and prolonged cardiopulmonary bypass.

Numerous factors contribute to the more common causes of acute parenchymal renal failure. Ischemic damage is the most important cause, and to a lesser extent sepsis and nephrotoxic medication.

Acute tubular necrosis (ATN) is a serious complication of cardiopulmonary bypass and is associated with increased mortality. It usually occurs after a period of prolonged hypotension that results in nephron ischemia and reduced renal cortical blood flow.

Metabolic abnormalities seen with acute renal failure include hyperkalemia, hypocalcemia, acidosis, and volume overload. Patients with acute renal failure in this setting will frequently require at least temporary (if not permanent) dialysis. Oliguric renal failure carries a worse prognosis than polyuric renal failure, and therefore many of these patients will be receiving therapy aimed at increasing urine output (diuretics, renal-dose dopamine, etc.).

The anesthetic management of these patients can be challenging. The course of the renal failure is often unpredictable, and, therefore, anesthetic agents and muscle relaxants with predominately renal excretion should be avoided. Hyperkalemia and acidosis may be present and thus may complicate anesthetic management. While volume overload should be avoided, dehydration may lead to a decline in urine flow and may worsen prerenal azotemia. Therefore, monitoring should include an accurate assessment of volume status, and a pulmonary artery catheter is recommended for all but the most minor surgical procedure.

Neurologic Complications

The incidence of stroke following cardiac surgery is estimated at 0.9 to 5.0 percent [28–30]. Etiology includes preexisting carotid disease [28], air and particulate emboli [31], hypotension, hypoxemia, cardiopulmonary bypass, and intracerebral hemorrhage.

Some patients will have temporary neurologic dysfunction related to any of the above causes. The patient may be disoriented, combative, or comatose. Hypotension during a subsequent anesthesia may worsen the neurologic injury. Long-acting anesthetics and muscle relaxants given during the subsequent noncardiac procedure may mask the neurologic examination and make evaluation of the patient's neurologic status difficult.

SURGICAL COMPLICATIONS AFTER CARDIOPULMONARY BYPASS

Though many complications can occur after cardiac surgery, most do not require surgical intervention. However, some problems that present in the postoperative period require emergency surgical intervention for either diagnosis or treatment. Additionally, on rare occasions unrelated coincidental surgical problems develop that require intervention. These problems primarily fall into two categories: intraabdominal and vascular catastrophes.

Intraabdominal Complications

General surgical complications that occur immediately after cardiac surgery are usually serious and difficult to assess. These complications tend to present in a different and more complex manner than usual. Postcardiac surgical patients may often be mildly febrile. In addition, laboratory values such as liver enzymes and white blood cell counts may be elevated and therefore mask the clinical picture. Abdominal air may be introduced during the cardiac procedure and therefore subdiaphragmatic air does not necessarily represent a ruptured viscus. Since the incidence of such complications is low, each physician's experience and therefore judgment may be limited. Finally, it is difficult to transport these patients for appropriate studies and therefore it is more likely that these complications will be missed by delaying the necessary evaluation.

Incidence and Etiology

The incidence of general surgical complications following cardiac surgery in both the early and late postoperative periods is low (0.9 and 1.6%, respectively) [32, 33]. General surgical complications that occurred within 6 weeks of cardiac surgery carried a mortality of 22 percent. General surgical complications that occurred more than 6 weeks after cardiac surgery had a mortality of 1.1 percent [32].

The most common cause of intraabdominal complications is visceral hypoperfusion [34–37]. It is more common to see these complications in patients who have had a prolonged period of cardiopulmonary bypass. This may be related to the fact that a greater percentage of these patients required reexploration of the chest for postoperative hypotension, low cardiac index, and bleeding, and many of them required continuous postoperative vasopressors, including the use of an IABP. Approximately 75 percent of patients in whom gastrointestinal complications developed had a prolonged bypass time or a depressed postoperative cardiac output, or both [34]. It is well known that end-organ hypoperfusion and ischemic damage can accompany the peripheral vasoconstriction and low cardiac output of cardiogenic shock [38, 39].

In a review of 2,500 cardiac procedures, Lawhorne and associates [40], found the incidence of postoperative abdominal complications to be 0.6 percent. In this group, 5 patients died, with an overall 30 percent mortality [40]. In 1982, Hanks and colleagues [1] reported that 37 of 4000 patients who underwent cardiopulmonary bypass had gastrointestinal complications (1% incidence rate). Multisystem failure was cited as the most common contributory factor leading to a 70 percent mortality. In one study, 50 percent of the patients with postoperative abdominal surgical complications had previously diagnosed gastrointestinal disease [35]. Although not all complications are preventable, recognition of preexisting disease may help to alert the physician at the onset of symptoms.

Gastroduodenal Ulcerations

Gastroduodenal ulcerations are well-recognized complications in "stressed" patients. The reported incidence in cardiac surgical patients has been 1 to 2 percent [39, 41–44]. Children appear to be more susceptible than adults [45]. Usually, symptoms of ulcer pain or bleeding respond to antacid and H_2-antagonist therapy, but if conservative measures fail, surgical intervention may be necessary. Using vagotomy, pyloroplasty, or resection, Taylor and associates [46] reported a 30 percent mortality in 26 patients undergoing surgery for gastroduodenal ulcers after cardiac surgery. Perhaps this mortality might be reduced by simply oversewing perforations and by attempts at controlling hemorrhage by fluoroscopically guided embolization techniques.

Significant gastroduodenal bleeding is defined as bleeding manifested by hematemesis or melena associated with an acute drop in the hemoglobin level of at least 2 gm. Regional blood flow alterations to the gastric mucosa are generally thought to be important in the development of stress ulcer–related gastrointestinal bleeding after cardiac surgery [41]. As was discussed earlier an increased incidence is found in older patients, in patients with histories of ulcer or gastrointestinal bleeding, in patients who require reoperation for excessive chest tube drainage, and in patients with other significant postoperative complications. Although cardiopulmonary bypass affects coagulation, gastroduodenal ulceration and bleeding are usually not the result of abnormalities of coagulation (see earlier in text). The sources of bleeding that were caused by "stress ulcerations" are typically multiple and superficial, and involve the stomach or duodenum, or both. Signs and symptoms may include hematemesis, which may occur as a result of any significant bleeding occurring at any site from the pharynx to the ligament of Treitz. The blood vomited may be fresh and red, indicating fairly rapid or recent bleeding, or it may be dark and "coffee ground," owing to the effect of stomach acid on the blood. Melena may persist for as long as 5 days after a significant gastrointestinal bleed, and occult blood may be detected for up to 3 weeks.

Endoscopy has become the favored technique for evaluating these patients [37, 44]. It has the advantage of being able to directly visualize such causes as ulcers and erosive gastritis. It can also be used therapeutically in electrocoagulation of bleeding sites.

Arteriography may pinpoint the site of bleeding in selected patients. For this to be possible, bleeding must be at a rate of approximately 5 ml per minute. Following the diagnostic phase of the study, the catheter can be left in place and used for therapeutic administration of vasopressin or embolic material.

Since most of these patients are sick, surgical treatment, when needed, should be as limited as possible. Suture ligation of the bleeding ulcer, vagotomy, and pyloroplasty are adequate for isolated duodenal ulcers, but partial gastrectomy with or without vagotomy is the preferred procedure whenever multiple duodenal or gastric ulcers are present [37, 44, 47].

The overall incidence of serious gastrointestinal bleeding after open heart surgery is small, and the routine use of postoperative antacids and H_2-receptor blockers is important in the prevention of this potentially devastating complication.

Acute Pancreatitis

The pancreas lies in a retroperitoneal position, draped across the vertebral column. Symptoms due to pancreatitis are on many occasions vague and nonspecific, and therefore hard to diagnose. Although the incidence of pancreatitis is less than 1 percent in patients undergoing cardiac surgery [37], pancreatitis in this setting usually occurs in conjunction with renal and other organ failure, with an aggressive, often fatal, course.

The diagnosis and treatment of acute pancreatitis after cardiac surgery is difficult. Symptoms may be atypical and misleading or may be obscured by other complications [37, 48]. The usual laboratory characteristics of pancreatitis, including hyperamylasemia, do not appear to be reliable indicators of the disease in patients after cardiopulmonary bypass. The diagnosis is often missed until autopsy, but even when it is made antemortem, the mortality of affected patients has been higher than in any other recognized form of pancreatitis. Clinically, we recognize two forms of pancreatitis, mild and fulminant necrotizing pancreatitis.

In mild pancreatitis, the patient has abdominal pain, decreased bowel sounds, nausea, and hyperamylasemia [37]. These symptoms often resolve with conservative treatment consisting of bowel rest and intravenous fluids. These patients usually do not experience hemodynamic instability, and their serum total and ionized calcium levels remain within normal limits.

Fulminating necrotizing pancreatitis appears in sick patients, and is marked by severe hemodynamic instability in the early postoperative period. Prolonged low cardiac output with a cardiac index of less than 2 liters per minute/m^2 and mean aortic pressure less than 80 mm Hg are common. These patients frequently require both α- and β-adrenergic support, as well as intraaortic balloon counterpulsation [37].

Etiology. A recent study pointed to the possible involvement of exogenously administered calcium in the pathogenesis of postcardiac surgery pancreatitis [49]. There is evidence that the pancreas, like the kidney, may be very sensitive to the effects of hypoperfusion. Experimental hypotension in dogs has been shown to cause a marked reduction in pancreatic blood flow, which in turn is associated with injury to the acinar cells, including lysosomal swelling, vacuolization, and the release of both proteolytic enzymes and a myocardial depressant factor. Bore and colleagues [50] demonstrated the production of severe edema in the isolated dog pancreas subjected to 2 hours of total ischemia.

Symptoms. The earliest and most common symptoms referable to pancreatitis are abdominal distention and hypoactive bowel sounds [51]. Significant abdominal pain and tenderness, however, are not noted until much later in the course of the disease. Total serum amylase levels are of little value in diagnosing or following progression of the disease in patients with necrotizing pancreatitis. Leukocytosis of more than 12,000 cells/mm^3 is usually present and decreased levels of serum ionized calcium are common. Frequently, these patients are thought to be septic and, despite negative blood cultures, they receive antibiotics. The diagnosis of necrotizing pancreatitis is usually made very late in its course. Persistence of fever, ileus, abdominal pain, and mild tenderness in a toxic patient may lead to an exploratory laparotomy where necrotizing pancreatitis is found.

The initial treatment of acute pancreatitis is supportive and includes fluids, electrolyte resuscitation, and respiratory support. Nasogastric decompression usually is instituted to relieve vomiting and perhaps to decrease pancreatic stimulation. Immediate laparotomy may be indicated diagnostically in order to exclude gangrenous cholecystitis, intestinal infarction, perforated ulcer, or some other intraabdominal problem. However, early therapeutic laparotomy in severe pancreatitis has a higher morbidity and mortality than does medical management.

The operative procedure in necrotizing pancreatitis is mobilization of the pancreas, debridement, and drainage, with concomitant gastrostomy, jejunostomy, and cholecystostomy. The prognosis of acute necrotizing pancreatitis is very poor and the mortality is very high.

Bowel Obstruction

The diagnosis of bowel obstruction is generally a clinical and radiographic one. Mild leukocytosis is commonly seen in uncomplicated mechanical obstruction. Moderate elevations of white cell count strongly suggest the presence of strangulation, and marked leukocytosis indicates primary mesenteric vascular occlusion. Another common laboratory finding is elevation of serum amylase, suggesting ischemic bowel.

Ogilvie's Syndrome. A specific form of adynamic colonic ileus is a form of colonic pseudo-obstruction [52–54]. On plain film, it appears similar to a mechanical obstruction of the left colon, and colonoscopy may be required to differentiate between the two. One must always consider underlying electrolyte abnormalities and drug effects as contributing to an adynamic ileus. The therapy is expectant relative to etiology, but includes nasogastric suction, rectal decompression, and correction of underlying fluid and electrolyte abnormalities.

Acute Cholecystitis

The patient with acute cholecystitis may have fever and leukocytosis but may lack localized physical findings. Persistent fever, leukocytosis, and hyperbilirubinemia should alert the physician to the possibility that extrahepatic biliary tract disease may be the cause. There may, however, be other causes of jaundice. Jaundice after heart surgery may also be related to chronic passive congestion, hemolysis, infection, vasoconstriction, obstruction by the venous cannula, and low cardiac output.

Fever is the abnormality most often noted initially, but because cholecystitis in the postoperative period is relatively rare, this diagnosis is not likely to head the list of possible causes of temperature elevation. The clinical diagnosis resides in repeated examinations of the right upper abdomen for a tender mass or for signs of local peritoneal irritation. The diagnostic evaluation includes radionucleotide scans and sonography. Causes of acute cholecystitis in the cardiac surgical setting include ischemia and a state of decreased perfusion leading to hypoxia of the gallbladder [55, 56]. This goes along with the higher incidence of acalculus cholecystitis that is seen in postoperative cardiac surgical patients, in comparison to the usual patient with cholecystitis. Cholecystitis in the postoperative period is a complication that is exceedingly serious [57].

In one series, acute cholecystitis occurred in 18 percent of patients with intraabdominal complications and carried a mortality of 73 percent [58]. In another series, the mortality was 66 percent [1]. The results of both studies suggest a higher mortality for postcardiopulmonary bypass cholecystitis compared with cholecystitis that occurs after noncardiac surgery (for which a mortality of 47% was reported). Though cholecystectomy is the preferred procedure, a cholecystostomy may provide a temporary solution in the gravely ill patient.

Intestinal Ischemia and Infarction

Patients with preexisting evidence of celiac or mesenteric artery disease are at an increased risk for development of bowel ischemia or infarction, secondary to prolonged postoperative low-output syndrome or embolic events. Common causes include emboli, microemboli, and preexisting atherosclerotic vascular disease. Functional hypoperfusion occurs with severe shock and with vasoconstriction, which is often accentuated by vasopressors used to treat the hypotensive patient. Bowel ischemia is suspected in patients who have generalized abdominal tenderness accompanied by a picture of persistent metabolic acidosis [1, 33, 34, 40, 58].

Diagnosis of ischemic bowel is made by endoscopy when possible. Barium enema will show the typical thumb-printing of the bowel wall. Surgical resection is the treatment for infarcted bowel; improvement in perfusion and, where possible, vasodilatation can be tried first if reversible bowel ischemia is suspected.

Vascular Complications

Iatrogenic arterial injuries can result from needles, catheters, or IABPs placed in the femoral artery. Arterial occlusion usually occurs as the result of thrombus in association with the intimal injury. Treatment consists of prompt exploration with arteriotomy and thrombectomy. Intimal and medial damage is usually treated by debridement back to the normal artery, with repair using a vein, Gortex patch, or interposition graft. Peripheral vascular complications are associated with preoperative evidence of peripheral vascular disease, prolonged peri- and postoperative low cardiac output syndrome, and cardiac emboli. If the cause is an IAPB, the device may have to be removed, and worsening of hemodynamic instability may follow. Early diagnosis allows for embolectomy or bypass procedures that can successfully salvage the limb. With late diagnosis, the patient may be toxic, myoglobinuric, and in real failure, and may require amputation. Surgery should not be delayed by attributing ischemia associated with arterial injury to arterial spasm.

When an extremity has been subjected to ischemia and muscle necrosis occurs, reperfusion can result in metabolic acidosis and profound hyperkalemia. Rhabdomyolysis releases myoglobin, which precipitates in acid urine, producing renal tubular obstruction and renal failure. Myoglobinuria produces a red urine that is free of red blood cells. Treatment requires prompt reversal of hyperkalemia to prevent cardiac arrest (IV insulin and glucose), administration of sodium bicarbonate to alkalinize the urine and to treat systemic metabolic acidosis, and osmotic diuresis with mannitol to prevent renal tubular obstruction.

Pulmonary Emboli

One must have a very low threshold for suspecting pulmonary emboli in postcardiac surgical patients. Eighty-five percent of pulmonary emboli arise from the lower extremity, 10 percent from the right atrium, and 5 percent from the pelvic veins, vena cava, or arms. Up to 30 percent of pulmonary embolic events are without symptoms, and only one third of patients with pulmonary emboli have physical evidence of deep-vein thrombosis at the time of diagnosis. Emboli produce symptoms either by the direct effect of pulmonary arterial obstruction or by secondary bronchospasm and vasoconstriction. The most common symptoms are dyspnea and chest pain, and the most common signs are tachycardia, tachypnea, and rales. The classic triad of dyspnea, pain, and hemoptysis is present in fewer than 25 percent of patients.

Pulmonary arteriograms are the most specific way to make the diagnosis. On ventilation-perfusion scans, areas of the lungs that are normally ventilated but not perfused and appear normal on chest x-ray are highly suspect for pulmonary emboli. The primary therapy for pulmonary emboli in most patients is anticoagulation. The precise role of thrombolytic agents is still in evolution. For certain patients, caval interruption may be indicated. These include patients in whom heparin therapy is contraindicated, those who have recurrent emboli while receiving anticoagulation therapy, and those with free-floating iliofemoral thrombi. Additionally, it includes some patients with septic pulmonary emboli that are refractory to heparin and antibiotics.

Patients with massive pulmonary emboli producing hypotension who survive the acute event are candidates for pulmonary embolectomy, using cardiopulmonary bypass and open clot extraction.

Multiorgan Failure

Multiple organ failure has become recognized as a clinical syndrome over the last 20 years. This is mostly a result of improved resuscitation, more aggressive operative intervention, advances in medical technology, and antibiotics, all of which have allowed patients to survive procedures that would have been fatal in previous decades [59–62].

The common initial event is relative or absolute hypoperfusion. Central to the systemic nature of this syndrome is a microcirculatory perfusion deficit and the resulting cellular injury in many or all body tissues, which in turn leads to the activation of the systemic inflammatory response. The clinical picture is heralded by acute lung injury and followed by renal and hepatic failure and often death.

The sequence of events usually starts from what appears to be a period of relative clinical stability. The patient begins to exhibit persistent hypermetabolism usually associated with some form of acute lung injury, which ranges from a mild capillary leak to fulminant adult respiratory distress syndrome. The persistent hypermetabolism may last for several weeks and is associated with progressive deterioration of renal and hepatic function.

This hypermetabolic stage is characterized by increased cardiac output and decreased systemic vascular resistance. The acute lung injury is characterized by arterial hypoxemia, decreased pulmonary compliance, increased intrapulmonary shunt, and diffuse infiltrates on the chest radiograph. In addition, oxygen uptake is compromised, a process related to the lung parenchymal injury. Peripheral oxygen utilization is also disturbed. Oxygen demands may be twice normal, and oxygen extraction may also be abnormal, similar to that which occurs in sepsis.

Repeated episodes of bacteremia and pneumonia, usually with gram-negative enteric organisms, and viral and fungal infection usually occur. Deterioration of gastrointestinal function is characterized by ileus, stress ulceration, bleeding, and diarrhea. Biliary dilatation and bile stasis are common and frequently occur in the absence of extrahepatic obstruction. The patient is frequently obtunded and comatose. With further multiorgan failure coagulopathy occurs, with a picture of impaired platelet function thrombocytopenia and DIC. Eventually, hyperbilirubinemia out of proportion to other hepatocellular enzyme elevation ensues. Mortality is extremely high (>80%) and surgical intervention is usually not helpful.

REFERENCES

1. Hanks, JB, Curtis, SE, Hanks, BB, et al. Gastrointestinal complications after cardiopulmonary bypass. *Surgery* 92:394–400, 1982.
2. Mangano, DT. Biventricular function after myocardial revascularization in humans: Deterioration and recovery patterns during the first 24 hours. *Anesthesiology* 62:571–577, 1985.
3. Lappas, DG, Powell, WMJ, Daggett, WM. Cardiac dysfunction in the perioperative period. *Anesthesiology* 47:117–137, 1977.
4. Krasna, MJ, Scott, GE, Scholz, PM, et al. Postoperative enhancement of urinary output in patients with acute renal failure using continuous furosemide therapy. *Chest* 89:294–295, 1986.
5. Tanaka, K, Takao, M, Yuasa, H, et al. Alterations

6. Kron, IL, Joob, AW, Van Meter, C. Acute renal failure in the cardiovascular surgical patient. *Ann Thorac Surg* 39:590–598, 1985.
7. Gardner, TJ, Horneffer, PJ, Manolio, TA, et al. Major stroke after coronary artery bypass surgery: Changing magnitude of the problem. *J Vasc Surg* 3:684–687, 1986.
8. Miller, DC, Stinson, EB, Oyer, PE, et al. Discriminant analysis of the changing risks of coronary artery operations; 1971–1979. *J Thorac Cardiovasc Surg* 85:197–213, 1983.
9. Breissblatt, WM, Stein, KL, Wolfe, CJ, et al. Acute myocardial dysfunction and recovery: A common occurrence after coronary bypass surgery. *J Am Coll Cardiol* 15:1261–1269, 1990.
10. Braunwald, E, Kloner, RA. The stunned myocardium: Prolonged, postischemic ventricular dysfunction. *Circulation* 6:1146–1149, 1982.
11. Kusuoka, H, Porterfield, JK, Weisman, HF, et al. Pathology and pathogenesis of stunned myocardium—depressed Ca^2 activation of contraction as a consequence of reperfusion-induced cellular calcium overload in ferret hearts. *J Clin Invest* 79:950–961, 1987.
12. Maccioli, GA, Lucas, WJ, Norfleet, EA. The intraaortic balloon pump: A review. *J Cardiothorac Anesth* 2:365–373, 1988.
13. Belo, SE, Mazer, CD. Effect of halothane and isoflurane on postischemic "stunned" myocardium in the dog. *Anesthesiology* 73:1243–1251, 1990.
14. Roberts, AJ, Niarchos, AP, Subramanian, VA, et al. Systemic hypertension associated with coronary artery bypass surgery. *J Thorac Cardiovasc Surg* 74:846, 1977.
15. Taylor, KM, Morton, IJ, Brown, JJ, et al. Hypertension and the renin-angiotensin system following open-heart surgery. *J Thorac Cardiovasc Surg* 74:840, 1977.
16. Ghia, J, Anderson, N. Pulmonary function and cardiopulmonary bypass. *JAMA* 212:593–597, 1970.
17. Jedrzejowicz, AM, Brophy, C, Moxham, J, et al. Assessment of diaphragm weakness. *Am Rev Respr Dis* 137:877–883, 1988.
18. Fedullo, AJ, Swinburne, AJ, Wahl, GW, et al. APACHE II score and mortality in respiratory failure due to cardiogenic pulmonary edema. *Crit Care Med* 16:1218–1221, 1988.
19. Byrick, RJ, Noble, WH. Postperfusion lung syndrome. *J Thorac Cardiovasc Surg* 76:685–693, 1978.
20. Mammen, EF, Koets, MH, Washington, BC, et al. Hemostasis changes during cardiopulmonary bypass surgery. *Semin Thromb Hemost* 11:281–292, 1985.
21. Karpatkin, S. Heterogenicity of human platelets. II. Functional evidence suggestive of young and old platelets. *J Clin Invest* 47:1083–1087, 1969.
22. Bick, RL, Frazier, BL, Saunders, CL, et al. Alterations of hemostasis during cardiopulmonary bypass: The potential role of factor XII activation in inducing primary fibrino(geno)lysis. *Blood* 64:926, 1984.
23. Bick, RL. Hemostasis defects associated with cardiac surgery, prosthetic devices, and other extracorporeal circuits. *Semin Thromb Hemost* 11:249–280, 1985.
24. Rush, B, Ellis, H. The treatment of patients with factor V deficiency. *Thromb Diasth Haemorrh* 14:74–82, 1965.
25. Salzman, EW, Weinstein, MJ, Weintraub, RM, et al. Treatment with desmopressin acetate to reduce blood loss after cardiac surgery—a double-blind randomized trial. *N Engl J Med* 314:1402–1406, 1986.
26. Gailiunas, P, Jr, Chawla, R, Lazarus, JM, et al. Acute renal failure following cardiac operations. *J Thorac Cardiovasc Surg* 79:241–243, 1980.
27. Hilberman, M, Myers, BD, Carrie, BJ, et al. Acute renal failure following cardiac surgery. *J Thorac Cardiovasc Surg* 77:880–888, 1979.
28. Reed, GL, III, Singer, DE, Picard, EH, et al. Stroke following coronary-artery bypass surgery—a case-control estimate of the risk from carotid bruits. *N Engl J Med* 319:1246–1250, 1988.
29. Breuer, AC, Furlan, AJ, Hanson, MR, et al. Central nervous system complications of coronary artery bypass graft surgery: Prospective analysis of 421 patients. *Stroke* 14:682–687, 1983.
30. Tufo, HM, Ostfeld, AM, Shekelle, R. Central nervous system dysfunction following open-heart surgery. *JAMA* 212:1333, 1970.
31. Slogoff, S, Girgis, KZ, Keats, AS. Etiologic factors in neuropsychiatric complications associated with cardiopulmonary bypass. *Anesth Analg* 61:903–911, 1982.
32. Pinson, CW, Alberty, RE. General surgical complications after cardiopulmonary bypass surgery. *Am J Surg* 146:133, 1983.
33. Beath, DB, Wolfgang, TC. General surgical complications following cardiac surgery. *Am Surg* 49:11, 1983.
34. Maneta, GC, Misback, GA, Ivey, TD. Hypoperfusion as a possible factor in the development of gastrointestinal complications after cardiac surgery. *Am J Surg* 149:648, 1985.
35. Welling, RE, Roth, R, Albers, JE, et al. Gastrointestinal complications after cardiac surgery. *Arch Surg* 121:1178, 1986.

36. Welsh, GF, Dozois, RR, Bartholomeo, LG, et al. Gastrointestinal bleeding after open heart surgery. *J Thorac Cardiovasc Surg* 65:738, 1973.
37. Hass, GS, Warshaw, AL, Paggett, WM, et al. Acute pancreatitis after cardiopulmonary bypass. *Am J Surg* 149:508, 1985.
38. Haber, MH, Brown, WT, Schneider, KA. Ischemic necrosis of multiple organs in prolonged shock. *JAMA* 163:7, 1963.
39. McNamara, JJ, Aisten, WG. Gastrointestinal bleeding occurring in patients with acquired valvular heart disease. *Arch Surg* 97:538, 1968.
40. Lawhorne, TW, David, JL, Smith, GW. General surgical complications after cardiac surgery. *Am J Surg* 136:254, 1976.
41. Stremph, JF, Mori, H, Lev, R, et al. The stress ulcer syndrome. *Curr Probl Surg* 2:64, 1973.
42. Katz, SE, Kornfeld, DS, Harris, PD, et al. Acute gastrointestinal ulceration with open heart surgery and aortic valve disease. *Surgery* 72:438, 1972.
43. Mead, J, Folk, F. Gastrointestinal bleeding after cardiac surgery. *N Engl J Med* 281:799, 1969.
44. David, E, Kelly, KA. Acute post-operative peptic ulceration. *Surg Clin North Am* 49:1111, 1969.
45. Kreel, I, Zaroff, LI. Acute gastrointestinal ulceration: Complications of cardiac surgery—a review with a report of five cases. *Mt Sinai J Med* 26:111, 1959.
46. Taylor, PC, Loop, FD, Hermann, RE. Management of acute ulcer syndrome after cardiac surgery. *Ann Surg* 178:1, 1973.
47. David, E, McGrath, DC, Higgins, JA. Clinical experience with acute peptic gastrointestinal ulcers. *Mayo Clin Proc* 46:15, 1971.
48. Smith, CR, Schwartz, S. Amylase: Creatinine clearance ratios, serum amylase and lipase after operation with cardiopulmonary bypass. *Surgery* 194:458, 1983.
49. Fernandez del Castillo, C, Harringer, W, Warshaw, AL, et al. Risk factors for pancreatic cellular injury after cardiopulmonary bypass. *NEJM* 325:382, 1991.
50. Bore, PJ, Zuidema, GD, Cameron, JC. The role of ischemia in acute pancreatitis: Studies with isolated perfused canine pancreas. *Surgery* 91:377–382, 1982.
51. Freiner, H. Pancreatitis after cardiac surgery. *Am J Surg* 131:684, 1976.
52. Norton, L, Young, D, Scribner, R. Management of pseudo obstruction of the colon. *Surg Gynecol Obstet* 138:595, 1974.
53. Geelhoed, GW. Colonic pseudo-obstruction in surgical patients. *Am J Surg* 149:258, 1985.
54. Wanebo, H, Nalhewason, C, Conolly, B. Pseudo-obstruction of the colon. *Surg Gynecol Obstet* 133:44, 1971.
55. Glen, F. Acute cholecystitis. *Surg Gynecol Obstet* 143:58, 1976.
56. Broc, PJ, Zuidema, GD, Cameron, JC. The role of ischemia in acute pancreatitis: Studies with an isolated perfused canine pancreas. *Surgery* 91:377, 1982.
57. Ohinger, LW. Acute cholecystitis as a post operative complication. *Ann Surg* 184:162, 1976.
58. Leitman, IM, Paul, DE, Barie, PS, et al. Intra abdominal complications of cardiopulmonary bypass operations. *Surg Gynecol Obstet* 165:251, 1987.
59. Barton, RG, Cerra, FB. The hypermetabolism–multiple organ failure syndrome. *Chest* 96:1153–1160, 1989.
60. Bawe, AE. Multiple, progressive or sequential organ failure: A syndrome of the 1970's. *Arch Surg* 110:779, 1975.
61. Cerra, FB. Multiple Organ Failure Syndrome. In DJ Bihari, FB Cerra, *New Horizon: Multiple Organ Failure*. California Society of Critical Care Medicine, 1989. Pp 1–24.
62. Cerra, FB, Negro, F, Abrams, JH. APACHE II score does not predict multiple organ failure or mortality in post-operative surgical patient. *Arch Surg* 125:519–522, 1990.

14
The Pregnant Patient with Cardiac Disease

DAVID WLODY

The anesthetic management of the patient with severe cardiac disease is a challenge under ideal circumstances. This challenge can be enormously compounded in pregnant patients. First and most importantly, the physiologic changes of pregnancy place significant stress on the cardiovascular system, and can lead to decompensation in patients who were previously asymptomatic, or only mildly so. Secondly, labor, delivery, and the puerperium add additional stresses to the maternal cardiovascular system. Finally, while maternal well-being must remain our paramount concern, our interventions must be influenced by the presence of the fetus, and every attempt must be made to maintain uteroplacental blood flow and fetal oxygen delivery.

THE EPIDEMIOLOGY OF CARDIAC DISEASE DURING PREGNANCY

The past half century has seen changes in both the absolute incidence of cardiac disease during pregnancy and the distribution of type of disease. The incidence of cardiac disease has decreased from 3.6 percent in the period from 1942 to 1951, to a current level of between 0.5 and 2.0 percent [1]. The primary cause for this is a significant decrease in the number of patients with rheumatic valvular heart disease, due to the widespread use of effective antibiotic treatment of streptococcal infections.

The most common rheumatic valvular disease seen in pregnancy is mitral stenosis, with an incidence of 90 percent. The next most common lesion is mitral insufficiency. Aortic disease is seen in fewer than 4 percent of pregnant women with rheumatic heart disease.

At the same time, the number of pregnant patients with congenital cardiac disease has increased significantly. This is due to the more effective medical treatment available, as well as advances in both corrective and palliative surgery. Thus, increasing numbers of patients with once fatal structural congenital cardiac disease are now reaching their childbearing years. Ventricular septal defect and atrial septal defect are the most common congenital lesions seen in pregnancy [1]. All told, the ratio of rheumatic heart disease to congenital heart disease has decreased from 25:1 to 3:1 [1] (Table 14-1).

While still uncommon, there is an ever increasing number of pregnant cardiac patients who have coronary artery disease [2]. Factors influencing this trend include the rising prevalence of cardiac disease in the population as a whole, as well as the increased incidence of smoking among women. The increasingly common postponement of preg-

Table 14-1. Incidence and mortality of rheumatic and congenital heart disease in pregnancy

Type of heart disease	Distribution (%)	Mortality (%) Maternal	Fetal
Rheumatic heart disease (75%)			
Mitral stenosis	90	1–17	3.5
Mitral insufficiency	6.5		
Aortic insufficiency	2.5		
Aortic stenosis	1.0		
	100		
Congenital heart disease (25%)			
Ventricular septal defect	7–26	7–40	2–16
Atrial septal defect	8–38	1–12	1–12
Patent ductus arteriosus	6–20	5–6	17
Tetralogy of Fallot	2–15	4–12	36–59
Eisenmenger's syndrome	2–4	12–33	30–54
Coarctation of the aorta	4–18	3–9	10–20
Aortic stenosis	2–10		22
Pulmonic stenosis	8–16		4
Primary pulmonary hypertension	1–2	53	7

Source: Reprinted with permission from DT Mangano, Anesthesia for the Pregnant Cardiac Patient. In SM Shnider and G Levinson (eds), *Anesthesia for Obstetrics* (2nd ed). Baltimore: Williams & Wilkins, 1987. P 346. © 1987, the Williams & Wilkins Co, Baltimore.

nancy until age 35 or beyond is undoubtedly another contributing factor to this increase.

MATERNAL PHYSIOLOGIC CHANGES DURING PREGNANCY

It is accurate to say that there is not a single organ system that is unaffected by pregnancy. A complete discussion of these changes is beyond the scope of this chapter. Instead, discussion is limited to those changes that are most pertinent to the pregnant patient with underlying cardiac disease.

Cardiovascular System

In normal pregnancy, numerous signs and symptoms may be erroneously ascribed to underlying cardiac disease [3] (Table 14-2). Decreased exercise tolerance, dyspnea, and orthopnea are not uncommon in uncomplicated pregnancy. These symptoms are primarily due to the mechanical effect of the uterus producing limitation of diaphragmatic excursion. Light-headedness or even syncope may occur. This is primarily a symptom of late gestation, and reflects the decreased cardiac output and hypotension that can be seen when venous return is impeded due to inferior vena cava compression by the gravid uterus (the supine hypotensive syndrome).

Table 14-2. Physical findings in normal pregnancy

Decreased exercise tolerance
Orthopnea
Dyspnea
Jugular venous distention and peripheral edema
Bibasilar rales
Systolic murmurs
ECG changes
QRS axis deviation
Q wave in lead III
ST segment depression

On physical examination, jugular venous distention is frequently seen after the 20th week of gestation. Ankle edema is also common, due to both increased femoral venous pressure secondary to caval compression and decreased colloid oncotic pressure. Bibasilar rales can be seen in the absence of cardiac disease; this is due to atelectasis, produced by the enlarged uterus compressing the lungs. In conjunction with the normal hyperventilation of pregnancy, this may be mistakenly interpreted as a sign of congestive heart failure. Auscultation of the heart demonstrates increased loudness of the first heart sound as early as the 12th week of gestation. Perloff [4] suggests that the cause of this increase is the hyperdynamic left ventricle. While less common, the second heart sound can also be increased in late pregnancy. Systolic murmurs are almost ubiquitous during pregnancy, with a reported incidence of as high as 96 percent [5]. These are generally grade 1 to 3/6, early to mid-systolic murmurs. They are believed to represent increased flow, due to increased cardiac output, as well as improved rheology of blood secondary to the normal dilutional anemia of pregnancy. A systolic murmur greater than 3/6, or any diastolic murmur, should be considered an abnormal finding.

Electrocardiographic changes are quite common during pregnancy. QRS axis deviation to the left and to the right have both been reported. Small Q waves in lead III have been reported to be a normal finding in pregnancy. ST segment depression has been shown in 14 percent of a group of normal women [6]. Finally, rhythm disturbances including supraventricular tachycardia, atrial premature contractions, ventricular premature contractions, and wandering atrial pacemaker are more common during pregnancy.

Pregnancy is associated with a significant increase in blood volume. This begins as early as the 6th week of pregnancy, and continues at a rapid rate until midpregnancy. Blood volume continues to increase, but at a slower rate, until the final weeks of pregnancy, when blood volume appears to plateau. Most studies show an increase in blood volume of approximately 50 percent at term. The cause of the hypervolemia of pregnancy is not known with certainty, but it has been hypothesized that estrogen increases the activity of the renin-angiotensin system, leading to hyperaldosteronism and sodium and water retention [7].

Cardiac output is known to increase in pregnancy, but the time of onset of these changes has not been studied extensively. Capeless and Clapp [8] studied eight women preconceptually and sequentially during pregnancy with M-mode echocardiography. They demonstrated a 22 percent increase in cardiac output by 8 weeks' gestation, which represented 57 percent of the total change seen at 24 weeks. This early change was due to an increase in stroke volume; heart rate was unchanged until 16 weeks, when it rose 11 percent above preconceptual values. Systemic vascular resistance (SVR) decreased 30 percent by 8 weeks' gestation; this represented 90 percent of the total decrease seen at 24 weeks. Thus, there is evidence that major hemodynamic changes occur during the earliest weeks of pregnancy [8] (Table 14-3; Fig. 14-1). After 24 weeks' gestation, cardiac output remains stable or increases slightly (Fig. 14-2). Older studies demonstrating a fall in cardiac output in the third trimester reflect measurements performed in the supine position. The vena caval compression produced by this positioning probably caused these decreases in cardiac output.

Table 14-3. Physiologic changes of pregnancy—hemodynamic

Blood volume increased 50% at term
Cardiac output increased 40% at term
Systemic resistance decreased 20% at term
Myocardial contractility unchanged
Cardiac output increased 80% above prelabor values during second stage

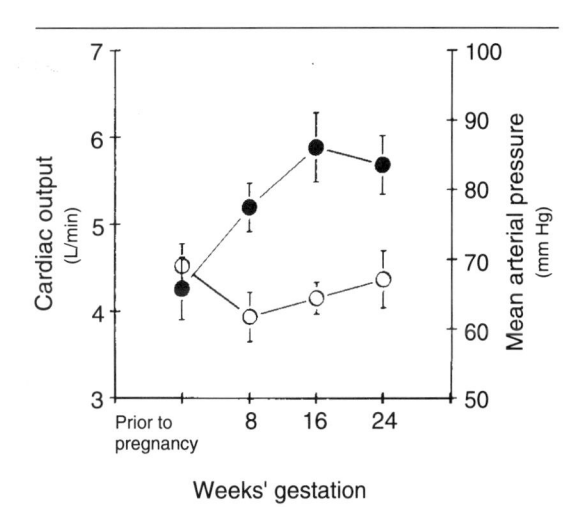

Fig. 14-1. Changes in cardiac output (*closed circles*) and mean arterial pressure (*open circles*) during early pregnancy. (Reprinted with permission from EL Capeless and JF Clapp, Cardiovascular changes in early phase of pregnancy. *Am J Obstet Gynecol* 161:1449–1453, 1989.)

It is only recently that hemodynamic assessment has been performed in normal pregnant women at term. Using pulmonary artery catheters in 10 such women, Clark and associates [9] demonstrated a 43 percent increase in cardiac output, a 17 percent increase in heart rate, and decreases in systemic and pulmonary vascular resistance of 21 and 34 percent, respectively (Fig. 14-3). The left ventricular stroke work index to pulmonary capillary wedge pressure ratio was unchanged; however, there is no intrinsic increase in myocardial contractility in late pregnancy [9].

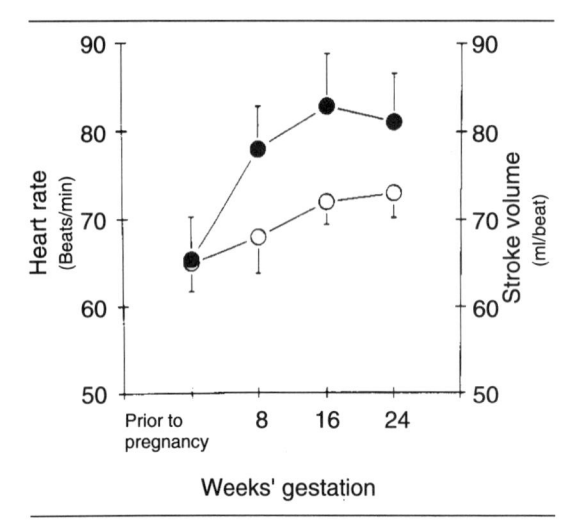

Fig. 14-2. Changes in heart rate (*closed circles*) and stroke volume (*open circles*) during early pregnancy. (Reprinted with permission from EL Capeless and JF Clapp, Cardiovascular changes in early phase of pregnancy. *Am J Obstet Gynecol* 161:1449–1453, 1989.)

Fig. 14-3. Maternal changes in hemodynamic variables at term. SVR = systemic vascular resistance; PVR = pulmonary vascular resistance; COP = colloid oncotic pressure; PCWP = pulmonary capillary wedge pressure; CO = cardiac output; HR = heart rate; MAP = mean arterial pressure; CVP = central venous pressure; PAP = pulmonary artery pressure; LVSWI = left ventricular stroke work index. (Reprinted with permission from SL Clark, DB Cotton, W Lee, et al. Central hemodynamic assessment of normal term pregnancy. *Am J Obstet Gynecol* 161:1439–1442, 1989.)

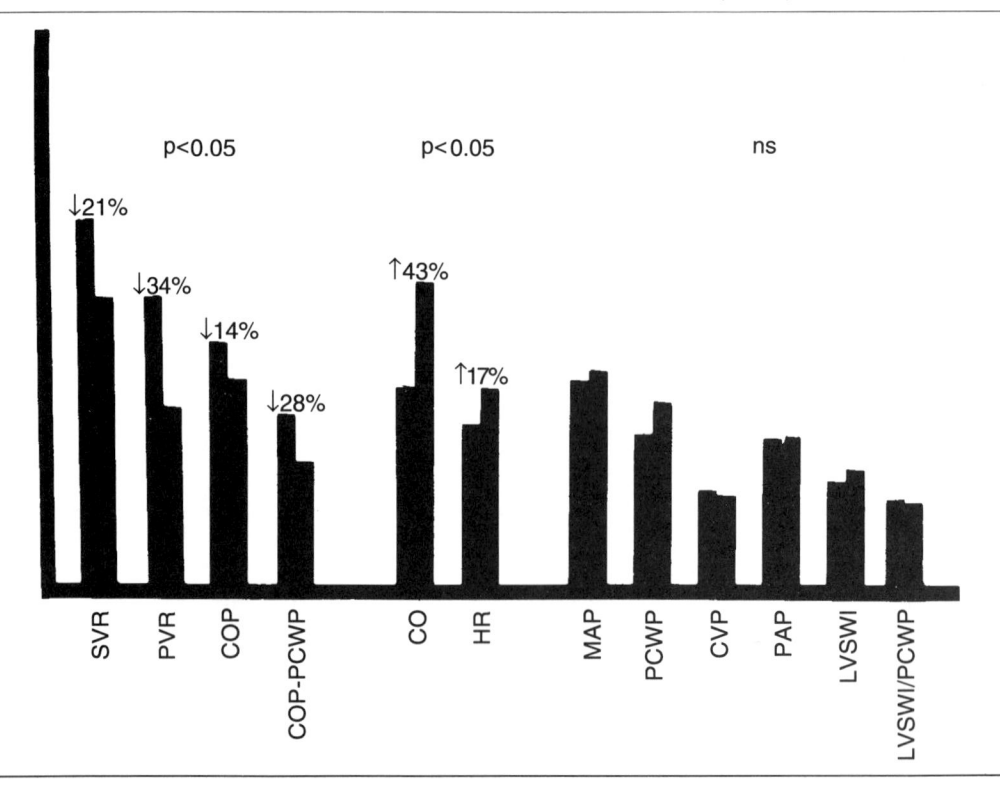

The mechanism for the decreased SVR during pregnancy has not been fully established. One contributing factor is the creation of a low-resistance vascular bed within the uterus, in parallel with the systemic circulation. In addition, elevated levels of estrogen, with its vasodilatory effects, decrease resistance in other vascular beds as well. Increased levels of prostacyclin (PGI_2) have a similar effect. Finally, the improved flow characteristics of blood secondary to the dilutional anemia of pregnancy produce a further decrease in resistance [7].

Labor produces increases in cardiac output as high as 60 percent above prelabor values. Part of this increase is due to the pain and apprehension associated with contractions, an increase that can be blunted by the provision of adequate analgesia [10]. There is a further increase in cardiac output, unaffected by analgesia, that is due to the "autotransfusion" of 300 to 500 ml blood from the uterus into the central circulation with each contraction.

Finally, cardiac output increases even further immediately postpartum, reaching levels 80 percent higher than prelabor values. This is again probably due to autotransfusion from the rapidly involuting uterus, as well as augmentation of preload secondary to alleviation of vena caval compression.

These changes lend credence to Elkayam and Gleicher's contention that "cesarean sections are often erroneously performed to avoid marked hemodynamic alterations that are associated with labor" [7]. It is clear that the operation itself, as well as the anesthetic required to perform it, can both have significant hemodynamic effects. The postpartum period will be marked by considerable hemodynamic fluctuation, whatever the route of delivery. Thus, in large measure the decision to perform cesarean section should be based on obstetric indications. Should vaginal delivery be performed in the patient with underlying cardiac disease, the provision of adequate analgesia will minimize the pain of labor and delivery, and thus the stress on the cardiovascular system.

Respiratory System

Capillary engorgement of the mucosa of the entire respiratory tract occurs during pregnancy, producing an increased tendency to bleeding if the mucosa is injured. This is particularly evident in the

Table 14-4. Physiologic changes of pregnancy—respiratory

Capillary engorgement
Minute ventilation increased 40%
Oxygen consumption increased 20%
Functional residual capacity decreased 20%
Low $PaCO_2$ (32 mm Hg)

nasal mucosa, and therefore nasotracheal intubation should be avoided whenever possible. This capillary engorgement can affect the larynx as well, sometimes requiring placement of a smaller endotracheal tube than predicted. In severe cases, laryngeal edema may make identification of the glottic opening almost impossible.

Minute ventilation is significantly increased during pregnancy, due to increases in both tidal volume and respiratory rate. Thus, normal arterial carbon dioxide tension ($PaCO_2$) in pregnancy is 30 to 32 mm Hg. Since serum bicarbonate level is decreased due to increased renal bicarbonate excretion, pH remains unchanged from nonpregnant levels (Table 14-4).

The most significant changes in the respiratory system revolve around oxygen supply and demand. Oxygen consumption is elevated 20 percent at term, due to the metabolic requirements of the fetus and placenta. At the same time, functional residual capacity (FRC) is decreased 20 percent. This combination of increased demand and decreased oxygen reserve produces the well-known propensity of pregnant women to rapidly become hypoxemic when made apneic at anesthetic induction. While this can be life threatening in any patient, it will only be worse in the cardiac patient, who may already be hypoxemic or who might have a hyperactive pulmonary vasculature. Thus, it bears repeating that adequate preoxygenation is essential before the induction of anesthesia during pregnancy.

Gastrointestinal System

Elevated levels of gastrin produced by the placenta will increase both the volume and acidity of gastric contents in pregnant women. The enlarged uterus can mechanically obstruct the pylorus, interfering with gastric emptying. The uterus may also cause a shift in the position of the stomach, impairing the pinch-valve mechanism at the gastroesophageal junction. Finally, progesterone will decrease gut motility through its smooth-muscle relaxant effects. These changes will all predispose pregnant women to the regurgitation and aspiration of gastric contents. Thus, the standard anesthetic induction for pregnant women includes cricoid pressure, avoidance of mask ventilation, and administration of thiopental and succinylcholine.

Unfortunately, such a technique may be highly undesirable in a patient with cardiac disease. As one example, a patient with poor left ventricular (LV) function might become severely hypotensive with such a regimen. Conversely, in a patient with good LV function and coronary artery disease, myocardial ischemia might develop as a result of the hypertension and tachycardia that such an induction technique can produce. These conflicting clinical imperatives are discussed under the headings of specific cardiac diseases later in this chapter. Suffice it to say that the risk of aspiration must be weighed against the risk posed by the underlying cardiac disease, as well as the risk that a particular anesthetic technique poses to the neonate, for example, prolonged respiratory depression after high-dose narcotic induction.

FETAL EFFECTS OF MATERNAL CARDIAC MEDICATIONS

Vasopressors

Adequate fluid preloading will usually minimize the hypotensive response to epidural and spinal blockade, but not in all cases. Rapid correction of hypotension is important because the uterine vasculature is maximally dilated, and uteroplacental blood flow therefore is dependent on the maintenance of an adequate perfusion pressure [11]. Additionally, the parturient with underlying cardiac disease may herself tolerate hypotension quite poorly.

The physiologic changes of regional anesthetic–induced sympathetic blockade must be understood before a particular vasopressor is selected. Butterworth and associates [12], using a dog model with cardiopulmonary bypass and a subarachnoid catheter, demonstrated that high spinal anesthesia reduced systemic resistance, decreased preload through dilation of venous capacitance beds, and reduced heart rate through blockade of cardiac sympathetics. Ephedrine administered intravenously increased SVR, decreased venous capacitance, and increased heart rate and contractility, thus reversing each of the changes produced by spinal anesthesia. Phenylephrine, on the other hand, increased blood pressure solely through its effect on SVR, and had no effect on venous capacitance or myocardial contractility [12].

If ephedrine appears to be a logical choice for reversing regional anesthetic–induced hypotension from a physiologic point of view, its effects on uteroplacental perfusion give further support to its use. In a now classic study, Ralston and associates [13] compared the effects of ephedrine, mephentermine, metaraminol, and methoxamine on uterine blood flow in the normotensive sheep model. Doses of ephedrine that raised mean arterial pressure 50 percent above control had no effect on uterine blood flow, whereas the predominantly alpha agents metaraminol and methoxamine lowered uterine blood flow at all doses [13]. Chestnut and colleagues [14] studied the effect of phenylephrine in gravid guinea pigs receiving ritodrine. They demonstrated a 50 percent decrease in umbilical blood flow velocity after the injection of phenylephrine, 10 μg/kg. Although this dose is considerably higher than the usual human dose, treatment with an equipotent dose of ephedrine had no such effect on uterine blood flow velocity [14]. Thus, ephedrine has become established as the vasopressor of choice in pregnancy, whereas the alpha agonists, including phenylephrine, have been avoided due to effects on uterine blood flow (Fig. 14-4).

Unfortunately, there are numerous maternal conditions, such as mitral stenosis with atrial fibrillation or coronary artery disease, in which the chronotropic response to ephedrine is undesirable. In addition, as Ramanathan and Grant [15] point out, the literature describing the effects of phenylephrine on uterine blood flow is based exclusively on animal studies. It is with these factors in mind that the use of phenylephrine in pregnancy has recently been investigated. Ramanathan and Grant compared the effects of phenylephrine and ephedrine on mothers in whom hypotension developed after the initiation of epidural anesthesia for

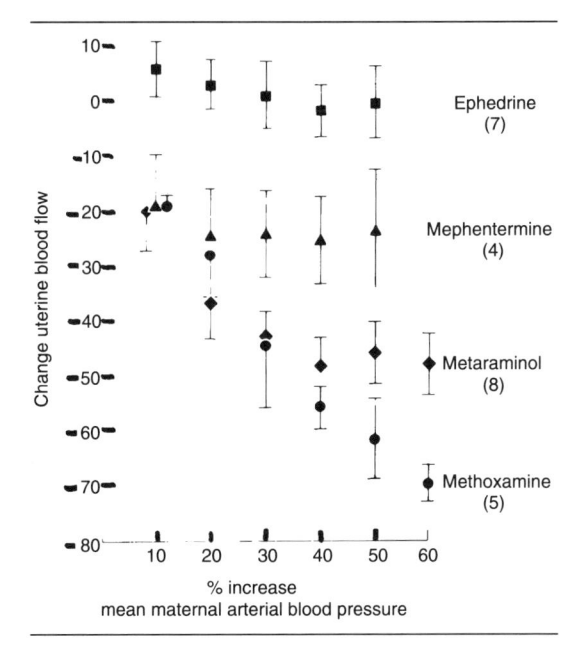

Fig. 14-4. Changes in uterine blood flow at equipotent doses of vasopressors. (Reprinted with permission from DH Ralston, SM Shniders, et al. Effect of equipotent ephedrine, metaraminol, mephentermine, and methoxamine on uterine blood flow in the pregnant ewe. *Anesthesiology* 40:354–370, 1974.)

elective cesarean section. Appropriate prehydration had been performed, and impedance cardiography was used to determine stroke volume, end diastolic volume, and ejection fraction. In both the ephedrine and phenylephrine groups, neonatal Apgar scores and umbilical cord gases were no different from those in infants whose mothers did not become hypotensive [15]. A similar study was reported by Moran and associates [16] in patients undergoing spinal anesthesia for cesarean section. Again, no differences were noted in Apgar scores or cord gases between infants whose mothers received either ephedrine or phenylephrine to maintain blood pressure [16].

Ramanathan and Grant [15] attempted to explain the difference between their clinical study and the previously reported animal work. They pointed out that the human subjects received adequate prehydration, and that aortocaval compression was carefully avoided. They also pointed out that the low doses of phenylephrine utilized (100 μg in divided doses to a maximum of 300 μg) primarily produced constriction in the venous capacitance bed, with little effect on SVR [15].

What recommendations, then, can be made regarding the use of phenylephrine to treat hypotension in pregnant women? First, while ephedrine remains the drug of choice for treating hypotension, phenylephrine is acceptable and in fact may be a good choice if the response to ephedrine is inadequate. Second, since phenylephrine has not been studied in women with diminished fetal reserve, and because there is at least the potential for decreasing uterine blood flow, phenylephrine is best avoided in this situation. Finally, when the maternal cardiovascular status is such that the chronotropic response to ephedrine is undesirable, phenylephrine is the pressor of choice.

Inotropes

Epinephrine can cause significant decreases in uterine blood flow. Chestnut and associates [17] studied the effects of epinephrine on uterine blood flow velocity (UBFV). UBFV was decreased to 72, 56, and 40 percent of baseline after boluses of 0.2, 0.5, and 1.0 μg/kg, respectively, despite significant increases in maternal blood pressure [17]. Hood and colleagues [18] demonstrated that a 5-μg bolus of epinephrine decreased uterine blood flow to 71 percent of control. They also showed that a 10-μg bolus of epinephrine, which is less than the standard epidural test dose, produced a statistically significant decrease in uterine blood flow that lasted more than 3 minutes [18].

Dopamine has been examined in both the normotensive [19] and hypotensive [20] pregnant ewe. Both these studies demonstrated decreased uterine blood flow despite increased maternal blood pressure. Fishburne and associates [21] compared dobutamine and dopamine in the pregnant ewe. Both agents resulted in significant decreases in uterine blood flow at all doses, although this was less marked with high-dose dobutamine [21].

Norepinephrine restores normal blood pressure in the hypotensive ewe without increasing uterine blood flow [22]. Similarly, infusion of norepinephrine in the normotensive ewe decreases uterine blood flow even while increasing maternal blood pressure [23].

Isoproterenol has no direct effect on the uterine

vasculature [24]. However, it can decrease uterine blood flow if maternal blood pressure decreases. There is also some concern that even in the presence of stable maternal blood pressure, vasodilation in other vascular beds may produce a steal phenomenon. However, a study of the use of isoproterenol as an epidural test dose showed no effect on fetal well-being, as assessed by fetal heart rate and beat-to-beat variability [25].

Vasodilators

In numerous situations, rapid-acting vasodilators may be of great utility in the parturient with cardiac disease. Before discussing individual agents, it should be reemphasized that uterine blood flow is primarily dependent on maternal blood pressure, and the blood pressure below which fetal oxygen delivery becomes insufficient cannot be predicted in a particular patient. Whenever possible, the fetal heart rate should be monitored in patients receiving vasodilators. In addition, measurements of the fetal scalp pH can provide invaluable information about the adequacy of uteroplacental perfusion and fetal well-being.

Hydralazine is the most commonly used vasodilator in pregnant patients. It has been shown to increase uterine blood flow in the pregnant ewe in both phenylephrine-induced hypertension [26] and surgically induced renovascular hypertension [27]. In a human study performed by Jouppila and associates [28], hydralazine did not alter intervillous blood flow measured by the xenon (Xe)-133 technique.

Craft and associates [29] have studied nitroglycerin in the pregnant ewe with phenylephrine-induced hypertension. Return of maternal blood pressure to control was associated with an improvement of uterine blood flow as well as increased fetal arterial pH [29]. In a human study, Hood and colleagues [30] administered 200 μg nitroglycerin immediately before induction of anesthesia for cesarean section in nine severe preeclamptic patients. This regimen blunted the hypertensive response to intubation, but it had no effect on Apgar scores or cord blood gases [30]. It may not be valid, however, to extend these findings to the use of nitroglycerin infusions.

Because of its reliable effect, sodium nitroprusside is frequently the agent of choice for the rapid control of hypertension. Ring and associates [26], however, were unable to demonstrate any improvement in uterine blood flow in the pregnant ewe with phenylephrine-induced hypertension. In addition, Naulty and colleagues [31] demonstrated fetal death due to cyanide intoxication in pregnant ewes receiving high-dose nitroprusside. Because of the apparent lack of fetal compromise in several case reports of the use of nitroprusside, it is generally believed that the short-term use of the drug during the induction of anesthesia is safe [32–34]. If longer-term use is contemplated, fetal heart rate monitoring should be utilized. In addition, the infusion must be stopped at the earliest signs of maternal tachyphylaxis.

The ganglionic blocker trimethaphan is believed to be more effective in the pregnant than in the nonpregnant patient. Its placental transfer is limited, due to its high molecular weight, and it appears to have no adverse fetal effects [35].

Digitalis Glycosides

In this chapter, discussion is limited to the use of digoxin. For complete information on the other digitalis glycosides, the reader is referred to the review by Mitani and associates [36].

Luxford and Kellaway [37] reported that 12 of 15 women receiving maintenance doses of digoxin had higher serum levels during pregnancy than 6 to 12 weeks postpartum. They postulated that increased drug bioavailability during pregnancy led to these increased drug levels [37]. These findings, however, may be due in part to the presence of digoxin-like immunoreactive substance (DLIS) in maternal serum. DLIS is detected in varying amounts by the different commercially available assays, and in fact it can be measured in patients not receiving digoxin (Fig. 14-5). It is not known if DLIS has any cardiovascular effects of its own, and its structure has not been determined. Graves and associates [38] demonstrated DLIS levels of 0.1 to 0.6 ng/ml in third-trimester pregnant women not receiving digoxin. These levels became undetectable in five of six women 1 day postpartum [38]. Thus, interpretation of serum digoxin levels during pregnancy must take into account the possibility of a significant contribution from DLIS.

Digoxin crosses the placenta quite readily. Saarikoski [39] demonstrated maternally administered

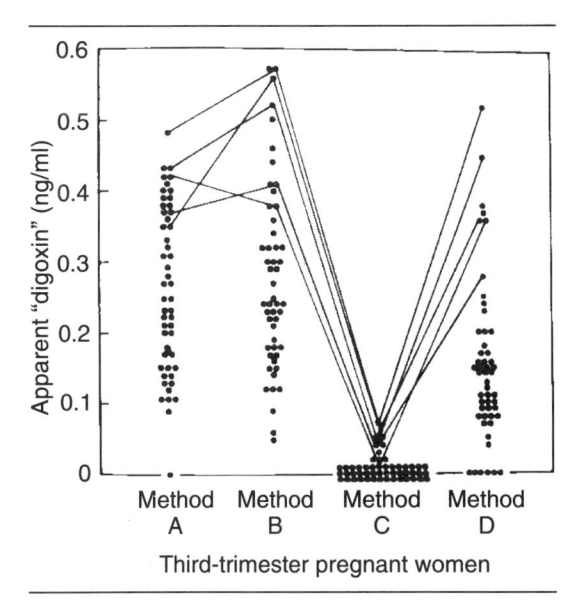

Fig. 14-5. Apparent plasma digoxin levels by four different assays in near-term pregnant women not receiving digoxin. (Reprinted with permission from SW Graves, R Valdes, and BA Brown, Endogenous digoxin–immunoreactive substance in human pregnancies. *J Clin Endocrinol Metab* 58:748–751, 1984. © The Endocrine Society.)

radiolabeled digoxin in cord blood within 5 minutes. Fetal plasma concentrations were identical to maternal levels within 30 minutes [39].

This rapid fetal transfer has been successfully exploited to treat fetal supraventricular tachycardia and congestive heart failure. The intravenous route is utilized to provide a maternal loading dose, and maternal drug levels are maintained at the upper levels of the therapeutic range, that is, 2.0 ng/ml.

Maternal digitalis toxicity has led to fetal death, secondary to fetal intoxication. There has also been a suggestion that maternal digitalis treatment leads to low birth weight. However, this may be due to a tendency for patients receiving digitalis to have an earlier onset of labor; when corrected for gestational age, these infants are of appropriate weight [40]. In general, appropriate maternal blood levels have no adverse effects on the fetus.

Anticoagulants

Because of the limited life span of bioprosthetic heart valves, women of childbearing age who have undergone valve replacement are much more likely to have received mechanical heart valves, which require prophylactic anticoagulation. Such therapy can also be used in patients with atrial fibrillation, dilated cardiomyopathy, and Eisenmenger's syndrome [2]. Aside from the anesthetic implications of such therapy, which are discussed later in this chapter, anticoagulation can have a significant impact on the developing fetus.

The use of warfarin (Coumadin) has been associated with a spontaneous abortion rate of between 10 and 50 percent. Coumadin therapy during the first trimester of pregnancy has been linked to the development of nasal bone hypoplasia and epiphyseal stippling (chondrodysplasia punctata). The use of oral anticoagulants has also been associated with optic nerve atrophy, deafness, and mental retardation. Finally, the anticoagulated fetus is at higher risk of intracranial hemorrhage, especially at the time of labor and delivery.

On the other hand, because of its high molecular weight and its polarity, heparin does not cross the placenta [41]. There is substantial evidence that the use of heparin has no effect on fetal morbidity or mortality [42, 43]. There is also good evidence that the use of adjusted-dose subcutaneous heparin (dose adjustment to maintain activated partial thromboplastin time [aPTT] at 1.5 to 2.25 times control) is effective prophylaxis for the patient with a prosthetic valve [44]. Therefore, heparin should be considered the anticoagulant of choice during pregnancy.

McGehee [45] has developed a schema for the management of the pregnant patient who requires anticoagulation. Its primary features are the cessation of warfarin before conception, or at the earliest time pregnancy is recognized; the use of adjusted-dose subcutaneous heparin during pregnancy; and the use of IV heparin near term, followed by the cessation of therapy at the onset of labor [45].

Antiarrhythmics

Antiarrhythmic therapy may be necessary in the pregnant patient with symptomatic or life-threatening disturbances of cardiac rate and rhythm. Unfortunately, most antiarrhythmic agents have not been studied in any systematic fashion with regard to their safety during pregnancy. There are numerous case reports describing the use of these drugs,

Table 14-5. Effects of antiarrhythmic agents used during pregnancy

Agent	Effect
Lidocaine	No apparent fetal effects
Quinidine	May produce preterm labor
Procainamide	No apparent fetal effects
Diisopyramide	Oxytocin-like effect
Verapamil	No apparent fetal effects
Phenytoin	Multiple congenital anomalies
Bretylium	No apparent fetal effects

however, and some guidelines can be provided [46] (Table 14-5).

Lidocaine has been studied in great detail due to its use as a local anesthetic. There is no evidence that it is teratogenic. Therapeutic blood levels have no effect on uterine activity or uterine blood flow. Although it readily crosses the placenta, there is no evidence that it causes neonatal depression in therapeutic doses.

Quinidine has been used extensively in the obstetric population. In therapeutic doses, it is essentially devoid of adverse effect on the fetus. It can, in rare instances, produce preterm labor, even at otherwise appropriate serum levels. Toxic doses can cause spontaneous abortion, as well as fetal auditory nerve damage.

Procainamide is not teratogenic, and despite transplacental passage it appears to have no fetal effects. Diisopyramide does not appear to be teratogenic. However, it has been reported to have an oxytocin-like effect [47].

Verapamil appears to be without teratogenic effect. It has been used to treat preterm labor and pregnancy-induced hypertension with no deleterious effect on the fetus.

Phenytoin has only rarely been used as an antiarrhythmic during pregnancy, but there is extensive experience with its use as an anticonvulsant. Fetal exposure during the first trimester can produce the fetal hydantoin syndrome, characterized by mental retardation, craniofacial malformations, and cardiac defects. Therefore, its use as an antiarrhythmic during pregnancy should only be for the immediate control of digitalis-induced arrhythmias that are unresponsive to other treatments.

The use of bretylium in the pregnant patient has not been investigated. There is evidence that it may be the treatment of choice for bupivacaine-induced ventricular fibrillation [48].

β-Adrenergic Blockers

The use of β-blockers during pregnancy has been controversial and indeed remains so. Before evaluating the effects of β-blockade on the fetus, it is first necessary to discuss adrenergic influences on the maternal-fetal system [49].

The myometrium responds to adrenergic stimulation. Stimulation of alpha receptors increases uterine activity, whereas beta stimulation decreases uterine contractility. This is, of course, exploited therapeutically through the use of beta agonists to suppress preterm labor. Conversely, β-blockade can increase both baseline uterine tone and the intensity of contractions. Theoretically, an increase in uterine tone could impair uteroplacental blood flow and cause intrauterine growth retardation. Such an effect on the myometrium might also induce preterm labor.

The fetus, too, responds to adrenergic influences. Oakes and associates [50] demonstrated that either maternal or fetal infusion of propranolol in the pregnant ewe produced significant decreases in fetal heart rate, as well as decreased umbilical blood flow secondary to increased umbilical vascular resistance. Again, these findings raise the concern that β-blockade might have significant adverse fetal effects. Have these concerns been borne out?

Propranolol is the β-blocker with which the most experience has been obtained. Neonatal bradycardia, respiratory depression, and hypoglycemia, as well as preterm labor and intrauterine growth retardation, have all been reported anecdotally or in retrospective studies. However, none of these findings have been consistently reported in prospective studies. Rubin [51] analyzed five studies of 94 pregnancies, which demonstrated an incidence of intrauterine growth retardation of 4 percent. However, two of the mothers subsequently delivered normal infants while receiving the same dose of propranolol. Thus, Rubin wrote that "it would therefore be inappropriate to conclude that beta-blockade during pregnancy is commonly associated with retardation of intrauterine growth" [51]. While β-blockade might impair the ability of the fetus to respond to stress, such a risk must be balanced against the maternal benefits of β-blockade.

Metoprolol, being a selective $β_1$-blocker, theoretically will not interfere with $β_2$ effects on uterine tone. Presumably, this would minimize the risk of growth retardation or initiation of preterm labor. At least one study demonstrates improved fetal growth in hypertensive women treated with metoprolol compared with hydralazine [52].

Labetalol, a nonselective β-blocker with $α_1$ blocking properties, has been found to provide excellent results as single-drug therapy for severe hypertension during pregnancy [53]. It is also quite effective when used acutely to control hypertensive crises in severe preeclampsia [54] and as a method of attenuating the hypertensive response to endotracheal intubation [55]. It neither decreases uterine blood flow [56] nor causes neonatal bradycardia or hypoglycemia [57]. Labetalol appears to be safe for both chronic use and for management of hypertensive emergencies in the pregnant patient, and in fact may be the drug of choice for the management of these emergencies.

There has been considerable interest in the use of the ultra–short-acting β-blocker esmolol in the preeclamptic patient undergoing cesarean section. Eisenach and Castro [58] studied the effects of esmolol infusions in the pregnant ewe. They showed no increase in uterine tone and no effect on uterine blood flow. They did demonstrate significant fetal hypoxemia and acidemia, as well as fetal bradycardia that persisted as long as 30 minutes after the infusion of esmolol was terminated [58] (Fig. 14-6). While a subsequent case report showed only small decreases in fetal heart rate after the maternal infusion of esmolol, it was suggested that its use be accompanied by continuous fetal heart rate monitoring whenever possible [59].

Despite the fetal complications that can be seen with the use of β-blockers, or indeed with any cardiac drug, it must be remembered that these drugs are not being administered to healthy women. In most cases, these women are being treated for conditions that may be life threatening, or at the very least associated with considerable fetal morbidity and mortality. As always, the risks of treatment must be weighed against the risks, to both mother and fetus, of failing to initiate treatment.

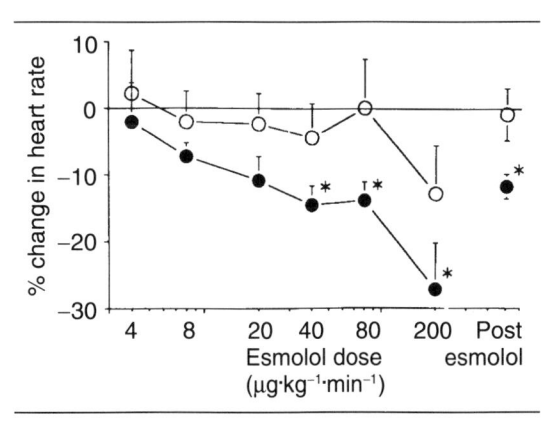

Fig. 14-6. Effects of maternally administered esmolol on fetal (*closed circles*) and maternal (*open circles*) heart rate. Note the persistently decreased fetal heart rate after termination of the infusion. (Reprinted with permission from JC Eisenach and MI Castro, Maternally administered esmolol produces fetal β-adrenergic blockade and hypoxemia in sheep. *Anesthesiology* 71:718–722, 1989.)

SPECIFIC CARDIAC DISEASES

Before discussing the management of specific disease states during pregnancy, it would be useful to discuss the logistics of caring for a laboring patient with significant cardiac disease. Except in the busiest labor and delivery suites in referral centers, the presence of a patient with severe cardiac disease is rare enough to produce a sense of unease, if not outright panic. However, if the underlying disease process is identified early enough in the pregnancy, there should be ample time to make plans for managing the patient during labor, and making these plans known to all the personnel who will be involved in the patient's care.

Identification of the patient with underlying cardiac disease will generally be quite straightforward. Occasionally, however, a patient may be asymptomatic or only mildly symptomatic. Symptoms may develop only with the progressive increase in cardiac workload that occurs during pregnancy. Thus, a careful history and physical examination are essential to detect potentially significant disease.

Once pregnancy is diagnosed, it is important to contact the patient's cardiologist or internist to establish her baseline function. In certain disease states, such as pulmonary hypertension, continuation of pregnancy to term may entail unacceptable risk. If this is the case, the patient must be made aware of this risk, and plans should be made for the possibility of pregnancy termination at the earliest opportunity, should the patient agree. In any event, the patient should be reevaluated at intervals throughout the pregnancy by a physician who is familiar with her history.

When it appears likely that the patient will carry the pregnancy to term, that is, to 20 to 24 weeks' gestation, it is appropriate for a member of the anesthesia team to become involved in her care. This can be in the setting of a high-risk obstetric clinic or as a visit scheduled with an anesthesiologist in a hospital setting. At this time, the anesthesiologist should have an opportunity to review the patient's records in their entirety and begin to formulate an anesthetic plan. It is also important at this time to establish contact with the patient's cardiologist and obstetrician to establish as great a degree of unanimity as possible. This may require a conference of all physicians involved, as well as the patient and perhaps the pediatrician who will be responsible for the neonate. It cannot be overemphasized how important it is for consensus to be arrived at before the patient presents in labor.

It is also important that there be communication between the anesthesiologist performing the initial evaluation and the other anesthesiologists who might be required to care for the patient. At a minimum, there should be a central location where the anesthetic consultation can be found, enabling the anesthesiologist responsible for the patient to quickly familiarize her- or himself with the previously formulated plan. Ideally, all the anesthesiologists who might care for the patient should have an opportunity to discuss the anesthetic plan before her arrival in labor. While there may be some differences in opinion, it is hoped that there will be reasonable agreement regarding major issues such as monitoring and choice of anesthetic technique.

A final series of decisions revolves around the location where the patient's labor, delivery, and recovery will occur. Ideally, the labor unit will be equipped with invasive monitors, and staffed with nursing personnel familiar with their use. Unfortunately, neither of these requirements can be guaranteed in every hospital. Thus, if permanent or portable monitors are not available, and if invasive monitoring is believed to be indicated, it will be necessary for the patient to labor in an intensive care setting. This will also be necessary if nurses familiar with invasive monitoring are not available on the labor and delivery unit. This obviously can lead to logistic problems of its own (for example, lack of proximity to an operating room should fetal distress develop, or the inability to provide epidural anesthesia). Therefore, whenever possible, a prior effort to provide monitors and nursing personnel should be made.

The site of the patient's recovery can be of critical importance as well. Due to the hemodynamic changes following delivery, the patient with cardiac disease may be at high risk for several days postpartum.

Valvular Heart Disease

Mitral Stenosis

Mitral stenosis is the most common valvular lesion seen during pregnancy, and is therefore the most common cardiac disease seen by the anesthesiologist in parturients (excluding mitral valve prolapse). The average age of onset of rheumatic fever is 12 years, and the latency period until the detection of a murmur is 19 years. Therefore, clinical signs of mitral stenosis can be expected to occur in the early thirties, with increasing symptomatology during the thirties and forties [60]. However, the physiologic changes of pregnancy interact unfavorably with the pathophysiology of mitral stenosis, leading to an earlier appearance and clinical deterioration.

The decreased mitral valve orifice leads to LV underloading and decreased cardiac output. Initially, left atrial contraction overcomes the obstruction, but as stenosis worsens, left atrial pressure and volume increase. This pressure increase is transmitted to the pulmonary circulation, where fluid transudation leads to decreased lung compliance and the symptoms of dyspnea and orthopnea. Eventually, obliterative changes occur in the pulmonary circulation, leading to right ventricular (RV) failure and tricuspid insufficiency.

It has been stated that mitral stenosis "protects" the left ventricle, but there is good evidence that left ventricular contractile abnormalities occur even in pure mitral stenosis. There is reason to believe that rheumatic myocarditis can cause persistent hypocontractility in the posterobasal wall of the left ventricle, secondary to calcific changes in the mitral valve apparatus or papillary muscles. These changes may cause persistent symptoms, even after successful valve replacement [61]. Secondly, the chronically underloaded left ventricle has inadequate wall thickness. By LaPlace's formula,

$$\text{Wall tension} = P \times R/2h$$

where P equals intraventricular pressure, R equals chamber radius, and h equals wall thickness. It is clear that inadequate wall thickness will lead to increased wall tension or afterload [61], which in turn can cause decreased ejection fraction, even in the absence of decreases in intrinsic myocardial contractility. A full discussion of the pathophysiology of mitral stenosis is presented in Chap. 7.

If the pathophysiology of mitral stenosis is understood, one can predict those factors that cause hemodynamic deterioration. Tachycardia is the most important of these factors. As tachycardia shortens diastole more than systole, the period during which LV filling occurs is shortened. Thus, to maintain cardiac output, the flow rate across the mitral valve must increase. However, the pressure gradient is proportional to the square of the flow rate; therefore, tachycardia can be associated with significant increases in left atrial and pulmonary venous pressure, leading to clinical deterioration [61]. Because it may lead to reflex tachycardia, decreased SVR can also worsen hemodynamics. Fluid overload is another factor that is poorly tolerated in patients with severe mitral stenosis. Finally, in the presence of significant RV dysfunction, those factors that worsen pulmonary hypertension (hypoxia, hypercarbia, acidosis, increased airway pressure) will lead to clinical deterioration.

It is not surprising that mitral stenosis is poorly tolerated during pregnancy, since the normal maternal response to pregnancy includes arteriolar vasodilation, tachycardia, and hypervolemia. Symptoms of pulmonary congestion typically occur by midgestation, and do not worsen after the 30th week of pregnancy [62]. Further deterioration may occur at the time of labor and delivery, secondary to maternal tachycardia. Sudden death in the puerperium has been reported; this has been hypothesized to be secondary to sudden blood loss in a patient who has depended on high atrial filling pressures to maintain adequate left ventricular preload [63]. All told, the maternal mortality in women with mitral stenosis is 1 percent. In New York Heart Association class III and IV, mortality is 4 to 5 percent and in women with superimposed atrial fibrillation, the mortality is 14 to 17 percent [64].

Patients with significant mitral stenosis should have invasive monitoring during labor and delivery. While a pulmonary artery catheter may not give an accurate measure of left ventricular filling pressure, it can be useful in determining the extent of pulmonary hypertension, and also in assessing the degree of left ventricular compromise.

Epidural anesthesia is recommended for labor and delivery. By eliminating maternal pain, it will prevent the sympathetic stimulation that can have such a deleterious effect on maternal hemodynamics. Epinephrine-containing local anesthetics should be avoided, because of their potential for producing tachycardia and vasodilation. Careful hydration is essential to prevent decreases in blood pressure that may lead to tachycardia. This is a situation in which phenylephrine may be preferable to ephedrine for the treatment of maternal hypotension, because of its lack of positive chronotropic effects; this will, of course, require careful fetal surveillance. Furthermore, in those patients with RV dysfunction, the increases in pulmonary vascular resistance (PVR) that can occur with phenylephrine may cause decompensation [61]. Finally, patients with significant left atrial enlargement may be receiving anticoagulants for prophylaxis of thromboembolic disease; if that is the case, adequate coagulation function must be confirmed before regional anesthesia is attempted.

For cesarean section, either epidural or general anesthesia is acceptable. Single-shot spinal anesthesia is less desirable, due to the exaggerated changes in maternal hemodynamics it can produce. If general anesthesia is selected, drugs such as ketamine, pancuronium, atropine, and meperidine, which produce tachycardia, should be avoided. Patients with mild disease will tolerate a standard rapid-sequence induction with thiopental and succinylcholine. In patients with more severe stenosis,

Table 14-6. Mitral stenosis in pregnancy

Most common valvular lesion
Pregnancy poorly tolerated
Pathophysiology: Increased left atrial (LA) pressure
                   Increased LA volume
                   Pulmonary venous hypertension
                   Fixed increases in PVR (late)
                   LV underloading
Avoid: Tachycardia, hypotension, increased PVR
Anesthetic choice for cesarean section: Epidural, general
Monitoring: Pulmonary artery catheter, arterial line

an inhalation induction with halothane will provide sufficient anesthetic depth to prevent a sympathetic response to intubation. Alternatively, a pure narcotic induction can be utilized, should significant ventricular dysfunction be present. Neither an inhalation nor a narcotic induction can be considered a rapid-sequence technique; thus, full pharmacologic aspiration prophylaxis, that is, histamine blocker, metoclopramide, and a nonparticulate antacid, should be used. Should atrial fibrillation occur intraoperatively, synchronized cardioversion, β-blockade, digitalization, or verapamil should be utilized to control the ventricular response. Finally, should pulmonary hypertension worsen, and if there is no response to correction of factors such as hypercarbia or hypoxia, inotropic support with dobutamine or dopamine and vasodilation with nitroglycerin are indicated (Table 14-6).

As stated previously, the puerperium is a time of increased maternal mortality. Therefore, all patients with moderate to severe mitral stenosis should be monitored in an intensive care setting for 24 to 48 hours postpartum.

Mitral Regurgitation

Mitral regurgitation (MR) is the second most common valvular lesion seen during pregnancy. Patients with MR are frequently asymptomatic for 30 to 40 years, and, as such, pregnancy is usually well tolerated. Nevertheless, a 5.5 percent incidence of pulmonary congestion and a 2.8 percent incidence of pulmonary embolism during pregnancy have been reported [1]. At one time, the predominant etiology of mitral regurgitation was rheumatic fever; at present, mitral valve prolapse is the most common cause of MR, followed by ischemic coronary artery disease [60].

In mitral regurgitation, a significant proportion of left ventricular output is ejected into the left atrium. During diastole, the left ventricle is filled by the normal systolic output of the right heart, as well as by the volume of blood that was ejected into the left atrium during the previous cardiac cycle. Thus, the left ventricle is subjected to a chronic volume overload. Because afterload is reduced in MR, the ejection fraction (which is afterload sensitive) may be normal or elevated. This conceals, however, the contractile abnormalities that chronic volume overload produces [61]. Because of the high compliance of the left atrium, the pulmonary capillaries are protected from elevated pressures until late in the course of the disease. When LV failure ensues, however, elevated pressures are transmitted to the pulmonary vasculature, and pulmonary hypertension can develop.

Several factors will cause decompensation in patients with mitral regurgitation. Increases in SVR will increase impedance to forward ejection, thus augmenting regurgitant flow. Bradycardia will also increase regurgitant flow, and in addition will decrease cardiac output, since stroke volume is fixed, thus making cardiac output rate dependent. Myocardial depressants are not well tolerated, even in the presence of a normal ejection fraction. Finally, factors that increase PVR can cause right ventricular failure in patients with pulmonary vascular disease.

Although the hypervolemia of pregnancy would be expected to worsen mitral regurgitation, the decreased SVR seen during gestation will improve forward flow. On the other hand, pain and anxiety during labor and delivery will lead to increased systemic resistance secondary to sympathetic stimulation.

Epidural anesthesia is recommended for labor and delivery, because it will prevent the increases in SVR that occur with painful contractions. The drop in SVR that accompanies the sympathetic blockade of epidural anesthesia may actually increase forward flow. Invasive monitoring is recommended. In particular, the degree of regurgitant flow can be quantitated by measuring the V wave of the pulmonary capillary wedge pressure (PCWP) trace. Should hypotension develop, the positive

Table 14-7. Mitral regurgitation in pregnancy

Second most common valvular lesion
Pregnancy well tolerated
Pathophysiology: LV volume overload
  Severe contractile abnormalities despite normal ejection fraction
Avoid: Increased afterload, bradycardia, myocardial depressants
Anesthetic choice for labor: Epidural
Anesthetic choice for cesarean section: Epidural
Monitoring: Pulmonary artery catheter allows determination of increased regurgitant flow

chronotropic effects of ephedrine will be beneficial.

Epidural anesthesia is likewise preferred for cesarean section. There is a theoretical concern that high epidural anesthesia may lead to bradycardia secondary to block of the cardiac accelerator fibers, but this is seldom a serious problem. Should general anesthesia be utilized, a standard rapid-sequence induction is appropriate, if an adequate depth of anesthesia is attained before intubation. Lidocaine, 1.0 mg/kg, will help blunt the sympathetic response to intubation; alternatively, nitroglycerin or nitroprusside can be effective in ameliorating the increase in systemic resistance. For maintenance of anesthesia, a nitrous oxide–narcotic technique is acceptable, but may require the concomitant use of a vasodilator. If LV function is well maintained, an inhalation agent can be used as a supplement (Table 14-7).

Patients with mitral regurgitation are not at any apparent increased risk in the postpartum period. Therefore, prolonged monitoring does not appear to be indicated.

Mitral Valve Prolapse

Mitral valve prolapse (MVP) is the most common structural cardiac lesion, seen in 5 to 10 percent of the general population, and perhaps in as many as 17 percent of women of childbearing age [65]. While most pregnant women tolerate this lesion quite well, it is so common that every anesthesiologist caring for pregnant women should be fully acquainted with its pathophysiology and management.

Mitral valve prolapse is defined as the pathologic protrusion of mitral valve tissue into the atrium during systole. Frequently, this is secondary to myxomatous degeneration of the valve leaflets or elongation of the chordae tendineae, although these histologic changes may be absent. The auscultatory finding that is pathognomonic for mitral valve prolapse, a mid-systolic click, is due to the sudden tensing of the prolapsed leaflets. If mitral regurgitation is present, this click may be accompanied by a late systolic murmur.

Clinically, the majority of patients with MVP are asymptomatic. Nevertheless, the disorder is associated with a wide array of symptoms, including anxiety attacks, palpitations, chest pain, lightheadedness, fatigue, and dyspnea. The elongated valve leaflet may act as a site for platelet aggregation, leading to cerebral embolization and stroke. There is a suggestion that patients with mitral valve prolapse are prone to coronary artery spasm [66, 67]. Finally, while exceedingly rare in patients with isolated mitral valve prolapse, sudden death due to ventricular arrhythmia is an important source of mortality in patients with significant mitral regurgitation.

There is a significant association between mitral valve prolapse and connective tissue disorders, including Marfan's syndrome, Ehlers-Danlos syndrome, osteogenesis imperfecta, and systemic lupus erythematosus. Interestingly, in those patients without underlying disease, that is, primary mitral valve prolapse, there is a high incidence of a marfanoid body habitus.

In the absence of significant mitral regurgitation, the hemodynamic alterations of MVP are relatively minor. The primary determinant of the degree of regurgitation is the LV end diastolic volume (LVEDV). Thus, conditions that decrease LVEDV, such as hypovolemia, venodilatation, tachycardia, and increased airway pressure, will increase regurgitation. Conversely, bradycardia, hypervolemia, afterload augmentation, and negative inotropes, which increase ventricular volume, will decrease the amount of regurgitant flow. It is important to realize, however, that in patients with significant preexisting mitral insufficiency, excessive increases in afterload will increase left ventricular pressures and therefore worsen regurgitant flow.

In those patients with the isolated finding of a mid-systolic click, no specific therapy is indicated. In those patients with palpitations, dysrhythmias, or chest pain, β-blockers can be quite effective. As discussed earlier in this chapter, β-blockade appears to be safe for the fetus, and should therefore be maintained throughout pregnancy if indicated for maternal well-being.

Pregnancy does not appear to worsen the symptoms of MVP, probably because of the expanded intravascular volume that is seen in normal pregnancy. In fact, a significant improvement may be seen during pregnancy. Rayburn [68] studied 21 women with echocardiographically confirmed mitral valve prolapse throughout pregnancy; 13 women had no evidence of prolapse at midgestation. Of the remaining 8 patients, symptoms disappeared in 5 by term. Thus, only 3 of 21 women with previously documented mitral valve prolapse had persistence of the disorder to term [68].

Mitral valve prolapse has not been demonstrated to have any adverse effects on pregnancy outcome, as measured by spontaneous abortion, premature labor, or congenital abnormalities [69, 70]. It has been hypothesized that labor might be shorter in women with mitral valve prolapse due to a generalized ligamentous laxity, but Shapiro and associates [71] could not demonstrate such an effect.

A source of controversy is whether patients with mitral valve prolapse require antibiotic prophylaxis for vaginal delivery or cesarean section. It is widely held that those patients with mitral regurgitation or thickened valve leaflets are at risk of developing infective endocarditis. What is less clearly defined is whether uncomplicated vaginal delivery or cesarean section leads to significant bacteremia, which would warrant prophylaxis. While the American Heart Association does not recommend prophylaxis for uncomplicated vaginal or cesarean delivery, some authorities have advised routine prophylaxis in women with documented MVP and thickened valve leaflets or mitral regurgitation [68]. At present, there is a wide range of clinical practice, which probably depends more on a given physician's willingness to accept a small risk of endocarditis than on empiric evidence.

Parturients who are asymptomatic, who have no evidence of mitral insufficiency, and whose murmur has remained unchanged during pregnancy do not require any specific alterations of their anesthetic management. Patients with either echocardiographic or clinical evidence of more severe prolapse should be managed with the goal of maintaining adequate left ventricular volume. In particular, decreased preload due to aortocaval compression, hemorrhage, or regional anesthetic–induced sympathetic blockade should be aggressively treated. In addition, since tachycardia will increase ventricular emptying, drugs that increase heart rate should be used with caution. Epidural anesthesia would be an appropriate choice for both vaginal delivery and cesarean section. Spinal anesthesia is less desirable due to the rapid onset of sympathetic block. Should hypotension develop after regional anesthesia, fluids and low-dose phenylephrine are the treatments of choice.

Should general anesthesia be required for cesarean section, a standard rapid-sequence induction with thiopental and succinylcholine can be performed in those patients with normal ventricular function. One should be prepared to treat the increases in heart rate that may accompany this technique. The negative inotropic and chronotropic properties of halothane make it a good choice for maintenance of anesthesia, since those characteristics would tend to maintain ventricular volume.

The management of patients with severe mitral regurgitation secondary to MVP is not unlike that of patients with rheumatic mitral valve disease and mitral regurgitation.

Aortic Insufficiency

Aortic insufficiency (AI) is uncommon in women of childbearing age, and is seen in roughly 2.5 percent of pregnant women with valvular heart disease. Typically, heart failure does not develop until the fourth or fifth decade of life. Pregnancy is therefore well tolerated; the incidence of congestive heart failure has been reported to be between 3 and 9 percent [1].

The primary pathophysiologic alteration of AI is left ventricular volume overload, since the ventricle receives blood from both the left atrium and the systemic circulation. This leads to the development of eccentric hypertrophy. This volume overload is tolerated for many years, but as the valve orifice enlarges and regurgitation worsens, contractile abnormalities become clinically evident. As the disease progresses, left ventricular compliance decreases, leading to increases in end diastolic and left atrial pressure, producing symptoms of congestive heart failure. An important characteristic of AI is the

Table 14-8. Aortic insufficiency in pregnancy

Seen in 25% of pregnant women with valve disease
Pregnancy well tolerated
Pathophysiology: LV volume overload
　　　　　　　　Long-term maintenance of stroke volume despite contractile dysfunction
Avoid: Increased SVR, bradycardia, myocardial depressants
Anesthetic choice for labor: Epidural
Anesthetic choice for cesarean section: Epidural
Invasive monitoring unnecessary in absence of significant symptoms

---

fact that preload reserve allows the maintenance of stroke volume even in the presence of severe depression of intrinsic contractility. Therefore, even patients who are totally asymptomatic may have already incurred irreversible ventricular dysfunction [61].

As in mitral regurgitation, the amount of regurgitant flow will depend on heart rate, the pressure gradient across the valve, and the dimension of the valve orifice. Thus, the increased heart rate and decreased SVR of pregnancy seem to counteract the increased blood volume, explaining why pregnancy is so well tolerated. Similarly, increases in systemic resistance associated with painful contractions can be expected to worsen regurgitation.

In the absence of significant symptoms, invasive hemodynamic monitoring should not be necessary. The anesthetic management of patients with AI is essentially comparable to that of patients with mitral regurgitation. Epidural anesthesia is recommended for both labor and cesarean section, bradycardia should be avoided, and increases in SVR should be aggressively treated, with either a rapid-acting vasodilator or, if LV function is adequate, an inhalation agent (Table 14-8).

Aortic Stenosis

Aortic stenosis (AS) is the least common valvular lesion seen during pregnancy, found in approximately 1 percent of parturients with valve disease. This is due to the prolonged latency period, 35 to 40 years, between the initial episode of rheumatic fever and the onset of symptoms. In pregnant women with AS, however, the mortality has been reported to be as high as 17 percent, with a fetal mortality of 32 percent [72].

The resistance to flow across the stenotic valve leads to an increase in intraventricular pressure, an increase that will be proportional to the degree of diminution of the area of the valve orifice. This chronic increase in LV pressure leads to the development of concentric hypertrophy. Although afterload-sensitive measures of cardiac performance such as ejection fraction may be depressed, intrinsic myocardial contractility is well maintained in aortic stenosis. However, ventricular hypertrophy does lead to significant alterations in ventricular compliance, and more importantly myocardial oxygen supply and demand [61].

Because of the decreased ventricular compliance, atrial contraction will play a major role in the maintenance of an adequate LVEDV. Thus, the maintenance of sinus rhythm is of great importance. Secondly, in the setting of increased wall stiffness, central venous pressure will only poorly estimate left ventricular end diastolic pressure (LVEDP). Therefore, a pulmonary artery catheter can be of great utility in the management of these patients. Finally, the poorly compliant left ventricle will be highly dependent on an appropriately elevated LVEDV; this necessitates careful replacement of intraoperative blood loss and the prevention or rapid treatment of those factors that decrease venous return.

There are alterations in both supply and demand of oxygen to the myocardium. On the supply side, epicardial coronary arteries do not enlarge proportionately to the increase in myocardial mass. Also, the elevated LVEDP will decrease coronary perfusion pressure (aortic diastolic pressure − LVEDP). On the demand side of the equation, the increased muscle mass of the left ventricle will increase basal myocardial oxygen consumption. Further, if ventricular hypertrophy is inadequate, that is, if h in LaPlace's law is inappropriately low, then wall tension and thus oxygen consumption will be elevated. It is therefore important to avoid significant increases in heart rate that may further alter oxygen supply and demand (see Chap. 6 for a more detailed discussion of myocardial supply-demand imbalances in aortic stenosis). It is similarly important to avoid decreases in SVR: first, because this may lead to diastolic hypotension and decreased coronary perfusion pressure, and second, because the fixed stroke volume means that blood pressure can only be maintained by increasing heart rate. (The fixed stroke volume implies that severe bradycardia will also be poorly tolerated.)

In view of the potential for myocardial ischemia, continuous ECG monitoring of lead V_5 is indicated during labor and delivery. Because of the sensitivity of the myocardium to decreased perfusion pressure, intraarterial pressure monitoring should be used in all patients with significant ventricular hypertrophy. For reasons described earlier, a pulmonary artery catheter will also be quite helpful.

It is often recommended that regional anesthesia be avoided in the parturient with AS, due to the potential for decreases in SVR and filling pressure [1, 2, 73]. On the other hand, Jackson and Thomas [61] have recommended that epidural and spinal anesthesia not be denied to patients with aortic stenosis if there are appropriate clinical indications for their use. Therefore, if appropriate monitoring and fluid replacement are ensured, a slowly titrated epidural anesthetic can be safely used for labor analgesia. Hypotension should be aggressively treated with fluids and an alpha agonist such as phenylephrine. Similarly, in the event that ECG changes consistent with ischemia occur, coronary perfusion pressure should be maintained with an infusion of phenylephrine or metaraminol. As was stated previously, this will require vigilant monitoring of the fetus to ensure adequacy of uteroplacental perfusion.

For cesarean section, general anesthesia is recommended. In patients with mild stenosis, a standard rapid-sequence induction with thiopental and succinylcholine followed by nitrous oxide–narcotic maintenance is acceptable. In the presence of normal LV contractile performance, low concentrations of an inhalation agent can be added for supplementation. On the other hand, in the presence of critical aortic stenosis, a standard rapid-sequence induction may lead to increases in heart rate that can cause significant myocardial ischemia. In such patients, a high-dose narcotic induction may be necessary.

As was stated previously, patients with AS are exquisitely sensitive to decreased preload. Invasive monitoring should therefore continue into the postpartum period, until the likelihood of excessive blood loss has diminished to an insignificant level (Table 14-9).

Table 14-9. Aortic stenosis in pregnancy

Extremely rare during pregnancy
Pathophysiology: Increased LV pressure
    Concentric ventricular hypertrophy
    Decreased LV compliance
    Altered oxygen supply-demand relationship
    Contractility well maintained
Avoid: Tachycardia, hypotension, decreased SVR
Anesthetic choice for labor: Epidural, slowly titrated
Anesthetic choice for cesarean section: General, may require high-dose narcotic
Monitoring: PA catheter, arterial line, V_5 lead

Congenital Heart Disease— Left-to-Right Shunts

Atrial Septal Defect

Atrial septal defect (ASD) is the most common form of congenital heart disease among adults, seen in 17.5 percent of adults with structural cardiac anomalies. However, it can be difficult to detect on physical examination, and patients with ASD may be asymptomatic until atrial arrhythmias, congestive heart failure, or pulmonary hypertension develop in the fourth or fifth decade of life [74]. Therefore, it may not be unusual for a pregnant woman to present with an uncorrected ASD.

As with other left-to-right shunts, an ASD increases right ventricular volume work and pulmonary blood flow. This eventually leads to right and left atrial distention, supraventricular arrhythmias, and signs of congestive heart failure (CHF). In addition, the increased pulmonary blood flow can on occasion lead to fixed increases in PVR and pulmonary hypertension [75]. As was stated above, however, these changes are seen relatively late in life. For this reason, pregnancy is well tolerated in the vast majority of patients with uncorrected ASD.

Those factors that increase the amount of left-to-right shunting will decrease left ventricular output and produce hypotension. The degree of shunting will depend, in turn, on the pressure gradient between the left and right atria. Therefore, the an-

Table 14-10. Atrial septal defect in pregnancy

Most common congenital lesion
Pregnancy generally well tolerated
Pathophysiology: Left-to-right shunt
                  Increased RV volume work
                  Increased pulmonary blood flow
                  Pulmonary hypertension develops rarely
Avoid: Increases in SVR
Anesthetic choice for labor: Epidural (low risk of shunt reversal)
Anesthetic choice for cesarean section: Epidural
Invasive monitoring not usually indicated

esthetic management of the patient with an ASD should seek to maintain that gradient at a normal level. An increase in SVR, or a decrease in PVR, will increase the gradient and augment shunt flow. Similarly, by impairing left atrial emptying, supraventricular tachycardia will increase left atrial pressure and thereby worsen left-to-right shunt. Even small amounts of intravenous air may cause "paradoxical left-sided air embolus" by crossing the ASD; therefore, all intravenous lines must be meticulously checked for air. This is true for any lesion in which an intracardiac right-to-left or left-to-right shunt exists.

Because epidural anesthesia will limit the increases in SVR that accompany painful contractions, it is the anesthetic of choice for labor in these patients. Similarly, for cesarean section, epidural anesthesia will avoid the increases in SVR that can accompany endotracheal intubation. Even with a small ASD, the potential may exist for shunt reversal if SVR drops precipitously; therefore, any decrease in oxygen saturation should be treated by increasing systemic resistance with small doses of phenylephrine.

General anesthesia can also be used for cesarean section if the interatrial pressure gradient is maintained at appropriate levels. Inhalation anesthesia can be used to control increases in SVR, although any preexisting degree of ventricular dysfunction mandates caution in its use. Antibiotic prophylaxis should be considered to prevent endocarditis. As was stated above, the great majority of patients with atrial septal defect tolerate pregnancy, labor, and delivery quite well, and seldom require invasive monitoring during the intrapartum or postpartum period (Table 14-10).

Ventricular Septal Defect

Ventricular septal defect (VSD) is the most common congenital cardiac defect; it is seen as an isolated lesion in 23 percent of infants and children with congenital heart disease. It occurs in 10 percent of adults with congenital cardiac malformations. While VSD may be associated with only minimal cardiopulmonary dysfunction, in its most severe form it can produce hemodynamic alterations that contraindicate pregnancy.

The pathophysiology of VSD is primarily dependent on the size of the defect [76]. In a small VSD, there is enough resistance to flow across the defect itself that right ventricular and pulmonary arterial pressures remain unchanged. There is only a minimal increase in pulmonary blood flow, and the only serious concern is the increased risk of infective endocarditis due to the jet effect of the blood ejected across the defect. With a moderate-sized VSD, pulmonary blood flow may be greatly increased, but right ventricular and pulmonary arterial pressures remain below systemic levels. These patients may develop left ventricular volume overload and CHF, but they are unlikely to develop pulmonary vascular disease. Finally, with large defects, there is no resistance to flow across the VSD, which permits right and left ventricular pressure to equalize. In such patients fixed increases in PVR are highly likely to develop, with eventual shunt reversal (Eisenmenger's syndrome).

Pregnancy is usually well tolerated in women with small VSDs. In one series of 50 patients having 98 pregnancies, no maternal deaths occurred. Some patients with fair to poor ventricular function developed CHF and arrhythmias, but these complications were not seen in women with excellent to good function [77]. On the other hand, the development of Eisenmenger's syndrome is associated with a much worse outcome (see later in text). Interestingly, the incidence of congenital heart disease has been estimated to be as high as 22 percent in children of women with VSD.

The anesthetic management of the parturient with VSD will be dependent on the size of the defect. As with ASD, intravenous air is a hazard. In patients with small defects and no evidence of pulmonary hypertension or ventricular dysfunction, invasive monitoring is not indicated, and the anesthetic management need not be altered in any substantial fashion. These patients are at risk of developing infective endocarditis, however, and should receive antibiotic prophylaxis.

In patients with larger defects and substantial increases in pulmonary blood flow, increases in heart rate and systemic vascular resistance can increase left-to-right shunting and produce congestive heart failure. Such patients will benefit from the provision of adequate pain relief during labor, and epidural anesthesia is the method of choice. Invasive monitoring is indicated in these patients. While shunt reversal is unlikely in the setting of normal pulmonary artery pressure, it is a possibility if SVR drops drastically; therefore, pulse oximetry should be utilized, and arterial desaturation should be treated by increasing SVR with small doses of phenylephrine.

Epidural anesthesia is recommended for cesarean section, again keeping in mind the potential for shunt reversal. Alternatively, stable hemodynamics can be maintained with a continuous spinal anesthetic. Should general anesthesia be required, increases in SVR and heart rate should be minimized by achieving an adequate depth of anesthesia before such noxious stimuli as endotracheal intubation and surgical incision. In patients with evidence of CHF or ventricular dysfunction, this may be best achieved by using small doses of thiopental and an inhalation agent, supplemented by narcotics (Table 14-11).

Table 14-11. Ventricular septal defect in pregnancy

Second most common congenital defect in adults
Pregnancy well tolerated with small shunt
Pathophysiology: Left-to-right shunt
    Hemodynamic alteration depends on size of shunt
    Moderate shunt—RV volume overload and CHF
    Large shunt—RV and LV pressures equalize, producing fixed increase in PVR
Pulmonary hypertension is a contraindication to pregnancy
In absence of large reversible shunt, epidural anesthesia is appropriate for both labor and cesarean section
Invasive monitoring not indicated

The management of the patient with Eisenmenger's syndrome secondary to ASD or VSD is discussed in the following section on right-to-left shunts.

Congenital Heart Disease—Right-to-Left Shunts

Tetralogy of Fallot

Tetralogy of Fallot (TOF) is the most common form of congenital cyanotic heart disease in both children and adults. Because of the increasing tendency toward correction of TOF rather than palliation, as well as the dismal prognosis of surgically untreated disease (95% mortality by age 25), it is rare to see a pregnant woman with uncorrected disease. Nevertheless, such women do exist; TOF remains the most common cyanotic congenital lesion in pregnancy. Furthermore, even after surgery, there may be residual anatomic defects that alter maternal cardiovascular function. Finally, a successful anatomic repair may be associated with residual myocardial dysfunction or conduction abnormalities. Despite the rarity of uncorrected TOF in the parturient, therefore, it is essential to have an understanding of its pathophysiology.

A full discussion of the pathophysiology of TOF is presented in Chap. 18; briefly, TOF is defined by four structural abnormalities: pulmonary stenosis, either infundibular, valvular, or supravalvular; ventricular septal defect; biventricular origin of the aorta; and right ventricular hypertrophy. Physiologically, the obstruction at the level of the pulmonary artery leads to right-to-left shunting across the VSD, producing arterial hypoxemia. This is manifested clinically by cyanosis, compensatory polycythemia, growth retardation, and hypercyanotic episodes ("tet spells"). These episodes, associated with exercise, are partially due to increased infundibular obstruction secondary to increases in myocardial contractility, similar to that seen in idiopathic hypertrophic subaortic stenosis (see later in text).

The medical management of TOF is primarily geared to the prevention and treatment of complications of the disease, for example, treatment of anemia to maintain oxygen-carrying capacity, early treatment of illnesses that might lead to dehydration and thrombotic complications, and β-blockade to prevent increases in myocardial contractility that might produce hypercyanosis [76]. In general, though, treatment is primarily surgical, and medical management is usually reserved for infants until they are large enough to undergo corrective surgery.

Pregnancy is poorly tolerated in women with uncorrected TOF. The maternal death rate has been reported to be as high as 12 percent [1]. This poor outcome is believed to be due to the decreased SVR seen during pregnancy, which will increase shunt flow and hypoxemia. A particularly dangerous period is during and immediately after delivery, when decreased blood pressure associated with blood loss can increase shunt flow and produce cardiovascular collapse. The fetal outcome in uncorrected TOF is similarly poor, with a mortality of 36 percent. In corrected TOF, maternal and fetal outcome are essentially normal, although the risk of congenital heart disease is increased in the infants of women with TOF.

The anesthetic management of the patient with TOF will be guided by the status of the repair. In patients with normal right ventricular function and no residual shunt, the usual anesthetic considerations apply, and invasive monitoring is not indicated. Some patients may have residual RV dysfunction after surgical repair, and should be managed in a fashion similar to that of patients with primary pulmonary hypertension, that is, maintain adequate filling pressures, prevent increases in pulmonary vascular resistance, and avoid myocardial depressants. The presence of conduction abnormalities may warrant continuous ECG monitoring during labor.

For patients with uncorrected TOF, invasive monitoring should be considered mandatory. Because of the risk of introducing a pulmonary artery catheter through the ventricular septal defect, and the lack of useful information regarding cardiac output in the presence of a shunt, a central venous catheter is preferred. The primary anesthetic goal should be the avoidance of those factors that increase right-to-left shunting. Therefore, decreases in SVR should be avoided, since they will lead to decreases in LV pressure that will promote shunt flow. In addition, the hypertrophied RV will require elevated filling pressures to maintain adequate flow through the stenotic pulmonary artery. Therefore, decreases in venous return and blood volume will be poorly tolerated. Finally, if significant dynamic infundibular obstruction is present, increases in myocardial contractility should be avoided.

Traditionally, systemic narcotics, paracervical block, and pudendal block have been recommended for labor analgesia. If epidural analgesia is utilized, extreme caution should be exercised to ensure that adequate filling pressures and systemic resistance are maintained. Pulse oximetry can be a useful tool for evaluating sudden changes in shunt flow. If extremely low concentrations of bupivacaine (0.03125–0.0625%) are used in combination with sufentanil or fentanyl, adequate analgesia can be attained with minimal changes in hemodynamics. Alternatively, a pure intrathecal or epidural opioid technique can be used, thus avoiding entirely the sympathetic block seen with local anesthetics, at the cost of somewhat less effective pain relief.

For cesarean section, general anesthesia is recommended. Ketamine, which causes an increased SVR, can be a very useful induction agent. In the absence of right ventricular dysfunction or significant infundibular stenosis, a routine rapid-sequence induction with ketamine is well tolerated, and anesthesia can be maintained with low concentrations of a volatile agent supplemented with narcotics. In patients with infundibular stenosis, drugs that increase heart rate and contractility should be avoided, and anesthesia should be maintained with halothane or enflurane. In these patients, increasing cyanosis should be treated with volume infusion, β-blockade, increased anesthetic depth, and increased SVR with phenylephrine. In patients with compromised RV function, the anesthetic should be primarily narcotic based. In this group, increasing cyanosis is usually due to decreased SVR or worsened right ventricular contractility, and should be treated by decreasing the depth of anesthesia (Table 14-12). Obviously, the management of these patients is in large part dependent on the nature of the right ventricular obstruction, and this information is essential to formulating an anesthetic plan.

Eisenmenger's Syndrome

Eisenmenger's syndrome has been defined as "pulmonary hypertension at systemic level, due to high pulmonary vascular resistance, with reversed or bidirectional shunt through a large VSD" [78]. The syndrome can also be seen with ASD, patent duc-

Table 14-12. Tetralogy of Fallot in pregnancy

Most common congenital cyanotic heart disease
Uncorrected disease tolerates pregnancy poorly
Pathophysiology: Dynamic obstruction to pulmonary blood flow
　　　Right-to-left shunt
　　　Peripheral cyanosis
Corrected disease may have residual RV dysfunction
Anesthetic choice for labor: Narcotics and paracervical block (epidural anesthesia requires extreme caution)
Anesthesia choice for cesarean section: High-dose narcotic or ketamine/halothane
Monitoring: Pulse oximetry, arterial line, central venous pressure (not pulmonary artery catheter)
Avoid increases in heart rate and contracility in patients with dynamic obstruction
Avoid decreases in SVR

---

tus arteriosus, or aorticopulmonary window. The inciting event is the exposure of the pulmonary circulation to high pressure due to left-to-right shunt. This leads to the production, over time, of obliterative changes in the pulmonary circulation, which causes fixed increases in PVR. This obstruction to RV outflow causes increases in RV pressure, and the direction of shunt flow reverses. Until the obliterative changes occur, closure of the systemic-pulmonary communication restores normal hemodynamics. Once fixed increases in PVR have occurred, however, closure of the communication is no longer indicated, because the risks of surgery outweigh any benefit that might accrue from closing the defect.

The degree of right-to-left shunt will depend on the relationship between SVR and PVR; as systemic resistance drops, left ventricular pressure will decrease, promoting right-to-left flow and cyanosis. Similarly, any increases in pulmonary resistance, secondary to acidosis, hypercarbia, or positive pressure ventilation, will also increase right-to-left shunt and cyanosis. Since systemic vascular resistance decreases during pregnancy, while PVR remains unchanged, one would suspect that pregnancy is a dangerous proposition in these patients. This was confirmed by Gleicher and associates [79], who demonstrated a 30 percent mortality in women with Eisenmenger's syndrome who became pregnant. Of the women studied, 52 percent died in connection with one of their pregnancies. In addition, neonatal outcome is quite poor; only 25 percent of all pregnancies are carried to term, and 30 percent of delivered infants show intrauterine growth retardation, presumably secondary to maternal hypoxemia. In total, fetal mortality has been reported to be between 30 and 50 percent [1]. Thus, it has been recommended that women with Eisenmenger's syndrome not become pregnant, and that abortion be performed should pregnancy occur.

The anesthetic management of these patients is similar to that of the patient with uncorrected TOF. Again, maintenance of adequate filling pressures and SVR will help maintain the appropriate relationship of right and left ventricular pressures and decrease right-to-left shunt. This will necessitate invasive monitoring with a central venous pressure catheter and arterial line, as well as pulse oximetry. Pulmonary artery catheters are not recommended because of the potential complications (i.e., crossing over to the left side) of their use and the lack of additional information provided. Factors that increase pulmonary resistance, such as hypercarbia, acidosis, hypoxia, and high ventilatory pressures, should be avoided, as should myocardial depressants due to the right ventricular failure. While systemic narcotics and paracervical block undoubtedly have the least effect on hemodynamics, epidural anesthesia can be used for analgesia during labor if hemodynamic changes are treated expeditiously. Low concentrations of local anesthetics combined with an opioid are recommended.

For cesarean section, the successful use of epidural anesthesia has been reported [80, 81], and some have recommended its use [82], but general anesthesia is usually recommended as the anesthetic of choice [1, 73]. High-dose fentanyl [82] or ketamine and modified high-dose fentanyl [73] have been recommended as induction techniques, with the caveat that aspiration prophylaxis be aggressively pursued and preparations made for prolonged mechanical ventilation of both the mother and the newborn. Nitrous oxide is avoided due to its potential effects on PVR, and potent inhalation agents are used sparingly to prevent myocardial depression.

There is a significant mortality seen in the postpartum period, due to thromboembolism, hypotension, or sudden increases in pulmonary resistance [2]. For this reason, observation in an intensive care setting should be routine for at least 48 hours postpartum.

Cardiomyopathies

Peripartum Cardiomyopathy

Peripartum cardiomyopathy is defined as the development of primary heart failure in a patient without previous evidence of heart disease in the last month of pregnancy, or the first 6 months postpartum [83]. It is a diagnosis of exclusion, in that nutritional, metabolic, toxic, infectious, or other secondary cardiomyopathies must be ruled out (Table 14-13). Peripartum cardiomyopathy is also known as cardiomyopathy of pregnancy, puerperal cardiomyopathy, or postpartal heart disease [1].

The incidence of peripartum cardiomyopathy has been reported to be as high as 1 in 1,300 live births [84], although a more recent survey showed an incidence of 1 in 15,000 [85]. Reported risk factors for development of the disease include maternal age greater than 30 years, multiparity, multiple gestation, toxemia, and obesity.

Despite intense investigation, there is as yet no consensus regarding the etiology of this disorder. In fact, it has been proposed that peripartum cardiomyopathy is no different, clinically or pathologically, from other idiopathic cardiomyopathies, and that pregnancy merely unmasks an underlying process that otherwise would have developed at a later time. Ribner and Silverman [86], however, point

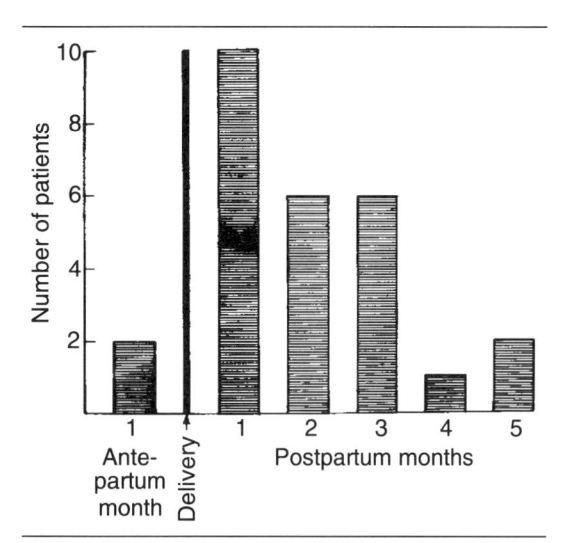

Fig. 14-7. Presentation of peripartum cardiomyopathy by month of gestation. Note that this disease most commonly presents in the first postpartum month. (Reprinted with permission from JG Demakis and SH Rahimtoola, Peripartum cardiomyopathy. *Circulation* 44: 964–968, 1971. By permission of the American Heart Association, Inc.)

out several facets of the disease that imply that it is unique. First, it is unusual for idiopathic cardiomyopathy to appear before middle age; when it does occur in young women, the great majority of patients relate the onset of symptoms to pregnancy. Second, a preexisting cardiomyopathy would be expected to be revealed in the second or third trimester, when the cardiac work load reaches a peak, whereas peripartum cardiomyopathy frequently presents after delivery (Fig. 14-7). The recurrence of cardiomyopathy with subsequent pregnancy appears to be unique to this disorder. Finally, spontaneous resolution of cardiac dilatation, while common in peripartum cardiomyopathy, is almost unheard of in other forms of idiopathic cardiomyopathy [86].

If one accepts that peripartum cardiomyopathy is a distinct disorder, then it is reasonable to ask whether it has a distinct etiology. There is certainly no shortage of suspected causative factors, but none have been proven beyond any reasonable doubt (Table 14-14).

Due to the high association between lower socioeconomic status and peripartum cardio-

Table 14-13. Secondary cardiomyopathies

Nutritional: Beriberi
Metabolic: Thyroid dysfunction, anemia
Toxic: Alcoholic, CCl_4, diphtheria
Infectious: Viral, rickettsial, protozoal
Ischemic
Infiltrative: Sarcoid, amyloid
Collagen-vascular disease: Lupus erythematosus
Neuromuscular: Muscular dystrophy, polymyositis
Peripartum: Cardiomyopathy

Source: Modified from MD Johnson and DH Saltzman, Cardiac Disease. In S Datta, *Anesthetic and Obstetric Management of High Risk Pregnancy.* St. Louis: Mosby, 1991. Pp 232–247.

Table 14-14. Putative causative factors of peripartum cardiomyopathy

Preeclampsia
Familial factors
Chronic hypertension
Viral infection
Inflammatory reaction
Autoimmune response

Source: Modified from HS Ribner and RI Silverman, Peripartal Cardiomyopathy. In LL Elkayam and N Gleicher (eds), *Cardiac Problems in Pregnancy* (2nd ed). New York: Alan R. Liss, 1990. Pp 115–127.

myopathy, nutritional factors have been suspected to play a role in development of the disorder. One study showed a high incidence of thiamine deficiency in a group of Korean women with peripartum cardiomyopathy, as well as a diminution of heart size when thiamine therapy was initiated [87]. However, most authors have been unable to document gross malnutrition or to demonstrate any evidence of a specific vitamin deficiency.

The role of preeclampsia in the development of peripartum cardiomyopathy was raised by Demakis and associates [88], who demonstrated a fourfold increase in the incidence of preeclampsia in women with cardiomyopathy compared with the overall obstetric population. However, this relationship has not been demonstrated in subsequent studies, which may reflect the rigor with which the diagnosis of preeclampsia is made [89, 90].

An immunologic basis for the disorder has been proposed. There is a higher incidence of peripartum cardiomyopathy in multiparas and in twin gestations, which suggests a reaction to the products of conception. Trophoblastic tissue may elicit a maternal antibody response that initiates an autoimmune reaction [91]. Interestingly, a similar immunologic mechanism has been proposed to be the triggering factor for preeclampsia.

While peripartum cardiomyopathy occurs by definition in the last month of pregnancy or within 6 months postpartum, it appears most commonly in the first 2 postpartum months [83]. Patients have the typical signs and symptoms of left ventricular failure, including orthopnea, dyspnea on exertion, paroxysmal nocturnal dyspnea, peripheral edema, jugular venous distention, and gallop rhythms. Both pulmonary and systemic thromboembolism are quite common, having been seen in 25 percent of Hull and Hidden's patients [92]. Chest radiography reveals biventricular enlargement, and echocardiography shows a dilated, hypokinetic ventricle. However, these findings are not specific to peripartum cardiomyopathy and are seen in any type of congestive cardiomyopathy. Nevertheless, these studies may be helpful in ruling out other causes of heart failure, such as valvular or pericardial disease [86].

Treatment of peripartum cardiomyopathy involves digitalization, sodium restriction, prophylactic anticoagulation, and bed rest. There may be a role for afterload reduction with angiotensin-converting enzyme inhibitors [93]. For severe intractable heart failure, cardiac transplantation may be the only remaining option.

As was alluded to previously, a substantial number of patients have spontaneous return of normal cardiac function, and these individuals have an excellent prognosis. On the other hand, patients with cardiomegaly that persists for greater than 6 months have a much worse outcome: 85 percent of patients with persistent cardiac enlargement died of cardiac failure, and the 5-year mortality was 55 percent [88].

Recurrence in subsequent pregnancies is not uncommon. Walsh and associates [94] described six patients who became pregnant after an episode of peripartum cardiomyopathy. All six had further deterioration of cardiac function postpartum [94]. Thus, several authors have recommended that an episode of peripartum cardiomyopathy represents a contraindication to further pregnancy [62, 90, 95]. Demakis and Rahimtoola [83], however, believed that deterioration of cardiac function is likely to occur with subsequent gestation only in those women who have persistent cardiac enlargement; they therefore suggested that women who have return of cardiac size to normal should not be advised against further pregnancies [83]. Interestingly, women who undergo successful cardiac transplantation for severe peripartum cardiomyopathy appear to tolerate subsequent pregnancy quite well [96].

The anesthetic management of the parturient with peripartum cardiomyopathy is not substantially different from that of any other patient with severe ventricular failure. Invasive hemodynamic monitoring should be used routinely. Anticoagulation should be suspended and the clotting status normalized before labor begins. Lumbar epidural anesthesia represents the anesthetic of choice for labor, as it prevents pain-induced increases in afterload that may lead to ventricular compromise. Fluid loading should be guided by the patient's wedge pressure.

Similarly, epidural anesthesia is a good choice for cesarean delivery, as it avoids the extreme increases in afterload that may accompany endotracheal intubation. Because of the more drastic hemodynamic alterations that may be seen with single-dose spinal anesthesia, it is probably best avoided in these patients. There may be a role, however, for the use of continuous spinal anesthesia, in that careful titration of the level of the block may prevent extreme alterations in hemodynamics.

If general anesthesia is utilized for cesarean section, myocardial depressants should be used with great care. High-dose narcotic induction may be necessary in patients with the most severe alterations in myocardial function, and will necessitate mechanical ventilation of the neonate. Vasodilators should be readily available in order to treat increases in afterload that may attend noxious surgical stimuli.

Idiopathic Hypertrophic Subaortic Stenosis

Idiopathic hypertrophic subaortic stenosis (IHSS), also known as asymmetric septal hypertrophy, is an autosomal dominant trait that produces hypertrophic changes in the interventricular septum and ventricular outflow tract. Hemodynamically, this hypertrophied muscle mass protrudes into the left ventricular cavity and produces obstruction to ejection of blood. Patients with IHSS complain of palpitations, dyspnea, chest pain, or syncope. In addition, they have an increased risk of sudden death (1–3% per year), probably secondary to ventricular arrhythmias [62].

IHSS produces a dynamic obstruction, that is, obstruction to ventricular ejection is worsened during systole, and is in fact further worsened by increases in myocardial contractility. Thus, β-blockade has become the mainstay of treatment for this disorder. The obstruction is also worsened when left ventricular volume decreases. Therefore, decreased preload, which will decrease LVEDV, is poorly tolerated. Similarly, afterload reduction will worsen the obstruction by increasing ventricular emptying. Supraventricular arrhythmias, which impair ventricular filling, will have a similar deleterious effect (Table 14-15).

The physiologic changes of pregnancy have mixed effects on IHSS. The increased blood volume will tend to maintain end diastolic volume and thus diminish obstruction. However, the increased cardiac output and decreased SVR would encourage ventricular emptying. Also, aortocaval compression would tend to worsen obstruction through its reduction of venous return. These variable effects are reflected in clinical studies, which have shown no consistent pattern to the course of the disease during pregnancy [97, 98].

The successful use of epidural anesthesia for cesarean section in a patient with IHSS has been reported [99], and some authorities have recommended epidural anesthesia for both cesarean and vaginal delivery [82]. If such a course is chosen, it is absolutely essential that every measure be taken to maintain SVR, filling pressures, and heart rate. Alternatively, a pure epidural or intrathecal narcotic technique can provide reasonable labor analgesia while leaving maternal hemodynamics unchanged. Paracervical block, inhalation analgesia, and systemic narcotics are least likely to have any effect on outflow obstruction.

Table 14-15. Factors that affect outflow obstruction in IHSS

Worsen obstruction
Beta agonists
Vasodilators
Digoxin
Pain
Ketamine
Hypovolemia
$CaCl_2$
Tachycardia and supraventricular arrhythmias
Aortocaval compression

Lessen obstruction
β-Blockers
Negative inotropes
Hypervolemia
Alpha agonists

For cesarean section, epidural anesthesia can be utilized if the protective measures discussed previously are taken. Due to its sudden and occasionally unpredictable effects on maternal hemodynamics, single-shot spinal anesthesia is not recommended, although a catheter technique may be acceptable if the level of block is titrated carefully. General anesthesia probably remains the anesthetic of choice for abdominal delivery. It is important to maintain an adequate depth of anesthesia to prevent cardiovascular stimulation. Lidocaine and small doses of narcotics will help blunt the response to intubation. A β-blocker should be readily available to control increases in heart rate and contractility that may worsen outflow obstruction. Halothane is a useful maintenance agent due to its beneficial effects on heart rate and contractility, and its minimal effect on SVR.

Whatever the route of delivery, and in fact whether or not anesthesia is administered, patients with IHSS should be monitored with an arterial line and a pulmonary artery catheter. This monitoring should be continued for 24 to 48 hours postpartum.

Miscellaneous Cardiac Disorders

Coronary Artery Disease

Coronary artery disease (CAD) remains a rare disorder in women of childbearing age. The incidence of myocardial infarction during pregnancy has been estimated to be less than 1 in 10,000 pregnancies [100]. Nevertheless, the anesthetic management of the pregnant patient with CAD is an important issue, not only because of its high mortality, but also because of certain trends that very likely will increase its incidence among pregnant women in the future.

The risk factors for CAD are well known. The increasingly common postponement of childbearing until the thirties and beyond has presumably increased the number of pregnant women with CAD. The growing incidence of cigarette smoking among young women undoubtedly has led to the acceleration of atherosclerotic heart disease in this age group. Through their effects on both blood pressure and serum cholesterol, oral contraceptives have been shown to be an independent risk factor for CAD. Finally, the use of cocaine, a potent coronary artery vasoconstrictor, has been suggested to be a contributing factor to the rising incidence of ischemic cardiac disease in pregnant women [82] (Table 14-16).

Table 14-16. Risk factors for coronary artery disease

Hypercholesterolemia
Hypertension
Cigarette smoking
Age
Sex
Family history
Diabetes
Lifestyles

The maternal mortality of myocardial infarction (MI) during pregnancy is reported to be between 30 and 40 percent [2]. Mortality is much higher when infarction occurs in the third trimester, and delivery within 2 weeks of MI is associated with a maternal mortality of 50 percent [101]. This is intuitively not unexpected; the mortality in patients undergoing surgery after acute MI is of a similar magnitude, and even uncomplicated vaginal delivery leads to physiologic trespasses that rival any surgical procedure. The mortality after MI during pregnancy is 14 percent for vaginal delivery and 23 percent for cesarean section [102]. This does not necessarily imply, however, that vaginal delivery is the preferred route.

The evaluation of the patient with CAD is not substantially different during pregnancy from that of the nonpregnant patient. A discussion of that workup is presented in Chap. 5. However, it is important to be aware of the risks of nuclear studies and angiography to the developing fetus. For example, a thallium stress test will expose the fetus to approximately 800 mrads, which can be expected to increase the risk of developing cancer by perhaps 40 percent [103]. Similarly, even careful shielding of the abdomen during coronary cineangiography exposes the fetus to 5.5 rads per minute, a level of exposure that would lead to severe structural abnormalities, if not fetal death, during the first trimester [103]. As always, maternal well-being must take precedence over the fetus, but diagnostic studies must be undertaken only if the fetal risk is understood, and only if there is a reasonable expectation that the results of those studies will significantly affect the management plan. Termination of pregnancy should be considered strongly if such studies are considered essential.

As in the nonpregnant patient, the treatment of CAD during pregnancy is predicated on the maintenance of an adequate balance of myocardial oxygen supply and demand. This will primarily involve the use of nitrates, β-blockers, and calcium channel antagonists.

Nitrates primarily produce venodilatation, which decreases left ventricular preload and thus wall tension, leading to decreased oxygen demand. Also, while routine doses of nitrates have little effect on arterial tone, the decreased preload will indirectly decrease ventricular volume during systole, which decreases systolic wall tension (afterload) and oxygen demand [102]. Finally, nitrates produce direct coronary vasodilatation, which will increase myocardial oxygen delivery. If excessive postural hypotension is avoided, there appears to be little risk to the use of nitrates during pregnancy [103].

β-Adrenergic blockers decrease oxygen demand through their negative inotropic and chronotropic effects. By slowing heart rate, they increase diastolic filling of the coronary arteries and thus augment oxygen delivery. As was discussed previously, despite anecdotal reports of fetal bradycardia, growth retardation, and neonatal depression, the use of β-blockers does not routinely lead to those effects, and their use, if indicated, should therefore not be avoided during pregnancy.

Calcium channel blockers decrease cardiac work through their negative inotropic and afterload-reducing effects. They also increase oxygen delivery through coronary artery vasodilation. Although experience during pregnancy is limited, no adverse fetal effects have been reported with the use of these drugs [46].

As was mentioned above, the maternal mortality appears to be somewhat lower when vaginal delivery is utilized than when cesarean section is performed. Also, in view of the similar hemodynamic changes seen postpartum, it seems unlikely that cesarean section spares the patient from the stress of labor, especially when that stress response can be effectively blunted with epidural anesthesia. Nevertheless, it has been argued that elective cesarean section should be performed preferentially, if only to prevent the scenario of a patient presenting emergently at a time of day when resources may be difficult to mobilize [81]. Unfortunately, while studies showing improved outcome with vaginal delivery might be criticized on a methodologic basis, there is no evidence that cesarean section has any such protective effect. Lacking such evidence, it is difficult to justify subjecting a woman to the additional stress of abdominal delivery unless it is obstetrically indicated.

Whether vaginal delivery or cesarean section is performed, the presence of significant CAD should be considered an indication for invasive hemodynamic monitoring. In view of the rapid changes in maternal hemodynamics that occur during labor, delivery, and the puerperium, accurate measurements of preload, afterload, and contractility are essential to maintain myocardial oxygen supply and demand.

For labor and delivery, epidural anesthesia will effectively blunt the increases in heart rate and afterload that are associated with contractions. Appropriate fluid loading and judicious use of vasopressors are essential to prevent the tachycardia and hypotension that can be seen with extensive sympathetic blockade. Phenylephrine may be a better choice than ephedrine for maintaining coronary perfusion pressure due to its lack of chronotropic effects. The use of epinephrine-containing local anesthetics should be avoided due to their potentially deleterious effects on heart rate.

For cesarean section, regional anesthesia is the preferred anesthetic technique. Epidural or continuous spinal anesthesia will produce gradual hemodynamic changes that are generally well tolerated. Because of the rapid onset of complete sympathetic blockade, single-dose spinal anesthesia is more likely to produce hypotension and ischemia, and is probably best avoided when cesarean section is performed.

If general anesthesia is performed for cesarean section, the primary goals are blunting the sympathetic response to noxious stimuli, particularly intubation, while at the same time avoiding excessive myocardial depression in those patients with impaired LV function. A standard rapid-sequence induction with thiopental and succinylcholine may fall short on both accounts. Induction with fentanyl, 5 to 10 μg/kg, and etomidate will produce stable hemodynamics, and can be followed by maintenance with nitrous oxide–relaxant anesthesia. In patients with good ventricular function, a volatile anesthetic can be added. In those patients with the most severe decrements in contractility, a high-dose narcotic-oxygen-relaxant technique may be necessary, at the obvious cost of requiring prolonged mechanical ventilation of the newborn.

After delivery, whether by the abdominal or vaginal route, monitoring in an intensive care setting for 24 to 48 hours is indicated. For patients who have undergone cesarean section, epidural opioids provide excellent analgesia while avoiding the sympathetic blockade attendant with local anesthetics.

Primary Pulmonary Hypertension

Pulmonary hypertension is defined as an elevation of pulmonary artery pressure above 30/15 mm Hg, or a mean pulmonary artery (PA) pressure greater than 25 mm Hg. This elevation is generally due to an obstructive lesion in the pulmonary circulation. These lesions can be broadly classified as being precapillary or postcapillary (Table 14-17).

In the overwhelming majority of cases, pulmonary hypertension is secondary to some other process. However, when a detailed and ongoing search fails to demonstrate any underlying cause for elevated pulmonary artery pressure, the diagnosis of primary pulmonary hypertension should be considered.

The etiology of primary pulmonary hypertension is by definition unknown. However, certain characteristics of the disease have suggested possible etiologic mechanisms. For example, in adults with primary pulmonary hypertension, the female-male ratio is 3:1. In childhood, however, the ratio is 1:1. There is also a frequent temporal relationship between the onset or worsening of the disease and a pregnancy. The frequent occurrence of antinuclear antibodies in patients with pulmonary hypertension suggests a possible autoimmune mechanism. Finally, familial clustering of some cases suggests a possible genetic predisposition to the disease [104].

It should be emphasized that primary pulmonary hypertension is a diagnosis of exclusion. Furthermore, the diagnosis may not actually be confirmed until postmortem examination, since a substantial proportion of these patients can be shown to have chronic thromboembolic disease that was unsuspected before death. Finally, even autopsy findings can be misinterpreted; up to one third of patients with supposedly autopsy-proven primary pulmonary hypertension were found on review to have another diagnosis [105].

Whatever the cause of pulmonary hypertension in a particular patient, the pathophysiology is similar. As PVR increases, right ventricular afterload and thus right ventricular stroke work increase. The right ventricle becomes hypertrophied and eventually fails. This is reflected by an increased central venous pressure and signs of hepatic congestion. Eventually, the right ventricle dilates and tricuspid insufficiency occurs. Left ventricular contractility is unimpaired, but cardiac output will fall due to LV underloading secondary to right ventricular failure.

Clinically, the initial manifestations of primary pulmonary hypertension are fatigue and exertional dyspnea, due to low cardiac output. Chest pain is not uncommon, secondary to right ventricular ischemia or pulmonary artery distention [106]. Palpitations are common, and indeed ventricular arrhythmias are frequently a terminal event. Dyspnea at rest, hemoptysis, and peripheral cyanosis may be seen with advanced disease. It is important to realize, however, that mild to moderate primary pulmonary hypertension is clinically silent, and that even mild exertional dyspnea usually reflects severe, long-standing disease [104].

Numerous vasodilators have been utilized in the

Table 14-17. Causes of pulmonary hypertension

Postcapillary obstructive lesions
Pulmonary veins (venocclusive disease)
Left atrium (myxoma)
Mitral valves (stenosis)
Left ventricle (hypertrophy or failure)

Precapillary obstructive lesions
Vascular disease secondary to increased pulmonary blood flow (VSD, PDA)
Primary pulmonary hypertension

Source: Modified from H Kuida, Primary and Secondary Pulmonary Hypertension: Pathophysiology, Recognition, and Treatment. In JW Hurst (ed), *The Heart* (2nd ed). New York: McGraw-Hill, 1990. Pp 1191–1219.

hope of relieving active pulmonary vasospasm, including isoproterenol, diazoxide, oxygen, hydralazine, phentolamine, nifedipine, and nitroglycerin. None of these agents has been an unqualified success. One of the difficulties with this approach is the fact that pulmonary hypertension due to vasospasm eventually produces irreversible structural changes in the pulmonary vasculature. Therefore, there is an undeniable advantage to initiating therapy while there is still a reversible, vasospastic component to the disease. The problem lies in diagnosing primary pulmonary hypertension at an early enough stage to take advantage of that reversible component [104].

Women with primary pulmonary hypertension who become pregnant have a mortality as high as 50 percent [107]. This apparently has little relation to previous functional status, since asymptomatic or mildly symptomatic women have a mortality of 30 percent or more [107]. Fetal wastage due to low cardiac output is quite high, even in women who survive the pregnancy. Finally, while not yet proven, there is at least a suggestion that pregnancy might accelerate the progress of the disease. For these reasons, it has been strongly recommended that women with primary pulmonary hypertension avoid pregnancy. If pregnancy occurs, termination under epidural anesthesia with full invasive monitoring should be performed as soon as possible [107].

If pregnancy is allowed to proceed to term, it is necessary to determine the extent of the patient's pulmonary hypertension and right ventricular failure. It is also essential to know which agents, if any, are effective in decreasing the patient's pulmonary resistance. Radial and pulmonary artery pressure monitoring should be used routinely during the intrapartum period, although passage of a PA catheter may be quite difficult due to right ventricular dilatation.

Management of these patients should be geared to maintenance of right ventricular function. Since myocardial contractility may already be impaired, negative inotropes should be used carefully, if at all. Factors increasing pulmonary resistance, such as hypoxia, hypercarbia, acidosis, hyperinflation, and untreated pain, should be scrupulously avoided. Since the failing right ventricle depends on an elevated central venous pressure (CVP) to maintain its output, any factors that decrease venous return, such as hypovolemia and aortocaval compression, should be corrected rapidly. Finally, since cardiac output is limited by the fixed right ventricular output, decreases in SVR may be poorly tolerated.

Because of their minimal effects on maternal hemodynamics, intravenous narcotics, paracervical block, and inhalation analgesia are all useful methods of providing pain relief during labor. Because of its potential effects on both preload and systemic resistance, epidural anesthesia must be utilized with extreme caution. This necessitates slow titration of the dermatomal level of anesthesia, as well as meticulous management of filling pressures and systemic resistance to maintain hemodynamic stability. Local anesthetics [108] and combinations of local anesthetics and narcotics [109] have both been used safely. Alternatively, intrathecal narcotics can be used to provide good labor analgesia for up to 18 to 24 hours, while having no effect on maternal hemodynamics [110].

If cesarean section is required, general anesthesia is preferred due to the drastic hemodynamic alterations that accompany major regional anesthesia. A standard induction of thiopental and succinylcholine followed by endotracheal intubation can lead to severe increases in pulmonary pressure and acute right ventricular failure. Induction with etomidate and small doses of fentanyl is more likely to maintain hemodynamic stability. Alternatively, a high-dose narcotic induction can be utilized, at the expense of neonatal respiratory depression that will require ventilatory support.

Anesthesia should be maintained with a combination of narcotics and low concentrations of a halogenated agent, if it is tolerated. Because of its deleterious effects on pulmonary artery pressure, nitrous oxide should be avoided. Ventilation should be controlled, using tidal volumes of 5 to 10 ml/kg to minimize the possibility of overinflation of the lungs. Should pulmonary artery pressure rise intraoperatively, hypoxia, hypercarbia, and acidosis must be ruled out. If pulmonary hypertension continues to worsen, isoproterenol or dopamine should be slowly titrated to maintain right ventricular output. It may become necessary to use nitroglycerin, phentolamine, or prostaglandis in the hope of producing pulmonary vasodilatation.

Unfortunately, delivery of the baby does not necessarily signify a good outcome, as the majority of maternal deaths occur immediately postpartum or in the first 7 days after delivery. This is usually due to thromboembolism or intractable heart failure, although the immediate cause of death frequently cannot be identified. There may therefore be an advantage to continued monitoring for at least several days into the postpartum period.

Marfan's Syndrome

Marfan's syndrome is an autosomal dominant trait, the primary characteristic of which is a generalized defect of connective tissue, secondary to an as yet unidentified abnormality of collagen synthesis [111]. There is also a significant sporadic appearance of the disease in patients with no family history, presumably due to a new mutation. Patient's with Marfan's syndrome have a distinct clinical presentation, consisting of greater than average height, disproportionately long limbs, sternal deformities, hyperextensibility of joints, subluxation of the lens, scoliosis, and an increased incidence of abdominal hernias [112]. Their anesthetic management can be complicated by difficulties with intubation and restrictive pulmonary disease. By far the most important abnormalities in these patients, however, are those involving the cardiovascular system.

The cardiovascular pathology in patients with Marfan's syndrome is initiated by degeneration of the elastic fibers in the media of the great vessels. They are replaced with collagen, which leads to weakness in the media, and in turn predisposes to the formation of saccular aneurysms. If such an enlargement involves the aortic root, aortic insufficiency may develop, which can lead to LV dilatation and eventual heart failure. The medial necrosis also predisposes to intimal tears, which may lead to aortic dissection [111]. This is, in fact, a common cause of death in patients with Marfan's syndrome. The medical therapy of these patients is based on chronic β-blockade. Presumably, by decreasing dp/dt, or shear stress, aortic root dilatation and dissection are less likely to occur, although long-term confirmation of this theory is lacking.

There is considerable controversy regarding both the effect of pregnancy on the progression of the cardiovascular lesions of Marfan's syndrome, and indeed whether pregnancy is contraindicated in these patients. Elkayam and associates [112] have surveyed the literature, and have found that early studies implying a poor outcome for women with Marfan's syndrome who became pregnant relied heavily on anecdotal data. They believe that a careful analysis of published data seems to show a small risk to women with Marfan's syndrome if they had no evidence of aortic root involvement [112]. On the other hand, McAnulty and colleagues [62] believe that, even in the absence of aortic root involvement, pregnancy is contraindicated in women with Marfan's syndrome. It seems prudent to follow Elkayam's recommendation that women with Marfan's syndrome be encouraged to complete their pregnancy if they have no evidence of aortic root involvement, if they are maintained on β-blockers, and if serial echocardiograms show no evidence of progressive aortic dilatation during the pregnancy. Should such dilatation occur, they recommend that strong consideration be given to terminating the pregnancy or repairing the aorta.

Another dilemma is the determination of the optimal route of delivery. Elkayam and associates [112] recommend that cesarean section be performed electively if there is evidence of aortic dissection, acute aortic insufficiency, or progressive dilatation of the aorta during pregnancy. Otherwise, cesarean section should be reserved for obstetric indications. They recommend that if vaginal delivery is chosen, bearing-down efforts should be avoided, and that forceps delivery should be performed to shorten the duration of the second stage.

In patients with an aortic dissection that has been well controlled medically, epidural anesthesia has obvious advantages. By providing a pain-free labor, it will minimize increases in blood pressure and heart rate that may lead to extension of the dissection. A normal to low-normal blood pressure should be maintained, and treatment of hypotension with large doses of vasopressors should be avoided to minimize the potential for rebound hypertension. Monitoring should include an arterial line and CVP catheter, and adequate large-bore peripheral lines should be placed to provide access for rapid resuscitation if rupture occurs. β-Blockers such as esmolol and labetalol should be readily available, as should a rapid-acting vasodilator. At the time of delivery, adequate perineal anesthesia should be provided in order to expedite forceps delivery and thereby shorten the second stage.

For cesarean section, epidural or continuous spinal anesthesia provides stable hemodynamics. Again, a β-blocker and a vasodilator should be readily available. If general anesthesia is selected, every effort must be made to minimize the sympathetic response to endotracheal intubation and surgical stimuli. Because of its negative inotropic and chronotropic effects, halothane is preferred for anesthetic maintenance.

For postoperative patients, epidural narcotics will minimize the sympathetic response that is seen with inadequately treated pain. Because of the hemodynamic changes that occur in the immediate postpartum period, monitoring should be continued whether vaginal or cesarean delivery was performed.

The Pregnant Patient with Corrected Cardiac Disease

An entirely new category of pregnant patients with cardiac disease has appeared with the development of cardiac surgical techniques: the patient with surgically corrected cardiac disease. Every cardiac abnormality, and in fact each patient with the same abnormality, must be individually evaluated. There are certain questions, however, that must be addressed in all patients who have undergone cardiac surgery before anesthesia can be administered (Table 14-18).

It must be determined whether the patient has required systemic anticoagulation. In general, anticoagulation will be withheld at the time the patient goes into labor. Before regional anesthesia is administered, however, it will be necessary to confirm that the coagulation profile has returned to normal. If this is not the case, regional anesthesia is contraindicated unless anticoagulation is actively reversed. Additionally, one must consider the possibility that reinstituting anticoagulation after the regional anesthetic has been administered may lead to the development of an epidural hematoma. Although the work of Rao and El-Etr [113] suggests that this is highly unlikely, case reports of this occurrence have been published. The safest course seems to be the avoidance of anticoagulation until the block has receded. This will permit the early recognition of motor and sensory changes that may herald the development of an epidural hematoma.

The need for antibiotic prophylaxis must be established. In general, the presence of any prosthetic material is an indication for prophylaxis, but the absence of such material does not mean that prophylaxis is not required.

Right and left ventricular contractility may be impaired, either due to residual effects of the structurally corrected lesion (e.g., aortic insufficiency), or as a consequence of the surgical approach (e.g., ventriculotomy for repair of tetralogy of Fallot). Any limitation of activity should be approached with a high index of suspicion, and should prompt an evaluation of ventricular function, in most cases by echocardiography, due to its lack of fetal effects.

Some surgical repairs are associated with a high incidence of arrhythmias or conduction abnormalities [114]. Symptoms such as syncope, dizziness, exercise intolerance, or palpitations should alert the physician to the possibility of significant arrhythmias. A baseline ECG is indicated in patients who have undergone cardiac surgery even in the absence of symptoms (Table 14-19).

Even after successful repair, a residual structural

Table 14-18. Questions to be addressed before administration of anesthesia in the patient with corrected cardiac disease

Is anticoagulation needed?
Is antibiotic prophylaxis needed?
Is ventricular function normal?
Are there residual electrocardiographic abnormalities?
Is there a residual structural defect?
Is the pulmonary vasculature normal?
What is the anatomy of the repair?

Table 14-19. Incidence of postoperative arrhythmias

Surgical procedure	Arrhythmia incidence (%)
Intraatrial repair of transposition	50–80
Tetralogy of Fallot repair	30–60
VSD repair	10
Secundum ASD repair	9

Source: Modified from VL Vetter, What every pediatrician needs to know about cardiac arrhythmias in children who have had cardiac surgery. Pediatr Ann 20:378–385, 1991.

defect may be present, for example, mitral stenosis after annuloplasty, small VSD, or residual infundibular obstruction after tetralogy repair. This information should be sought out, particularly in patients who have any limitation of functional capacity.

There may be persistent structural changes in the pulmonary vasculature after repair of longstanding left-to-right shunts. It is vital to determine whether the PVR is normal, elevated, or hyperreactive.

It is essential to know the precise anatomy of the repair, particularly if the procedure was palliative. For example, a patient with pulmonary atresia may have undergone a Fontan procedure. In these patients, pulmonary blood flow is entirely provided by passive flow from the right atrium through the pulmonary artery. Unless one was familiar with the procedure, the need for high right-sided filling pressures and low PVR might not be appreciated, with potentially disastrous results.

These factors should serve to confirm the need for maintaining close contact with the patient's cardiologist, or sometimes her surgeon, throughout her pregnancy. The safe conduct of anesthesia may be difficult, if not impossible, if such contact is not maintained.

REFERENCES

1. Mangano, DT. Anesthesia for the Pregnant Cardiac Patient. In SM Shnider, G Levinson (eds), *Anesthesia for Obstetrics* (2nd ed). Baltimore: Williams & Wilkins, 1987. Pp 345–369.
2. Joyce, TH, Palacios, QT. Cardiac Disease. In FM James et al. (eds), *Obstetric Anesthesia: The Complicated Patient* (2nd ed). Philadelphia: Davis, 1988. Pp 159–177.
3. Elkayam, U, Gleicher, N. Changes in Cardiac Findings During Normal Pregnancy. In U Elkayam, N Gleicher (eds), *Cardiac Problems in Pregnancy* (2nd ed). New York: Alan R. Liss, 1990. Pp 31–38.
4. Perloff, JK. Pregnancy and Cardiovascular Disease. In E. Braunwald (ed), *Heart Disease* (3rd ed). Philadelphia: Saunders, 1988. Pp 1848–1869.
5. Cutforth, R, MacDonald, CB. Heart sounds and murmurs in pregnancy. *Am Heart J* 71:741–747, 1966.
6. Oram, S, Holt, M. Innocent depression of the ST segment and flattening of the t-wave during pregnancy. *J Obstet Gynaecol Br Commonw* 68:765–770, 1961.
7. Elkayam, U, Gleicher, N. Hemodynamics and Cardiac Function During Normal Pregnancy and the Puerperium. In U Elkayam, N Gleicher (eds), *Cardiac Problems in Pregnancy* (2nd ed). New York: Alan R. Liss, 1990. Pp 5–24.
8. Capeless, EL, Clapp, JF. Cardiovascular changes in early phase of pregnancy. *Am J Obstet Gynecol* 161:1449–1453, 1989.
9. Clark, SL, Cotton, DB, Lee, W, et al. Central hemodynamic assessment of normal term pregnancy. *Am J Obstet Gynecol* 161:1439–1442, 1989.
10. Ueland, K, Hansen, JM. Maternal cardiovascular dynamics. III. Labor and delivery under local and caudal analgesia. *Am J Obstet Gynecol* 103:8–18, 1969.
11. Parer, JT. Uteroplacental Circulation and Respiratory Gas Exchange. In SM Shnider, G Levinson (eds), *Anesthesia for Obstetrics* (2nd ed). Baltimore: Williams & Wilkins, 1987. P 18.
12. Butterworth, JF, Piccione, W, Berrizbeitia, LD, et al. Augmentation of venous return by adrenergic agonists during spinal anesthesia. *Anesth Analg* 65:612–616, 1986.
13. Ralston, DH, Shnider, SM, et al. Effects of equipotent ephedrine, metaraminol, mephentermine, and methoxamine on uterine blood flow in the pregnant ewe. *Anesthesiology* 40:354–370, 1974.
14. Chestnut, DH, Ostman, LG, Weiner, CP. The effect of vasopressor agents upon uterine artery blood flow velocity in the gravid guinea pig subjected to ritodrine infusion. *Anesthesiology* 68:363–366, 1988.
15. Ramanathan, S, Grant, GJ. Vasopressor therapy for hypotension due to epidural anesthesia for cesarean section. *Acta Anaesthesiol Scand* 32:559–565, 1988.
16. Moran, DH, Perillo, M, et al. Phenylephrine in treating maternal hypotension secondary to spinal anesthesia. *Anesthesiology* 71:A857, 1989.
17. Chestnut, DH, Weiner, CP, Martin, JG, et al. Effect of intravenous epinephrine on uterine artery blood flow velocity in the pregnant guinea pig. *Anesthesiology* 65:633–636, 1986.
18. Hood, DD, Dewan, DM, James, FM. Maternal and fetal effects of epinephrine in gravid ewes. *Anesthesiology* 64:610–613, 1986.
19. Callender, K, Levinson, G, Shnider, SM, et al. Dopamine administration in the normotensive pregnant ewe. *Obstet Gynecol* 51:586–589, 1978.
20. Rolbin, SH, Levinson, G, Shnider, SM. Dopamine treatment of spinal hypotension decreases uterine

blood flow in the pregnant ewe. *Anesthesiology* 51: 36–40, 1978.
21. Fishburne, J, Meis, P, Urban, R, et al. Vascular and uterine responses to dobutamine and dopamine in the gravid ewe. *Am J Obstet Gynecol* 137:944–951, 1980.
22. Greiss, FC, Crandell, DL. Therapy for hypotension induced by spinal anesthesia during pregnancy. *JAMA* 191:793–796, 1965.
23. Greiss, FC, Pick, JR. The uterine vascular bed: Adrenergic receptors. *Obstet Gynecol* 23:209–213, 1964.
24. Krasnow, N, Rolett, EL, Yurchak, PM, et al. Isoproterenol and cardiovascular performance. *Am J Med* 37:514–525, 1964.
25. Baker, BW, Longmire, S, Jones, MM, et al. The epidural test dose in obstetrics reconsidered. *Anesthesiology* 67:A625, 1987.
26. Ring, C, Krames, E, Shnider, SM, et al. Comparison of nitroprusside and hydralazine in hypertensive pregnant ewes. *Obstet Gynecol* 50:598–602, 1977.
27. Brinkman, CR, Assali, NS. Uteroplacental Hemodynamic Response to Antihypertensive Drugs in Hypertensive Pregnant Sheep. In MD Lindheimer, AI Katz, et al. (eds), *Hypertension in Pregnancy*. New York: Wiley, 1976. Pp 363–375.
28. Jouppila, P, Kirkinen, P, Koivula, A, et al. Effects of dihydralazine infusion on the fetoplacental blood flow and maternal prostanoids. *Obstet Gynecol* 65:115–118, 1985.
29. Craft, JB, Co, EG, Yonekura, ML, et al. Nitroglycerin therapy for phenylephrine induced hypertension in pregnant ewes. *Anesth Analg* 59:494–499, 1980.
30. Hood, DD, Dewan, DM, James, FM. The use of nitroglycerin in preventing the hypertensive response to tracheal intubation in severe pre-eclampsia. *Anesthesiology* 63:329–332, 1985.
31. Naulty, J, Cefalo, RC, Lewis, PE. Fetal toxicity of nitroprusside in the pregnant ewe. *Am J Obstet Gynecol* 139:708–711, 1981.
32. Donchin, Y, Amirav, B, Sahar, A, et al. Sodium nitroprusside for aneurysm surgery in pregnancy. *Br J Anaesth* 50:849–851, 1978.
33. Rigg, D, McDonogh, A. Use of sodium nitroprusside for deliberate hypotension during pregnancy. *Br J Anaesth* 53:985–987, 1981.
34. Willoughby, JS. Sodium nitroprusside, pregnancy, and multiple intracranial aneurysms. *Anaesth Intensive Care* 12:351–357, 1984.
35. Santos, AC, Petrikovsky, BM, Kaplan, GP. Neurologic and Muscular Diseases. In S Datta (ed), *Anesthetic and Obstetric Management of High Risk Pregnancy*. St. Louis: Mosby, 1991. P 142.
36. Mitani, GM, Harrison, EC, Steinberg, I. Digitalis Glycosides in Pregnancy. In U Elkayam, N Gleicher (eds), *Cardiac Problems in Pregnancy* (2nd ed). New York: Alan R. Liss, 1991. Pp 417–427.
37. Luxford, AME, Kellaway, GSM. Pharmacokinetics of digoxin in pregnancy. *Eur J Clin Pharmacol* 25:117–121, 1983.
38. Graves, SW, Valdes, R, Brown, BA. Endogenous digoxin–immunoreactive substance in human pregnancies. *J Clin Endocrinol Metab* 58:748–751, 1984.
39. Saarikoski, S. Placental transfer and fetal uptake of 3H-digoxin in humans. *Br J Obstet Gynaecol* 83:879–884, 1976.
40. Weaver, JB, Pearson, JF. Influence of digitalis on time of onset and duration of labor in women with cardiac disease. *Br Med J* 3:519–520, 1973.
41. Flesa, HC, Kapstrom, AB, Glueck, HI, et al. Placental transport of heparin. *Am J Obstet Gynecol* 93:570–573, 1965.
42. Hall, J, Pauli, RM, Wilson, KM. Maternal and fetal sequelae of anticoagulation during pregnancy. *Am J Med* 68:122–140, 1980.
43. Ueland, K, McAnulty, J, Ueland, F, et al. Special considerations in the use of cardiovascular drugs. *Clin Obstet Gynecol* 24:809–823, 1981.
44. Lee, PK, Wang, RY, Chow, JS, et al. Combined use of warfarin and adjusted subcutaneous heparin during pregnancy in patients with an artificial heart valve. *J Am Coll Cardiol* 8:221–224, 1986.
45. McGehee, W. Anticoagulation in Pregnancy. In U Elkayam, N Gleicher (eds), *Cardiac Problems in Pregnancy* (2nd ed). New York: Alan R. Liss, 1991. Pp 397–415.
46. Rotmensch, HH, Pines, A, Donchin, Y. Antiarrhythmic Drugs in Pregnancy. In U Elkayam, N Gleicher (eds), *Cardiac Problems in Pregnancy* (2nd ed). New York: Alan R. Liss, 1991. Pp 361–379.
47. Leonard, RF, Braun, TE, Levy, AM. Initiation of uterine contractions by disopyramide during pregnancy. *N Engl J Med* 299:84–85, 1978.
48. Kasten, GW, Martin, ST. Bupivacaine cardiovascular toxicity: Comparison of treatment with bretylium or lidocaine. *Anesth Analg* 64:911–916, 1985.
49. Frishman, WH, Chesner, M. Use of Beta-adrenergic Blocking Agents in Pregnancy. In U Elkayam, N Gleicher (eds), *Cardiac Problems in Pregnancy* (2nd ed). New York: Alan R. Liss, 1991. Pp 351–359.
50. Oakes, GK, Walker, AM, Ehrenkranz, RA, et al. Effect of propranolol infusion on the umbilical and

uterine circulations of pregnant sheep. *Am J Obstet Gynecol* 126:1038–1042, 1976.
51. Rubin, PC. Beta-blockers in pregnancy. *N Engl J Med* 305:1323–1326, 1981.
52. Sandstrom, B. Antihypertensive treatment with the adrenergic beta-receptor blocker metoprolol during pregnancy. *Gynecol Obstet Invest* 9:195–204, 1978.
53. Michael, CA. Use of labetalol in the treatment of severe hypertension during pregnancy. *Br J Clin Pharmacol* 8 (Suppl 2):211–215, 1979.
54. Michael, CA. Intravenous labetalol and intravenous diazoxide in severe hypertension complicating pregnancy. *Aust NZ J Obstet Gynaecol* 26:26–29, 1986.
55. Ramanathan, J, Sibai, BM, Mabie, WC, et al. The use of labetalol for attenuation of the hypertensive response to endotracheal intubation in pre-eclampsia. *Am J Obstet Gynecol* 159:650–654, 1988.
56. Jouppila, P, Kirkinen, P, Koivula, A, et al. Labetalol does not alter the placental and fetal blood flow or maternal prostanoids in pre-eclampsia. *Br J Obstet Gynaecol* 93:543–547, 1986.
57. MacPherson, M, Broughton Pipkin, F, Rutter, N. The effect of maternal labetalol on the newborn infant. *Br J Obstet Gynaecol* 93:539–542, 1986.
58. Eisenach, JC, Castro, MI. Maternally administered esmolol produces fetal beta-adrenergic blockade and hypoxemia in sheep. *Anesthesiology* 71:718–722, 1989.
59. Losasso, TJ, Muzzi, DA, Cucchiara, RF. Response of fetal heart rate to maternal administration of esmolol. *Anesthesiology* 74:782–784, 1991.
60. Rackley, CE, Edwards, JE, Karp, RB. Mitral Valve Disease. In JW Hurst (ed), *The Heart* (2nd ed). New York: McGraw-Hill, 1990. Pp 820–851.
61. Jackson, JM, Thomas, SJ. Valvular Heart Disease. In JA Kaplan (ed), *Cardiac Anesthesia* (2nd ed). Orlando, FL: Grune & Stratton, 1987. Pp 596–623.
62. McAnulty, JH, Metcalfe, J, Ueland, K. Cardiovascular Disease. In GN Burrow, TF Ferris (eds), *Medical Complications During Pregnancy* (3rd ed). Philadelphia: Saunders, 1988. Pp 180–203.
63. McAnulty, JH, Metcalfe, J, Ueland, K. Heart Disease and Pregnancy. In JW Hurst (ed), *The Heart* (2nd ed). New York: McGraw-Hill, 1990. Pp 1465–1478.
64. Ueland, K. Rheumatic Heart Disease and Pregnancy. In U Elkayam, N Gleicher (eds), *Cardiac Problems in Pregnancy* (2nd ed). New York: Alan R. Liss, 1990. P 101.
65. Savage, DD, Garrison, RJ, Devereux, RD, et al. Mitral valve prolapse in the general population. I. Epidemiologic features: The Framingham Study. *Am Heart J* 106:571–576, 1983.

66. Chesler, E, Matisonn, RE, Lakier, JB, et al. Acute myocardial infarction with normal coronary arteries: A possible manifestation of the billowing mitral leaflet syndrome. *Circulation* 54:203–209, 1976.
67. Sakuma, T, Kakihana, M, Togo, T, et al. Mitral valve prolapse syndrome with coronary artery spasm: A possible cause of recurrent ventricular arrhythmia. *Clin Cardiol* 8:306–308, 1985.
68. Rayburn, WF. Mitral Valve Prolapse and Pregnancy. In U Elkayam, N Gleicher (eds), *Cardiac Problems in Pregnancy* (2nd ed). New York: Alan R. Liss, 1990. P 186.
69. Rayburn, WF, Fontana, ME. Mitral valve prolapse and pregnancy. *Am J Obstet Gynecol* 141:9–11, 1981.
70. Tang, LCH, Chan, SYW, Wong, VCW, et al. Pregnancy in patients with mitral valve prolapse. *Int J Gynaecol Obstet* 23:217–221, 1985.
71. Shapiro, EP, Trimble, EL, Robinson, JC, et al. Safety of labor and delivery in women with mitral valve prolapse. *Am J Cardiol* 56:806–807, 1985.
72. Arias, F, Pineda, J. Aortic stenosis in pregnancy. *J Reprod Med* 20:229–231, 1978.
73. Ferguson, JE, Wyner, J, Albright, GA. Maternal Health Complications. In GA Albright (ed), *Anesthesia in Obstetrics* (2nd ed). Boston: Butterworth, 1986. Pp 384–388.
74. Elkayam, U, Cobb, T, Gleicher, N. Congenital Heart Disease and Pregnancy. In U Elkayam, N Gleicher (eds), *Cardiac Problems in Pregnancy* (2nd ed). New York: Alan R. Liss, 1990. P 78.
75. Hickey, PR, Wessel, DL. Anesthesia for Treatment of Congenital Heart Disease. In JA Kaplan (ed), *Cardiac Anesthesia* (2nd ed). Orlando, FL: Grune & Stratton, 1987. P 699.
76. Nugent, EW, Plauth, WH, Edwards, JE. The Pathology, Abnormal Physiology, Clinical Recognition, and Medical and Surgical Treatment of Congenital Heart Disease. In JW Hurst (ed), *The Heart* (2nd ed). New York: McGraw-Hill, 1990. P 666.
77. Whittenmore, R, Hobbins, JC, Engle, MA. Pregnancy and its outcome in women with and without surgical treatment of congenital heart disease. *Am J Cardiol* 50:641–651, 1982.
78. Wood, P. The Eisenmenger syndrome or pulmonary hypertension with reversed shunt. *Br Med J* 2:701–709, 755–762, 1958.
79. Gleicher, N, Midwall, J, Hochberger, D, et al. Eisenmenger's syndrome and pregnancy. *Obstet Gynecol Surv* 34:721–741, 1979.
80. Rosenberg, B, Simon, K, Peretz, BA, et al. Eisen-

80. menger's syndrome in pregnancy. Controlled segmental epidural block for cesarean section. *Reg Anaesth.* Vol 7. 131–133, 1984.
81. Spinnato, JA, Kraynack, BJ, Cooper, MW. Eisenmenger's syndrome in pregnancy. Epidural anesthesia for elective cesarean section. *N Engl J Med* 304: 1215–1217, 1981.
82. Johnson, MD, Saltzman, DH. Cardiac Disease. In S Datta (ed), *Anesthetic and Obstetric Management of High Risk Pregnancy.* St. Louis: Mosby, 1991. Pp 232–247.
83. Demakis, JG, Rahimtoola, SH. Peripartum cardiomyopathy. *Circulation* 44:964–968, 1971.
84. Meadows, WR. Idiopathic myocardial failure in the last trimester of pregnancy and the puerperium. *Circulation* 15:903–914, 1957.
85. Cunningham, FG, Pritchard, JA, Hankins, GDV, et al. Peripartum heart failure: Idiopathic cardiomyopathy or compounding cardiovascular events? *Obstet Gynecol* 67:157–168, 1986.
86. Ribner, HS, Silverman, RI. Peripartal Cardiomyopathy. In U Elkayam, N Gleicher (eds), *Cardiac Problems in Pregnancy* (2nd ed). New York: Alan R. Liss, 1990. Pp 115–127.
87. Blegen, SD. Postpartum congestive heart failure: Beri-beri heart disease. *Acta Med Scand* 178:515–524, 1965.
88. Demakis, JG, Rahimtoola, SH, Sutton, GC, et al. Natural course of peripartum cardiomyopathy. *Circulation* 44:1053–1061, 1971.
89. Burch, GE, Giles, TD, Tsui, C-Y. Postpartal cardiomyopathy. *Cardiovasc Clin* 4:270–282, 1972.
90. Burch, GE, McDonald, CD, Walsh, JJ. The effect of prolonged bed rest on postpartal cardiomyopathy. *Am Heart J* 81:186–201, 1971.
91. Melvin, KR, Richardson, PJ, Olsen, EGJ, et al. Peripartum cardiomyopathy due to myocarditis. *N Engl J Med* 307:731–734, 1982.
92. Hull, E, Hidden, E. Postpartal heart failure. *South Med J* 31:265–270, 1938.
93. Julian, DG, Szekely, P. Peripartum cardiomyopathy. *Prog Cardiovasc Dis* 27:223–240, 1985.
94. Walsh, JJ, Burch, GE, Black, WC, et al. Idiopathic myocardiopathy of the puerperium (postpartal heart disease). *Circulation* 32:19–31, 1965.
95. Ueland, K. Cardiac Diseases. In RK Creasy, R Resnik (eds), *Maternal-Fetal Medicine* (2nd ed). Philadelphia: Saunders, 1989. P 755.
96. Camann, W, Goldman, G, Johnson, M, et al. Cesarean delivery of a patient with a transplanted heart. *Anesthesiology* 71:618–620, 1989.
97. Brown, AK, Doukas, N, Riding, WD, et al. Cardiomyopathy and pregnancy. *Br Heart J* 29:387–393, 1967.
98. Turner, GM, Oakley, CM, Dixon, HG. Management of pregnancy complicated by hypertrophic obstructive cardiomyopathy. *Br Med J* 4:281–284, 1968.
99. Boccio, RV, Chung, IH, Harrison, DM. Anesthetic management of cesarean section in a patient with idiopathic hypertrophic subaortic stenosis. *Anesthesiology* 65:663–665, 1986.
100. Sullivan, JM, Ramanathan, KB. Management of medical problems in pregnancy—severe cardiac disease. *N Engl J Med* 313:304–309, 1985.
101. Hankins, GD, Wendel, GD. Myocardial infarction during pregnancy: A review. *Obstet Gynecol* 65: 139–146, 1985.
102. Kates, RA. Antianginal Drug Therapy. In JA Kaplan (ed), *Cardiac Anesthesia* (2nd ed). Orlando, FL: Grune & Stratton, 1987. P 455.
103. Goldman, ME, Meller, J. Coronary Artery Disease in Pregnancy. In U Elkayam, N Gleicher (eds), *Cardiac Problems in Pregnancy* (2nd ed). New York: Alan R. Liss, 1990. Pp 153–165.
104. Kuida, H. Primary and Secondary Pulmonary Hypertension: Pathophysiology, recognition, and treatment. In JW Hurst (ed), *The Heart* (2nd ed). New York: McGraw-Hill, 1990. Pp 1191–1219.
105. Wagenvoort, CA, Wagenvoort, N. Primary pulmonary hypertension: A pathologic study of the lung vessels in 156 clinically diagnosed cases. *Circulation* 42:1163–1184, 1970.
106. Ross, RS. Right ventricular hypertension as a cause of precordial pain. *Am Heart J* 61:134–135, 1961.
107. Elkayam, U, Gleicher, N. Primary Pulmonary Hypertension and Pregnancy. In U Elkayam, N Gleicher (eds), *Cardiac Problems in Pregnancy* (2nd ed). New York: Alan R. Liss, 1990. Pp 189–197.
108. Sorenson, BM, Korshin, JD, Fernandes, A, et al. The use of epidural analgesia for delivery in a patient with pulmonary hypertension. *Acta Anaesthesiol Scand* 26:180–182, 1982.
109. Robinson, DE, Leicht, CH. Epidural analgesia with low-dose bupivacaine and fentanyl for labor and delivery in a parturient with severe pulmonary hypertension. *Anesthesiology* 68:285–288, 1988.
110. Abboud, TK, Raya, J, Noueihed, R. Intrathecal morphine for relief of labor pain in a parturient with severe pulmonary hypertension. *Anesthesiology* 59:477–479, 1983.
111. Millar, WL. Other Hereditary Disorders. In J Katz, JL Benumof, LB Kadis (eds), *Anesthesia and Uncommon Diseases* (3rd ed). Philadelphia: Saunders, 1990. Pp 144–145.

112. Elkayam, U, Rose, J, Jamison, M. Vascular Aneurysms and Dissections in Pregnancy. In U Elkayam, N Gleicher (eds), *Cardiac Problems in Pregnancy* (2nd ed). New York: Alan R. Liss, 1990. Pp 215–229.
113. Rao, TL, El-Etr, AA. Anticoagulation following placement of epidural and subarachnoid catheters. An evaluation of neurologic sequelae. *Anesthesiology* 55:618–620, 1981.
114. Vetter, VL. What every pediatrician needs to know about cardiac arrhythmias in children who have had cardiac surgery. *Pediatr Ann* 20:378–385, 1991.

15
The Patient with Systemic Disease Affecting the Cardiovascular System

SHELDON GOLDSTEIN
MICHAEL S. TARAGIN

The presence of cardiac disease in patients with medical disorders adds an extra element of concern when anesthetizing these patients. Knowledge of the cardiac problems associated with particular systemic medical diseases will help the anesthesiologist focus attention where necessary. Dividing these concerns into categories will help the anesthesiologist formulate an appropriate anesthetic plan. A suggested division of cardiovascular problems is listed in Table 15-1.

The purpose of our discussion is to review the relationship of these problems to the associated systemic disease and the effects on cardiovascular function. A detailed discussion of anesthetic management of patients with all of these diseases is beyond the scope of this chapter. However, we discuss hemodynamic goals and the cardiovascular considerations for the various disease states as well as some detailed anesthetic management where necessary. To avoid repetition the reader may be referred to other chapters where anesthetic management of particular problems is discussed in greater detail (e.g., pericardial disease). Although our focus is on patients undergoing noncardiac surgery, much of the research in the literature has been performed on patients undergoing cardiac surgery. While the situations may not be synonymous, we frequently refer to the cardiac anesthesia literature for the information it affords.

PREOPERATIVE TESTING

Preoperative testing for patients with systemic diseases includes the entire range of cardiovascular studies, performed as indicated. We discuss them here briefly, as they have been reviewed in depth in Chap. 5. Preoperative evaluation of contractility is indicated in patients with signs and/or symptoms of decreased left ventricular function (LVF), regardless of the etiology. Most frequently this will consist of echocardiographic or multigated radionuclide measurement of ejection fraction. In patients with a history consistent with increasing ischemia, electrocardiographic or thallium stress testing should probably be performed preoperatively if at all possible. Some patients are unable to achieve their predicted maximum heart rate due to fatigue, shortness of breath, or a physical handicap such as arthritis. Dipyridamole thallium testing may be appropriate in such patients. Gerson and associates [1] have suggested that the inability to increase heart rate above 90 beats per minute after 2 minutes of supine bicycle exercise predicts perioperative myocardial infarction with an 80 percent sensitivity [1]. Although this test has a specificity of only 53 percent, the increased incidence of perioperative ischemic events in those who are unable to exercise to a heart rate greater than 90 beats per minute suggests that these patients should receive

Table 15-1. Cardiovascular abnormalities associated with systemic diseases

Abnormal conduction
Abnormal contractility
Abnormal loading conditions
Abnormalities of the coronary arteries
Abnormalities of the cardiac valves
Abnormalities of the myocardium
Abnormalities of the right ventricle
Abnormalities of the left ventricle
Abnormalities of the pericardium
Abnormalities of the pulmonary circulation
Abnormalities of the autonomic nervous system
Abnormalities of metabolism that affect the cardiovascular system (e.g., acidosis, hyperglycemia, hypokalemia, etc.)

further preoperative evaluation. Systolic hypotension (a decrease ≥10 torr), unrelated to hypovolemia or medication, an increase in diastolic pressure greater than 110 torr, and an inability to exercise for longer than 3 minutes are also associated with an increased risk of severe coronary disease [2].

While ejection fraction is not a gold standard, it does offer useful information. Certainly, patients with an ejection fraction of less than 40 percent are at an increased perioperative risk and should be monitored appropriately, bearing in mind the surgical procedure. However, in patients with a history strongly suggestive of ischemia we consider invasive monitoring even with a normal ejection fraction, as intraoperative ischemia can result in rapid deterioration of left ventricular function. For patients with a history and physical examination consistent with severe ischemia, coronary angiography may be the preferred route, as coronary artery bypass grafting or coronary angioplasty may be chosen to precede the scheduled surgical procedure.

Patients with cardiomegaly and a pericardial friction rub should have preoperative echocardiography to assess the size of the effusion and its effects on right and left ventricular function. Chronic pericardial effusions may occur in association with a number of systemic diseases, including chronic renal failure, myxedema, systemic lupus erythematosus, rheumatoid arthritis, and severe chronic anemia (see Chap. 8).

Patients with ventricular ectopy identified on preoperative ECG frequently have Holter monitoring performed before elective surgery; in patients with malignant arrhythmias, however, we believe it is important to know left ventricular function as well. Certainly, if they have decreased exercise tolerance, at minimum an ejection fraction should be measured, as ectopy in patients with decreased ventricular function is associated with an increased incidence of adverse cardiovascular events [3-6].

Though many signs and symptoms may identify the presence of ischemic heart disease, some patients manifest silent ischemia, as detected by preoperative Holter monitoring. Similarly, some patients with decreased LVF exert themselves less, either intentionally or without even realizing it. Some attribute their decreased exercise tolerance to old age or other diseases such as arthritis. It is therefore important to take a careful history to document the patient's exercise tolerance. If it has decreased, one should seek subtle signs and symptoms of congestive heart failure (CHF), as noted in Table 15-2.

Patients with poor ventricular function should probably be monitored with a pulmonary artery (PA) catheter for all but minor surgical procedures. Although a full preoperative workup may define the functional state of the patient's heart, time does not always allow this before urgent surgery. For patients in whom vital signs, history, or physical or laboratory studies do not clarify what seems to be poor cardiac function, we prefer to place a PA catheter before the induction. If the history and physical examination indicate severe ventricular

Table 15-2. Subtle signs and symptoms of congestive heart failure

Fatigue
Irritability
Right upper quadrant discomfort
Nocturnal cough
Insomnia
Nocturia
Unexplained tachycardia
Unexplained sweating

Source: Adapted from NJ Clark and TH Stanley, Anesthesia for Vascular Surgery. In RD Miller, RF Cucchiara, et al. (eds), *Anesthesia* (3rd ed). New York: Churchill Livingstone, 1990. Pp 1693-1736.

dysfunction, we prefer to admit the patient to the intensive care unit for preoperative placement of a PA catheter and construction of their Frank-Starling curve.

MANAGEMENT OF MEDICAL THERAPY

Many of the disorders discussed are treated with chronic medical therapy. As a general rule we prefer to continue therapy for systemic medical diseases up until the time of surgery. While we may hold off treatment for minor conditions, in order to decrease the number of pills and amount of water swallowed immediately before operation, we certainly continue all medications used to treat cardiovascular disease.

Though case reports have been published documenting bradycardia and hypotension perioperatively in patients receiving antihypertensive therapy, this reflected a lack of understanding of the sympatholytic effects of these agents as well as the decreased anesthetic requirement associated with them [7]. It is currently recommended that all antihypertensive agents be administered the morning of surgery, with the possible exception of diuretics as patients are NPO.

For patients receiving chronic steroid therapy, it has become common practice to administer 100 mg hydrocortisone the night before surgery, 100 mg the morning of surgery, and 100 mg intraoperatively. The dose is then tapered gradually over the next several days. It should be noted that these recommendations were made based on the maximal daily output of the adrenal glands [8]. Work in adrenalectomized monkeys supports the necessity for administration of glucocorticoids to chronically treated patients. Adrenalectomized monkeys who received subphysiologic cortisol replacement were hemodynamically unstable before, during, and after cholecystectomy and had a significantly higher mortality than the control group. They manifested decreased arterial blood pressure, systemic vascular resistance (SVR) index, cardiac index, and left ventricular stroke work index, consistent with decreased contractility and decreased vascular tone. Those who received physiologic replacement did the same as animals that received suprahysiologic doses of cortisol [9], underlining the importance of replacement therapy, but also raising the issue of whether suprahysiologic doses of perioperative glucocorticoids are necessary. While such large doses certainly protect against adrenal atrophy, they may result in significant hyperglycemia, and diabetics may require careful treatment of hyperglycemia for several days. In addition, hyperglycemia may result in decreased responsiveness to inotropic therapy, as subsequent control of glucose with insulin has been shown to improve responsiveness to inotropes [10].

Although we are concerned about suppression of the adrenal axis, this occurrence is actually quite rare. Chernow and associates [11] have reported that perioperative catecholamine levels correspond to the level of surgical stress, and that hormonal levels return to normal within 24 hours of uncomplicated surgery. While catecholamine levels may remain elevated for several days after major surgery, maximal steroid output from the adrenal glands almost never occurs, except perhaps in patients in whom severe hemodynamic instability develops for reasons unrelated to the adrenal axis. Therefore, we administer the patient's usual morning dose of steroid. Then, taking into account the dose and length of time the patient has been receiving steroid therapy as well as the type of surgery, we adjust our dose of intravenous perioperative steroid accordingly. In patients with cardiac disease or hypertension, it may be useful to choose a steroid preparation with minimal sodium-retaining properties. The relative glucocorticoid and mineralocorticoid potencies of various steroid preparations and their relative potencies are listed in Table 15-3.

APPROACH TO THE PATIENT WITH CARDIOVASCULAR MANIFESTATIONS OF SYSTEMIC DISEASE

We find it helpful to categorize patients preoperatively into those who have mild, moderate, or severe cardiac disease. Initially, we review the special conditions inherent to the surgical procedure. We then choose our anesthetic technique and monitors based on the requirements of the procedure

Table 15-3. Glucocorticoid preparations

Commonly used name[a]	Estimated potency (mg)[b] Gluco-corticoid	Mineralo-corticoid
Short acting		
Cortisol	1	1
Cortisone	0.8	0.8
Intermediate acting		
Prednisone	4	0.25
Prednisolone	4	0.25
Methylprednisolone	5	<0.01
Triamcinolone	5	<0.01
Long acting		
Paramethasone	10	<0.01
Betamethasone	25	<0.01
Dexamethasone	30–40	<0.01

[a] The steroids are divided into three groups according to the duration of biologic activity. Short-acting preparations have a biologic half-life of less than 12 hours; long-acting, greater than 48 hours; and intermediate, between 12 and 36 hours. Triamcinolone has the longest half-life of the intermediate-acting preparations.
[b] Relative milligram comparisons with cortisol, setting the glucocorticoid and mineralocorticoid properties of cortisol as 1. Sodium retention is insignificant in usual doses employed of methylprednisolone, triamcinolone, paramethasone, betamethasone, and dexamethasone.
Source: Reproduced with permission of McGraw-Hill, Inc. From GH Williams and RG Dluhy, Diseases of the Adrenal Cortex. In JD Wilson, E Braunwald, et al. (eds), *Harrison's Principles of Internal Medicine* (12th ed). New York: McGraw-Hill, 1991. P 1733.

and the pathophysiology of the patient's particular abnormalities. For a patient who is to undergo a near total pancreatectomy who is 60 years old but has no cardiovascular disease, we frequently place a PA catheter for management of fluids intraoperatively as well as in the postoperative period. Some would place only a central venous catheter. Certainly, if a patient with moderate mitral stenosis and a dilated cardiomyopathy secondary to alcoholism were to undergo the same procedure, the combination of the procedure and the patient's medical problems would influence us to place a PA catheter even if the patient were but 40 years of age. Whether to place monitors before induction or afterward is dependent on the patient's cardiovascular status and the likelihood of hemodynamic instability during induction. Probably all patients with mild disease can have their monitors placed after the induction, especially because most patients in this category will be receiving invasive monitors solely because of the procedure, not the severity of their underlying disease. Most patients with moderate disease states can have their invasive lines safely placed after the induction of anesthesia, whereas most patients with severe underlying disease should have invasive monitoring placed before induction.

Many patients who present for noncardiac surgery have cardiac problems secondary to systemic diseases. It is important to appreciate these processes and the impact they have on the cardiovascular system and its response to anesthetics. Additionally, patients may have concomitant coronary or valvular disease. The preoperative history and physical examination will identify those patients at increased risk and guide appropriate evaluation. For emergency procedures, when there is no time for further studies, the history and physical examination can be used as a basis for choosing appropriate anesthetic management. Classifying patients as having mild, moderate, or severe disease will make the decision process regarding monitor placement a more objective one. It is important to remember that the clinical status of the patient may change intraoperatively or in the recovery room and if so additional monitors or therapy, or both, may be appropriate.

Monitoring

Although it has been difficult to show that placement of a PA catheter improves outcome, most agree that patients with severe cardiac disease often warrant such monitoring. We believe patients do better with a PA catheter when it is used appropriately. This entails measurement of filling pressures, determination of cardiac indices, and deriving a complete profile of hemodynamic parameters. Mixed venous oxygenation can be used to calculate shunt fraction, and catheters are now available that calculate right ventricular ejection fraction (RVEF). If therapy results in an increase in oxygen consumption, it is likely that additional circulatory beds have been opened that perfuse relatively hypoxic tissues, which then extract more oxygen. Indeed, decreased mixed venous oxygen saturation results in a debt that must be repaid in order for the patient to survive [12]. This suggests that use of the PA catheter to calculate and optimize oxygen consumption helps direct appropriate therapy in the critical care setting, thereby leading to improved outcome.

Complications from the use of PA catheters are uncommon and they tend not to be life threatening [13] (see Chap. 4). Regrettably, it has been shown that many physicians may not use the PA catheter as well as they should [14] and this may account for the difficulty in proving better outcome with its use.

Transesophageal echocardiography (TEE) is uniquely suited as a valuable monitor of cardiovascular function in the operating room. While many believe that TEE is a valuable monitor for ischemia, London and associates [15] reported a low incidence of new systolic wall motion abnormalities and found that most occurred transiently and were not specifically associated with ischemic changes on the electrocardiogram or with postoperative infarction. Nevertheless, many believe that TEE can detect ischemia before the ECG. It is also useful to monitor patients for abnormalities of ventricular contraction and atrioventricular (AV) valve function. A particularly beneficial use for TEE is in patients with abnormal compliance in whom the pulmonary capillary wedge pressure (PCWP) may not accurately reflect left ventricular end diastolic volume. This can be confirmed when a PCWP of 20 or 22 mm Hg is associated with decreased filling of the left ventricle as seen on transesophageal echocardiography. In the absence of TEE, such patients would frequently be started on inotropes when volume would have solved the problem, thereby unnecessarily increasing myocardial oxygen consumption, and possibly resulting in ischemia.

SPECIFIC DISEASE STATES

Hypertension

Epidemiology

Hypertension is a multisystem disease that may produce end-organ damage involving the heart, vasculature, kidneys, and brain. Since patients are frequently asymptomatic, the disorder may manifest itself when end-organ damage appears. The level of end-organ damage may help to measure the severity of the disease in a given patient. Additionally, blood pressure itself may be indicative of outcome. A blood pressure of less than 110/70 mm Hg is associated with a long life span, while blood pressure greater than 160/95 mm Hg is associated with an increased risk of death due to cardiovascular, cerebrovascular, and kidney disease [16].

Primary or essential hypertension is that with no known etiology and accounts for greater than 90 percent of cases of hypertension in the United States. Mild hypertension is frequently defined as a diastolic blood pressure between 90 and 104 mm Hg, moderate hypertension as a diastolic pressure between 105 and 114, and severe hypertension as a diastolic pressure greater than 115. Occasionally, patients who present for surgery with a minimal elevation of blood pressure, such as 145/88 mm Hg, will behave perioperatively in a manner similar to that of known hypertensives. This is referred to as labile hypertension [17]. Since an acute elevation of blood pressure may occur secondary to stress in an otherwise normal patient, such as that associated with visiting a doctor's office or being admitted to a hospital, blood pressure should be checked several times to ensure the accuracy of the reading.

Pathophysiology

The pathophysiology of hypertension may be broken down into two main areas of concern, cardiac effects and vascular effects. Left ventricular hypertrophy (LVH) is the response of the myocardium to maintain cardiac output against the increased resistance to ejection [18]. Increased production of the V3 form of myosin results in a slower, more sustained contraction that requires less energy [19]. However, hypertrophy decreases the ability of the ventricle to relax and therefore impairs diastolic filling, resulting in a decreased ventricular volume for any given pressure [20]. Although this maintains cardiac output against the increased afterload, the trade-off is that any decrease of filling pressures such as that due to hypovolemia or a dysrhythmia may produce significant hypotension and decreased cardiac output. The presence of LVH is even more damaging in that it increases myocardial oxygen demand and decreases supply. The geometric changes in the ventricle as well as histologic abnormalities may result in stiffening of the ventricle with classic signs and symptoms of diastolic dysfunction. These include signs and symptoms of congestive failure in patients with an ejection fraction documented to be normal (≥45%). Myocardial oxygen demand is increased due to the increased muscle mass, and the possible subsequent ischemia may aggravate the already present diastolic dysfunction [21]. Myocardial oxygen supply may be endangered as well because in order to maintain normal coronary blood flow in the presence of LVH intramyocardial resistance vessels remain vasodilated, particularly in the subendocardium [22, 23]. Since these vessels cannot increase their diameter significantly, myocardial ischemia, especially subendocardial, may occur even in the absence of stenoses of the coronary arteries. There also exist a group of hypertensive patients with ischemia in the absence of epicardial coronary disease that may be due to an abnormally high resistance of the coronary microvasculature [24].

With time hypertension compromises the ability of the heart to supply the tissues because decreased compliance compromises appropriate filling. Chronic exposure of the heart to excessive work such as that caused by hypertension eventually decreases the ability of the heart to contract, thus compromising systolic function and eventually leading to CHF [25, 26]. The right ventricle as well as the left has been shown to manifest abnormal diastolic function, which is not surprising considering the shared septum. This may manifest as increased right atrial and right ventricular (RV) diastolic pressures, associated with a lower RV ejection fraction [27]. In addition to the direct cardiac effects of hypertension, hypertrophy of vascular smooth muscle increases the response to vasomotor stimuli, causing vascular hyperreactivity [28]. Patients with significant diastolic hypertension manifest transcapillary shift of salt, water, and albumin into the interstitial compartment [29, 30]. The result of these changes in circulating volume is that they contribute to the large fluctuations in blood pressure in the perioperative period. Besides being vasoconstricted and chronically volume depleted due to their disease process, many hypertensive patients are receiving diuretic therapy, although there has been a recent movement away from diuretics and increasing usage of β-blockers, calcium channel blockers, and arterial dilators. Chronic antihypertensive therapy, with the possible exception of thiazide diuretics and propranolol, is important because it promotes repletion of the intravascular volume [28].

Clinical Manifestations

While hypertension may cause symptoms such as headache or neurologic changes, this is uncommon and tends to happen only when the elevation in blood pressure is severe. Most symptoms in the hypertensive patient are those related to end-organ damage, such as dyspnea due to congestive failure, fluid retention due to end-stage renal disease, deteriorating vision due to retinopathy, or mental status changes due to cerebrovascular disease. Most patients with this extent of end-organ damage will have been diagnosed as hypertensive before contact with the anesthesiologist.

Similarly, the physical findings related to hypertension are essentially those related to end-organ damage. The exception, of course, is the measurement of elevated blood pressure itself. Some of the cardiovascular effects of hypertension are listed in Table 15-4.

The history may reveal dyspnea, on exertion, at rest, or after a period of recumbency. These complaints are often attributable to left ventricular dysfunction. Hypertension predisposes to coronary artery disease, and, therefore, patients may complain of chest or upper-extremity pain with exertion, or even at rest. The sudden tearing pain associated with aneurysmal dissection is classic and ominous.

Physical findings related to the cardiovascular system may include an exaggerated precordial apical impulse, an S_4 gallop indicating decreased left ventricular compliance, or an S_3 gallop indicating left ventricular failure. Hypertrophy of the myocardium may distort the mitral valve apparatus, producing a systolic murmur heard best at the apex. The history and physical examination are particu-

Table 15-4. Cardiac effects of systemic hypertension

Myocardium: left ventricular hypertrophy
Coronary arteries: increased risk of atherosclerosis
Left ventricle: decreased compliance
Congestive heart failure
Myocardial infarction and sudden death
Contributes to ruptured aortic aneurysm

larly important to evaluate risk because clinical signs of uncompensated heart failure may be better predictors of postoperative cardiac deaths than even a prior myocardial infarction [31]. Orthopnea, dyspnea due to heart disease, peripheral edema, rales, pulmonary edema, and cardiomegaly have all been reported to be associated by themselves with an increased risk of cardiac deaths, and when none of these signs or symptoms were present a history of heart failure was not associated with a greater risk of cardiac complications [32].

Patients with a history of heart failure who do not have an S_3 gallop or jugular venous distention have an incidence of fatal complications of about 5 percent, even if they manifest orthopnea, rales, cardiomegaly, or a history of CHF. However, patients undergoing vascular or major aortic surgery who have a left ventricular ejection fraction (LVEF) of 35 percent or less do have an increased incidence of perioperative cardiac morbidity, even if signs of decompensated heart failure are not present. Signs and symptoms of early heart failure may be subtle (see Table 15-2) and patients who exhibit them should probably be studied to determine ejection fraction, either by echocardiography or radionuclide ventriculography.

The physical examination may reveal signs of LVH such as a prominent or laterally displaced point of maximal impulse (PMI). The chest x-ray may reveal cardiomegaly (Fig. 15-1). If a patient has deteriorated to the point of congestive failure, pulmonary vascular redistribution or pleural effusions may be present. Still, no signs on the chest x-ray are specific for hypertension. Many ECG findings are associated with hypertension, but none is pathognomonic. Criteria of LVH may be met, indicating the effort of the heart to maintain ejection against an increased afterload. The electrocardiogram may show a pattern of LVH with strain (Fig. 15-2). Strain pattern refers to the development of ST segment and T- and U-wave abnormalities. Detection of LVH is important because

Fig. 15-1. Chest x-ray showing cardiomegaly and pleural effusions in a patient with congestive heart failure.

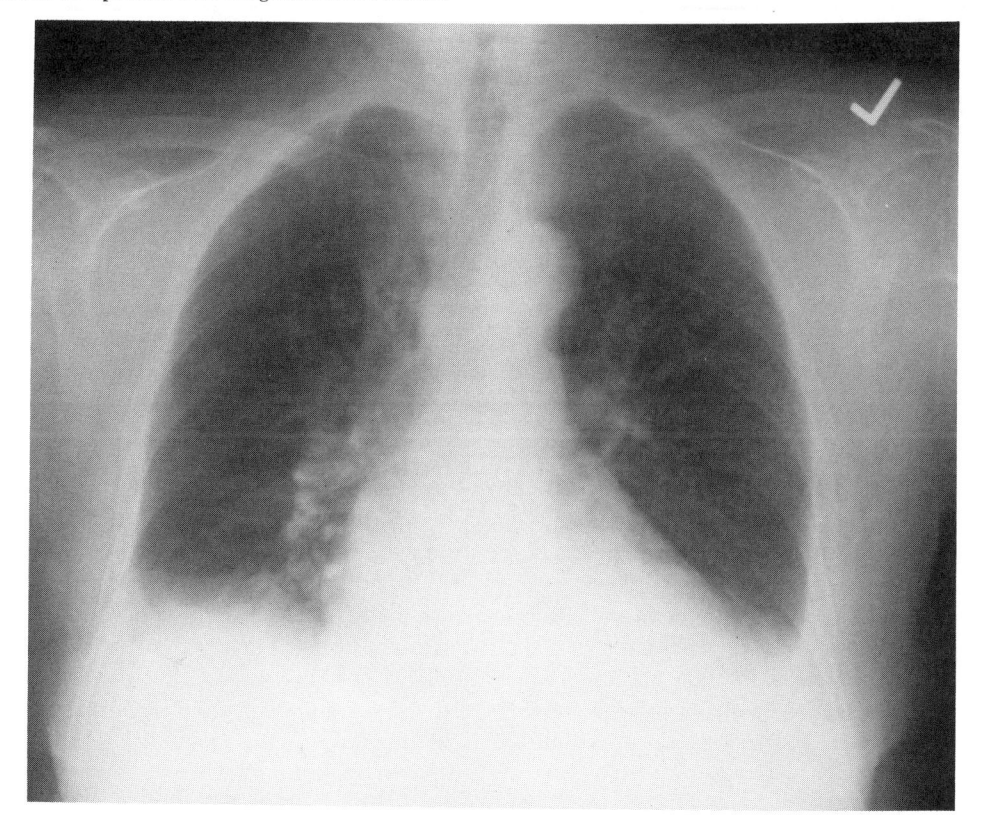

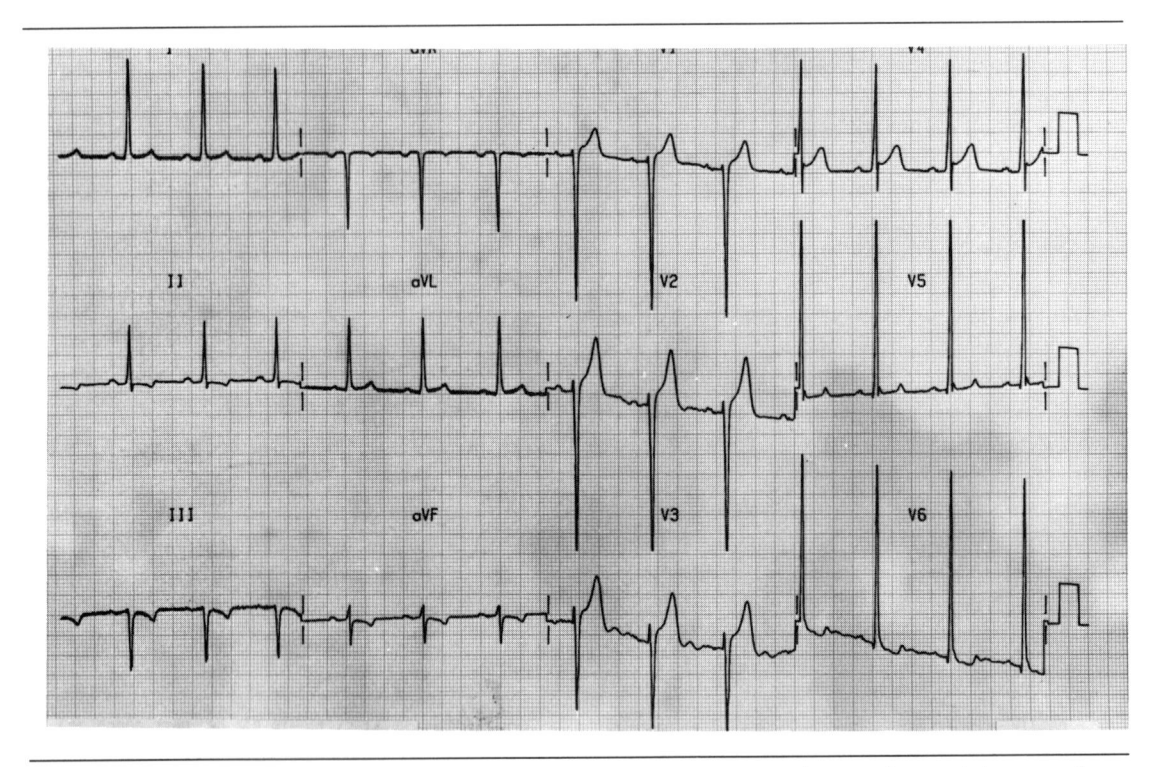

Fig. 15-2. Electrocardiogram showing left ventricular hypertrophy with strain pattern.

patients with this abnormality have a higher incidence of complex ventricular ectopy [33] and morbid cardiovascular events [34]. Since LVH is most easily detected by echocardiography [35], patients with hypertension who have not been studied echocardiographically should be carefully evaluated preoperatively to detect other signs of organ involvement that would indicate the presence of significant chronic hypertension. T-wave changes may also develop as a result of digitalis effect or hypokalemia secondary to diuretics. ST and T-wave changes consistent with ischemia may be present. The presence of premature ventricular contractions may reflect underlying ischemia. Conduction disturbances that may be present include first-degree heart block, unifascicular block, or bifascicular block.

Cardiac arrhythmias are a potentially dangerous problem during the perioperative period. Although hypertension does not predispose to specific arrhythmias, hypertensive patients often manifest many of the risk factors for arrhythmias (Table 15-5).

Table 15-5. Risk factors for arrhythmias

Hypertension
Myocardial ischemia
Congestive heart failure
Blood gas abnormalities
Electrolyte disturbances

Source: Adapted from RL Katz and JT Bigger, Cardiac arrhythmias during anesthesia and operation. Anesthesiology 33:193, 1970.

Hypertensive patients are often on diuretics. Though this may lead to hypokalemia, it may not be a risk factor for perioperative arrhythmias, except in patients receiving digitalis therapy [36]. Though intravenous potassium can be administered at rates up to 0.5 mEq/kg/hr with ECG monitoring, this may be associated with life-threatening arrhythmias and cardiac arrest during subsequent anesthesia [37, 38]. Apparently, it is the rate of change in potassium level that may increase risk.

It is therefore preferable for potassium repletion to proceed orally over several days before surgery whenever possible.

If cardiac function deteriorates to the point of active congestive failure, delivery of oxygen to the tissues is significantly impaired [26]. These patients may approach a 15 to 20 percent incidence of cardiac complications resulting in death [28]. Acute elevations of blood pressure, as occur in poorly controlled hypertensive patients, may acutely compromise cardiac function, resulting in the back-up of blood into the pulmonary circulation and compression of small airways [39]. Patients who are in severe congestive failure probably should not be operated on at that time, for this may be particularly dangerous, but if they must undergo operation for emergent procedures they may require awake intubation, as any period of apnea may result in severe hypoxemia and possibly cardiac arrest. Intraoperative CHF may be particularly dangerous as the decreased cardiac output may rapidly deepen the anesthetic level.

Anesthetic Concerns

Preoperative measurement of blood pressure identifies those patients at increased risk for anesthesia and surgery. While there are no fixed rules, we prefer not to begin an anesthetic if the systolic pressure is greater than 200 torr or the diastolic pressure is greater than 110 torr. However, these numbers are only guidelines, as we certainly would proceed with emergency surgery with appropriate monitoring.

It is preferable for blood pressure to be well controlled before elective surgery. Complications of hypertension affecting the cardiovascular, renal, and central nervous systems, and associated deaths, have been lessened by chronic antihypertensive therapy in a group of patients with mild to moderate hypertension [40]. It has even been shown to be beneficial to treat patients with a diastolic pressure of 90 to 104 mm Hg [41]. Berglund and associates [42] documented a decrease in deaths due to myocardial infarction in patients treated for mild and moderate hypertension. Treatment of hypertension may not only attenuate hypertrophy of the heart but may alleviate abnormalities of autonomic function as well [43].

Fluctuation in hemodynamic parameters is common in uncontrolled hypertensive patients during the perioperative period. Prys-Roberts and associates [44] reported that patients with elevated preoperative blood pressure manifested greater falls in blood pressure and SVR than did patients who were normotensive and receiving chronic antihypertensive therapy, whether or not patients in the elevated blood pressure group were being treated. The group with higher starting blood pressures also had more frequent hypotensive episodes associated with ECG changes consistent with subendocardial ischemia. Mauney and colleagues [45] reported an increased incidence of postoperative infarction and death in hypertensive patients. Significant fluctuation of vital signs may itself increase the risk of ischemia [45–47] and even vital signs that are unchanging may predispose to ischemia if significant tachycardia, hypotension, or hypertension is present. Indeed, Stone and coworkers [48] reported that one oral dose of a β-blocker preoperatively can significantly decrease the incidence of perioperative myocardial ischemia. However, such therapy does not permit time for restoration of intravascular volume, and since large fluctuations of heart rate and blood pressure may increase morbidity and mortality [44, 45, 49–51] it is preferable to control hypertension preoperatively. Additionally, positive pressure ventilation aggravates the tendency toward hypotension even further in the group with higher baseline pressures, because of large decreases in stroke volume and cardiac output [52]. Patients who are hypertensive are also more likely to develop large blood pressure reductions after the administration of lumbar or thoracic epidural blockade, whether or not it is combined with general anesthesia [53].

Despite the tendency for treated hypertensive patients to have fewer and less significant episodes of hypotension with either general or regional anesthesia than their uncontrolled counterparts, they may be just as likely to develop significant episodes of hypertension in response to laryngoscopy and intubation [49, 54], and preoperative β-blockade does not fully prevent this exaggerated sympathetic response [55].

Management of Blood Pressure in the Perioperative Period

While it is preferable for all patients to arrive in the operating room with normal blood pressure, patients may not be adequately controlled because of poor medical follow-up, poor patient compliance, or unknown secondary forms of hypertension. Additionally, the use of estrogen-containing contraceptives or sympathomimetics found in over-the-counter medications may prevent adequate control. When administering anesthesia to hypertensive patients, it is important to evaluate them preoperatively for control of blood pressure as well as volume status. Orthostatic pulse and blood pressure changes may not adequately reflect their state of hydration, as many will be receiving β-blockers or have autonomic dysfunction. Still, these maneuvers may be useful. It may be helpful to review the ratio of blood urea nitrogen (BUN)–creatinine, as a ratio greater than 20:1 is consistent with dehydration. A significant change in recent laboratory values (if available) may confirm the diagnosis of dehydration, bearing in mind that if the patient's condition prevents him or her from eating, the BUN may be decreased irrespective of the state of hydration, while gastrointestinal bleeding will increase BUN.

Roizen [2] has suggested that recording vital signs several times preoperatively offers safe guidelines within which to control vital signs intraoperatively. While this approach has not been formally studied, it does offer the benefit of bringing to the operating room blood pressure and heart rates that the patient has tolerated without adverse effect during the preoperative period. Our only concern with this approach is that silent myocardial ischemia is not an uncommon finding in patients undergoing 24-hour preoperative Holter monitoring. Perhaps a study recording vital signs during preoperative Holter monitoring will help us determine whether we need to control blood pressure and heart rate at a level better than the patient's inherent range.

If patients present to the operating room with elevated pressure but a diastolic pressure less than 110 mm Hg, it is usually safe to proceed. We are careful to treat these patients with antihypertensive agents and not to simply "deepen" the anesthesia. Such a practice may result in significant myocardial depression, especially when inhalational agents are used to control blood pressure. Also of concern is the increase in blood pressure that is likely to occur when the inhalation anesthetic is removed and the patient awakens in pain. Our primary goal when choosing an antihypertensive agent is control of blood pressure that will continue into the postoperative period. We prefer diastolic blood pressure to be less than 90 torr before the induction of anesthesia, while morbidity or mortality is probably not increased with diastolic pressure up to 110 torr. These patients may have enough intraoperative fluctuation of pressure to require placement of an arterial line. We choose our antihypertensive agent based on the hemodynamics preferred for that particular patient's cardiac disease.

Although treatment of hypertension frequently entails decreasing an elevated SVR, the only short-acting α-blocker available, phentolamine, produces tachycardia and occasionally tachyphylaxis because of its ability to block the α_2 receptor. The appropriate treatment of hypertension preoperatively, either a β-blocker [56] or clonidine [57–59], has been shown to decrease intraoperative blood pressure fluctuations. If hypertension is first noted the night before surgery or on a preadmission visit, a calcium channel blocker such as nifedipine is another good choice. Sublingual nifedipine has been reported in a small study to be efficacious for the treatment of moderately severe hypertension in elderly patients undergoing eye surgery [60]. Since withdrawal of many of the available antihypertensive agents may lead to rebound hypertension, we prefer to continue treatment into the postoperative period and ask our medical colleagues to adjust the antihypertensive medications before discharge, or at outpatient follow-up examination.

When intravenous agents are required, we often use nitroglycerin as our first choice of antihypertensive in the patient with known coronary disease. However, since it is predominantly a venodilator, a second agent is often required. We prefer labetalol for its combined alpha and beta effects as well as its duration of several hours. If these agents are not effective, we use a systemic arterial dilator, either nitroprusside for a short duration or hydralazine for a long duration of action. Recently, esmolol has been used for perioperative blood pressure control, with good results [61, 62]. Its short duration of action makes it particularly suitable in unstable situations in which it is unclear how much β-blockade a given patient can tolerate. Esmolol can be used as an infusion and titrated to effect. Since many antihypertensive agents are available, we choose therapy for a given patient based on several concerns, listed in Table 15-6. Consideration should be given to whether the patient has the syndrome of ventricular diastolic dysfunction. If so, nitrates, β-blockers, and calcium channel blockers are preferable to digitalis and especially arterial dilators, which may result in precipitous hypotension [21]. Table 15-7 presents guidelines that can be used in the perioperative management of the hypertensive patient.

Table 15-6. Considerations for choosing an antihypertensive agent

Severity of blood pressure elevation
Preferred duration of action
Ability of patient's myocardium to tolerate β-blockade
Preference for decreased heart rate with coronary artery disease
Preference for decreased heart rate with stenotic valvular lesions
Preference for increased heart rate with regurgitant valvular lesions
Current cardiac output and SVR
History of supraventricular tachycardia
History of bradycardia or sinus node dysfunction
History of conduction defects (e.g., Wolff-Parkinson-White syndrome)

Table 15-7. Guidelines for anesthetic management of the hypertensive patient

Ensure adequate preoperative blood pressure control whenever possible
Patients should receive all preoperative antihypertensive agents with the possible exception of diuretics
Measure urine output during all but short procedures
Consider placement of an arterial pressure monitoring line
Consider placement of a central venous pressure monitoring line
In poorly controlled patients, consider placement of a pulmonary artery catheter to construct hemodynamic profiles at frequent intervals
Choose an anesthetic technique that will afford good control of blood pressure and heart rate
Choose an anesthetic that has minimal effects on contractility for patients with decreased ventricular function
Use regional anesthesia with caution since the patient may be hypovolemic
Have pharmacologic means available to adjust heart rate and blood pressure changes when appropriate doses of anesthetic agents are not sufficient to do so
Continue to monitor and treat hypertension into the postoperative period

Anesthetic Management of the Hypertensive Patient with Cardiac Disease

The choice of anesthetic for the hypertensive patient with cardiac disease will be influenced by the type of cardiac disease. The main concerns are the increased risk of ischemia and the possibility that decreased compliance will result in abnormally elevated filling pressures in the face of decreased systemic perfusion. It is also preferable to prevent labile blood pressure. A narcotic base is a good starting point, as this will offer some blunting of the sympathetic response to noxious stimuli as well as some pain relief in the immediate postoperative period. Inhalational anesthesia can be titrated to blood pressure for minute-to-minute control, as well as to produce an amnestic effect. Nitrous oxide or intravenous benzodiazepines can also be used, although they may worsen ventricular function, especially if given in addition to an inhalation agent. Although halothane is the most cardiac depressant of the three inhalation agents, it can be used in patients with good ventricular function, as it slows the heart rate and decreases myocardial oxygen demand. Enflurane and isoflurane also have myocardial depressant effects but are more likely to cause tachycardia. Isoflurane in particular may result in significant reflex tachycardia because of the decrease in SVR. Additionally, it may produce coronary steal. Droperidol may be a useful anesthetic adjunct due to its α-adrenergic blocking properties. Ketamine should probably be avoided in these patients since it is likely to cause hypertension tachycardia and is also a myocardial depressant. The newer nondepolarizing agents may be preferable to pancuronium, which may precipitate tachycardia as a result of its vagolytic properties. Arrhythmogenic effects of the various anesthetics should be considered in patients known to have dysrhythmias. Partial pressure of carbon dioxide should be maintained in the normal range to prevent iatrogenic arrhythmias. The reader is referred to Chaps. 2 and 3 for a more complete discussion of the cardiovascular effects of the various anesthetic agents.

More important than the particular agent chosen is the maintenance of the balance between myocardial oxygen supply and demand. Monitoring urine output will help assess tissue perfusion. The presence of decreased urine output in the face of increased central venous or pulmonary capillary wedge pressure should raise the possibility of decreased ventricular compliance. Nitroglycerin or other vasodilators can be used to decrease filling pressures when administered to maintain tissue perfusion.

Regional anesthesia can be used in these patients if they are not severely hypovolemic. Epidural blockade may be preferable since the sympathetic blockade has a slower onset. If there is doubt about the patient's volume status and a regional anesthetic is preferred, central monitoring can be placed before administration of the block. Postoperative use of the epidural catheter can provide excellent pain relief and will help prevent hypertension secondary to incisional pain.

Summary

The combination of direct cardiac effects and vascular effects of hypertension results in patients who tend to be hypovolemic and vasoconstricted. They may have decreased ventricular compliance underscoring their requirement for adequate filling volumes. Loss of sinus rhythm may also compromise filling pressures. With time systolic function may be decreased. Hypertrophy of the myocardium may increase the myocardial oxygen demand. If the hypertension is long-standing, the patient may have coronary artery disease or poor left ventricular function. All of these considerations must be taken into account when choosing an anesthetic for the hypertensive patient. It is important to determine the severity and form of cardiac disease in the particular patient. With this knowledge an appropriate anesthetic can be chosen. We have a preference for a narcotic-based technique, with an inhalational agent superimposed. The narcotic provides some blunting of the hemodynamic response to stress, while the inhalational anesthetic allows titration of the agent to blood pressure. However, there is no best anesthetic agent for any particular patient.

As long as the anesthesiologist maintains hemodynamic parameters appropriately and chooses the anesthetic based on the functional status of the patient's cardiovascular system, most of these patients will have a good outcome. Finally, knowledge and clinical use of antihypertensive agents in the operating suite should become a routine part of modern anesthetic care.

Diabetes Mellitus

Epidemiology

Diabetes mellitus affects between 1 and 2 percent of the population. It has numerous end-organ effects, mediated via damage to blood vessels, nerves, and the basement membrane. Organs frequently involved include the eyes, kidneys, and heart. The diagnosis is made by a fasting plasma glucose concentration of 140 mg/dl or greater on at least two occasions. Alternatively, plasma glucose greater than or equal to 200 mg/dl at 2 hours and on one other sample within 2 hours of the ingestion of 75 gm glucose confirms the diagnosis [63]. Although the classification of type I and type II diabetes discerns those patients who require insulin from those who do not, this division is not always distinct. While type I diabetics require insulin to prevent ketoacidosis, type II diabetics may with time come to require insulin. Also, ketoacidosis may develop in type II diabetics when under stress, such as that due to surgery, as a result of endogenous release of glucagon and catecholamines. If hyperosmolar coma develops in a type II diabetic, insulin is used to help restore the normal metabolic state. It is therefore preferable to refer to these patients as insulin dependent and non–insulin dependent.

Insulin-dependent patients are usually thin and are genetically susceptible to the disease as determined by HLA antigens. Destruction of islet cells in the pancreas is believed to occur as an autoimmune phenomenon, perhaps triggered by viral infection [63].

Non–insulin-dependent diabetics display abnormal insulin secretion as well as insulin resistance. Most of these patients are overweight. Accumulation of amylin, a 37–amino acid peptide, in the islet cells may contribute to the development of the disease. No HLA pattern has been identified in patients with non–insulin-dependent diabetes mellitus [63].

Studies separating the effects of diabetes from organ dysfunction reveal that diabetics may not be at increased risk perioperatively. The fact that they have a 3 to 5 times increased incidence of perioperative mortality lends support to the importance of cardiac disease in those diabetic patients who experience morbidity or mortality. Though diabetics without heart disease may have no increased risk, diabetics of any age are more likely to have cardiac disease than their nondiabetic peers. This is due to several factors, including hypertension, increased atherosclerosis, small-vessel disease, systolic and diastolic dysfunction, and metabolic effects of diabetes on the cardiovascular system.

Pathophysiology
Diabetics, whether insulin dependent or non–insulin dependent, have an increased incidence of hypertension, variably reported between 29 and 54 percent, and they may lose elasticity of the arterial wall prematurely [64]. Others have reported the incidence of hypertension in diabetics to be as much as twice that in the general population. This contributes to their increased risk for coronary artery disease [65]. Non–insulin dependent diabetics are also at increased risk for the development of hypertension. Hyperinsulinemia present in non–insulin-dependent diabetes mellitus (NIDDM) may increase blood pressure via sodium retention and sympathetic nervous system stimulation [66]. There is a tendency to angiopathy of myocardial vessels as well as a generalized increase in atherosclerosis, which tends to be more widespread and more severe than that in the general population [2]. This tendency may be related to both increased glucose and increased insulin levels. Although the level of hyperglycemia has not been specifically correlated with the severity of coronary disease, the increased frequency of large-vessel disease in diabetics and the increased occurrence of hyperglycemia in patients with coronary disease make the association clear [65]. Additionally, many diabetics are overweight, and insulin resistance, common in overweight people, leads to hyperinsulinemia. This results in increased production of triglyceride-rich lipoproteins, so that plasma triglyceride and cholesterol levels increase. In fact, many patients with hyperlipidemias or hypertriglyceridemia manifest elevated glucose as the initial problem that results in identification of their lipid abnormality [67]. The metabolic effects of insulin that promote atherosclerosis are: stimulated proliferation of arterial–smooth-muscle cells, enhanced binding of low-density and very-low-density lipoprotein, and decreased binding of high-density lipoprotein to cells [Adapted with permission from 67a].

Several other abnormalities in addition to insulin effects contribute to vascular disease. Dysfunctional endothelium interacts with monocytes and platelets to deposit subintimal plaque. Platelets have increased adhesiveness, possibly due to increased synthesis of thromboxane A2. Sorbitol accumulates in the arterial wall of diabetic patients, producing increased cell water content and decreased oxygenation. Diabetics who smoke carry an even greater risk of vascular disease [63].

Clinical Manifestations
Classic symptoms of hyperglycemia include polyuria, polydipsia, and sometimes blurring of vision. Changes in mental status may occur during ketoacidosis and usually do occur in patients in hyperosmolar coma. On physical examination patients may be found to have diabetic ulcers or peripheral neuropathy. Skin and joint abnormalities also occur. Cardiac, renal, and cerebrovascular disease are due to underlying abnormalities of the vasculature. Cerebrovascular accidents are approximately twice as common in diabetic as in nondiabetic patients [68]. The cardiac abnormalities that occur secondary to diabetes affect myocardial oxygenation, contractility, and conduction.

Coronary Artery Disease in Diabetes
The increased tendency among diabetics to atherosclerosis is manifested clinically in both insulin-dependent and non–insulin-dependent diabetics, who have at least a twofold increased incidence of myocardial infarction compared to nondiabetic control subjects. This risk is even more prominent among younger diabetics, and diabetic women are more prone to coronary ischemia than diabetic men, perhaps because their coronary arteries are smaller. Not only is myocardial infarction twice as likely in diabetic patients [69], but reinfarction and mortality are higher in diabetics after infarction

and especially among diabetic women, who carry an increased risk of severe CHF [70].

Diabetic patients are also more likely to have had a past infarction, and diabetics with angina have more severe coronary disease than nondiabetics [2]. Diabetics may also develop an ischemic cardiomyopathy in which chronic ischemic damage may be silent, and congestive failure is the first manifestation. The tendency of diabetics to develop silent myocardial ischemia is more prominent in those patients with microvascular disease [71] or signs of autonomic neuropathy, such as an attenuated heart rate response to changing respiration or upon standing, lack of sweating, or impotence [72, 73].

Preoperative stress testing may identify those diabetics at risk for cardiac events. Gerson and Khoury [74] reported that of 69 diabetic patients who were asymptomatic and had normal resting and exercise radionuclide ventriculograms 97 percent were free of coronary disease in a follow-up evaluation 29 months later. In contrast, 40 percent of patients with abnormal radionuclide findings developed clinical coronary artery disease and were found to have coronary artery stenoses of 50 percent or more [74].

Small-Vessel Disease. In addition to large-vessel disease, diabetics also have small-vessel disease, which by itself can produce ischemia by limiting flow reserve [75]; and has been touted as the cause of pulmonary edema as well as positive stress tests in patients with normal epicardial coronary arteries. Metabolic changes may impair the ability of the diabetic to respond to vasoconstrictor or vasodilator stimuli. In addition to atherosclerosis, diabetics may manifest proliferative changes with wall thickening and narrowing of the vascular lumen [76, 77].

Ventricular Function Abnormalities in the Diabetic Patient

Subclinical deterioration of cardiac function in diabetic patients is common and affects both systolic and diastolic function. These abnormalities may be caused by abnormal contractility due to changes in myosin isoenzyme content, abnormalities of contractile proteins, increased tissue calcium, and abnormalities in the sarcoplasmic reticulum that affect calcium uptake and metabolism of adenosine triphosphate (ATP) [78, 79]. Diabetics may have a decreased ejection fraction in response to exercise as an early manifestation of underlying cardiac disease. Arvan and associates [80] reported that in a group of young patients without other systemic disease diabetics had significantly poorer responses to exercise, manifested as a smaller increase in ejection fraction and heart rate as compared to a nondiabetic control group. It has also been shown in diabetics who have neither hypertension nor coronary artery disease that even when systolic function is unimpaired they may manifest abnormal diastolic function [81]. The amount of diastolic dysfunction in diabetics may correlate with the severity of microangiopathy. Jermendy and colleagues [82], using apexcardiography, reported normal systolic function in 27 insulin-dependent diabetics without overt cardiac disease, but with abnormal diastolic function during exercise. They noted no relationship between the diastolic dysfunction and the control of blood sugar, but did find that the presence of the diastolic abnormality was correlated with the length of time the patient had diabetes [82]. Although Jermendy's group purports the problem to be abnormal diastolic relaxation, Borow and coworkers [83] reported that diabetics have left ventricular systolic dysfunction as seen on radionuclide angiography and that this abnormality demonstrated during exercise may be due to decreased preload reserve secondary to an autonomic neuropathy. Similarly, Danielson and colleagues [84] have reported that subclinical ventricular dysfunction, demonstrated during exercise with M-mode echocardiography, is due to impaired diastolic filling, but not the result of decreased contractility or increased afterload.

Some diabetics manifest increased left ventricular filling pressures in the absence of large-vessel coronary disease, consistent with myocardial dysfunction due to a restrictive cardiomyopathy. Under histologic examination these patients show abnormalities of the myocardial interstitium, including increased deposits of collagen, glycoprotein, triglycerides, and cholesterol, while some patients manifest changes of the intima and small intramural arteries as well.

In addition to the abnormalities present without coronary disease, diabetics who have coronary disease and are insulin dependent seem to have stiffer

Table 15-8. Signs of diabetic autonomic neuropathy

Diminished variation of heart rate with respiration
Decreased sweating
Early satiety
Decreased or absent pulse rate changes with orthostatic maneuvers
A decrease in blood pressure of more than 30 torr with standing
Tachycardia at rest
Nocturnal diarrhea
Notable peripheral neuropathy
Impotence

Source: Adapted with permission from MF Roizen, Anesthetic Implications of Concurrent Diseases. In RD Miller, RF Cucchiara, et al. (eds), *Anesthesia* (3rd ed). New York: Churchill Livingstone, 1990. Pp 799–800.

ventricles, with higher elevation of left ventricular end diastolic pressure than nondiabetic control subjects [10].

Autonomic Neuropathy

Autonomic neuropathy has been reported in up to 40 percent of diabetic patients and may result in hemodynamic instability even in those without coronary disease. Reported problems include bradycardia, lability of blood pressure, and even cardiac arrest. The baroreflex may be significantly attenuated. Cardiac vagal neuropathy may be detected by evaluation of heart rate response to respiration, orthostatic blood pressure changes, or heart rate changes with the Valsalva maneuver, and a combination of tests may be required to identify patients with cardiovagal neuropathy [85]. Signs of autonomic neuropathy are listed in Table 15-8 [2].

Hypertension seems to serve as a marker of autonomic neuropathy in diabetics, as half the patients in this study who were hypertensive displayed autonomic neuropathy, whereas fewer than 10 percent of the patients without neuropathy were hypertensive [86]. The importance of documenting neuropathy is that it may identify a group of patients who require more invasive monitoring, such as placement of an arterial line.

Burgos and associates [87] reported that diabetics with signs of autonomic abnormalities were more likely to have hypotension during the induction of anesthesia and more likely to have a diminished blood pressure increase in response to laryngoscopy and tracheal intubation. Thirty-five percent of diabetic patients required vasopressors intraoperatively, versus just 5 percent of the control subjects ($p < .05$). It is important to note that the diabetics who required vasopressors had significantly greater abnormalities of autonomic function than those diabetics who did not need intraoperative vasopressors [87]. Additionally, bradycardia and hypotension that did not respond to atropine and ephedrine have been reported in diabetic patients who were known to have advanced autonomic neuropathy [73, 88, 89]. Page and Watkins [73] reported that the diabetics in whom cardiorespiratory arrest developed all displayed a pulse difference of 5 beats per minute with deep inspiration, as opposed to a normal difference of 15 beats per minute.

Metabolic Effects of Diabetes on the Cardiovascular System

As stated earlier, the increased incidence of perioperative complications in diabetics is primarily due to end-organ dysfunction rather than the absolute level of glucose control [90]. However, metabolic derangements of significant magnitude may adversely affect cardiovascular function even in diabetics without significant end-organ disease. Metabolic abnormalities, which tend to occur in diabetics and may adversely affect cardiovascular function, are listed in Table 15-9. While these abnormalities tend to occur in insulin-dependent diabetics, and in this group of patients specifically during ketoacidosis or hyperosmolar states, it should be noted that non–insulin-dependent diabetic patients may be clinically similar to insulin-dependent diabetics during periods of stress. Addi-

Table 15-9. Metabolic abnormalities in diabetes and their cardiovascular effects

Metabolic abnormality	Cardiovascular effect
Hyperglycemia and acidosis	Decreased responsiveness to inotropes
Acidosis	Decreased myocardial contractility
Ketosis	Decreased myocardial contractility
Hypokalemia	Increased risk for arrhythmias
Hypophosphatemia	Increased risk for arrhythmias

tionally, hyperosmolar states are significantly more common among non–insulin-dependent diabetics.

Metabolic abnormalities may also affect cardiac function. Fitzovich and Randall [91] reported that left ventricular contractility in chronically instrumented dogs decreased with carotid occlusion only in those animals with both high glucose and high insulin levels. Frater and associates [10] have reported that in patients who were in sinus rhythm, and had acceptable filling pressures, electrolytes, and blood gases, poor responses to inotropic therapy were noted in the presence of hyperglycemia. After insulin adequately controlled the blood sugar, the response to inotropes was improved [10]. Additionally, patients who are also acidotic due to ketosis are at an even greater risk for myocardial dysfunction. Perhaps control of blood glucose is more important than previously thought. This may be especially true in the diabetic who begins with decreased ventricular function. However, while there is some evidence to suggest that insulin therapy decreases the severity of myocardial dysfunction [92], tight control is controversial, as chronic hyperinsulinemia may worsen the arteriosclerotic tendency [93].

Electrolyte abnormalities increase the risk of arrhythmias. Patients in ketoacidosis may be hyperkalemic due to shift of potassium extracellularly. In addition, treatment of ketoacidosis with insulin promotes intracellular movement of potassium and phosphorus so that patients are frequently hypokalemic and hypophosphatemic within hours of the institution of therapy.

Diabetic Ketoacidosis

Ketoacidosis is a metabolic state that tends to occur in insulin-dependent diabetics whose disease is significantly out of control. Signs and symptoms may include nausea, vomiting, tachypnea, and dyspnea, all of which may bring these patients to a physician. If they are hyperglycemic and ketotic for many hours, they may be severely dehydrated, often by as much as three or four liters. This may manifest as fatigue, lethargy, or mental status changes. Physical examination may reveal orthostatic changes. The absence of such changes in an uncontrolled diabetic who otherwise appears clinically dry may indicate the presence of autonomic abnormalities as well. Although most patients with ketoacidosis recover, about 10 percent do not and myocardial infarction is a significant cause of death. The tendency to infarction may be due to thrombosis, brought on by volume depletion, dehydration, increased viscosity of blood, and changes in clotting factors [63].

Hyperosmolar Coma

Though non–insulin-dependent diabetics sometimes develop classic ketoacidosis, they usually do not. Rather, they may dehydrate and become severely hypernatremic before they come to the attention of a physician. Insulin-dependent diabetics may also become hyperosmolar if they are receiving enough insulin to prevent ketosis but not enough to treat their hyperglycemia. Patients with hyperosmolar coma are usually severely dehydrated. Their serum glucose will often approach 1,000 mg/dl and the serum osmolarity frequently measures greater than 370 mOsm per liter. It is important to monitor serum sodium as well as glucose. The hypertonic state in these patients causes dehydration of cells in the central nervous system, which may result in neurologic deterioration when the sodium is normalized too rapidly [94].

Management of Hyperglycemia in the Perioperative Period

Many regimens for perioperative control of blood glucose have been proposed and have been reviewed elsewhere [2]. As long as monitoring of glucose is done at regular intervals and appropriate insulin therapy is instituted, we have no preferred regimen.

All patients with a glucose greater than 300 mg/dl should be evaluated for acidosis, ketosis, or hypernatremia preoperatively, and if any of these are present elective surgery should be postponed until the metabolic state is normalized, to avoid the aforementioned added stress to the cardiovascular system.

When patients present in a hyperglycemic state for emergency surgery, measurement of serum glucose becomes an important part of anesthetic monitoring. If serum glucose is not readily available, fingerstick glucose levels will guide therapy with intravenous or subcutaneous insulin, though these levels should be confirmed at reasonable intervals.

Patients who are ketotic or in hyperosmolar coma should not undergo elective operation, but if surgery is emergent, such as exploration for a ruptured appendix, we would measure glucose every half hour. Regular intravenous insulin can be administered every hour. If patients are acidotic, ketotic, or even just poorly controlled (glucose ≥ 300 mg/dl), we frequently begin a continuous insulin drip. For patients with glucose of 400 mg/dl or greater, the stress of surgery often makes the glucose extremely difficult to control, even in the absence of ketoacidosis, and thus all the aforementioned effects on the myocardium will come into play.

Serum electrolytes should be measured at least every 2 hours in patients who are ketotic or hyperosmolar. Potassium supplements should be given if the potassium level approaches 3.0 mEq per liter, or 3.5 mEq per liter in patients receiving digitalis preparations. Hypophosphatemia should be treated if the serum level approaches 2.5 mg/dl. When the inorganic phosphorus level nears 1 mg/dl, patients are at serious risk for ventricular arrhythmias. These are easily treated with intravenous administration of the ion, usually potassium phosphate. If the patient is in renal failure, sodium phosphate may be a better alternative. The importance of such therapy must be emphasized. In addition to arrhythmias, severe phosphorus depletion can result in a cardiomyopathy if left untreated. This can result in hypotension, a decreased cardiac output, and a decreased pressor response to catecholamines. A decreased threshold to arrhythmias can be seen acutely and may be present with a phosphorus concentration of 1.0 mg/dl (normal, 3.0–4.5 mg/dl) [95].

Anesthetic Management of the Diabetic Patient with Cardiac Disease

Anesthetic management of the diabetic patient must take into account the presence and severity of any cardiac abnormalities. These are usually determined by history and physical examination, though testing may be necessary as diabetics often have silent processes. The management of ischemia is essentially the same as that of coronary disease (see Chap. 5). However, because diabetic patients may have small-vessel disease it is important to monitor them for ischemia, even in the absence of epicardial coronary disease. We adjust our ECG leads accordingly. Ventricular dysfunction is also managed in such a manner because of the presence of other pathophysiologic processes (see Chaps. 5 and 9). Metabolic abnormalities in the diabetic need to be followed serially, as they can compromise cardiac function. It is important in both ketotic and hyperosmolar patients to optimize preload for that patient's Starling curve. A drainage catheter to measure urine output is essential. If the patient has any history of ventricular dysfunction, either systolic or diastolic, central monitoring is indicated for surgical procedures of any significant length of time. The decision to use a central venous or pulmonary artery catheter is one best made by considering the patient's history of ischemic symptoms, exercise tolerance, and whether or not there is a history of a recent myocardial infarction. Objective data, such as an ejection fraction or echocardiography documenting wall motion, will obviously be helpful if they are available. It is important to measure arterial blood gases in those patients with a decreased serum bicarbonate level, as patients with a pH of less than 7.2 are likely to manifest a decreased response to inotropic agents.

The choice of particular anesthetic agent should be made bearing in mind the patient's cardiovascular function. Since the primary pathophysiologic problems are ischemia and abnormal compliance, anesthetic regimens discussed for hypertension will usually be good choices for the diabetic patient as well. However, the presence of autonomic neuropathy may mask such helpful preoperative indicators as orthostatic changes in the hypovolemic patient. Additionally, the presence of small-vessel disease or abnormal responses to vasodilator stimuli may result in myocardial ischemia in a diabetic patient whose preoperative history and physical examination did not support the presence of myocardial ischemia. It is therefore of the utmost importance in these patients to maintain the balance between myocardial oxygen supply and demand, and to monitor these patients carefully. It is more important to maintain preload, afterload, heart rate, and contractility within an appropriate range than to use any particular anesthetic agent. However, in patients with known poor ventricular function, a narcotic-based technique is preferable to a deep-inhalation anesthetic. The ability of isoflurane to cause both tachycardia and coronary steal should make one cautious when using this agent in high doses. The newer nondepolarizing agents may be preferable to pancuronium, which may precipitate tachycardia due to its vagolytic properties. Ketamine may not be a good choice as the tachycardia it produces may precipitate myocardial ischemia. Droperidol may be useful to decrease abnormally high afterload due to its ability to block alpha receptors. In patients in whom unexpected myocardial ischemia develops, a TEE probe can be used to assess wall motion and volume status. A pulmonary artery catheter may be especially helpful in critically ill diabetic patients in whom optimization of oxygen consumption serves as a useful end point for hemodynamic therapy to ensure normal tissue perfusion into the postoperative period.

Regional anesthesia may be a good choice in these patients. As with hypertensive patients, placement of an epidural catheter may be preferable to use of a spinal anesthetic. An epidural technique will have a slower, more controlled onset and the catheter can be used for pain management in the postoperative period. Diabetic patients frequently undergo vascular bypass procedures, and an epidural anesthetic is an especially good choice for those patients in whom major vessels will not be crossclamped. For those who will require clamping of the aorta or iliac vessels, consideration should be given to combining an epidural technique with a light general anesthetic.

Hemochromatosis

Although hemochromatosis is actually a separate disorder with a genetic predisposition we discuss it briefly here, as many patients with hemochromatosis have diabetes, as a result of deposition of iron in the pancreas, and in about 15 percent of these patients cardiac disease is the initial manifestation of their disease. Congestive failure may be the presenting problem in young patients and, if untreated, death may rapidly ensue. The heart is enlarged diffusely and arrhythmias may occur. These may include supraventricular arrhythmias, such as atrial flutter or fibrillation, as well as varying amounts of atrioventricular block [96]. Diagnosis of the primary problem in these patients is important for treatment, which entails removal of excessive iron from the body and supportive treatment of the organs involved. If such patients present to the operating room for surgery, they should be recognized as a population with the potential for severe ventricular dysfunction. They may require invasive monitoring, especially if signs of congestive failure are present (see Chap. 9).

Renal Failure

Epidemiology

The three most common causes of chronic renal failure are diabetes, hypertension, and glomerulonephritis. Glomerulonephritis, once the leading cause of renal failure, now accounts for only 21 percent of cases as a result of improved treatment of this disease. Diabetic nephropathy causes about 28 percent of end-stage renal disease, while hypertension causes approximately 25 percent. Polycystic kidney disease causes about 4 percent and unknown processes account for the rest of the cases. Considering the frequency of these processes, it is not surprising that many cities maintain their own dialysis programs, and patients with chronic renal failure are therefore commonly seen by the anesthesiologist.

Acute renal failure may be caused mechanically, as by obstruction and hydronephrosis, or by hemodynamic instability, resulting in decreased cardiac output and renal blood flow. Ischemic insults may occur intraoperatively, such as those associated with placement of an aortic crossclamp, resulting in acute tubular necrosis. Other causes include transfusion reactions, interstitial nephritis such as that due to drugs, or the effect of toxins. Radiographic dyes are quite safe in normal patients, but in those with underlying kidney disease, especially diabetics, they may precipitate renal failure in more than 10 percent of patients [97]. Finally, renal failure may occur following crush injury as a result of rhabdomyolysis and myoglobinuria.

Pathophysiology

Destruction of nephrons by systemic diseases results in functional hypertrophy of remaining nephrons. This causes increased glomerular capillary pressures and flows, ultimately resulting in destruction of these nephrons. Acute tubular necrosis is primarily due to renal ischemia, especially that associated with long periods of hypoperfusion. Nephrotoxic agents can also cause acute tubular necrosis, with the most common agents today being aminoglycoside antibiotics and intravenous contrast.

When evaluating patients preoperatively the serum creatinine should be noted, as it correlates with glomerular filtration rate (GFR). For each decrease of 50 percent in GFR, the serum creatinine will approximately double [98]. A serum creatinine concentration of 5.5 mg/dl correlates with a GFR of 15 to 20 ml per minute and is the level at which the body becomes incapable of excreting an unlimited amount of ingested substances. This may result in increases in sodium, potassium, and phosphate; fluid retention; and increased blood urea nitrogen. Since serum creatinine of approximately 1.3 mg/dl represents a 50 percent reduction in creatinine clearance, it can be appreciated that even a small increase in serum creatinine may represent a cause for concern and for optimal management of those parameters that determine renal function, such as cardiac index, renal perfusion pressure, and adequate preload. This is particularly important in patients undergoing repair of an abdominal aortic aneurysm or other major vascular surgery that requires aortic crossclamping. In these patients a serum creatinine of 2 mg/dl or greater is associated with a significantly increased risk of postoperative renal failure, and those patients in whom renal failure develops have a high incidence of sepsis and death.

Cardiac Manifestations and Concerns in Renal Failure

Though our discussion focuses primarily on chronic renal failure (CRF), patients with acute renal failure manifest many of the same cardiovascular problems, including hypertension, fluid overload, pericarditis, hyperkalemia, and arrhythmias. The effects of chronic renal failure on the cardiovascular system are summarized in Table 15-10.

Hypertension. Arterial hypertension is the complication most frequently seen in CRF, and the patient is usually receiving antihypertensive therapy. The hypertension is usually due to fluid overload. Still, some patients are hypertensive even when euvolemic, probably due to increased levels of circulating renin. When severe hypertension ac-

Table 15-10. Cardiovascular effects of chronic renal failure

Hypertension
Fluid retention
Congestive heart failure
High-output failure (especially in the presence of AV grafts)
Euvolemic pulmonary congestion
Accelerated atherosclerosis
Myocardial and vascular calcification
Pericarditis

companies CRF, it is best treated aggressively with agents such as nifedipine, captopril, enalapril, or minoxidil. When acute intravenous therapy is required for severe hypertension, nitroglycerin can be tried but nitroprusside is usually required.

Fluid Retention and Pulmonary Edema. Fluid retention may result in pulmonary edema. This is more common in the elderly when chronic hypertension has taken its toll on the left ventricle. Still, pulmonary congestion may occur even in euvolemic patients in association with normal or mildly increased intracardiac and pulmonary capillary wedge pressures. This is due to increased permeability of the alveolar capillary membrane. The chest x-ray reveals a perihilar vascular congestion. This form of pulmonary edema usually responds quickly to hemodialysis, as do the other forms of fluid overload in renal failure [99].

Patients receiving chronic dialysis have a high incidence of accelerated atherosclerosis, partly due to hypertension; chronically increased cardiac output; and vascular and myocardial calcification [99].

Pericarditis. Pericarditis is no longer a frequent occurrence due to early treatment with dialysis, as uremic pericarditis is believed to be caused by retained metabolic toxins. When pericarditis occurs in a well-dialyzed patient, it is more likely due to viral infection or another underlying systemic disease. Clinical manifestations of uremic pericarditis, when it does occur, are essentially the same as those due to other diseases. The cardinal manifestations of pericarditis are listed in Table 15-11.

The ECG changes of acute pericarditis can

Table 15-11. Cardinal manifestations of pericarditis

Chest pain
Pericardial friction rub
ECG showing low-voltage and flat or inverted T waves
ST elevation acutely
Atrial fibrillation
Cardiomegaly on chest x-ray
Pericardial effusion
Cardiac tamponade
Pulsus paradoxus

be differentiated from those of infarction by the features described in Table 15-12. In chronic pericarditis the ECG changes are relatively fixed, frequently including low-voltage and inverted T waves. Flat or inverted T waves are present in essentially all cases, with abnormal P waves present in about 75 percent of cases and low voltage occurring in more than half of cases. Usually, such changes are noted in many if not all leads. Interestingly, the depth of inversion of the T waves is usually related to the degree of adherence of the pericardium to the myocardium, so that deep T waves frequently occur in patients in whom surgical stripping of the pericardium proves difficult or impossible. Atrial fibrillation occurs in more than 30 percent of patients in whom chronic constrictive pericarditis develops [100]. Figure 15-3 displays a typical ECG in a patient with pericarditis.

Pericarditis due to CRF may be differentiated at pericardiocentesis from that due to other causes by the tendency for uremic pericarditis to cause hemorrhagic fluid. Vigorous dialysis will usually result in clinical improvement in the pericarditis. A full discussion of the anesthetic management of patients with pericardial disease is presented in Chap. 8.

Arrhythmias. Patients in renal failure have an increased incidence of arrhythmias for several reasons, which are listed in Table 15-13. Acute renal failure may be especially associated with supraventricular arrhythmias.

It is common for these patients to have nonspecific ST and T-wave changes perioperatively, and it may be difficult to determine their significance, especially in patients who are also diabetic. These changes may be related to shifts in vascular volume, electrolytes, or pH.

Cardiomyopathy in Chronic Renal Failure. Myocardial calcification may result in a cardiomyopathy and congestive failure. It tends to occur in patients with hypocalcemia and hyperphosphatemia and may be more likely to be seen in patients who are noncompliant with phosphate binders. In addition, a calcium-phosphorus product of 60 may be indicative of patients who are likely to develop this disorder. The occurrence of AV block in a patient with a high calcium-phosphorus product may be a sign of impending heart failure within a few months' time [101]. In addition, proliferation of vascular intima and medial calcification may occur in medium-sized coronary arteries [102].

Anemia and Chronic Renal Failure. In addition to the above considerations, anemia commonly accompanies CRF, as a result of depressed erythropoiesis, hemolysis, gastrointestinal blood loss, and possibly aluminum intoxication. This confuses the preoperative evaluation as these patients often complain of easy fatigability. Additionally, in those patients with coronary disease, severe anemia may worsen ischemia and compromise contractile function even more. Erythropoietin therapy results in a significant rise in hematocrit in patients with CRF. However, this leads to increased viscosity and

Table 15-12. Differentiation of acute pericarditis and acute infarction

ECG finding	Acute pericarditis	Acute infarction
ST reciprocity (between limb leads I and III)	Absent, elevation in both I and III	Present, elevated in one lead, depressed in the other
ST shape	Concave upward	Convex upward
Q waves	Absent	Present

Source: Adapted with permission from HJL Marriott, Miscellaneous Conditions. In HJL Marriott, *Practical Electrocardiography* (8th ed). Baltimore: Williams & Wilkins, 1988. P 519.

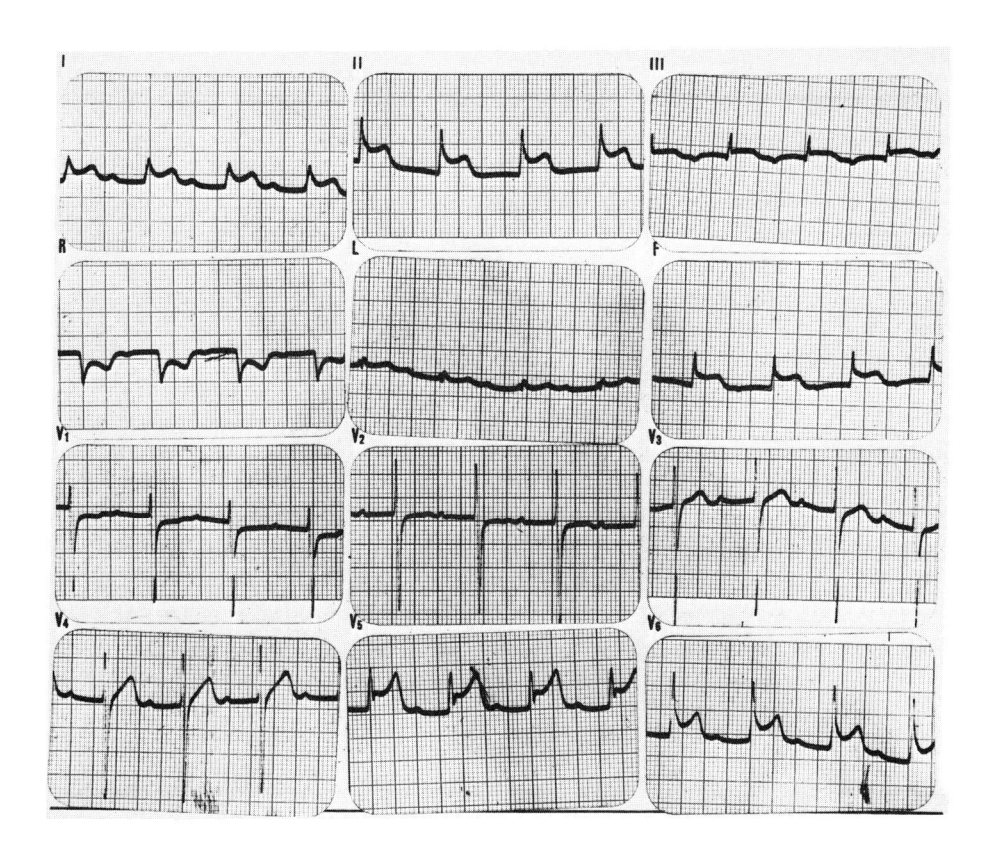

Fig. 15-3. Electrocardiogram of a patient with ST and T-wave changes due to pericarditis.

Table 15-13. Etiologies of arrhythmias in renal failure

Congestive heart failure
Electrolyte abnormalities
Digitalis intoxication
Pericarditis
Anemia

Source: Adapted with permission of McGraw-Hill, Inc. From RJ Anderson and RW Schrier, Acute Renal Failure. In JD Wilson, E Braunwald, et al. (eds), *Harrison's Principles of Internal Medicine* (12th ed). New York: McGraw-Hill, 1991. Pp 1144–1150.

blood pressure. These changes are most severe in patients who were previously hypertensive. Therefore, the use of erythropoietin may result in an increased requirement for antihypertensive therapy [103].

Cardiac output (CO) rises in response to anemia in order to maintain perfusion to the tissues. The resting cardiac output is usually increased when the hemoglobin is 7 gm or less. The increased cardiac output is generally due to increased stroke volume [104] without significant changes in heart rate. In response to exercise, patients with anemia also respond primarily with an increase in stroke volume, whereas normal patients increase their heart rate more than their stroke volume [105]. When hemoglobin decreases to approximately 3 gm, CO is usually still above normal but does not rise any further, perhaps due to a decrease in myocardial oxygen supply. Patients with underlying heart disease may not be able to increase their CO in response to anemia. During exercise normal patients increase CO 550 to 800 ml per 100 ml increase in oxygen consumption per minute. In patients with chronic anemia, the increase in cardiac output with exercise is usually 1,000 to 1,500 ml or more per 100 ml increase in oxygen consumption per minute [105].

Circulation time is usually increased but not always. Generally, plasma volume is slightly increased while total blood volume and central blood volume are decreased. The proportion of central to peripheral blood volume may be abnormal and in some anemic patients transfusion may greatly increase central blood volume resulting in pulmonary congestion. In addition, the right atrial pressure before transfusion does not predict whether or not transfusion will result in pulmonary congestion [105].

Although many signs and symptoms accompany anemia, few are specific. Still, clinicians who frequently examine the conjunctiva and nail beds may reliably diagnose anemia by examination of these areas. The arterial pulse may be bounding as a result of a hyperkinetic state. The precordial impulse may be prominent and displaced to the left. On auscultation S_1 and S_2 may be louder than usual and both S_3 and S_4 gallops are common in anemia, even in the absence of congestive failure [105].

Anesthetic Management of the Renal Failure Patient with Cardiac Disease

Since many patients with renal failure have hypertension and diabetes, many of the same anesthetic considerations apply. However, ischemia and abnormal compliance are only some of the problems that affect patients with renal failure. Volume status may fluctuate rapidly in these patients, both due to abnormal central blood volume and the rapid changes induced by dialysis. In patients with poor ventricular function who are also hypovolemic, the use of inhalation anesthetics may compromise the patient's hemodynamic status. Electrolyte abnormalities may result in arrhythmias, and hyperkalemia or acidosis should be treated, preferably with dialysis, before elective surgery is performed. Partial pressure of carbon dioxide should be maintained in an appropriate range in order to prevent wide fluctuations of serum potassium. Placement of an arterial line will facilitate measurement of hematocrit, electrolytes, and arterial blood gases.

The difficulties inherent in the management of patients with renal failure are partially due to problems with contradictory anesthetic implications. Though these patients are frequently hypovolemic, if they miss a dialysis treatment they may present in pulmonary edema. Though a small amount of blood loss may compromise them hemodynamically, rapid blood transfusion may not be tolerated. Therefore, these patients frequently require measurement of central venous or pulmonary capillary wedge pressures.

The presence of a significant pericardial effusion is of particular concern, as the anesthetic management differs from that for coronary disease. Tachycardia is frequently necessary to maintain blood pressure, and ketamine may be chosen for induction. In the patient who is undergoing pericardial drainage, ketamine may be the preferred induction agent, although there is a risk of precipitating myocardial ischemia. A large pericardial effusion decreases diastolic filling and results in abnormally elevated filling pressures for any given end diastolic volume. Both preload and afterload should be maintained. It is important to maintain contractility and the inhalation anesthetics may not be a good choice in this situation. A narcotic technique combined with intravenous benzodiazepines may be preferable. The benzodiazepines should be carefully titrated, as their administration combined with narcotics may result in significant myocardial depression. If the patient displays critically abnormal hemodynamics, pericardial drainage can be performed using a local anesthetic (see Chap. 8).

Regional anesthesia can be used in these patients if their coagulation status is normal. An epidural or regional nerve block may be preferable to a spinal block due to the slower onset of sympathetic blockade. However, both spinal and epidural techniques may precipitate severe hypotension in patients who have been recently dialyzed. Placement of central monitoring before performing these techniques may be helpful. When a large pericardial effusion is present, epidural and spinal block are best avoided, as they may precipitate severe hypotension, since blood pressure in these patients depends on maintenance of both preload and afterload.

Chronic Obstructive Pulmonary Disease

The term *chronic obstructive pulmonary disease* (*COPD*) includes those disorders that cause cough,

Table 15-14. Chronic obstructive pulmonary diseases

Emphysema
Chronic bronchitis
Bronchiectasis secondary to cystic fibrosis
Bronchiectasis secondary to pneumonitis
Asthmatic bronchitis

Table 15-15. Common signs and symptoms of emphysema

Dyspnea
Airway obstruction
Decreased diffusion capacity
Increased residual volume
Increased total lung capacity
Hyperlucent lung field on chest x-ray

Table 15-16. Clinical and laboratory findings in chronic bronchitis

Dyspnea
Cough
Chronic or recurrent bacterial infections
Hypoxia
Hypercapnia
Secondary erythrocytosis
Cardiomegaly
Pulmonary hypertension
Right-sided heart failure

dyspnea, sputum production, and irreversible airway obstruction. The latter criterion is important, as it differentiates asthma that manifests reversible airway obstruction from asthmatic bronchitis. Asthmatic bronchitis describes a reversible component of airway reactivity that is present in some patients with COPD. Disorders included under the heading COPD are listed in Table 15-14.

Pathophysiology and Clinical Manifestations

Patients with asthma or COPD will display a decreased FEV_1:FVC ratio characteristic of airway obstruction. Patients with COPD may manifest a decreased or normal vital capacity. Emphysema is a disorder characterized by loss of alveolar structure. This results in loss of elastic recoil and airways that are compliant and collapsible. Although it is a pathologic diagnosis, certain clinical features are common, as noted in Table 15-15.

Patients with pure emphysema are frequently dyspneic and have been referred to as pink puffers. They have minimal cough and may have normal arterial blood gases at rest. They tend to be thin, and on chest x-ray display hyperlucent lung fields and a small cardiac silhouette. Patients with pure chronic bronchitis have been referred to as blue bloaters. Dyspnea may be mild or moderate. They tend to have prominent secretions and coughing, often aggravated by chronic or recurrent bacterial infections. Laboratory and clinical findings in chronic bronchitis are summarized in Table 15-16. Not all of these findings need be present early in the disease or at any given time. However, patients with severe disease that has progressed to right-sided heart failure will usually manifest most or all of these features of the disease. It should be noted that several items on this list specifically involve the cardiovascular system, or can affect it adversely.

Patients with COPD include those with emphysema or chronic bronchitis. Some of these patients have a reversible component to their disease, as is present in asthma. In patients with COPD nocturnal episodes of desaturation due to hypoventilation elevate pulmonary artery pressure and may result in pulmonary hypertension and cor pulmonale [106].

Cardiac Effects of Chronic Obstructive Pulmonary Disease. Steele and associates [107] reported that LVEF as measured by bedside radionuclide scan was normal in patients with severe COPD. However, in those with stable COPD and coronary artery disease (CAD), LVEF was significantly lower (42+/−3.5%) than LVEF in those without CAD (55+/−2.1%). In patients with acute obstructive pulmonary disease, LVEF was 28+/−10.4 percent in those with CAD, which was significantly different than the LVEF of 61+/−1.9 percent in those without CAD [107]. LVEF is generally normal in severe chronic obstructive lung disease and in acute ventilatory failure. In patients with respiratory failure, LVEF of less than 40 percent was associated with an increase in mortality and was usually associated with evidence of CAD. Though depression of LVEF may be seen in patients with CAD and COPD severe enough to result in significantly low arterial oxygen tensions ($PaCO_2$), these patients do not have improved LVEF when given sufficient oxygen to normalize the PaO_2. However,

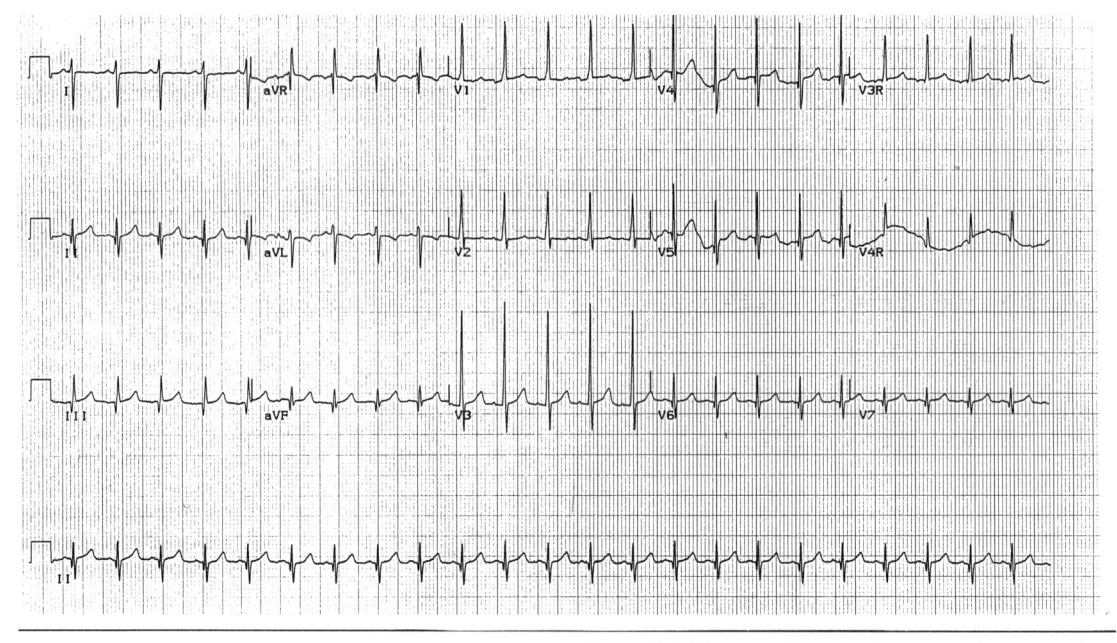

Fig. 15-4. Electrocardiogram showing right ventricular hypertrophy.

this does not prove that low arterial oxygen tensions may not contribute to the depression of LVEF, as it may take time to correct cellular and/or myocardial abnormalities. Certainly, patients with severe chronic hypoxemia may have depressed LVEF on that basis alone. Left ventricular end diastolic pressure (LVEDP) has been variably reported as normal or elevated, while LVH has been reported as present or absent. Perhaps some of these results are attributable to underlying CAD, especially since many patients with COPD are smokers [107]. Indeed, a normal LVEDP has been documented at rest and during exercise in patients with COPD [108], and Williams and colleagues [109] documented a normal left ventricular response to increased afterload produced with methoxamine in patients with COPD. Therefore, it is our impression that patients with COPD have normal left ventricular function in the absence of other cardiac disease processes.

Despite the presence of normal ventricular function, many patients with COPD have limited exercise tolerance that would not be predicted by their arterial blood gases. Burrows and associates [110] have shed light on this issue by describing cardiac and pulmonary abnormalities and the relationship between them in three groups of patients. Patients with mild obstructive pulmonary disease displayed CO values in the low-normal range and pulmonary artery pressures within the normal range at rest. These patients did not have severe hypoxemia (oxygen saturation no less than 84%) or significant arterial carbon dioxide retention. There was no clinical evidence of right ventricular hypertrophy (RVH), although 2 of 36 patients displayed RVH on the electrocardiogram. A second group of patients with more severe obstructive pulmonary disease had blood gas values not significantly different than those of the first group, but pulmonary vascular resistance (PVR) was increased moderately and cardiac index (CI) was decreased to less than 2.5 liters/min/m^2. Pulmonary artery

Table 15-17. Clinical findings in patients with COPD, grouped by PVR and blood gas values

Clinical finding	Group A[a] (mean)	Group B[b] (mean)	Group C[c] (mean)
Arterial oxygen saturation (%)	91	88	69
Pulmonary vascular resistance (dynes/sec/cm^5)	379	670	740
Arterial CO_2 tension (mm Hg)	42	42	54
Cardiac index (liters/min/m^2)	2.5	1.9	3.5
Definite RVH on ECG (% of group)	6	33	100
Emphysema on chest x-ray (%)	47	33	0
Inflammatory change on chest x-ray (%)	39	33	100

[a] Patients with mild obstructive pulmonary disease.
[b] Patients with more severe obstructive pulmonary disease.
[c] Patients with clinical signs of cor pulmonale.
Source: Adapted with permission of the *New England Journal of Medicine.* From B Burrows, LJ Kettel, et al. Patterns of cardiovascular dysfunction in chronic obstructive lung disease. *N Engl J Med* 286:912, 1972.

pressure was minimally elevated, yet remained within the normal range. However, PVR increased significantly even at rest, with pulmonary hypertension clearly manifested during exercise. The third group included five patients who had clinical signs of cor pulmonale. Four of the five were markedly hypoxemic and chronically hypercapnic. All five had ECG changes consistent with RVH (Fig. 15-4) and chest x-ray signs of chronic inflammation. All of these patients had PVR values exceeding 500 dynes/sec/cm^{-5} with cardiac indices greater than 2.8 liters/min/m^2 (Table 15-17).

Among 10 patients culled from all groups with PVR greater than 550 dynes/sec/cm^{-5}, there were no survivors at 3 years. The importance of elevated PVR as a marker of cardiovascular disease should be noted. Interestingly, the third group had higher cardiac indices than the second, but perhaps that was due to the RVH, which developed in order to pump against the increased PVR. When right-sided heart failure occurs secondary to COPD, the primary goal of therapy is to increase the arterial oxygen tension. A goal of 60 torr is a useful guideline. If diuresis does not occur with improvement in arterial oxygen tension, diuretics may be necessary. Digoxin or a short course of intravenous inotropes may be useful but should be used cautiously in the presence of hypoxemia. If the hematocrit is greater than 60 percent, phlebotomy is indicated. Certainly, if a patient in right-sided failure who is hypoxic presents to the operating room for emergency surgery, placement of a pulmonary artery catheter is recommended.

It is useful to place a pulmonary artery catheter in patients with hypoxemia or hypercapnia due to pulmonary disease, in order to measure and treat PVR and CI in the perioperative period. A more difficult decision is what to do with patients in the second group, who may or may not have a clear history of shortness of breath. Their blood gases may not draw our attention and they do not manifest RVH. Still, with increased PVR and decreased CI some of these patients would benefit from a pulmonary artery catheter.

Asthma

Epidemiology

Asthma affects approximately 5 percent of the adult population and 7 to 10 percent of children. It is found more commonly in younger age groups, with about 50 percent of cases developing before age 10 and another 30 percent before age 40. The disease is twice as common among male children as female children, but develops equally between the sexes by age 30 [111].

Pathophysiology

Patients with asthma display a narrowed airway diameter due to smooth-muscle contraction, bronchial wall edema, and the presence of thick secretions. During an acute attack this causes an increase in airway resistance, which manifests as decreased forced expiratory flow rates, increased residual volume and functional residual capacity, and hypoxemia. Hypocapnia and respiratory alkalosis are common findings, but due to the increased work of breathing patients may tire, and if untreated may suffer a respiratory arrest. Most patients who present for treatment have a forced vital capacity of 50 percent or less of normal, and when asthmatics report that their attack is over, the FEV_1 is usually at least 50 percent of normal [111].

Clinical Manifestations

Asthma is a disorder characterized by increased reactivity of the bronchial musculature. Symptoms include cough, dyspnea, and wheezing. Attacks are precipitated by numerous stimuli such as grasses and dust, though some are brought on by exercise, especially if the air being breathed is cold. Patients with upper respiratory tract infections may have an increased incidence of bronchospasm. During acute attacks patients may hyperventilate to overcome hypoxemia. If a normal arterial carbon dioxide tension is present, the patient should be considered at risk for impending respiratory failure. Such patients are seriously ill, and should not undergo anesthesia and surgery if at all possible. An acute asthma attack, in our opinion, is an absolute contraindication to anesthesia and surgery, except for the most emergent procedures. Even then, we prefer to treat the patients aggressively for their asthma with pharmacologic agents before the induction of anesthesia. Such treatment may include inhaled bronchodilators, anticholinergics, steroids, aminophylline preparations, and systemic glucocorticoids. The use of regional anesthesia to avoid airway manipulation should be considered.

Cardiac Manifestations

An acute asthma attack may affect the cardiovascular system by increasing intrathoracic pressures, thus decreasing venous return. Also, bronchoconstriction increases right ventricular afterload, which not only decreases RVEF but also shifts the intraventricular septum, thereby compromising left ventricular output. If severe bronchospasm and hypoxemia develop, severe pulmonary hypertension may rapidly ensue, even if PVR and PA pressures were normal before the hypoxia. It is therefore of the utmost importance to treat asthmatics with their usual bronchodilating medications up until the time of surgery. As was discussed earlier, those receiving steroid therapy should receive appropriate perioperative adjustment of their dose.

Most patients with asthma who present for surgery will have their asthma reasonably well controlled, so that the hemodynamic changes mentioned above will not be paramount. However, many agents used to treat asthma have cardiovascular side effects, including tachycardia, increased myocardial contractility, and precipitation of arrhythmias. Additionally, agents used to treat arrhythmias such as β-blockers may aggravate bronchospasm, although the new short-acting β-blocker esmolol has been used in small groups of patients with relative safety in this population. Even if a rare patient does develop bronchospasm, with a half-life of just 7 minutes the effect of the drug will be short lived. Aminophylline prevents the metabolism of cyclic adenosine monophosphate (cAMP) and thereby increases cardiac contractility in a fashion similar to that of phosphodiesterase inhibitors.

Anesthetic Management of the Patient with COPD or Asthma and Cardiac Disease

Patients with asthma frequently have episodic dyspnea. However, patients with COPD may have chronic dyspnea, and it may be quite difficult to differentiate from that due to left ventricular dysfunction. Chest crackles and wheezing may be heard in both disease states. Although COPD causes signs of right-sided heart failure such as peripheral edema, jugular venous distention, or hepatojugular reflux, left-sided failure can cause these symptoms as well. Pulmonary function tests (PFTs) may help distinguish which problem is causing the dyspnea. CHF results in a decrease in FVC but rarely is the FEV_1 less than 70 percent of the FVC. Patients with COPD may have a decreased FVC, although the ratio of FEV_1 to FVC will often be less than 70 percent. However, heart disease develops in many patients as a consequence of smoking and the presence of both processes may make it difficult to distinguish which is causing the symptoms. It may therefore be necessary to perform noninvasive testing of left ventricular function. If surgery must proceed urgently, the only course may be to place a PA catheter preoperatively to measure the PCWP. Still, a high PCWP does not rule out COPD for, as we have already stated, it is not uncommon for the two to coexist.

In patients with COPD or asthma, our primary concern is to prevent bronchoconstriction, hypoxemia, or hypercarbia, as these may result in right-sided heart failure, arrhythmias, or pulmonary hypertension. We prefer the inhaled agents for their bronchodilating effects. Though we would use halothane for an inhalation induction, we prefer to maintain asthmatics with either enflurane or isoflurane, because of the risk of arrhythmias if aminophylline or epinephrine is required to treat asthma in patients receiving halothane. For induction in patients who are wheezing and who must undergo emergency surgery, ketamine is our induction agent of choice.

The presence of decreased ventricular function should be considered when choosing an anesthetic agent for those patients with concomitant CAD. Patients with acute respiratory failure who also have CAD may have severely compromised ventricular function. The use of myocardial depressants such as the inhalation anesthetics may be detrimental in these patients and in patients with severe cor pulmonale. Although nitrous oxide can be safely used in patients with asthma or COPD whose lung function is stable, use of nitrous oxide during an acute respiratory event prevents administration of high concentrations of oxygen. While patients who are actively wheezing are not brought to surgery electively, if bronchospasm develops intraoperatively it is best to discontinue nitrous oxide and administer 100 percent oxygen until the pulmonary status has stabilized and blood gases document acceptable partial pressures of oxygen. Oxygenation and ventilation are of primary importance, as hypoxemia and hypercarbia may result in myocardial ischemia and increased sympathetic tone, respectively. In patients with cor pulmonale, nitrous oxide may elevate pulmonary artery pressure; if it is used, the pulmonary artery pressure should be monitored. Ketamine is a good induction agent for patients who present for emergency surgery and are wheezing. However, the associated sympathetic nervous system stimulation, mediated via release of endogenous catecholamines, may precipitate myocardial ischemia in the susceptible patient. It is preferable to treat patients who are wheezing with inhaled beta agonists, steroids, and anticholinergics before the induction of anesthesia. Such therapy results in minimal cardiovascular effects. If a patient develops severe bronchospasm during general anesthesia and does not respond to such therapy via the ventilator circuit, we prefer to administer small doses of epinephrine intravenously. Titration of 2.5-μg increments followed by a low-dose continuous drip of epinephrine will usually result in significant improvement of the patient in bronchospasm, without precipitating myocardial ischemia. Though the risk of ischemia is there, arterial desaturation is the more dangerous of the two. If ischemia occurs, appropriate therapy can then be administered. Although isoproterenol (Isuprel) has been recommended for the treatment of bronchospasm, we prefer not to administer this agent to patients with cardiac disease, as the combination of tachycardia and decreased SVR may seriously impair the balance between myocardial oxygen supply and demand.

Alcoholism

Epidemiology

Alcohol abuse refers to a physiologic dependence such that alcohol is necessary for adequate function, combined with occasional heavy consumption. The term *alcohol dependence* implies, in addition, evidence of an increased tolerance to alcohol or physical signs of withdrawal with abstinence. Using strict criteria, the risk of developing alcoholism in one's lifetime in Western countries is approximately 10 percent for men and between 3 and 5 percent for women. The average alcoholic is a blue-collar or white-collar worker or housewife. Alcoholism is present in all races, ethnic groups, and socioeconomic classes. Alcoholism refers to continued use until it adversely affects one's job or relationships, or results in significant physical effects, such as cardiomyopathy, cirrhosis, or alcoholic hepatitis.

The first major problem caused by alcohol tends to occur in most patients between the ages of 25 and 50. There is strong evidence that alcoholism is a multifactorial disorder. That biologic and genetic factors are involved is supported by a fourfold increased risk of alcoholism in children of alcoholics, even if adopted at birth and raised without knowledge of their biologic parents' problem. Also, the risk of an identical twin of an alcoholic becoming an alcoholic is much greater than that of a fraternal twin [112]. Recently, it has been learned that two to three drinks per day are likely to decrease the

Table 15-18. Pathophysiologic effects of alcohol on the cardiovascular system

Hypertension
Arrhythmias
Cardiomyopathy
Decreased left ventricular function
Right-sided heart failure

---

risk of cardiovascular morbidity and mortality. This is likely due to the associated increase in high-density lipoprotein levels or effects on clotting [112]. However, the risk of death from cardiovascular disease increases with consumption of more than five drinks a day [113].

Manifestations of Cardiac Disease in Patients who Abuse Alcohol

The signs and symptoms of alcohol abuse vary with the stage of the disease and the organ system affected. Patients may manifest signs of hepatitis, cirrhosis, or cardiomyopathy. We focus our discussion here primarily on those signs consistent with alcohol-induced cardiac disease.

The effects of alcohol on the heart are significant. Pathophysiologic alterations that result in signs and symptoms of heart disease in alcoholic patients are listed in Table 15-18.

Pathophysiology

Some of the cardiac effects may be mediated by hypertension, which is associated with alcohol intake; significant elevations of systolic and diastolic pressures have been shown to occur in patients imbibing more than 20 ml per day. This hypertension may be mediated in part through calcium depletion [114]. No particular pattern of drinking is associated with the onset of cardiac failure. Though some patients report worsening of their drinking before the onset of heart failure, others have recrudescence of their CHF while abstinent [115]. Still, the negative effects of alcohol are clear, as those patients who stop drinking have a decreased mortality compared to those who continue [116].

There are two subclinical forms of alcoholic heart disease. Early on, there is increased wall thickness but normal internal diameter in diastole; later, internal diameter is enlarged without abnormality of wall dimensions [117]. Up to 50 percent of asymptomatic alcoholics have LVH as documented by M-mode echocardiography. Early in the process, diastolic compliance of the left ventricle is decreased [118]. After a number of years, left ventricular contractility may decrease [118, 119]. It is believed that contractility is decreased because of decreased availability of calcium to the contractile proteins in the absence of a change of total calcium [119]. Chronic ethanol abuse has an inhibitory effect on myosin adenosine triphosphatase (ATPase) and calcium-activated myofibrillar ATPase [119]. Histologically, there are no features of alcoholic heart disease to differentiate it from other congestive cardiomyopathies [120]. An increased amount of fibrous tissue is commonly found and may replace myocardial fibers [115]. Not only is alcoholic cardiomyopathy associated with decreased contractility, but alcohol can also cause acute changes, as demonstrated by decreased stroke volume associated with increased LVEDPs after ethanol ingestion in patients without heart disease [121]. Among sudden death victims with documented moderate alcohol levels, many did not have myocardial hypertrophy, and liver examination revealed fatty liver changes significantly more frequently than cirrhosis [122]. This implies that even moderate levels of drinking can result in malignant arrhythmias, and cardiac examination at autopsy does in fact reveal foci of fibrosis and necrosis.

The Electrocardiogram in Alcoholic Heart Disease. The electrocardiogram may be normal at the onset of disease or may have nonspecific changes. However, arrhythmias are frequently the first sign of heart disease. It may be concluded in error that the arrhythmia is idiopathic as the patient may significantly downplay the amount of alcohol consumption. After a few days in the hospital and resolution of the arrhythmia, the patient frequently has no evidence of heart disease by history, physical examination, or diagnostic studies. The holiday heart syndrome, manifested primarily by arrhythmias, frequently occurs over holidays or weekends and is related to heavy alcohol ingestion in a chronic alcohol abuser. Frequently, the patient has no other signs of heart disease. The arrhythmias are predominantly supraventricular, with atrial fibrillation being the most common [115]. Although pharmacologic intervention or cardioversion may be required, it is not uncommon for normal sinus rhythm to return spontaneously. Electrolytes are usually normal, and moderate conduction delays documented by high-speed ECG are thought to be the underlying cause of the arrhythmias [123]. Although patients may be acutely intoxicated when they present, many are not. Occasionally, onset of the disorder may be preceded by a prolonged sleepless period. In a study of 100 consecutive patients with new-onset atrial fibrillation, one third were thought not to have clinical heart disease. Compared with control subjects, their alcohol intake for the 2 days before presentation was significantly greater. This was even more apparent in those who drank more than 30 gm alcohol per day [124]. When intoxicated subjects were studied with Holter monitors but excluded if they had evidence of ischemic heart disease, a population with significant arrhythmias including premature ventricular contractions (PVCs) was revealed. Increased circulating catecholamines were documented and propranolol decreased the incidence of arrhythmias.

Although magnesium deficiency is common in alcoholics, there is no evidence that this predisposes to arrhythmias [115]. Cardiac arrest has been reported in alcoholics without CAD and in fact a decreased fibrillation potential has been documented in an animal model of chronic alcoholism [125].

Malnutrition, Alcoholism, and the Heart. Malnutrition, as is seen in cirrhotics, is usually not present in patients with alcoholic cardiomyopathy unless concomitant hepatic disease is present [115].

Still, some alcoholics do have dietary deficiencies and in those with decreased intake of protein, calories, or both, a malnourished state with thiamine deficiency may develop. Thiamine deficiency is associated with arteriolar vasodilation and an increased cardiac output; a thin, pale flabby heart; and interstitial changes. Clinically, cardiac output has been variably described as increased and decreased and may therefore reflect underlying cardiac disease. Patients with increased outputs may reflect a decreased systemic resistance. With time cardiac function worsens until patients with severe cardiac failure develop hypoperfusion of the intestine and venous congestion, resulting in anorexia and malabsorption, which aggravates the already poor nutritional status [92]. Generalized edema is caused by decreased oncotic pressure as well as decreased cardiac output. Although it is generally believed that right ventricular failure is predominant when symptoms occur, there are in fact significant elevations of left ventricular end diastolic and pulmonary capillary wedge pressures. These signs of right and left ventricular compromise can be reversed with thiamine therapy [115]. Although cardiac disease due to full-blown thiamine deficiency may be seen in alcoholics, usually other signs of the disease are present, such as peripheral neuropathy, glossitis, and anemia [92]. The classic cardiac disorder is characterized by high-output failure with tachycardia, increased cardiac output, and elevated filling pressures of both the left and right sides of the heart [92]. Vasomotor depression is believed to be responsible for the high-output failure, due to a reduction in SVR. These patients are tachycardic, have an increased pulse pressure, an S_3, and frequently an apical systolic murmur. Chest x-ray usually shows cardiomegaly as well as the classic signs of congestive failure. Changes on ECG include decreased voltage, a prolonged QT interval, and abnormal T waves. These patients frequently do not respond to treatment with digitalis or diuretics. However, these agents may be quite useful during therapy, when the heart may have difficulty adjusting to the increased work load. Thiamine therapy may result in a decrease in cardiac output and heart size, as well as an increase of SVR and clearance of pulmonary congestion, all within 24 to 48 hours of administration [92].

Vitamin C–deficient diets are associated with complaints of chest pain and shortness of breath, as well as a prolonged PR interval and abnormal ST segments. These ECG changes are rapidly reversed with parenteral vitamin C [115].

Clinical Manifestations of Alcoholic Heart Disease. Manifestations of alcoholic cardiomyopathy may include chest pain, congestive failure, or arrhythmias. The major diagnostic feature is a history of ingesting intoxicating amounts of alcohol for many years. Denial is common and the history may need to be taken several times until the amount of alcohol abuse is apparent. Patients who drink may not volunteer this information. It has been shown that the two most reliable questions to ask in order to obtain the history of alcohol abuse are: (1) Have you had a drink in the past 24 hours? and (2) Have you ever had a drinking problem? [126]. The patient may have a family history of alcoholism, social problems, and accident-proneness. The particular beverage makes no difference. In contrast to other forms of myocardial disease, CHF manifests initially in fewer than half of patients with alcoholic cardiomyopathy. Many patients have arrhythmias without CHF. Classic anginal chest pain is a relatively common symptom reported, yet many of these patients have normal coronary arteries on angiography.

Alcoholics not infrequently delay medical evaluation and therefore may present initially with signs of advanced disease such as right-sided heart failure. As myocardial function decreases, low cardiac output will eventually result in dyspnea with exertion and subsequently at rest or when lying down. Cardiomegaly may be moderate with the onset of disease and yet return to normal when CHF resolves. With time cardiomegaly may become severe. At this time right-sided failure is often present, with clinical signs including distended jugular neck veins; a large, tender liver; and dependent edema.

Anesthetic Management of the Alcoholic Patient with Cardiac Disease

Anesthetic management of the alcoholic patient with cardiac disease will be determined by the degree of right- or left-sided failure. The history and physical examination are particularly important in these patients since abstinence may return heart function toward normal. Therefore, a patient with a history of congestive failure one year ago may now have normal exercise tolerance and ventricular function. The presence or absence of cardiomegaly on chest x-ray will help support or rule out severe cardiac dysfunction. The presence of tachycardia, arrhythmias, and clinical signs of failure will determine which monitors to place and which anesthetics would be most appropriate.

The choice of monitors is made with the usual considerations in mind. With mild cardiac dysfunction a central venous line may be adequate. If significant arrhythmias or electrolyte disturbances are present, an arterial line for frequent blood sampling will be useful. This will also assist in assessing the hemodynamic consequences of arrhythmias. Patients with a history of dyspnea, significant cardiomegaly, or signs of left-sided failure should have a pulmonary artery catheter placed preoperatively. The same applies for patients with signs of right-sided failure.

The first concern when choosing an anesthetic agent is the status of ventricular function. If ventricular function is compromised, the inhalational anesthetics should be used cautiously, as they may further depress the myocardium. Halothane should be avoided in those patients with arrhythmias. Ketamine may also aggravate the arrhythmogenic tendency of these patients. Hypertension due to peripheral vasoconstriction may be the first compensatory mechanism in the presence of myocardial dysfunction. Tachycardia may be present as well. Isoflurane in low doses may be appropriate in these patients, as it maintains forward flow due to decreased SVR and will maintain or increase the heart rate. The benefits of this agent should be carefully weighed, however, in patients known to have CAD. Droperidol may be a useful adjunct to anesthesia as it decreases systemic resistance and will maintain the compensatory tachycardia. Narcotics and benzodiazepines are usually well tolerated, although in the presence of severe ventricular dysfunction the combination of these agents may result in significant myocardial depression. Still, benzodiazepines are usually tolerated in patients with ventricular dysfunction when titrated in small doses and are useful adjuncts to anesthetic management, as they generally prevent the signs of alcohol withdrawal, which may begin as soon as 5 hours after the patient's last drink and usually peak in severity within 24 to 72 hours. These include agitation, tremors, and generalized seizures as well as autonomic dysfunction. The last two are obviously a problem in the perioperative period, but of most concern are the arrhythmias, which may occur even if the patient is presently sober. Since the sympathetic nervous system is probably related to their occurrence, β-blockers may be useful if the patient is found to have frequent PVCs and does not have severely compromised ventricular dysfunction.

Cardiac Disease in the Obese Patient

Epidemiology
Obesity is defined as a weight greater than 20 percent above ideal body weight. Between 20 and 30 percent of adult men and 30 to 40 percent of adult women are obese. Morbid obesity defines those patients who weigh more than 45 kg above ideal body weight and may be associated with increased perioperative morbidity [127].

Pathophysiology
Obese patients often have hypertension, which may contribute to cardiomegaly and left ventricular failure. The association with NIDDM and cardiovascular disease relates to patients with abdominal obesity and not gluteal-femoral obesity. This may be explained by the very sensitive free fatty acid mobilization system present in abdominal adipose tissue [128]. This may result in increased levels of glucose and insulin, and may be related to the increased incidence of hypertension, as the hyperinsulinemia of obesity contributes to activation of the sympathetic nervous system, resulting in increased cardiac output, SVR, and reabsorption of sodium by the kidneys. Obese patients are at an increased risk for coronary ischemia, primarily because of the increased incidence of hypertension, diabetes, and hyperlipoproteinemia. However, obesity itself represents a mild independent risk factor for ischemia [129]. In addition to all these factors that predispose to heart disease, it is important to understand that cardiac output needs to increase 100 cc per minute to perfuse each kilogram of adipose tissue. The perioperative period places an even greater stress on the already overworked cardiovascular system of the morbidly obese patient.

Obesity Hypoventilation Syndrome. The obesity hypoventilation syndrome is characterized by a decreased functional residual capacity (FRC), especially when the patient is in the supine position. This results in underventilation of the lung bases as some of these airways will be closed during part or even all of the respiratory cycle. Most obese patients increase their central respiratory drive sufficiently to maintain a normal arterial CO_2 tension. However, in a small percentage of obese patients hypercarbia develops, which in turn results in pulmonary hypertension, cor pulmonale, and right-

Table 15-19. Signs and symptoms seen in the obesity hypoventilation syndrome

Morbid obesity
Pedal edema
Cyanosis
Hepatomegaly
Increased S_2
Jugular venous distention
Alveolar hypoventilation (which can be voluntarily overcome)
Hypoxemia
Polycythemia
Cor pulmonale
Right ventricular failure

sided heart failure. The decreased FRC resulting in early airway closure also contributes to hypoxemia. The hypercarbia and hypoxemia are aggravated during sleep, when cortical influences to breathe are decreased even further. The most beneficial therapy is weight reduction. In patients who are to undergo surgery, a few days of oxygen therapy to prevent hypoxemia may decrease PA pressures somewhat. Progesterone, a respiratory stimulant, has been used as well. Signs and symptoms that may occur in the obesity hypoventilation syndrome are listed in Table 15-19.

Pickwickian Syndrome. Patients with the Pickwickian syndrome have cardiovascular problems similar to those seen in the obesity hypoventilation syndrome. Specifically, central apnea, hypoxemia, pulmonary hypertension, and cor pulmonale tend to develop, in addition to the classic symptom of this disorder, daytime somnolence [92]. If the history or physical examination suggests ischemia or left ventricular dysfunction, appropriate preoperative studies should be undertaken.

Hemodynamic Concerns in the Obese Patient
Obese patients have characteristic hemodynamic abnormalities of the cardiovascular system, including increased central and total blood volume, cardiac output, and left ventricular filling pressures [92]. Left ventricular filling pressures are frequently at the upper limits of normal and rise further with exercise, placing the patient at risk of alveolar

edema. Chronic volume and pressure overload produce eccentric hypertrophy, resulting in cardiac dilation and possibly decreased left ventricular function. At pathologic examination, obese patients may have not only left but also right ventricular hypertrophy. A small percentage of obese patients are also hypercapnic and hypoxemic, and may display pulmonary hypertension and right-sided heart failure. However, these signs and symptoms are more common in the obesity hypoventilation syndrome and the Pickwickian syndrome.

For patients with known ischemia or pulmonary hypertension, the pulmonary artery catheter will be helpful. It is important to understand that since these patients have increased cardiac indices and filling pressures, documentation of these should not trigger therapeutic diuresis, but rather the understanding that such values are necessary to perfuse the large body mass. However, if filling pressures are increased and cardiac index is not, pharmacologic means may be necessary to improve the patient's hemodynamics. The cardiac manifestations of obesity may respond to conventional therapy such as diuretics and digitalis, or in the acute setting inotropes and vasodilators.

Anesthetic Management of the Obese Patient with Cardiac Disease

For patients with a normal exercise tolerance, adequate fluid replacement and maintenance of good urine output are indicative of acceptable cardiac function. In such patients essentially any anesthetic technique can be used; there are no significant cardiovascular advantages for one inhalation anesthetic agent over another in such patients. If the history reveals a decreased exercise tolerance, preoperative assessment of cardiac function is in order. If time does not permit, central monitoring may be useful. If there are no signs of congestive failure, a central venous catheter may be adequate, bearing in mind that these patients may require elevated filling pressures. If fluid loading does not maintain urine output and/or blood pressure, a pulmonary artery catheter is required. Patients who require intraoperative inotropic therapy usually have a history and physical examination consistent with decreased ventricular function. However, occasional patients may not, and a borderline cardiac index in the face of elevated filling pressures is enough basis on which to initiate inotropic or vasodilator therapy, or both, as guided by hemodynamic parameters obtained from the pulmonary artery catheter. Such therapy may need to be continued into the postoperative period as well.

If urine output or blood pressure is compromised, inhalation agents can be discontinued and a narcotic technique substituted. Nitrous oxide is usually well tolerated but should be used cautiously in those patients with pulmonary hypertension. Arterial blood gas analysis is helpful to detect hypoxemia in those patients receiving low concentrations of oxygen. There are no specific contraindications to ketamine in obese patients with reasonable ventricular function, and it can be used if the situation calls for it.

While regional anesthesia may be technically difficult to perform, it can be safely used in obese patients. Since these individuals may require elevated filling pressures, adequate volume loading should precede performance of a regional technique. There are advantages and disadvantages to regional blockade in obese patients. If the surgical procedure is to be performed on the lower extremities, a regional technique will provide good anesthesia while avoiding the difficulties inherent in intubation and positive pressure ventilation. However, if an intraabdominal procedure is to be performed, the required level of blockade may compromise ventilatory function in an obese patient. Monitoring of end-tidal carbon dioxide and oxygen saturation is therefore imperative. A good alternative is the combination of a light general anesthetic and endotracheal intubation with regional blockade via an epidural catheter. Postoperatively, a continuous epidural narcotic infusion will aid respiratory status by providing good pain relief, thereby assisting deep breathing and the use of incentive spirometry.

Rheumatoid Arthritis

Epidemiology

Rheumatoid arthritis (RA) is a multisystem disease characterized by synovial inflammation of peripheral joints. It occurs in approximately 1 percent of the general population, with women being affected three times more often than men. It presents most frequently between the ages of 30 and 50, with 80 percent of patients developing the disease between 35 and 50 years. It is more common with increasing age and the tendency to affect women decreases with age. There is a genetic predisposition to the disease, as severe RA is about four times more common among first-degree relatives of patients with seropositive disease [130].

Pathophysiology

Rheumatoid arthritis is an immunologic disease. Activation of T cells, B cells, and complement results in a chronic inflammatory process that affects not only the joints but other tissues as well, including the heart. There may be a systemic arteritis, resulting in leg ulcers, peripheral neuropathy, and cardiac ischemia.

Clinical Manifestations

Patients often complain of generalized weakness, fatigue, anorexia, and vague musculoskeletal symptoms before the onset of synovitis. Such a prodrome may last weeks or months before the diagnosis is made. The diagnosis becomes easier to make as several joints gradually become involved, usually in a symmetric fashion. Though symmetric joint involvement is typical, occasional patients will have an asymmetric pattern. While some have mild disease, severe polyarthritis with severe deformity develops in others.

In about 30 percent of patients, only one or a few joints will be involved. In about 10 percent of patients, the onset is acute with rapid development of polyarthritis, frequently accompanied by fever, lymphadenopathy, and splenomegaly. Approximately 15 percent of patients will have remission of the disease and no significant remaining deformity [130]. Deforming bony changes may be evident on both physical and radiographic examination. Subcutaneous rheumatoid nodules are characteristic of the disease.

Though no tests specifically diagnose rheumatoid arthritis, certain laboratory findings such as rheumatoid factor, LE cells, antinuclear antibody, thrombocytosis, and neutropenia, as part of Felty's syndrome, are found with the disease [Adapted with permission from 130a]. Though rheumatoid factor may be present in up to 80 percent of patients with rheumatoid arthritis, it is present in many other diseases as well. Lupus erythematosus cells may be noted in up to 25 percent of patients, but the number of cells seen in a preparation is fewer than in patients with systemic lupus erythematosus (SLE). Antinuclear antibody is present in 10 to 50 percent of patients with RA, though usually in low titer. The exceptions are patients with long-standing and destructive RA, or those with vasculitis or Felty's and Sjögren's syndromes.

Cardiac Disease in Patients with Rheumatoid Arthritis

Cardiac problems seen in patients with rheumatoid arthritis include pericarditis, valvular disease, and conduction abnormalities. However, these problems are rarely of clinical significance. There may be an increased incidence of ischemic heart disease, which may be attributable to steroid use [131].

The most frequent clinical problem is pericarditis. It is more common in males with seropositive disease and is unrelated to the duration of the arthritis. It is present in 30 to 50 percent of patients with rheumatoid arthritis and is more common in those with subcutaneous nodules or a systolic murmur [132]. It is usually asymptomatic and detected by echocardiography or on postmortem examination. Only a small percentage of patients develop clinical manifestations of pericarditis and usually the course is benign, though some patients do develop constrictive pericarditis or tamponade resulting in death.

Treatment is that of the underlying disease with antiinflammatory agents or steroid preparations, or both. Corticosteroids are usually effective but chronic effusion or constriction may nevertheless follow [133, 134]. Though pericarditis often responds to treatment, it may recur and pericardiectomy may become necessary [135].

Though 20 percent of patients have coronary arteritis with inflammation of the intima and edema, only rarely does this result in angina or infarction. Myocarditis may occur but only rarely does it produce significant dysfunction. Inflammation and granuloma formation may affect the valves, most commonly involving the mitral and aortic. Occasionally, enough deformity may occur to produce significant regurgitation [92].

Complete AV block with a ventricular rhythm has been reported in a patient who underwent autopsy examination of the conduction system. Fibrotic patches believed to be healed granulomas were present and impinging on the conduction system. In addition there was narrowing of arterioles and small arteries leading to the conduction system. These changes occurred in the absence of cortisone administration and were therefore believed to be due to the rheumatoid process itself [136].

Anesthetic Management of the Rheumatoid Patient with Cardiac Disease

As noted above, significant cardiac disease is uncommon in patients with rheumatoid arthritis. However, the possibility of ischemia or conduction abnormalities should be borne in mind during the preoperative evaluation. The most significant concern is the patient with pericarditis and a large pericardial effusion; anesthetic management of such patients has been described in Chap. 8.

Thyroid Disease

Thyroid disease is most common among women between the ages of 20 and 60, but occurs in other populations as well. Since grossly abnormal thyroid function may have a significant effect on the cardiovascular system, it is important to understand these disease states, their diagnosis, and their treatment. One can then decide on an appropriate anesthetic for the clinical setting.

There are no clear data to document increased risk among patients with thyroid disease who are undergoing surgery. Still, it is challenging to manage myxedematous patients and it may be frightening to manage a patient in whom thyroid storm develops. It has therefore been recommended that patients be treated until they are in a euthyroid state before elective surgery is performed. However, urgent surgery should proceed and some have advocated that at least hypothyroidism should not delay urgent revascularization procedures [137].

Hypothyroidism

Epidemiology

Hypothyroidism is a common adult disease, being present in 3 to 6 percent of patients, depending on the population studied [2]. It may also present as depression in postpartum patients [138] and is not uncommon among the elderly, who may be asymptomatic.

Pathophysiology

The cause of hypothyroidism is thyroid disease 95 percent of the time. In 5 percent of cases, the etiology is suprathyroid in origin. The most common cause of thyroid hypothyroidism is that induced by radioactive ablation of the gland. Primary hypothyroidism is frequently associated with circulating antibodies directed against the thyroid. It may occur in association with other diseases in which autoantibodies are present, such as SLE, rheumatoid arthritis, and chronic hepatitis. Hypothyroidism may also occur as a multiglandular deficient state. The inability to synthesize thyroid hormone results in abnormally elevated thyroid-stimulating hormone (TSH) levels and the result is seen grossly as a goiter [139].

Suprathyroid hypothyroidism is most often due to postpartum pituitary necrosis or a tumor in the region of the pituitary, which results in decreased production of TSH. Hypothalamic hypothyroidism is less common, and produces the syndrome as a result of decreased secretion of thyrotropin releasing hormone (TRH) [139].

Laboratory Evaluation

The diagnosis of hypothyroidism is confirmed chemically. Since screening tests are often performed, most hypothyroid patients are diagnosed when asymptomatic, with elevated TSH levels being their only biochemical abnormality [137]. Patients with more apparent disease will have decreased levels of thyroid hormones as well as a decreased free thyroid index. Hypothyroidism in patients with severe systemic illness is at least partially due to poor conversion in the periphery of T4 to T3. Simons and associates [140] reported a direct correlation between level of illness as appraised by the American Society of Anesthesiologists (ASA) classification and the level of hypothyroidism. Patients who have been adequately treated should have serum T4, T3, TSH, and free thyroxine index within normal limits. In addition to abnormalities of thyroid hormones, hypothyroid patients may have increased creatine phosphokinase (CPK), serum glutamic oxaloacetic transaminase (SGOT), and lactic dehydrogenase (LDH), and if they present in congestive failure may be mistakenly diagnosed as suffering an acute myocardial infarction.

Clinical Manifestations

Since more attention has been focused on occult hypothyroidism, hypothyroid states are being diagnosed earlier. It is therefore rare for all the manifestations to develop and some patients may complain only of dyspnea or fatigue. Physical findings that correlate well with hypothyroidism are limited to delayed ankle reflexes, huskiness of the voice, and dry skin [141]. Mild hypothyroidism is not associated with major cardiac problems. One third of hypothyroid patients have a pericardial effusion but this produces tamponade only rarely. The pericardial as well as pleural effusions are caused by increased capillary permeability. Many signs and symptoms normally ascribed to cardiac disease are present in patients with moderate to severe hypothyroidism. Patient complaints may include fatigue, dyspnea, orthopnea, and paroxysmal nocturnal dyspnea. Table 15-20 lists the cardiovascular effects that may be present in hypothyroidism.

Patients with severe hypothyroidism may present in myxedema coma. They frequently have bradycardia and hypothermia, and may have a pericardial effusion and CHF. Impaired water excretion and vasoconstriction may contribute to the congestive failure. They may also be hypothermic.

The chest x-ray in hypothyroidism may show cardiomegaly and bilateral pleural effusions, as well as other signs of congestive failure. Though hypothyroid patients may have ECG changes, the disease has no specific ECG abnormalities. Low-voltage, prolonged AV conduction and decreased P-wave voltage may occur. ST segment and T-wave changes are nonspecific but may mimic ischemia. Though the QT interval is invariably prolonged, it is often difficult or impossible to measure due to the T-wave changes [92]. These changes as well as sick sinus syndrome may be particularly likely to occur in hypothyroid patients with associated amyloidosis [142].

Preoperative Preparation of the Hypothyroid Patient

Though the T4 can be used as a guide to treatment, patients who have been adequately treated should have serum T4, T3RU, T3, and TSH within normal limits. Ideally, patients should be chemically euthyroid before being brought to the operating room. However, urgent or emergent procedures may make it necessary to proceed in patients who are significantly hypothyroid. These patients should receive their usual daily dose of thyroid replacement. Patients who are myxedematous and in failure will require more aggressive therapy, possibly including intravenous hormone replacement. Obviously, myxedematous patients should only be brought to the operating room for lifesaving surgery. L-Thyroxine can be given in a dose of 200 to 500 μg followed by oral replacement. This will frequently result in an improvement in cardiovascular function within 24 to 72 hours. However, this is potentially dangerous, as asymptomatic CAD is a significant problem in the general adult population and aggressive treatment with hormone replacement can precipitate acute coronary ischemia. The risk of rapidly inducing the euthyroid state and perhaps inducing angina should be considered, taking into account whether the patient has signs of cardiac disease from hypothyroidism, such as congestive failure [143]. The decision seems more difficult in patients with known symptomatic CAD, in whom treatment may result in a significant increase in anginal symptoms. However, the combined use of thyroid replacement and β-blockade may be an appropriate course before urgent noncardiac surgery. Deaths from arrhythmias, congestive failure, cardiogenic shock, and myocardial infarction have occurred in nontreated hypo-

Table 15-20. Cardiovascular effects of hypothyroidism

Bradycardia
ECG abnormalities
Decreased pulse pressure
Decreased blood pressure
Weak arterial pulses
Distant heart sounds
Decreased stroke volume
Decreased cardiac output (as much as 40%)
Increased systemic vascular resistance
Prolonged circulation time
Cardiomegaly
Pericardial effusions
Pleural effusions
Congestive heart failure

thyroid patients who were awaiting bypass surgery [2]. Delaying elective surgery for treatment in patients with less severe coronary disease may be appropriate.

In addition to thyroid replacement, some administer perioperative steroids to patients who are significantly hypothyroid because of the association with Addison's disease and its relative steroid deficiency [2].

After replacement, the lack of signs of congestive failure and normal thyroid function tests are reassuring. However, it should be noted that Lee and associates [144] have reported that hypothyroid patients have depressed systolic ejection force that improves with return to the euthyroid state, though this may take up to 6 months on average. It is important to realize this when administering anesthesia to a patient who was recently rendered euthyroid with replacement therapy. We would probably not place invasive monitoring in the absence of history and physical findings of heart disease.

Anesthetic Management of the Hypothyroid Patient

Care should be taken not to overventilate hypothyroid patients. Because of their decreased metabolic rate, they may have a decreased ventilatory requirement [145]. Decreased $PaCO_2$ may result in decreased sympathetic tone. The reduction in pH and associated decrease in ionized calcium may also decrease the inotropic state. Also, hypocapnia may increase tissue oxygen demand [146, 147], while decreasing supply due to increased hemoglobin affinity for oxygen. Several mechanisms have been proposed to explain the increased oxygen demand, but the underlying cause seems to be decreased H^+ concentration.

Hypothyroid patients may manifest pronounced responses or side effects when administered usual doses of digoxin [148, 149], nitrates [150, 151], or propranolol [152, 153]. Hypothyroid patients taking propranolol have also been reported to require significantly less narcotics than expected [145, 154]. Also, it should be noted that the administration of ketamine to patients receiving thyroid replacement may precipitate severe tachycardia and hypertension, as well as arrhythmias, even in patients who are clinically euthyroid [155].

Anesthetic Management of the Hypothyroid Patient with Cardiac Disease

Hypothyroid patients may be particularly difficult to manage since various concerns need to be addressed simultaneously. Mild hypothyroidism will probably not have a significant impact on anesthetic management. However, it should be borne in mind that ventricular function may not have returned to normal in patients who have recently been rendered chemically euthyroid, and severe hemodynamic stress may place such patients at risk for congestive failure. Patients with a good exercise capacity will likely tolerate most anesthetics well. However, in patients with signs and symptoms of decreased ventricular function anesthetics need to be chosen more judiciously, and monitoring requirements will increase. Poor ventricular function may preclude the use of myocardial depressants such as the inhalation anesthetics. Myxedematous patients will likely have received intravenous L-thyroxine and though ventricular function may begin to improve within hours this may precipitate coronary ischemia. Even narcotic-based techniques may result in borderline hemodynamic function in the myxedematous patient and inotropic therapy may be necessary. Myxedematous patients will require an arterial line and a pulmonary artery catheter. Less severe states of hypothyroidism with more reasonable ventricular function will require less monitoring. In patients with significant hypothyroidism, one of the newer nondepolarizing muscle relaxants may be preferable to pancuronium, the vagolytic effects of which may precipitate tachycardia and myocardial ischemia.

Hyperthyroidism

Epidemiology

Graves' disease has a classic triad that includes diffuse goiter, exophthalmos, and dermopathy. These signs need not appear at the same time and, in fact, frequently do not. Although Graves' disease may occur at any age, it is most common between the ages of 20 and 40. It is more common in women, with the ratio of women to men possibly being as high as 7:1. HLA haplotypes are associated with the disease, which explains its familial occurrence. Clinical syndromes that may occur in the same patient over time include Graves' disease, Hashimoto's thyroiditis, and primary myxedema. All three are believed to be autoimmune diseases.

An unusual but potentially problematic form of hyperthyroidism is the Jod-Basedow phenomenon, in which patients with multinodular goiter are administered iodine for x-ray studies. These patients may develop full-blown hyperthyroidism due to uptake of the iodine into the gland and if elderly may manifest severe cardiovascular manifestations. It is recommended that if elderly patients with multinodular goiter need x-ray studies they should receive therapy with propylthiouracil, 450 to 600 mg per day, before and for 1 week after the administration of iodine to prevent this phenomenon from occurring. More unusual forms of hyperthyroidism may be due to secretion of thyroid hormone or TSH from ectopic tissue and have been described elsewhere [139].

Pathophysiology
Hyperthyroidism is most frequently due to overproduction of thyroid hormones by the gland itself. It is called Graves' disease when immunologically mediated or toxic nodular goiter is due to inherent glandular function. Excessive release of hormones may also occur in patients with inflamed glands such as in thyroiditis [156]. In the elderly, hyperthyroidism may be referred to as apathetic because of a paucity of clinical findings.

An excess of thyroid hormone does not increase sympathetic nervous system activity as norepinephrine levels are normal in thyrotoxic patients, so a normal amount of sympathetic activity seems to evoke an exaggerated physiologic effect. Perhaps the best explanation for the ability of thyroid hormone to exert effects on the sympathetic nervous system, independently of catecholamines, is the fact that thyroid hormone can induce the Na^+/K^+ ATPase pump and its messenger ribonucleic acids (RNAs). The effect of thyroid hormone in target tissues may not be a direct effect on the sodium-potassium pump, but rather augmentation of passive Na^+ influx and potassium efflux [157].

Increased levels of thyroid hormones increase total body oxygen consumption, thereby increasing the work load on the heart, and possibly leading to high-output failure. Thyroid hormone increases the density of beta receptors in the heart and has direct inotropic, chronotropic, and dromotropic effects [92, 158].

The cardiac hypertrophy associated with hyperthyroidism is mediated via myosin isoenzyme V1, which results in more rapid contraction [19]. Thyroid hormone also increases myocardial concentrations of actin and myosin, as well as the basal state of contractility and adenylate cyclase activity. Muscular dilatation and hypertrophy commonly result. Hyperthyroidism also enhances responses of the beta receptor. In some tissues thyroid hormone causes an increase in receptor number. In other tissues even if the number is not increased the coupling of receptors to the cAMP system is augmented, thus enhancing or amplifying the response to catecholamines.

Although it is not clear whether a hyperadrenergic state results in the cardiac effects, or whether a specific pathologic entity is associated with hyperthyroidism, it is clear that the use of β-blocking agents attenuates most of the cardiovascular effects of hyperthyroidism [159]. This may be particularly important for an elderly patient with underlying cardiac disease, in whom a persistent tachycardia may result in ischemia, congestive failure, or death. A decrease in heart rate is a good sign that the β-blocker is attenuating the cardiac effects of the excess thyroid hormone [160]. However, it is important to remember that total body oxygen consumption is not decreased, as it depends on direct effects of thyroid hormone on the sodium pump [161].

Laboratory Evaluation
The diagnosis of hyperthyroidism is usually easily made by an elevated T4, resin T3 uptake, T3, and free T4 index. Alternatively, some laboratories measure free thyroxine directly, which establishes the diagnosis. Sometimes there will be a normal T4 and RT3U but increased T3 and FT3I indicating T3 toxicosis. There are no clinical signs or symptoms that distinguish T3 toxicosis from that due to thyroxine. While some patients with T3 toxicosis never manifest an increased T4, with time many patients display elevations of both hormones. For this reason some believe T3 toxicosis is a prodrome of thyrotoxicosis [162]. Finally, in mild hyperthy-

roidism both thyroid hormones may be in the upper range of normal, and a basal TSH as well as a TRH stimulation test may be necessary to make the diagnosis.

Clinical Manifestations

Presenting signs often include systolic hypertension, systolic murmur, palpitations, and fatigue, as well as angina or symptoms of heart failure in those with underlying heart disease. Elderly patients may have cardiac manifestations as the only sign of their hyperthyroid state. Though hyperthyroidism can cause myocardial dysfunction, angina and congestive failure are unusual unless underlying heart disease is present, and frequently angina and congestive failure resolve with treatment of the hyperthyroid state. In apathetic hyperthyroidism sympathomimetic signs may be absent and symptoms or signs may be limited to only one organ system. On physical examination a hyperactive precordium may be noted as well as an increase in S_2 and P_2, and the presence of an S_3. An increased incidence of mitral valve prolapse occurs in hyperthyroid patients, which may be heard as a mid-systolic murmur, with or without a click at the left sternal border or apex. The Means-Lerman scratch, described as a scratchy systolic sound heard at the second left intercostal space during exhalation, is thought to be caused by the rubbing of hyperdynamic pericardium against pleura. Cardiac manifestations involving the cardiovascular system are listed in Table 15-21.

Generalized signs and symptoms of hyperthyroidism include tremors, nervousness, inability to sleep, heat intolerance, excessive sweating, and weight loss. Proximal muscle weakness may present as difficulty in climbing stairs. The skin is often warm and moist, and the hair fine and silky. Hyperreflexia is frequently present. Some patients have an ocular stare due to wide palpebral fissures and lid lag while those with Graves' disease have exophthalmos [139].

Electrocardiographic Changes

Electrocardiographic changes in hyperthyroidism are essentially those of rate and rhythm. Both sinus tachycardia and atrial fibrillation occur. The PR interval will be prolonged. More serious abnormalities of AV conduction may occur including complete heart block, even in the absence of cardiomegaly or congestive failure [163]. Hyperthyroidism is associated with hypomagnesemia and if it occurs in combination with hypokalemia may result in conduction abnormalities, arrhythmias, and even ventricular fibrillation [164].

Treatment

Though treatment regimens for many systemic diseases are managed by the internist, the anesthesiologist should be knowledgeable regarding those for hyperthyroidism. The severe effects of hyperthyroidism on the cardiovascular system are such that, in the event of perioperative thyrotoxicosis, such knowledge may have a significant impact on the outcome of the patient.

Treatment of hyperthyroidism usually includes radioactive iodine although during the acute phase hyperthyroidism may be controlled with antithyroid agents such as propylthiouracil or methimazole, which inhibit the formation of thyroid hormones by interfering with the uptake of iodine into tyrosyl residues of thyroglobulin. The usual dose of propylthiouracil is 75 to 150 mg every 8 hours, although up to 1,200 mg per day may be required. When more than 300 mg per day is needed, it is best to divide the doses to be given every 6 or even every 4 hours, as its half-life in plasma is approximately 2 hours. The initial dose of methimazole is 5 or 10 mg every 8 hours, with a half-life of 6 to 13 hours. Though either agent can be used, propylthiouracil also inhibits the peripheral deiodination of thyroxine to triiodothyronine, and therefore results in more rapid improvement in symptoms. Although some patients with severe hyperthyroidism show a response within one day, it is more common

Table 15-21. Cardiac manifestations of hyperthyroidism

Sinus tachycardia
Atrial fibrillation
Angina
Congestive failure
Increased cardiac output
Increased stroke volume
Increased pulse pressure
Increased left ventricular contractility

---

for the initial response to take several days and sometimes up to 2 weeks.

Frequently, it is necessary to control the manifestations of hyperthyroidism with β-blockers during the initial period of treatment. The usual dose of oral propranolol required is 20 to 40 mg every 6 hours. It is important to remember that since intravenous propranolol avoids first-pass hepatic metabolism, the equivalent intravenous dose is just 1 mg, and even this should be administered in small increments. Propranolol also has some ability to decrease the peripheral conversion of T4 to T3. Still, for the most part, β-blockade only controls the manifestations of the disease, and therapy to control the underlying disease is required to prevent thyroid crisis during the stress of the perioperative period. The use of β-blockers may adversely affect adrenergic support of myocardial contractility and may result in congestive failure in patients with underlying cardiac disease. In this latter group, it may be helpful to place a pulmonary artery catheter during the preparation for surgery to construct Starling curves at different points in therapy.

While thyrotoxicosis has been controlled historically with β-blockers or sodium iodide, or both, a case has been reported in which the clinical signs of muscle rigidity and pyrexia responded immediately to dantrolene, which was given because of a mistaken diagnosis of malignant hyperthermia. The clinical scenario was subsequently proven to be thyrotoxicosis. Increased calcium flux at the sarcoplasmic reticulum has been associated with increased thyroxine levels, which offers an explanation for the benefits of dantrolene in this disorder [165].

Interestingly, a paradoxical response occurs with the administration of iodide. Iodide's ability to acutely inhibit synthesis of iodotyrosine and iodothyronine is known as the Wolff-Chaikoff effect, but its most important effect is inhibition of the release of thyroid hormone. Lugol's solution contains iodine, which is reduced to iodide in the intestine before it is absorbed. Sodium iodide is also available as a 10 percent solution for intravenous use. It is primarily for patients with severe manifestations of the disease, such as thyroid storm, or for patients with severe thyrocardiac disease [166]. Better control of the hyperthyroid state is achieved if antithyroid agents are begun before the administration of iodide preparations [167].

Anesthetic Management of the Hyperthyroid Patient with Cardiac Disease

Certainly, it is preferable that all patients presenting for surgery be chemically euthyroid. However, the need for emergency surgery may preclude this possibility. During preoperative evaluation of the patient with hyperthyroidism, a careful history and physical examination should focus on identifying signs and symptoms of cardiovascular disease. By taking into account the current manifestations of hyperthyroidism, the anesthesiologist should be able to choose appropriate monitors and anesthetics. The main concerns are to avoid myocardial depressants in those patients in congestive failure and to avoid arrhythmogenic agents in general. In addition to agents used to treat the hyperthyroid state itself, β-blockers can be administered to control tachycardia, angina, or systolic hypertension. Because of the tendency to arrhythmias, we prefer not to administer halothane or ketamine to these patients. In the face of good ventricular function, enflurane, isoflurane, or intravenous anesthetics may all be acceptable. However, heart rate should be considered when choosing the anesthetic, as isoflurane or droperidol may aggravate tachycardia. A nondepolarizing muscle relaxant with minimal cardiovascular effects may be preferable to pancuronium, which may worsen tachycardia.

While regional anesthesia can be used for these patients, monitoring for signs and symptoms of angina and congestive failure is important. The occurrence of an arrhythmia with hemodynamic compensation may require cardioversion. An arterial line may be appropriate for monitoring hyperthyroid patients receiving a regional anesthetic if they are hypertensive and have a history of arrhythmias.

Systemic Lupus Erythematosus

Epidemiology

Systemic lupus erythematosus is an autoimmune disease that most commonly affects women of childbearing age, particularly during the second and third decades of life. However, it also may affect men, children, and the elderly. In the United

States it occurs in between 15 and 50 patients in 100,000. It is both more common and more severe in blacks than in whites.

Pathophysiology

Lupus results in the deposition of antibodies and immune complexes to tissues, thereby damaging them. Involved organs include the heart, brain, kidneys, joints, and skin, so that arthralgias, fever, pleuritis, and rashes are frequent presenting symptoms.

Laboratory Evaluation

Complement levels are decreased in most patients with SLE but are usually normal or increased in patients with other connective tissue disorders [168]. Most patients have a positive LE preparation at some point during their illness. Antinuclear antibodies and rheumatoid factor are often detected. Although the LE cell and anti-DNA antibodies are present in SLE, they are not diagnostic of the disease, as they are also present in other autoimmune diseases. However, levels of anti-DNA antibody do correlate with the severity of the disease.

Lupus usually follows a chronic course, with more than 80 percent of patients alive at 10 years. Most patients die of infections, renal failure, or disease of the central nervous system. Rarely, the course is acute and severe. Stress such as that due to pregnancy, surgery, or infection may exacerbate lupus. A lupus-like syndrome may be produced by hydralazine, procainamide, isoniazid, penicillamine, or nonbarbiturate anticonvulsants. Patients who are slow acetylators of hydralazine or procainamide are more likely to manifest the lupus-like syndrome. The drug-induced syndrome is similar to the spontaneous disease but the manifestations and progression of the disease are usually milder [169].

Nonspecific symptoms may include fatigue, fever, anorexia, and weight loss. A characteristic malar rash may occur. Renal manifestations may include proteinuria and the nephrotic syndrome and even renal failure [170]. Pulmonary disease may develop and patients may complain of a dry cough and shortness of breath. Blood gases may demonstrate arterial hypoxemia and the chest x-ray may reveal diffuse infiltrates and pleural effusions. Pulmonary function tests frequently reveal a restrictive pattern of disease.

Cardiovascular Effects

The cardiovascular system may be affected by SLE in many ways. Still, it is uncommon for SLE to cause significant morbidity or mortality due to cardiac disease. Myocarditis is common on histologic examination but rarely results in congestive failure. However, it does parallel the course of the disease and congestive failure may occur especially in association with hypertension. The myocarditis may also cause conduction abnormalities. Patients with SLE have an increased incidence of atherosclerosis of the coronary arteries. It is unknown if this is an effect of the disease or the commonly associated hypertension or treatment with glucocorticoids. Arteritis of the coronary arteries may occur but rarely produces ischemia [92]. Hypertension is the most common cause of myocardial hypertrophy and congestive failure in patients with SLE, and it is more common in patients who have renal disease or are taking steroid preparations.

Systemic lupus erythematosus may cause a pancarditis with involvement of the pericardium, endocardium, myocardium, and the coronaries. The pericardium is the region most involved, both clinically and at postmortem examination [171, 172]. A benign pericarditis with no apparent etiology may be the first manifestation of SLE, and more than half of patients with active lupus have a pericardial effusion at some time during their disease [171]. In most SLE patients the pericardial involvement is clinically silent. Rarely, lupus pericarditis may result in constrictive pericarditis [171, 173] or acute tamponade [174]. The pericarditis that occurs with lupus is most commonly diffuse and fibrinous. In patients with a long history of lupus who have responded to anti-inflammatory drugs, pericarditis occurs in more than half of patients, but a postmortem examination is more likely to reveal a healed fibrous lesion as opposed to a more active fibrinous pericarditis [172]. A rare patient with lupus pericarditis will develop a purulent pericarditis. This tends to occur in those who have severe systemic disease and renal failure, especially those who are immunosuppressed. This form of pericarditis is life threatening [175].

The pericarditis seen with lupus may present with only a pericardial friction rub or a very large pericardial effusion. Patients may have transient signs of ischemia on the ECG and are frequently tachycardic. Patients who have pericarditis usually have myocardial disease as well. It is rare for SLE to result in large enough effusions to require drainage [176]. In rare cases of cardiovascular inflammation due to SLE, it may be necessary to administer nonsteroidals, steroids, or even cytotoxic agents to these patients.

The most well-known cardiac lesion associated with SLE is Libman-Sacks or "verrucous" endocarditis. The lesions are fibrinous sterile vegetations that may occur anywhere on the valve surfaces but most commonly on the left side, especially the undersurface of the mitral valve. Although up to 40 percent of patients with SLE have evidence of endocarditis at autopsy, the endocarditis of SLE is usually clinically silent with no associated valvular dysfunction. Although it is unusual for valvular dysfunction to occur in the acute stage, the healed form of the disease results in formation of fibrous scar, which may lead to valvular dysfunction, most commonly mitral or aortic insufficiency. Patients who have been treated with corticosteroids may have smaller and fewer endocardial lesions. Those treated with steroids may also have univalvular lesions rather than multivalvular and have them predominantly on the left side of the heart, with the mitral valve most frequently affected [177–179]. The verrucous lesions also present a risk of endocarditis and patients with this history should receive prophylactic antibiotics (see Chap. 17).

A mild cardiomyopathy may occur in lupus patients. This is supported by hemodynamic and echocardiographic studies that suggest decreased systolic and diastolic function during exercise [173]. The myocardial abnormalities are due to autoimmune disease of the myocardium. It is usually difficult to differentiate small changes in cardiac function secondary to an abnormal myocardium from those due to hypertension, ischemia, or pericarditis.

Chest X-ray and Electrocardiographic Findings

Cardiomegaly may be present if a significant pericardial effusion is present. If coronary disease or myocarditis has resulted in poor left ventricular function, classic signs of congestive failure may be present as well.

Arteritis may result in occlusive arterial lesions or scarring involving the sinoatrial (SA) and AV nodes. Localized fibrosis or collagen degeneration may be present as well. These changes, as well as pericarditis, are likely responsible for the ECG abnormalities, which may be present in up to 50 percent of patients with SLE [180]. Most patients, but especially those with pericarditis, have ST or T-wave changes. Other abnormalities that may occur include abnormal P waves, varying degrees of bundle branch block, and signs of right and left ventricular hypertrophy. In a study of ECG changes in 137 patients over a 5-year period, Hejtmancik and associates [171] reported sinus tachycardia to be the most frequent abnormal rhythm. Others included paroxysmal nodal tachycardia in one patient and atrial fibrillation in another, each occurring in patients who were neither in congestive failure nor receiving digitalis. One patient who was not digitalized developed ventricular fibrillation, which was the cause of death [171].

Anesthetic Management for the Lupus Patient with Cardiac Disease

Anesthetic preoperative evaluation should take the usual approach, looking for signs of conduction abnormalities, pericardial disease, ischemia, or ventricular abnormalities. Treatment of hypertension, congestive heart failure, and arrhythmias should be with the usual appropriate agents. Patients who manifest various degrees of heart block should probably not receive halothane or sufentanil. Pancuronium may be preferable for these patients due to its vagolytic properties. Enflurane or isoflurane can be used as long as contractility is not severely impaired. A narcotic-based technique with superimposed inhalation anesthetic may be ideal for hemodynamic stability with good blood pressure control. The presence of symptoms that suggest coronary ischemia should lead one to choose agents that will not cause tachycardia. A paradox may be present in the patient with a large pericardial effusion and hemodynamic instability. The benefits of ketamine in this situation will need to be weighed against the possibility of inducing coronary ischemia.

The use of regional anesthesia for these patients is acceptable, bearing in mind the usual concerns for patients with ischemic disease or conduction abnormalities. The presence of a large pericardial effusion would preclude a regional technique, as such patients may develop severe hemodynamic instability with loss of vascular tone and decreased cardiac filling.

Acquired Immunodeficiency Syndrome

Patients with AIDS are known to have frequent opportunistic infections of the lungs. Since these infections may result in large A-a gradients, anesthesiologists have learned to be aware of these problems. However, cardiac disease also occurs in AIDS patients and may be life threatening. It is therefore important to be aware of the cardiovascular effects of this disease.

Epidemiology

The acquired immunodeficiency syndrome has reached epidemic proportions on the global scale. It is believed that between 1 and 1.5 million people are infected within the United States. The disease is not limited to adults. By mid-1990, approximately 2,000 cases had been reported in children below the age of 13.

Sexual contact is the most common mode of transmission of the human immunodeficiency (HIV) virus. Transmission occurs between homosexual and heterosexual partners. During heterosexual contact women are much more likely to contract the virus than men. It is also transmitted via the blood, a common mechanism among intravenous drug users who share their needles with others. Similarly, the virus can be transmitted via blood transfusion. Despite routine testing, there is approximately a 1 in 40,000 incidence of a false-negative test, thus resulting in contamination of the blood supply. Clearly, the incidence of false-negative tests varies in different geographic locations. Finally, the virus can also be spread from mother to fetus, as well as via breastfeeding [181].

Pathophysiology

Acquired immunodeficiency virus produces a state of generalized immunosuppression. Cell-mediated immunity is the most compromised. The result is a high incidence of opportunistic infections and cancers. Neoplasms that may occur include Kaposi's sarcoma, Hodgkin's disease, some B-cell lymphomas, and some carcinomas. The Epstein-Barr virus may play a role in causing some of the B-cell lymphomas. The opportunistic infections may result in significant cardiac effects, which are discussed in the following section.

The primary defect of the immune system is due to abnormalities of the T_4 population of thymus-derived lymphocytes. These abnormalities are of both a qualitative and quantitative nature. The HIV virus transcribes its RNA to DNA by utilizing the host's reverse transcriptase. Several factors may result in conversion from a latent process to active infection, and have been discussed elsewhere [181].

Signs and symptoms of AIDS are well known. These patients may complain of chronic fatigue and weight loss. Dyspnea, due to pulmonary disease, is common. These patients are at risk for pneumonia from the usual as well as opportunistic infections.

Cardiovascular Effects

It is now becoming evident that AIDS patients are also at risk for cardiac disease. Lewis [183] reported on autopsy findings of cardiac problems in AIDS patients. Lesions found included dilated cardiomyopathy, marantic (thrombotic, nonbacterial) endocarditis, right ventricular hypertrophy, pericardial effusions, and fibrinous pericarditis. Several patients also had findings of Kaposi's sarcoma invading the pericardium and myocardium [182]. In 58 consecutively autopsied patients with AIDS, Reilly and associates [183] reported that of the 32 patients without histopathologic myocarditis, none had clinical left ventricular (LV) dysfunction, congestive failure, or ventricular tachycardia. Twenty-six patients in this study had histopathologic myocarditis, and, of these, 15 had more than one clinical abnormality. These included 10 with abnormal ECGs; 4 with abnormalities of the pericardium; 6 with LV dysfunction, congestive failure, or both; and 4 who had experienced ventricular tachycardia [183]. Monsuez and colleagues [184] reported that pericardial tamponade was the most common abnormality in their series of AIDS patients, and in 8 of the 11 patients with tamponade, studies of the fluid yielded the causative agent.

Myocarditis in patients with AIDS is usually due to opportunistic infection or metastatic involvement by Kaposi's sarcoma. Patients with AIDS often have a mild focal myocarditis, but occasionally, a patient will manifest four-chamber cardiac enlargement and severe congestive failure that does not respond to therapy [185].

Cardiac effects of the disease may affect all parts of the heart. Right ventricular dilatation has been reported in 17 percent of AIDS patients, biventricular dilatation in 9 percent, and pericardial effusion in 21 percent [186].

Opportunistic Infections and the Cardiovascular System. Opportunistic infections may result in pericarditis, myocarditis, or endocarditis, each with its associated signs and symptoms. Candidiasis, cryptococcosis, toxoplasmosis, and mycobacterial disease are some of the agents responsible for cardiac manifestations of AIDS. Bacterial infections that are most frequently encountered in AIDS patients include *Salmonella*, *Haemophilus influenzae*, and *Streptococcus pneumoniae*. *Salmonella* may result in myocarditis, *Haemophilus influenzae* infections may cause pericarditis and rarely endocarditis, and *Streptococcus pneumoniae* endocarditis can be particularly destructive to valves.

Since these patients often have indwelling catheters, *Staphylococcus aureus* and *epidermidis* septicemia are not uncommon and bring with them their attendant risk of endocarditis. The presence of a murmur should make one consider the possibility of endocarditis, and the value of a preoperative echocardiogram should be weighed.

Anesthetic Concerns in the Patient with AIDS-Induced Cardiac Disease

Though it is clear that myocarditis and its associated problems occur in critically ill AIDS patients who die, the incidence of cardiac problems in AIDS patients who are less ill is not known. It is therefore best to consider the history and physical examination when evaluating these patients preoperatively. One should consider the diagnosis of congestive failure in AIDS patients who are dyspneic and have rales on examination or pulmonary infiltrates on chest x-ray, and such patients may warrant measurement of ejection fraction preoperatively, as well as placement of invasive lines [183].

In addition to cardiac disease, additional causes of hemodynamic instability that may occur in AIDS patients include autonomic neuropathy and adrenal insufficiency. Autonomic neuropathy has been reported as a cause of vasovagal reactions in five AIDS patients undergoing fine-needle aspiration of the lung, and one of these patients died. Craddock and associates [187] discussed tests of autonomic function, which may predict risk of this problem in AIDS patients.

Anesthetic Management of the AIDS Patient with Cardiac Disease

Cardiovascular function in AIDS patients varies greatly. Among those who are young and have no other medical problems, cardiac function may be preserved even late in the course of the disease. In older patients with other contributory factors as well as in some young patients, severe cardiovascular dysfunction may occur. For those patients in congestive failure, arterial pressure and pulmonary artery pressure should be continuously monitored. The possibility of ventricular arrhythmias should be borne in mind. Halothane is best avoided in these patients, though enflurane or isoflurane may be an acceptable choice in patients who do not have severely compromised ventricular function. A narcotic-based technique may offer stability of both rhythm and blood pressure. Patients with large pericardial effusions may be critically ill. Though ketamine can be considered for anesthetic induction, drainage of pericardial fluid is perhaps best performed under local anesthesia.

Other concerns notwithstanding, a regional technique can be chosen if cardiovascular status permits. The usual concerns regarding volume shifts in patients with cardiovascular compromise apply. For patients with large pericardial effusions, vasodilation secondary to sympathetic blockade may result in severe hemodynamic compromise.

Our discussion has focused on several of the more common systemic diseases. However, we approach all systemic diseases in a similar fashion. During the preoperative evaluation, we concentrate history-taking and physical examination skills in those areas that reflect manifestations of cardiac disease. Further preoperative testing may be indicated when the history and physical examination do not adequately define the nature of the patient's problems. The manifestations of cardiac disease may be classified into one of several categories, such as ischemia, ventricular hypertrophy, congestive failure, arrhythmias, and so forth. An appropriate monitor and anesthetic can then be chosen based on such evaluation. By using such an approach, today's anesthesiologists will be able to provide their patients with the highest standard of care.

REFERENCES

1. Gerson, MC, Hurst, JM, et al. Cardiac prognosis in noncardiac geriatric surgery. Ann Intern Med 103: 832, 1985.
2. Roizen, MF. Anesthetic Implications of Concurrent Diseases. In RD Miller, RF Cucchiara, et al. (eds), Anesthesia (3rd ed). New York: Churchill Livingstone, 1990. Pp 793–893.
3. Trappe, H-J, Brogada, P, et al. Prognosis of patients with ventricular tachycardia and ventricular fibrillation: Role of the underlying etiology. J Am Coll Cardiol 12:166, 1988.
4. Buxton, AE, Marchlinski, FE, et al. Prognostic factors in nonsustained ventricular tachycardia. Am J Cardiol 53:1275, 1984.
5. Schulze, RA, Jr, Strauss, HW, Pitt, B. Sudden death in the year following myocardial infarction: Relation to ventricular premature contractions in the late hospital phase and left ventricular ejection fraction. Am J Med 62:192, 1977.
6. Swerdlow, CD, Winkle, RA, Mason, JW. Determinants of survival in patients with ventricular tachyarrhythmias. N Engl J Med 308:1436, 1983.
7. Miller, RD, Way, WL, Eger, EI, II. The effects of alpha-methyldopa, reserpine, guanethidine, and iproniazid on minimum alveolar anesthetic requirement (MAC). Anesthesiology 29:1153, 1968.
8. Lewis, L, Robinson, RF, et al. Fatal adrenal cortical insufficiency precipitated by surgery during prolonged continuous cortisone treatment. Ann Intern Med 39:116, 1953.
9. Udelsman, R, Ramp, J, et al. Adaptation during surgical stress; a reevaluation of the role of glucocorticoids. J Clin Invest 77:1377, 1986.
10. Frater, RWM, Oka, Y, et al. Diabetes and coronary artery surgery. Mt Sinai J Med 49:237, 1982.
11. Chernow, B, Alexander, R, et al. Hormonal responses to graded surgical stress. Arch Intern Med 147:1273, 1987.
12. Shoemaker, WC, Appel, PL, Kram, HB. Tissue oxygen debt as a determinant of lethal and nonlethal postoperative organ failure. Crit Care Med 16:1117, 1988.
13. Shah, KB, Rao, TLK, et al. A review of pulmonary artery catheterization in 6,245 patients. Anesthesiology 61:271, 1984.
14. Iberti, TJ, Fischer, EP, et al. A multicenter study of physicians' knowledge of the pulmonary artery catheter. JAMA 264:2928, 1990.
15. London, MJ, Tubau, JF, et al. The "natural history" of segmental wall motion abnormalities in patients undergoing noncardiac surgery. Anesthesiology 73: 644, 1990.
16. Whelton, PK, Russell, RP. Systemic Hypertension. In AM Harvey, RJ Johns, et al. (eds), The Principles and Practice of Medicine (22nd ed). Norwalk: Appleton & Lange, 1988. Pp 127–144.
17. MC Fishman, AR Hoffman, et al. Medicine (2nd ed). Philadelphia: Lippincott, 1985. Pp 75–85.
18. Folkow, B. Structure and function of the arteries in hypertension. Am Heart J 114:938, 1987.
19. Braunwald, E. Cellular and Molecular Biology of Cardiovascular Disease. In JD Wilson, E Braunwald, et al. (eds), Harrison's Principles of Internal Medicine (12th ed). New York: McGraw-Hill, 1991. Pp 835–841.
20. Inouye, I, Massie, B, et al. Abnormal left ventricular filling: An early finding in mild to moderate systemic hypertension. Am J Cardiol 53:120, 1984.
21. Stauffer, JC, Gaasch, WH. Recognition and treatment of left ventricular diastolic dysfunction. Prog Cardiovasc Dis 32:319, 1990.
22. Strauer, BE. Ventricular function and coronary hemodynamics in hypertensive heart disease. Am J Cardiol 44:999, 1979.
23. Opherk, D, Mall, G, et al. Reduction of coronary reserve: A mechanism for angina pectoris in patients with arterial hypertension and normal coronary arteries. Circulation 69:1, 1984.
24. Brush, JE, Jr, Cannon, RO, III, et al. Angina due to coronary microvascular disease in hypertensive patients without left ventricular hypertrophy. N Engl J Med 319:1302, 1988.
25. Parmley, WW. Pathophysiology of congestive heart failure. Am J Cardiol 56:7A, 1985.
26. Weber, KT, Janicki, JS, et al. Pathophysiology of acute and chronic cardiac failure. Am J Cardiol 60: 3C, 1987.
27. Chakko, S, de Marchena, E, et al. Right ventricular diastolic function in systemic hypertension. Am J Cardiol 65:1117, 1990.
28. Clark, NJ, Stanley, TH. Anesthesia for Vascular Surgery. In RD Miller, RF Cucchiara, et al. (ed.), Anesthesia (3rd ed). New York: Churchill Livingstone, 1990. Pp 1693–1736.
29. Tarazi, RC, Dustan, HP, et al. Plasma volume and chronic hypertension. Relationship to arterial pres-

sure levels in different hypertensive diseases. *Arch Intern Med* 125:835, 1970.
30. Parving, HH, Gyntelberg, F. Transcapillary escape rate of albumin and plasma volume in essential hypertension. *Circ Res* 32:643, 1973.
31. Goldman, L, Caldera, DL, et al. Multifactorial index of cardiac risk in noncardiac surgical procedures. *N Engl J Med* 297:845, 1977.
32. Goldman, L, Caldera, DL, et al. Cardiac risk factors and complications in non-cardiac surgery. *Medicine* 57:357, 1978.
33. McLenachan, JM, Henderson, E, et al. Ventricular arrhythmias in patients with hypertensive left ventricular hypertrophy. *N Engl J Med* 317:782, 1987.
34. Casale, PN, Devereux, RB, et al. Value of echocardiographic measurement of left ventricular mass in predicting cardiovascular morbid events in hypertensive men. *Ann Intern Med* 105:173, 1986.
35. Savage, DD. Overall risk of left ventricular hypertrophy secondary to systemic hypertension. *Am J Cardiol* 60:8-1, 1987.
36. Vitez, TS, Soper, LE, et al. Chronic hypokalemia and intraoperative dysrhythmias. *Anesthesiology* 63:130, 1985.
37. Surawicz, B, Gettes, LS. Two mechanisms of cardiac arrest produced by potassium. *Circ Res* 12:415, 1963.
38. Fisch, C. Relation of electrolyte disturbances to cardiac arrhythmias. *Circulation* 47:408, 1973.
39. Murray, JF. The lungs and heart failure. *Hosp Pract* 20:55, 1985.
40. Veterans Administration Cooperative Study Group on Antihypertensive Agents. Effects of treatment on morbidity in hypertension: Results in patients with diastolic blood pressure averaging 90 through 114 mm Hg. *JAMA* 213:1143, 1970.
41. Hypertension, Detection and Follow-up Program Cooperative Group. The effect of treatment on mortality in "mild" hypertension. *N Engl J Med* 307:976, 1982.
42. Berglund, G, Wilhelmsen, L, et al. Coronary heart disease after treatment of hypertension. *Lancet* 1:1, 1978.
43. Ayobe, MH, Tarazi, RC. Reversal of changes in myocardial B-receptors and inotropic responsiveness with regression of cardiac hypertrophy in renal hypertensive rats (RHR). *Circ Res* 54:125, 1984.
44. Prys-Roberts, C, Meloche, R, Foex, P. Studies of anesthesia in relation to hypertension. I: Cardiovascular responses of treated and untreated patients. *Br J Anaesth* 43:122, 1971.
45. Mauney, FM, Ebert, PA, Sabiston, DC. Postoperative myocardial infarction: A study of predisposing factors, diagnosis and mortality in a high risk group of surgical patients. *Ann Surg* 172:497, 1970.
46. Eerola, M, Eerola, R, et al. Risk factors in surgical patients with verified preoperative myocardial infarction. *Acta Anaesthesiol Scand* 24:219, 1980.
47. Slogoff, S, Keats, AS. Further observations on perioperative myocardial ischemia. *Anesthesiology* 65:539, 1986.
48. Stone, JG, Foex, P, et al. Myocardial ischemia in untreated hypertensive patients. Effect of a single small oral dose of a beta-adrenergic blocking agent. *Anesthesiology* 68:495, 1988.
49. Goldman, L, Caldera, DL. Risks of general anesthesia and elective operation in the hypertensive patient. *Anesthesiology* 50:285, 1979.
50. Bedford, RF, Feinstein, B. Hospital admission blood pressure: A predictor for hypertension following endotracheal intubation. *Anesth Analg* 59:367, 1980.
51. Schneider, AJL, Knoke, JD. Morbidity prediction using pre- and intraoperative data. *Anesthesiology* 51:4, 1979.
52. Prys-Roberts, C, Foex, P, et al. Studies of anaesthesia in relation to hypertension. IV: The effects of artificial ventilation on the circulation and pulmonary gas exchange. *Br J Anaesth* 44:335, 1972.
53. Dagnino, J, Prys-Roberts, C. Studies of anaesthesia in relation to hypertension. VI. Cardiovascular responses to extradural blockade of treated and untreated hypertensive patients. *Br J Anaesth* 56:1065, 1984.
54. Prys-Roberts, C, Green, LT, et al. Studies of anaesthesia in relation to hypertension. II. Haemodynamic consequences of induction and endotracheal intubation. *Br J Anaesth* 43:531, 1971.
55. Prys-Roberts, C, Foex, P, et al. Studies of anaesthesia in relation to hypertension. V: Adrenergic beta-receptor blockade. *Br J Anaesth* 45:671, 1973.
56. Kahn, AH. Beta adrenoreceptor blocking agents. Their role in reducing chances of recurrent infarction and death. *Arch Intern Med* 143:1759, 1983.
57. Ghignone, M, Calvillo, O, Quintin, L. Anesthesia and hypertension: The effect of clonidine on perioperative hemodynamics and isoflurane requirements. *Anesthesiology* 67:3, 1987.
58. Flacke, JW, Bloor, BC, et al. Reduced narcotic requirement by clonidine with improved hemodynamic and adrenergic stability in patients undergoing coronary bypass surgery. *Anesthesiology* 67:11, 1987.
59. Ghignone, M, Noe, C, et al. Anesthesia for ophthalmic surgery in the elderly. The effects of clonidine on intraocular pressure, peri-operative hemodynamics and anesthetic requirement. *Anesthesiology* 68:707, 1988.

60. Adler, AG, Leahy, JJ, Cressman, MD. Management of perioperative hypertension using sublingual nifedipine. Experience in elderly patients undergoing eye surgery. Arch Intern Med 146:1927, 1986.
61. Newsome, LR, Roth, JV, et al. Esmolol attenuates hemodynamic responses during fentanyl-pancuronium anesthesia for aortocoronary bypass surgery. Anesth Analg 65:451, 1986.
62. Harrison, L, Ralley, FE, et al. The role of an ultrashort-acting adrenergic blocker (esmolol) in patients undergoing coronary artery bypass surgery. Anesthesiology 66:413, 1987.
63. Foster, DW. Diabetes Mellitus. In JD Wilson, E Braunwald, et al. (eds), Harrison's Principles of Internal Medicine (12th ed). New York: McGraw-Hill, 1991. Pp 1739–1759.
64. Bell, DSH. Hypertension in the person with diabetes. Am J Med Sci 297:228, 1989.
65. Bierman, EL. Atherosclerosis and Other Forms of Arteriosclerosis. In JD Wilson, E Braunwald, et al. (eds), Harrison's Principles of Internal Medicine (12th ed). New York: McGraw-Hill, 1991. Pp 992–1001.
66. O'Hare, JA. The enigma of insulin resistance and hypertension. Insulin resistance, blood pressure and the circulation. Am J Med 84:505, 1988.
67. Brown, MS, Goldstein, JL. The Hyperlipoproteinemias and Other Disorders of Lipid Metabolism. In JD Wilson, E Braunwald et al. (eds), Harrison's Principles of Internal Medicine (12th ed). New York: McGraw-Hill, 1991. Pp 1814–1825.
67a. Bierman, EL. Atherosclerosis and other forms of arteriosclerosis. In JD Wilson, E Braunwald, et al. (eds), Harrison's Principles of Internal Medicine (12th ed). New York: McGraw-Hill, 1991. Pp 992–1001.
68. Saudek, CD. Diabetes Mellitus. In AM Harvey, RJ Johns, et al. (eds), The Principles and Practice of Medicine (22nd ed). Norwalk: Appleton & Lange, 1988. Pp 956–968.
69. Herlitz, J, Malmberg, K, et al. Mortality and morbidity during a five-year follow-up of diabetics with myocardial infarction. Acta Med Scand 224:31, 1988.
70. Savage, MP, Krolewski, AS, et al. Acute myocardial infarction in diabetes mellitus and significance of congestive heart failure as a prognostic factor. Am J Cardiol 62:665, 1988.
71. Murray, DP, O'Brien, T, O'Sullivan, DJ. Silent myocardial ischemia in diabetes mellitus. J Am Coll Cardiol 11:23A, 1988.
72. Kannel, WB, McGee, DL. Diabetes and cardiovascular disease. JAMA 241:2035, 1979.
73. Page, MM, Watkins, PJ. Cardiorespiratory arrest and diabetic autonomic neuropathy. Lancet 1:14, 1978.

74. Gerson, MC, Khoury, JC. Prospective prediction of clinical coronary disease in patients with type I diabetes mellitus by exercise radionuclide ventriculography. J Am Coll Cardiol 11:215A, 1988.
75. Zoneraich, S. Small-vessel disease, coronary artery vasodilator reserve and diabetic cardiomyopathy. Chest 94:5, 1988.
76. Blumenthal, HT, Alex, M, Goldenberg, S. A study of lesions of the intramural coronary artery branches in diabetes mellitus. Arch Pathol 70:27, 1960.
77. Zoneraich, S, Silverman, G, Zoneraich, O. Primary myocardial disease, diabetes mellitus, and small-vessel disease. Am Heart J 100:754, 1980.
78. Schaffer, SW, Mozaffari, MS, et al. Basis for myocardial mechanical defects associated with non-insulin dependent diabetes. Am J Physiol 256:E25, 1989.
79. Dillmann, WH. Diabetes and thyroid-hormone–induced changes in cardiac function and their molecular basis. Ann Rev Med 40:373, 1989.
80. Arvan, S, Singal, K, et al. Subclinical left ventricular abnormalities in young diabetics. Chest 93:1031, 1988.
81. Takenaka, K, Sakamoto, T, et al. Left ventricular filling determined by Doppler echocardiography in diabetes mellitus. Am J Cardiol 61:1140, 1988.
82. Jermendy, G, Khoor, S, et al. Left ventricular diastolic dysfunction in type 1 (insulin-dependent) diabetic patients during dynamic exercise. Cardiology 77:9, 1990.
83. Borow, KM, Jaspan, JB, et al. Myocardial mechanics in young adult patients with diabetes mellitus: Effects of altered load, inotropic state and dynamic exercise. J Am Coll Cardiol 15:1508, 1990.
84. Danielsen, R, Nordrehaug, JE, Vik-Mo, H. Left ventricular performance during exercise in long-term type 1 diabetic men: An echocardiographic study. Clin Physiol 8:475, 1988.
85. Wieling, W. Impaired vagal heart rate control in diabetics: Relationship to long term complications. Neth J Med 33:260, 1988.
86. Maser, RE, Pfeifer, MA, et al. Diabetic autonomic neuropathy and cardiovascular risk: Pittsburgh epidemiology of diabetes complications study III. Arch Intern Med 150:1218, 1990.
87. Burgos, LG, Ebert, TJ, et al. Increased intraoperative cardiovascular morbidity in diabetics with autonomic neuropathy. Anesthesiology 70:591, 1989.
88. Ciccarelli, LL, Ford, CM, Tsueda, K. Autonomic neuropathy in a diabetic patient with renal failure. Anesthesiology 64:283, 1986.
89. Triantafillou, AN, Tsueda, K, et al. Refractory bradycardia after reversal of muscle relaxant in a diabetic with vagal neuropathy. Anesth Analg 65:1237, 1986.

90. MacKenzie, CR, Charlson, MR. Assessment of perioperative risk in the patient with diabetes mellitus. *Surg Gynecol Obstet* 167:293, 1988.
91. Fitzovich, DE, Randall, DC. Modulation of baroreflex by varying insulin and glucose in conscious dogs. *Am J Physiol* 258:R624, 1990.
92. Colucci, WS, Braunwald, E. Cardiac Tumors, Cardiac Manifestations of Systemic Disease, and Traumatic Cardiac Injury. In JD Wilson, E Braunwald, et al. (eds), *Harrison's Principles of Internal Medicine* (12th ed). New York: McGraw-Hill, 1991. Pp 988–991.
93. Gwinup, G, Elias, AN. The physiologic replacement of insulin (letter). *N Engl J Med* 322:333, 1990.
94. Levinsky, NG. Fluids and Electrolytes. In JD Wilson, E Braunwald, et al. (eds), *Harrison's Principles of Internal Medicine* (12th ed). New York: McGraw-Hill, 1991. Pp 278–289.
95. Knochel, JP. Disorders of Phosphorus Metabolism. In JD Wilson, E Braunwald, et al. (eds), *Harrison's Principles of Internal Medicine* (12th ed). New York: McGraw-Hill, 1991. Pp 1933–1935.
96. Powell, LW, Isselbacher, KJ. Hemochromatosis. In JD Wilson, E Braunwald, et al. (eds), *Harrison's Principles of Internal Medicine* (12th ed). New York: McGraw-Hill, 1991. Pp 1825–1829.
97. Anderson, RJ, and Schrier, RW. Acute Renal Failure. In JD Wilson, E Braunwald, et al. (eds), *Harrison's Principles of Internal Medicine* (12th ed). New York: McGraw-Hill, 1991. Pp 1144–1150.
98. Alfrey, AC. Chronic Renal Failure: Manifestations and Pathogenesis. In RW Schrier (ed), *Renal and Electrolyte Disorders* (2nd ed). Boston: Little, Brown, 1980. Pp 409–441.
99. Brenner, BM, Lazarus, JM. Chronic Renal Failure. In JD Wilson, E Braunwald, et al. (eds), *Harrison's Principles of Internal Medicine* (12th ed). New York: McGraw-Hill, 1991. Pp 1150–1157.
100. Dalton, JC, Pearson, RJ, White, PD. Constrictive pericarditis: A review and long term follow-up of 78 cases. *Ann Intern Med* 45:445, 1956.
101. Arora, KK, Lacy, JP, et al. Calcific cardiomyopathy in advanced renal failure. *Arch Intern Med* 135:603, 1975.
102. Lewin, K, Trautman, L. Ischaemic myocardial damage in chronic renal failure. *Br Med J* 4:151, 1971.
103. Raine, AEG. Hypertension, blood viscosity, and cardiovascular morbidity in renal failure: Implications of erythropoietin therapy. *Lancet* 1:97, 1988.
104. Bishop, JM, Donald, KW, Wade, OL. Circulatory dynamics at rest and on exercise in the hyperkinetic states. *Clin Sci* 14:329, 1955.
105. Varat, MA, Adolph, RJ, Fowler, NO. Cardiovascular effects of anemia. *Am Heart J* 83:415, 1972.
106. Boysen, PG, Block, AJ, et al. Nocturnal pulmonary hypertension in patients with chronic obstructive pulmonary disease. *Chest* 76:536, 1979.
107. Steele, P, Ellis, JH, Jr, et al. Left ventricular ejection fraction in severe chronic obstructive airways disease. *Am J Med* 59:21, 1975.
108. Khaja, F, Parker, JO. Right and left ventricular performance in chronic obstructive lung disease. *Am Heart J* 82:319, 1971.
109. Williams, JF, Jr, Childress, RH, et al. Left ventricular function in patients with chronic obstructive pulmonary disease. *J Clin Invest* 47:1143, 1968.
110. Burrows, B, Kettel, LJ, et al. Patterns of cardiovascular dysfunction in chronic obstructive lung disease. *N Engl J Med* 286:912, 1972.
111. McFadden, ER, Jr. Asthma. In JD Wilson, E Braunwald, et al. (eds), *Harrison's Principles of Internal Medicine* (12th ed). New York: McGraw-Hill, 1991. Pp 1047–1053.
112. Schukit, MA. Alcohol and Alcoholism. In JD Wilson, E Braunwald, et al. (eds), *Harrison's Principles of Internal Medicine* (12th ed). New York: McGraw-Hill, 1991. Pp 2146–2151.
113. Dyer, AR, Stamler, J, Paul, O, et al. Alcohol consumption, cardiovascular risk factors, and mortality in two Chicago epidemiologic studies. *Circulation* 56:1067, 1977.
114. Criqui, MH, Langer, RD, Reed, DM. Dietary alcohol, calcium, and potassium: Independent and combined effects on blood pressure. *Circulation* 80:609, 1989.
115. Regan, TJ. The Heart, Alcoholism, and Nutritional Disease. In JW Hurst, RC Schlant, et al. (eds), *The Heart* (7th ed). New York: McGraw-Hill, 1990. Pp 1533–1538.
116. Demakis, JG, Proskey, A, et al. The natural course of alcoholic cardiomyopathy. *Ann Intern Med* 80:293, 1974.
117. Mathews, EC, Jr, Gardin, JM, et al. Echocardiographic abnormalities in chronic alcoholics with and without overt congestive heart failure. *Am J Cardiol* 47:570, 1981.
118. Thomas, G, Haider, B, et al. Progression of myocardial abnormalities in experimental alcoholism. *Am J Cardiol* 46:233, 1980.
119. Sarma, JSM, Shigeaki I, et al. Biochemical and contractile properties of heart muscle after prolonged alcohol administration. *J Mol Cell Cardiol* 8:951, 1976.
120. Olsen, EGJ. The pathology of cardiomyopathies: A critical analysis. *Am Heart J* 98:385, 1979.
121. Regan, TJ, Levinson, GE, et al. Ventricular func-

tion in noncardiacs with alcoholic fatty liver: Role of ethanol in the production of cardiomyopathy. *J Clin Invest* 48:397, 1969.
122. Vikhert, AM, Tsiplenkova, VG, Cherpachenka, NM. Alcoholic cardiomyopathy and sudden cardiac death. *J Am Coll Cardiol* 8:3A, 1986.
123. Ettinger, PO, Wu, CF, et al. Arrhythmias and the "holiday heart": Alcohol-associated cardiac rhythm disorders. *Am Heart J* 95:555, 1978.
124. Koskinen, P, Kupari, M, et al. Alcohol and new onset atrial fibrillation: A case control study of a current series. *Br Heart J* 57:468, 1987.
125. De La Cruz, CL, Jr, Haider, B, et al. Effects of ethanol on ventricular electrical stability in the chronic alcoholic animal. *Alcoholism* 1:158, 1977.
126. Cyr, MG, Wartman, SA. The effectiveness of routine screening questions in the detection of alcoholism. *JAMA* 259:51, 1988.
127. Buckley, FP. Anesthesia and Obesity and Gastrointestinal Disorders. In PG Barash, BF Cullen, RK Stoelting (eds), *Clinical Anesthesia*. Philadelphia: Lippincott, 1989. Pp 1117–1131.
128. Sperry, RJ, Stanley, TH. Metabolic disease, alcohol-related problems and gross obesity. *Curr Opin Anaesth* 4:399, 1991.
129. Olefsky, JM. Obesity. In JD Wilson, E Braunwald et al. (eds), *Harrison's Principles of Internal Medicine* (12th ed). New York: McGraw-Hill, 1991. Pp 411–417.
130. Lipsky, PE. Rheumatoid Arthritis. In JD Wilson, E Braunwald, et al. (eds), *Harrison's Principles of Internal Medicine* (12th ed). New York: McGraw-Hill, 1991. Pp 1437–1443.
130a. Stevens, MB. Differential diagnosis of multisystem disease. In AM Harvey, RJ Johns, et al. (eds), *The Principles of Medicine* (2nd ed). Norwalk: Appleton & Lange, 1988. Pp 517–521.
131. Pincus, T, Callahan, LF, Vaughn, WK. Questionnaire, walking time and button test measures of functional capacity as predictive markers for mortality in rheumatoid arthritis. *J Rheum* 14:240, 1987.
132. Nomeir, A, Turner, R, et al. Cardiac involvement in rheumatoid arthritis. *Ann Intern Med* 79:800, 1973.
133. Kirk, J, Cosh, J. The pericarditis of rheumatoid arthritis. *Q J Med* 38:397, 1969.
134. Franco, AE, Levine, HD, Hall, AP. Rheumatoid pericarditis. *Ann Intern Med* 77:837, 1972.
135. Thadani, U, Iveson, JMI, Wright, V. Cardiac tamponade, constrictive pericarditis and pericardial resection in rheumatoid arthritis. *Medicine* 54:261, 1975.
136. Lev, M, Bharati, S, et al. The conduction system in rheumatoid arthritis with complete atrioventricular block. *Am Heart J* 90:78, 1975.
137. Weinberg, AD, Brennan, MD, et al. Outcome of anesthesia and surgery in hypothyroid patients. *Arch Intern Med* 143:893, 1983.
138. Amino, N, Mori, H, et al. High prevalence of transient postpartum thyrotoxicosis and hypothyroidism. *N Engl J Med* 306:849, 1982.
139. Wartofsky, L, Ingbar, SH. Diseases of the Thyroid. In JD Wilson, E Braunwald, et al. (eds), *Harrison's Principles of Internal Medicine* (12th ed). New York: McGraw-Hill, 1991. Pp 1692–1712.
140. Simons, RJ, Simon, JM, et al. Thyroid dysfunction in elderly hospitalized patients. Effect of age and severity of illness. *Arch Intern Med* 150:1249, 1990.
141. RK Stoelting, SF Dierdorf, RL McCammon. *Anesthesia and Co-Existing Disease* (2nd ed). New York: Churchill Livingstone, 1988. Pp 473–515.
142. Surawicz, B, Mangiardi, ML. Electrocardiogram in endocrine and metabolic disorders. *Cardiovasc Dis* 8:243, 1977.
143. Bough, EW, Crowley WF, et al. Myocardial function in hypothyroidism: Relation to disease severity and response to treatment. *Arch Intern Med* 138:1476, 1978.
144. Lee, RT, Plappert, M, St. John Sutton, MG. Depressed left ventricular systolic ejection force in hypothyroidism. *Am J Cardiol* 65:526, 1990.
145. Gyermek, L, Henderson, G. Low ventilatory and anesthetic drug requirements during myocardial revascularization in a hypothyroid patient. *J Cardioth Anesth* 2:70, 1988.
146. Karetzky, MS, Cain, SM. Effect of carbon dioxide on oxygen uptake during hyperventilation in normal man. *J Appl Physiol* 28:8–12, 1970.
147. Cain, SM. Increased oxygen uptake with passive hyperventilation of dogs. *J Appl Physiol* 28:4–7, 1970.
148. Doherty, JE, Perkins, WH. Digoxin metabolism in hypo- and hyperthyroidism. *Ann Intern Med* 64:489, 1966.
149. Croxson, MS, Ibbertson, HK. Serum digoxin in patients with thyroid disease. *Br Med J* 3:566, 1975.
150. Ellis, LB, Mebane, JG, et al. The effect of myxedema on the cardiovascular system. *Am Heart J* 43:341, 1952.
151. Paine, TD, Rogers, WJ, et al. Coronary arterial surgery in patients with incapacitating angina pectoris and myxedema. *Am J Cardiol* 40:226, 1977.
152. Schoolmeester, WL, Jackman, WM. Variant angina in the setting of hypothyroidism and beta-

blockade: A proposed mechanism. *South Med J* 72: 776, 1979.
153. Shenfield, GM. Influence of thyroid dysfunction on drug pharmacokinetics. *Clin Pharmacokinet* 6:275, 1981.
154. Stanley, TH, De Lange, S, et al. The influence of chronic preoperative propranolol therapy on cardiovascular dynamics and narcotic requirements during operation in patients with coronary artery disease. *Can Anaesth Soc J* 29:319, 1982.
155. Kaplan, JA, Cooperman, LH. Alarming reactions to ketamine in patients taking thyroid medication—treatment with propranolol. *Anesthesiology* 35:229, 1971.
156. Ladenson, PW. Disorders of the Thyroid Gland. In AM Harvey, RJ Johns, et al. (eds), *The Principles and Practice of Medicine* (2nd ed). Norwalk: Appleton & Lange, 1988. Pp 901–918.
157. Gick, GG, Ismail-Beigi, F. Thyroid hormone induction of Na^+-K^+-ATPase and its mRNAs in a rat liver cell line. *Am J Physiol* 258:C544, 1990.
158. Grossman, W, Robin, NI, et al. The enhanced myocardial contractility of thyrotoxicosis: Role of the beta adrenergic receptor. *Ann Intern Med* 74: 869, 1971.
159. Landsberg, L, Young, JB. Physiology and Pharmacology of the Autonomic Nervous System. In JD Wilson, E Braunwald, et al. (eds), *Harrison's Principles of Internal Medicine* (12th ed). New York: McGraw-Hill, 1991. Pp 380–392.
160. Levey, GS. The heart and hyperthyroidism: Use of beta-adrenergic blocking drugs. *Med Clin North Am* 59:1193, 1975.
161. Edelman, IS. Thyroid thermogenesis. *N Engl J Med* 290:1303, 1974.
162. MC Fishman, AR Hoffman, et al. *Medicine* (2nd ed). Philadelphia: Lippincott, 1985. Pp 209–221.
163. Muggia, AL, Stjernholm, M, Houle, T. Complete heart block with thyrotoxic myocarditis. *NEJM* 283:1099, 1970.
164. Knochel, JP. Disorders of Magnesium Metabolism. In JD Wilson, E Braunwald, et al. (eds), *Harrison's Principles of Internal Medicine* (12th ed). New York: McGraw-Hill, 1991. Pp 1935–1938.
165. Bennett, MH, Wainwright, AP. Acute thyroid crisis on induction of anaesthesia. *Anaesthesia* 44:28, 1989.
166. Haynes, RC, Jr, Murad, F. Thyroid and Antithyroid Drugs. In AG Gilman, LS Goodman, et al. (eds), *The Pharmacological Basis of Therapeutics* (7th ed). New York: Macmillan, 1985. Pp 1389–1411.
167. Davidson, B, Soodak, M, et al. The irreversible inactivation of thyroid peroxidase by methylmercaptoimidazole, thiouracil, and propylthiouracil in vitro and its relationship to in vivo findings. *Endocrinology* 103:871, 1978.
168. Harvey, AM, Shulman, LE, et al. Systemic lupus erythematosus: Review of the literature and clinical analysis of 138 cases. *Medicine* 33:291, 1954.
169. RK Stoelting, SF Dierdorf, RL McCammon. *Anesthesia and Co-Existing Disease* (2nd ed). New York: Churchill Livingstone, 1988. Pp 620–622.
170. Hahn, BH. Systemic Lupus Erythematosus. In JD Wilson, E Braunwald, et al. (eds), *Harrison's Principles of Internal Medicine* (12th ed). New York: McGraw-Hill, 1991. Pp 1432–1437.
171. Hejtmancik, MR, Wright, JC, et al. The cardiovascular manifestations of systemic lupus erythematosus. *Am Heart J* 68:119, 1964.
172. Bulkley, BH, Roberts, WC. The heart in systemic lupus erythematosus and the changes induced in it by corticosteroid therapy: A study of 36 necropsy patients. *Am J Med* 58:243, 1975.
173. Doherty, NE, Siegel RJ. Cardiovascular manifestations of systemic lupus erythematosus. *Am Heart J* 110:1257, 1985.
174. Ansari, A, Larson, PH, Bates, HD. Cardiovascular manifestations of systemic lupus erythematosus: Current perspective. *Prog Cardiovasc Dis* 27:421, 1985.
175. Klacsmann, PG, Bulkley, BH, Hutchins, GM. The changed spectrum of purulent pericarditis: An 86 year autopsy experience in 200 patients. *Am J Med* 63:666, 1977.
176. GP Rodnan, HR Schumacher. *Primer on the Rheumatic Diseases* (8th ed). Atlanta: The Arthritis Foundation, 1983. Pp 49–59s.
177. Bulkley, BH, Roberts, WC. Systemic lupus erythematosus as a cause of severe mitral regurgitation: New problem in an old disease. *Am J Cardiol* 35: 305, 1975.
178. Paget, SA, Bulkley, BH, et al. Mitral valve disease of systemic lupus erythematosus: A cause of severe congestive heart failure reversed by valve replacement. *Am J Med* 59:134, 1975.
179. Seningen, RP, Borer, JS, et al. Libman-Sacks endocardoma: Diagnosis during life with radiographic, fluoroscopic and angiocardiographic findings. *Radiology* 113:597, 1974.
180. James, TN, Rupe, CE, Monto, RW. Pathology of the cardiac conduction system in systemic lupus erythematosus. *Ann Intern Med* 63:402, 1965.
181. Fauci, AS, Lane, C. The Acquired Immunodeficiency Syndrome (AIDS). In JD Wilson, E Braunwald, et al. (eds), *Harrison's Principles of Internal*

Medicine (12th ed). New York: McGraw-Hill, 1991. Pp 1402–1410.
182. Lewis, W. AIDS: Cardiac findings from 115 autopsies. *Prog Cardiovasc Dis* 32:207, 1989.
183. Reilly, JM, Cunnion, RE, et al. Frequency of myocarditis, left ventricular dysfunction and ventricular tachycardia in the acquired immune deficiency syndrome. *Am J Cardiol* 62:789, 1988.
184. Monsuez, JJ, Kinney, EL, et al. AIDS heart disease: Results in 85 patients. *J Am Coll Cardiol* 11:195A, 1988.
185. Wynne, J, Braunwald, E. The Cardiomyopathies and Myocarditides. In JD Wilson, E Braunwald, et al. (eds), *Harrison's Principles of Internal Medicine* (12th ed). New York: McGraw-Hill, 1991. Pp 975–981.
186. Coplan, NL, Bruno, MS. Acquired immunodeficiency syndrome and heart disease: The present and the future. *Am Heart J* 117:1175, 1989.
187. Craddock, C, Bull, R, Pasvol, G, et al. Cardiorespiratory arrest and autonomic neuropathy in AIDS. *Lancet* 2:16, 1987.

The Pediatric Patient

16
Pediatric Monitoring

ROBERT H. MCDOWALL, JR.

The child with heart disease requires a thorough, physiologically directed management in the perioperative period. A clear understanding of the pathophysiology of congenital lesions and the influence of surgical correction or palliation is essential. Careful monitoring allows prompt recognition and management of related occurrences such as arrhythmia, heart failure, and pulmonary hypertension. Knowledge of the limitation of any monitoring modality is critical and must be considered together with the clinical assessment of the patient.

RESPIRATORY MONITORING

Changes in respiratory parameters, oxygenation, and CO_2 status can have rapid and serious hemodynamic effects in the child with congenital heart disease. Despite the proliferation of clinical monitoring and alarm systems, there are still those who advocate continuous ascultation of the heart and breath sounds through a precordial or esophageal stethoscope [1]. Intraoperative respiratory complications, although usually correctable, are more common in children than adults. This is not only due to smaller airway anatomy and equipment but also to the relatively rapid rate of oxygen consumption. The quality of breath sounds is a parameter that cannot otherwise be monitored, although alarmed capnography, spirometry, and airway pressure also serve as early warnings of potentially catastrophic events such as airway disconnection or obstruction.

Pulse Oximetry

Pulse oximetry, in addition to providing standard anesthesia safety monitoring, allows detection of circulatory changes such as dangerous reductions in pulmonary blood flow in children with cyanotic heart disease or alteration in shunt flow through a patent ductus arteriosus.

Optical differences between oxygenated and deoxygenated hemoglobin molecules are responsible for changes in the color and absorption spectrum of blood. The absorbance of near infrared light is greater for oxyhemoglobin, while visible red light is absorbed more by reduced hemoglobin. The absorption spectra of various hemoglobin species can be compared in Fig. 16-1. The pulse oximeter uses two light-emitting diodes, which emit at 940 nm (infrared) and 660 nm (visible red) while a photodiode measures the transmitted light [2]. Functional oxygen saturation is then determined as the ratio of oxyhemoglobin to the sum of oxyhemoglobin and reduced hemoglobin. This calculation excludes dysfunctional hemoglobin species such as

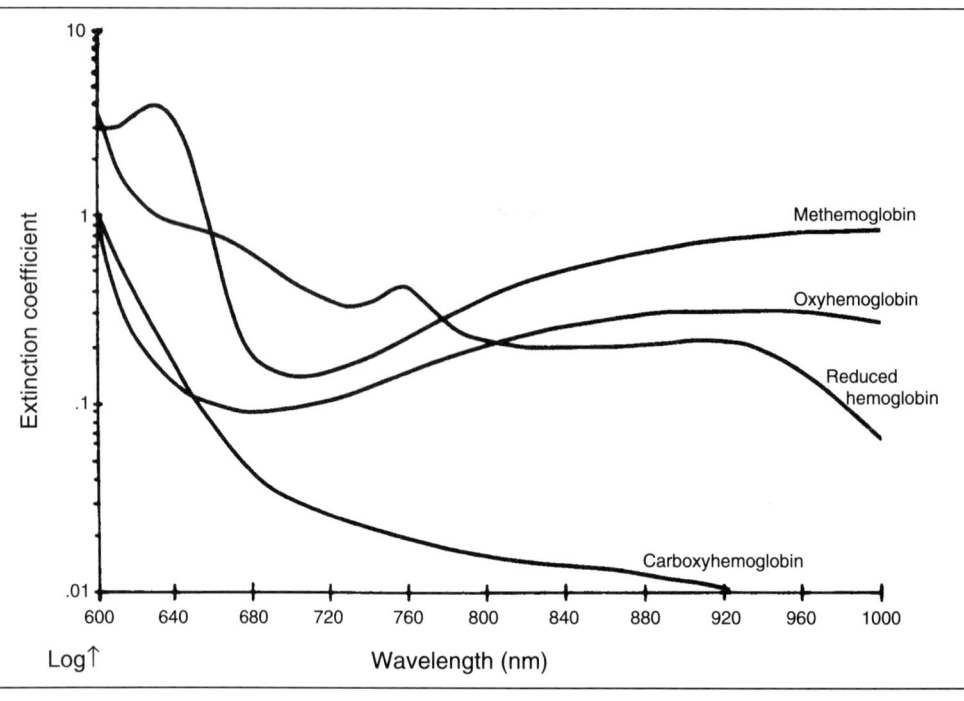

Fig. 16-1. Hemoglobin extinction curves showing the absorption spectra of hemoglobin, oxyhemoglobin, carboxyhemoglobin, and methemoglobin. (Reprinted with permission from *Journal of Clinical Monitoring*. From MW Wukitsch, MT Petterson, DR Tobler, et al., Pulse oximetry: Analysis of theory, technology, and practice. *J Clin Monit* 4:290, 1988.)

carboxyhemoglobin and methemoglobin from the denominator, which would otherwise be included for determination of total oxygen saturation measured in vitro [3]. Pulse oximetry therefore overestimates total oxygen saturation in the presence of abnormal hemoglobins [2]. Fetal hemoglobin is a functional hemoglobin and its saturation measurement compares favorably with that of adult hemoglobin [4], although one must remember the difference in the relationship between oxygen saturation and arterial oxygen tension (PaO_2) in the presence of hemoglobin F.

To eliminate interference by absorbance of venous blood and surrounding tissues and to isolate arterial blood measurement, the oximeter electronically subtracts the reference signal obtained during diastole from the arterial pulsation of blood occurring during systole [5]. Saturation cannot be determined without adequate arterial pulsation and therefore the instrument may fail during hypotension, vasopressor therapy, hypothermia, or severe peripheral vasoconstriction from any cause. A plethysmographic display allows examination of the shape of each wave form, to confirm that oxygen saturation measurement is based on true arterial blood flow. Alternatively, the oximeter pulse signal and heart beat indicator from either the electrocardiograph or invasive arterial pressure monitor should maintain one-to-one correlation during a perfusing rhythm. When placed on a well-perfused arterial bed, pulse oximetry correlates very well with both transcutaneous oxygen tension (PO_2) and in vitro measurement of arterial oxygen saturation (SaO_2) in neonates, children, and adults [3, 4, 6, 7]. With a mean difference from in vitro measurements of only 1 to 3 percent [6, 8], oxygen saturation measured by pulse oximetry is very sensitive to changes in arterial oxygen content (CaO_2). Indeed, true CaO_2 can be assessed despite shifts of the hemoglobin-oxygen dissociation curve due to perioperative changes in temperature, 2,3–diphosphoglyceric acid (2,3-DPG) levels, or acid-base status. In children with respiratory failure or cyanotic heart disease, who fall on the steep portion of the hemoglobin-oxygen dissociation curve, SaO_2 is more sensitive to changes than PaO_2. Unfortunately, some pulse oximeters are less reliable at SaO_2 below 60 to 70 percent [9, 10]. Preductal placement of an oximeter sensor on the right upper extremity measures oxygenation of cerebral blood supply. By comparison a postductal sensor will allow monitoring of right-to-left shunting, as it varies in conditions such as heart disease associated with pulmonary hypertension, and a patent ductus.

Although the pulse oximeter is accurate at higher oxygen levels, it becomes less sensitive to changes in PaO_2 above 100 mm Hg because of the flat slope of the hemoglobin-oxygen dissociation curve in this region. This becomes clinically relevant in eliminating hyperoxia in patients at risk for retinopathy of prematurity or pulmonary toxicity, and in the assessment of CaO_2 in profoundly anemic patients [11].

Interference with the photodetector may occur with ambient light from fluorescent, infrared, solar, and other sources. The absorption spectra of some intravascular dyes, including methylene blue, indocyanine green, and indigo carmine, may also introduce artifact [12]. Anesthetic gases and hyperbilirubinemia do not interfere [4, 6, 13]. An oximeter probe that is too large in relation to a child's finger allows light to reach the sensor without passing through the tissues. A variety of pediatric probe designs allows placement over any tissue with arterial flow, including the foot, palm, ear, cheek, nose, or penis. Attachment circumferentially or with a clamp must not occlude blood flow. A probe should be used only with the unit for which it is specifically designed, as variation in light source energy can burn the skin.

Surveillance is enhanced by monitors that vary the pitch of the audible pulse signal directly with SaO_2. Arterial desaturation is not uncommon during any phase of anesthetic induction, maintenance, emergence, or transport, particularly in young children. Its rapidity and severity relate to higher oxygen consumption per body mass, lower functional residual capacity, and higher pulmonary arterial reactivity. Visual recognition of cyanosis varies with perfusion, hemoglobin concentration, and ambient light and is very insensitive for detection of arterial desaturation. Detectable hemodynamic changes such as bradycardia and hypotension occur late and significant hypoxemia is much more likely to go unnoticed unless SaO_2 is continually monitored [14].

Transcutaneous Oxygen Monitoring

The interpretation of transcutaneously measured PO_2 ($PtcO_2$) requires an understanding of the anatomy and physiology of the skin and its blood supply. The dermis, which contains a rich blood supply, is covered by the epidermis. The dermal capillary loops, strata papillare, extend to the basal layer of epidermis and are more dense in newborns than in adults. Vascular plexuses in the dermis have numerous arteriovenous anastomoses and are important in the control of peripheral blood flow and thermoregulation. Heating of the skin increases local blood flow [15].

When tissue oxygen consumption ($\dot{V}O_2$) is in steady state, there is a hyperbolic relationship between blood flow (Q) and the difference between arterial and venous oxygen content (CaO_2 and CvO_2, respectively), defined by:

$$Q = \frac{\dot{V}O_2}{(CaO_2 - CvO_2)}$$

Rearranging the equation:

$$CaO_2 - CvO_2 = \frac{\dot{V}O_2}{Q}$$

or:

$$CaO_2 = CvO_2 + \frac{\dot{V}O_2}{Q}$$

By increasing flow to its maximum, the quotient $\dot{V}O_2/Q$ becomes very small, and CaO_2 is thereby flow independent. Thus, with local hyperemia CaO_2 can be approximated by measuring CvO_2 at the skin surface, and this is the basis for transcutaneous monitoring [15]. This simplified linear relationship will not apply if low cardiac output or peripheral vasoconstriction diminishes blood flow. In such circumstances CaO_2 would revert to its normally flow-dependent state and no longer be reliably measured by CvO_2. Transcutaneous PO_2 is therefore a nonspecific indicator of alteration in either arterial PO_2 or perfusion.

The transcutaneous PO_2 monitoring device uses locally applied heat to cause vasodilation and hyperemia. Oxygen flows by diffusion from the dermal capillaries to the skin surface and across a semipermeable membrane, where it is reduced on contact with platinum-yielding electrons from a Clark polarographic electrode. The current that is generated is proportional to oxygen tension [5]. When circulation is adequate there is very good correlation between $PtcO_2$ and PaO_2 over a wide range of oxygen tensions in respiratory failure or cyanotic heart disease [16–18]. However, this relationship is nullified if circulation is diminished. Since it is actually a measure of oxygen delivery, $PtcO_2$ will fall with a decrease in either cardiac output or CaO_2 [5]. Thus, a further diagnostic step is necessary to determine whether decreased $PtcO_2$ results from hypoxia, shock, or both.

More commonly used in infants, the transcutaneous PO_2 monitoring device has been applied to older children and adults as well, although beyond infancy correlation is more sensitive to circulatory effects [18, 19]. Because the electrode can burn the skin, application should be limited to 2 hours at 43°C for premature infants, 4 hours at 44°C for term neonates, and 6 hours at 45°C for older children. Other disadvantages include periodic calibration requirements, warm-up equilibration time, and response time, although the delay is minimal in neonates. Interference from anesthetic gases, which are reduced at the electrode, may be minimized by the use of a less permeable Mylar membrane and a polarization voltage of −600 mV [20, 21].

Transcutaneous Carbon Dioxide Monitoring

Unlike transcutaneous PO_2 monitoring, in which oxygen is actually measured, the transcutaneous carbon dioxide tension (PCO_2) sensor utilizes the Stowe-Severinghaus principle. Carbon dioxide diffuses from the skin through a permeable membrane and alters the pH of an electrolyte solution. The electrical potential between glass pH and Ag/AgCl reference electrodes is thereby changed and converted to torr [22].

Transcutaneously measured PCO_2 ($PtcCO_2$) is always higher than arterial PCO_2 ($PaCO_2$). The gradient between the two parameters is probably related to increased local metabolism by the heated sensor, a tissue-capillary carbon dioxide gradient, and the anaerobic heating coefficient of blood, which directly relates PCO_2 with temperature [22]. One must remember that $PtcCO_2$ is not physiologically the same as $PaCO_2$ and the numerical difference varies between individuals, hemodynamic state, and calibration technique. Thus, $PtcCO_2$ should be interpreted as an absolute number and not "corrected" to equal an assumed $PaCO_2$. Despite the difference between arterial and transcutaneous PCO_2, there is a close linear correlation in infants [22–25] and adults [26]. However, when tissue oxygenation is impaired by hypoxemia or shock, causing local acidosis or impaired carbon dioxide clearance, $PtcCO_2$ rises significantly and no longer correlates with $PaCO_2$. This is observed clinically in a low cardiac output state (cardiac index < 1.5 liters/min/m²), hypoxemia (PaO_2 < 40 torr), and acidosis (pH < 7.3) [25, 26]. Hypotension alone, with mean arterial pressure as low as 15 to 30 mm Hg in neonates, does not necessarily affect accuracy [23, 25]. Thus, $PtcCO_2$, like $PtcO_2$, is a nonspecific indicator of oxygen delivery. Changes indicate the need for further clinical assessment and the determination of true $PaCO_2$.

Although nonheated electrodes are available, the response time and correlation with $PaCO_2$ are enhanced by using higher-electrode temperature [27]. Anesthetic gases do not significantly influence the pH of the electrolyte layer surrounding the AgCl reference electrode and therefore do not interfere with $PtcCO_2$ measurement [21, 26]. Electrosurgical units will interfere with the signal, and perioperative utility is limited by a response time of several minutes [27].

Combined oxygen and carbon dioxide transcutaneous sensors are available that offer greater convenience and nearly the same accuracy [28].

Capnography

Analysis of end-tidal carbon dioxide ($PetCO_2$) by either mass spectrometry or infrared absorption is possible in small children. Sidestream or mainstream sampling can be used provided the airway portion of the equipment is of low dead space, resistance, and weight.

Correlation between end-tidal and arterial PCO_2 is adequate in healthy supine individuals when measuring gas from perfused alveoli [29]. However, the difference between the two is inconsistent when there is redistribution of ventilation relative to perfusion [30], as may occur during anesthesia, positive pressure ventilation, changes in position, and any variation in pulmonary blood flow from altered cardiac output or intracardiac shunting. It has recently been demonstrated that a changing difference between arterial $PaCO_2$ and $PetCO_2$ correlates with changing SaO_2 in children with cyanotic congenital heart disease [31]. In small infants additional error is introduced by relatively greater equipment dead space, rapid respiratory rate, and dilution of end-tidal gas with fresh gas. These problems can be minimized by using low–dead space equipment, higher sample flow rates, and non-rebreathing circuits [32, 33]. Obvious dilution artifact in a child is shown in Fig. 16-2, rendering end-tidal measurement of CO_2 unreliable. In the absence of significant artifact, qualitative analysis of the capnogram allows detection of airway obstruction; equipment disconnection or extubation; rebreathing; alteration of pulmonary blood flow, including embolic phenomena; and malignant hyperthermia. However, despite a normal appearance, a wave form with a flat alveolar plateau phase may underestimate $PaCO_2$ [33]. Accurate quantitative determination of $PaCO_2$ therefore requires arterial sampling. In cardiac arrest $PetCO_2$ is not a reliable indicator of $PaCO_2$, but does correlate with improved pulmonary blood flow, indicating either a perfusing rhythm or effective cardiopulmonary resuscitation [34, 35].

Monitoring the capnograph in children with cyanotic heart disease is imperative to aid in recognition of hypoventilation, in which hypercapnia increases the ratio of pulmonary to systemic vascular resistance and enhances right-to-left shunt. Likewise, mild hypoventilation may be beneficial when congestive heart failure is associated with excessive pulmonary blood flow, as in patients with ventricular septal defect.

The concentration of inspired and expired anesthetic gases can also be monitored by either mass spectrometry or an infrared device. Although usually only of theoretic concern, the speed of anesthetic induction may be affected by right-to-left or mixed shunting [36]. Mass spectrometry offers the advantage of measuring nitrogen in the expiratory gas, a sensitive indicator of venous air embolism that may have catastrophic consequences in patients with intracardiac shunts.

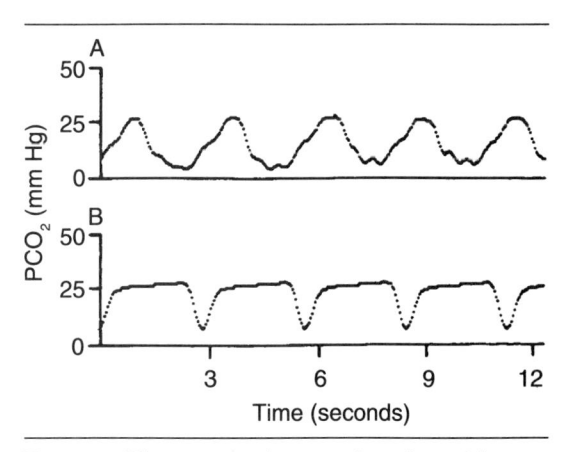

Fig. 16-2. The capnographic wave form for an 8-kg child during ventilation with: (A) a partial rebreathing circuit and (B) a non-rebreathing circuit. (Reprinted with permission from JM Badgwell, JE Heavner, WS May, et al., End-tidal PCO_2 monitoring in infants and children ventilated with either a partial rebreathing or a non-rebreathing circuit. *Anesthesiology* 66:405, 1987.)

HEMODYNAMIC MONITORING

Electrocardiography

As one cannot maintain constant visual contact with any monitoring system, audible confirmation of the heartbeat should be continuous. This is particularly important in children, in whom a bradyarrhythmia can occur rapidly and may indicate a critical decrease in cardiac output. Typical ranges of heart rate for normal children are given in Table 16-1. While the heart rate decreases with age, it is highly dependent on activity, excitement, temperature, intravascular volume, perioperative changes in autonomic tone, and drugs. Thus, it is the trend or sudden change from a baseline rate, rather than an isolated absolute value, that must be interpreted in the context of clinical conditions.

Most ECG monitors are ill equipped to diagnose a serious arrhythmia reliably in the pediatric car-

Table 16-1. Heart rate and increasing age

Age	Heart rate (bpm)
Preterm	150 ± 20
Term	133 ± 18
6 mo	120 ± 20
12 mo	120 ± 20
2 yr	105 ± 25
3 yr	101 ± 15
5 yr	90 ± 10
12 yr	70 ± 17
23 yr	77 ± 5

Source: Reprinted with permission from GA Gregory, *Pediatric Anesthesia.* In RD Miller (ed), *Anesthesia* (2nd ed). New York: Churchill Livingstone, 1986.

diac patient due to the rapid intrinsic heart rate, congenital or surgically acquired conduction abnormalities, and intraoperative signal artifact. An audible heart rate signal is essential for immediate detection of rhythm disturbance not only during high-risk periods such as laryngoscopy, but also for unexpected events during an otherwise smooth intraoperative course. Auscultation of heart sounds through a precordial or esophageal stethoscope offers real-time monitoring of heart rate that is usually free from artifact. While diagnostic information is limited, it allows vigilance when more sophisticated systems are rendered inoperable by patient movement, electrocautery, or equipment failure.

Placement of ECG leads at nondependent sites away from the surgical field may be difficult in a small child. A variety of infant electrodes are available that minimize trauma to neonatal skin. Beyond infancy larger electrodes will suffice, providing adequate gel and adhesive to maintain contact despite patient movement during induction, positioning, emergence, and transport. Using a basic three-lead system, the negative electrode is placed near or on the right arm, the positive electrode on the left arm or leg, and the ground at any caudal site. The ability to monitor additional leads allows enhanced recognition of rhythm and conduction abnormality as well as changes in configuration that might represent ischemic or metabolic events. Diagnosis of complex arrhythmias may require careful examination of the electrocardiogram, and the monitor should have the ability to print an accurate tracing. In the patient with normal cardiac anatomy, lead II generally detects sinoatrial activity, allowing diagnosis of varying degrees of heart block or atrioventricular dissociation. This is particularly important in children with sick sinus syndrome or a propensity for any nonsinus rhythm. Immediate detection of atrioventricular conduction abnormality in a patient dependent on synchronized atrial contraction, such as after the Fontan procedure, may be essential for rapid intervention to maintain cardiac output. In the presence of an ectopic atrial rhythm or malposition of the atria, the P-wave morphology and orientation will be altered. For example, atrial situs solitus creates a normal sinus impulse that in turn creates a positive P wave in leads I and AVF, while situs inversus results in a P wave that is negative in lead I and positive in lead AVF.

Simultaneous monitoring of a combination of limb and precordial leads will aid in detection of ventricular conduction abnormalities or myocardial ischemia. Interpretation of QRS morphology and orientation depends on knowledge of the ventricular position, which may be independent of atrial situs. For example, three variants of ventricular position are shown in Fig. 16-3. Dextrocardia and levocardia refer only to the position of the ventricular mass in the right or left chest, respectively; orientation of ventricular left-right relation varies. In mirror-image dextrocardia the ventricles are reversed and a recording of the right precordial leads (V_1 and V_3R-V_7R) produces "normal" QRS morphology on the electrocardiogram. Dextrocardia without anatomic reversal of the ventricles is known as dextrorotation. A varying degree of rightward shift and slight counterclockwise rotation of the heart move the voltage transition to a right precordial lead. Finally, in ventricular inversion without dextrocardia the anatomic left and right ventricles are reversed and positioned side by side. Septal depolarization is reversed, resulting in a Q wave in lead V_1 that is absent from lead V_6 (Fig. 16-4).

While ST segment analysis of leads II and V_5 or leads V_4 and V_5 is a sensitive indicator of ischemic episodes in the adult with coronary artery disease [37], ischemia detection in pediatrics has not been systematically evaluated. Other causes of ST seg-

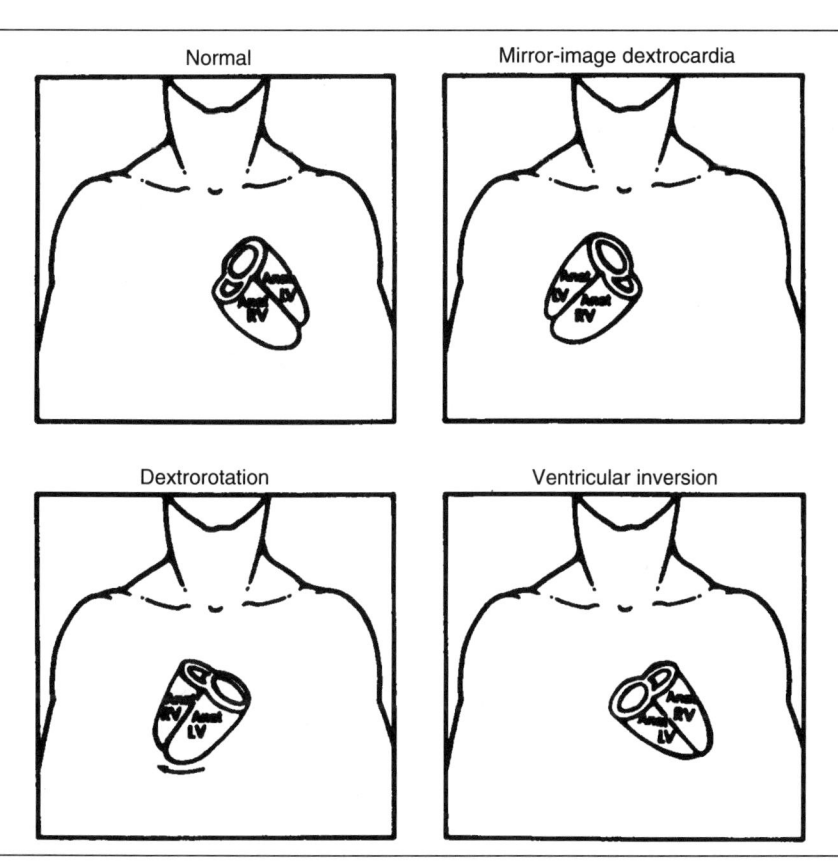

Fig. 16-3. Ventricular position. The normal heart is in the left chest, with the anatomic right ventricle to the right of and anterior to the anatomic left ventricle. Ventricular malposition refers to displacement of the cardiac mass to the right chest and/or changes in the relative position of the anatomic left and right ventricles. (Reprinted with permission from A Garson, Jr, Electrocardiography. In A Garson, Jr, JT Brickner, and DG McNamara (eds), *The Science and Practice of Pediatric Cardiology*. Philadelphia: Lea & Febiger, 1990. Pp 713–767).

ment changes include increased sympathetic tone, tachyarrhythmia, change in position or lead placement, altered cardiothoracic dimensions by thoracotomy or sternotomy, retraction of pericardial structures, pericarditis, and secondary repolarization changes caused by abnormal depolarization occurring with conduction abnormalities or hypertrophy [38, 39]. The electrocardiogram will be altered predictably by metabolic derangements such as potassium, calcium, or sodium imbalance, and by the effects of drugs such as digitalis and other antiarrhythmics. Although rare in children there are clinical situations in which ischemia or injury is known to occur, including aortic or pulmonary stenosis, patent ductus arteriosus, anomalous left coronary artery, Kawasaki's disease, and myocarditis. Prompt diagnosis and management may be facilitated by analysis of the ST segment and T wave. In mixing lesions with a high pulmonary-systemic flow ratio with or without congestive heart failure, such as truncus arteriosus and hypoplastic left heart, intraoperative detection of inadequate coronary perfusion by ST-segment depression has allowed intervention such as ventilatory adjustment to increase pulmonary vascular resistance, thereby enhancing systemic diastolic blood pressure [40]. Postmortem evidence of myocardial ischemia following ductus arteriosus ligation or Blalock-Taussig shunt placement [41] suggests that perioperative ST segment analysis may be beneficial.

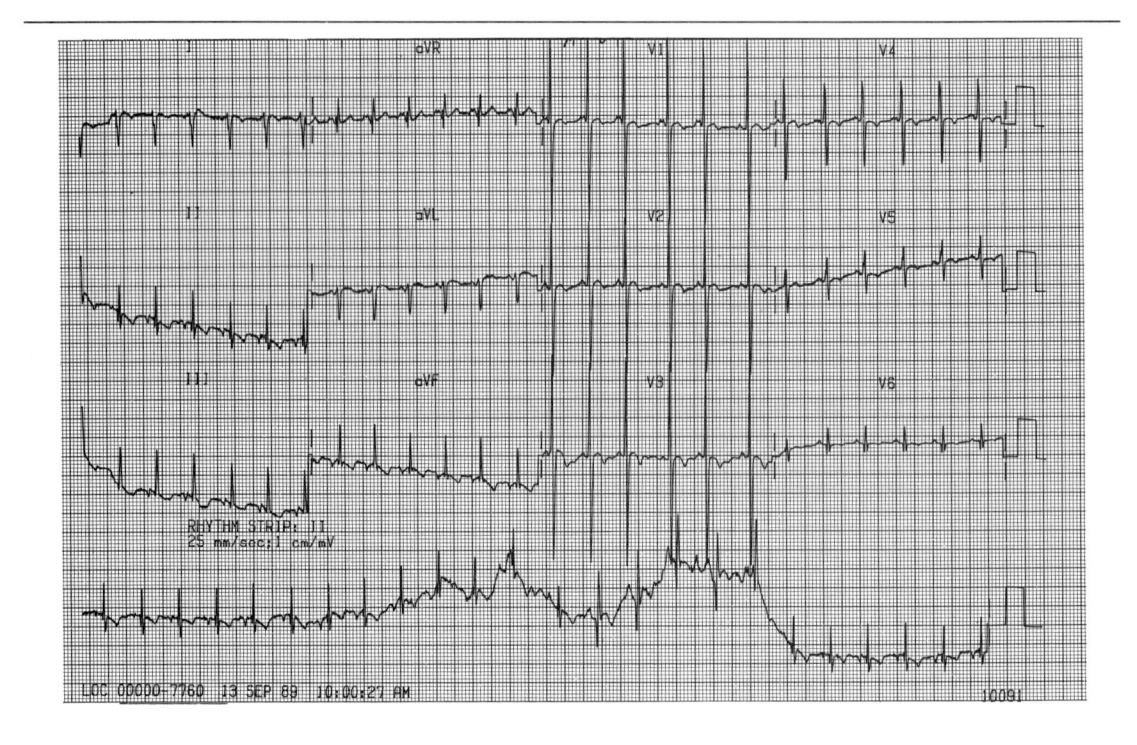

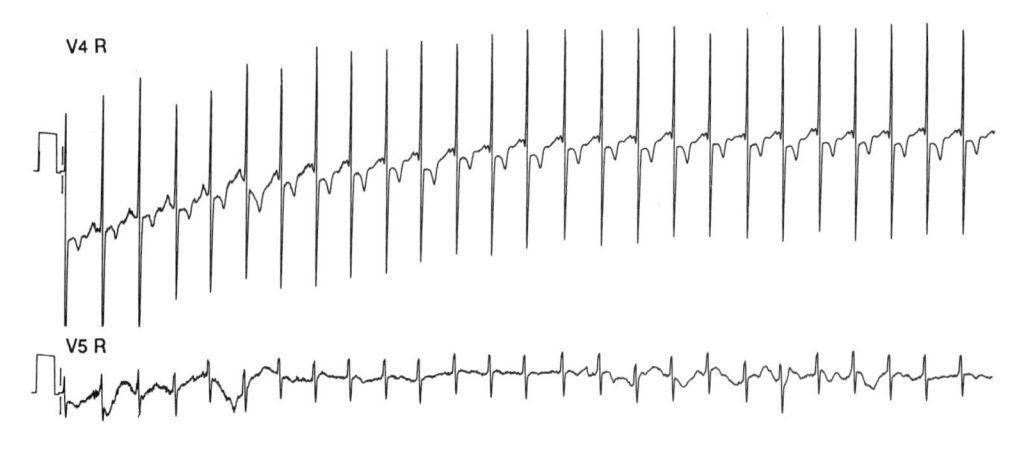

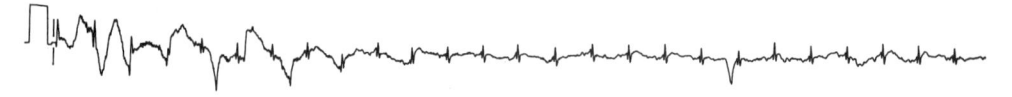

Fig. 16-4. Right-axis deviation with mirror-image P wave in this child with dextrocardia, L-transposition, pulmonic atresia, and a ventricular septal defect.

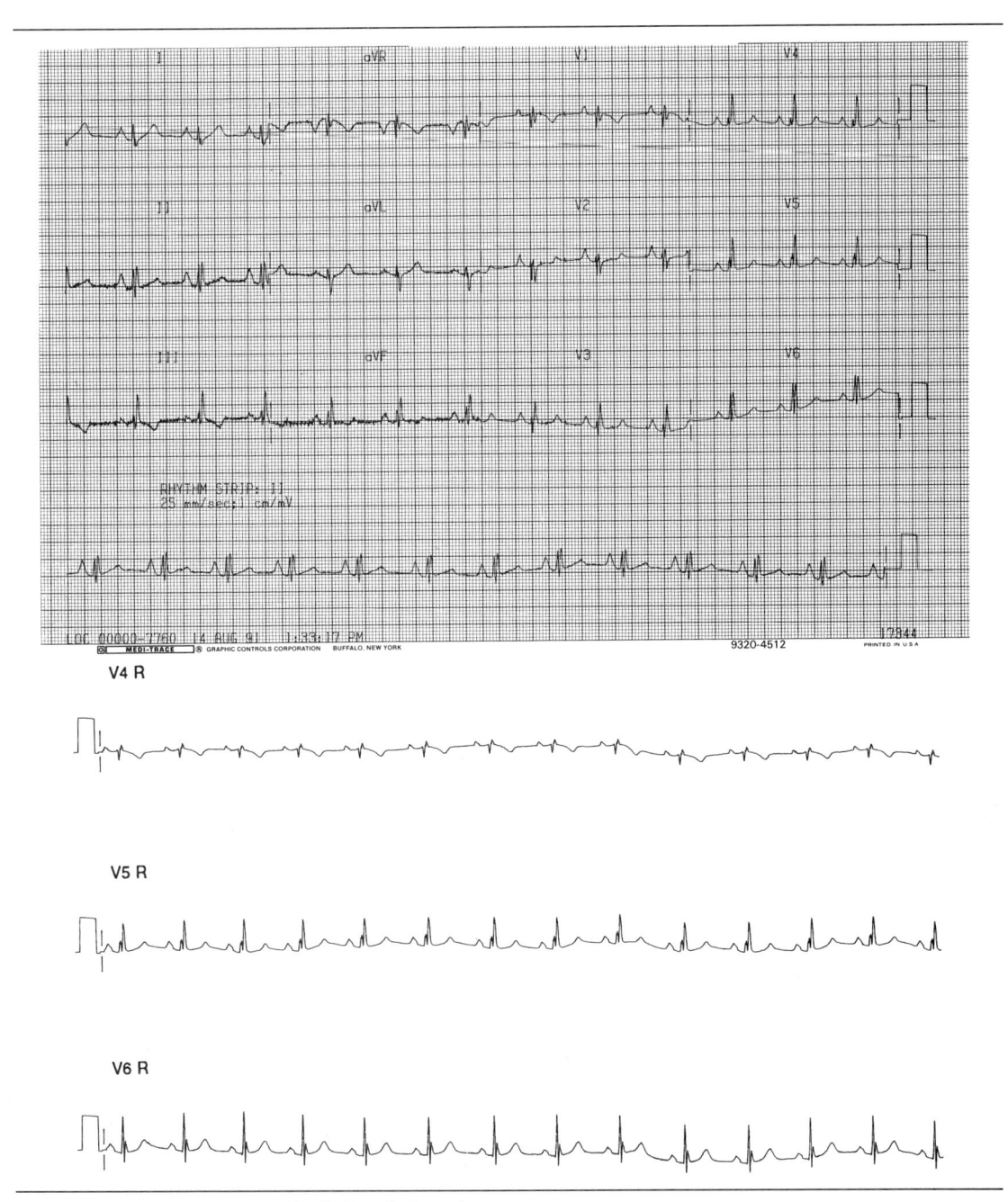

Fig. 16-5. Note large P wave and right bundle branch block pattern in this child with Epstein's anomaly.

Variable abnormalities of atrioventricular (AV) conduction can persist after open heart surgery and can be seen when these patients subsequently present for noncardiac surgery. They range from first-degree heart block to AV dissociation, which is commonly seen following surgery near the AV node. Heart block is more common after repair of complete AV canal, ventricular septal defect, or tetralogy of Fallot. Bundle branch block can also be associated with intrinsic myocardial disease (Fig. 16-5); some of these patients are at risk for progression to complete heart block. The risk may be complicated further by drugs such as digoxin or metabolic derangements such as hypocalcemia and hypokalemia.

In a child with a cardiac pacemaker, the ECG monitor should be able to distinguish between the pacemaker stimulus and the patient's QRS complex. Several factors influence the detection of a pacemaker stimulus, and monitored but undetected cardiorespiratory arrest has been reported. To minimize the risk of a monitor interpreting pacemaker stimuli as QRS complexes, it is recommended that ECG electrode placement should maximize QRS and minimize pacemaker amplitude; monitor sensitivity should be set as low as possible and filter settings should maximize the monitor band width [42]. The importance of multimodality monitoring in these patients is obvious.

Systemic Blood Pressure Monitoring

Multiple methods for the measurement of blood pressure are available, and some lend themselves in particular to the small vessels and blood flow of pediatric patients. A range of blood pressures that are considered normal, which increase with age, is given in Table 16-2. Whether using an invasive or noninvasive modality, it is essential to understand what each pressure represents for a given method, location of measurement, and circulatory status.

Table 16-2. Blood pressure and increasing age

Age	Arterial blood pressure (mm Hg)	
	Systolic	Diastolic
Preterm	50 ± 3	30 ± 2
Term	67 ± 3	42 ± 4
6 mo	89 ± 2	60 ± 10
12 mo	96 ± 30	66 ± 25
2 yr	99 ± 25	64 ± 25
3 yr	100 ± 25	67 ± 23
5 yr	94 ± 14	55 ± 9
12 yr	109 ± 16	58 ± 9
23 yr	122 ± 30	75 ± 20

Source: Reprinted with permission from GA Gregory, Pediatric Anesthesia. In RD Miller (ed), *Anesthesia* (2nd ed). New York: Churchill Livingstone, 1986.

Indirect Noninvasive Arterial Pressure Measurement

With noninvasive methods for determination of blood pressure, the most common source of error is inappropriate cuff size. Determined by the size of the limb being used for measurement, rather than the age of the patient, the width of the inflatable bladder should equal 40 percent of the circumference of the midpoint of the limb [43]. Although earlier practice related cuff size to acromion-olecranon distance or limb diameter [44], circumference has become a simple and acceptable standard of reference. When the cuff is of sufficient width, the pressure indicated by the manometer extends undiminished to the artery, as illustrated in Fig. 16-6. A bladder that is too narrow will yield a pressure reading that is erroneously high, while a wide cuff will reveal an erroneously low pressure.

Indirect, nonautomatic measurement of blood pressure requires observation of a mercury or aneroid sphygmomanometer. While the manometer can be placed at any level, the artery at the point of measurement must be at the phlebostatic axis. A correction for hydrostatic pressure is otherwise necessary, equal to 0.8 mm Hg for each centimeter vertical distance from the right midatrial level [45]. Any limb can be used provided the size of the cuff is appropriate. In normal children there is no difference in pressure measured on the left or right [46] but discrepancies will exist when anatomic anomalies result in obstruction or shunt. An unaffected limb must be used for pressure measurement in patients with congenital obstruction, such as coarctation of the aorta; following any procedure using a supply artery, such as the subclavian for repair of aortic coarctation; or with redirected flow, such as following the creation of a systemic to pulmonary artery shunt. Modification of the Blalock-Taussig procedure, avoiding takedown of the subclavian artery, may maintain systolic pressure in the ipsilateral arm, but diastolic pressure will be inaccurate.

The simplest measurement technique is the direct palpation method of Riva-Rocci, but it is relatively inaccurate [46] and reveals no diastolic pressure. The Korotkov auscultatory method yields blood pressures that are very close to direct measurement [47] (see Chap. 4). As the cuff deflates below systolic pressure, turbulent arterial blood

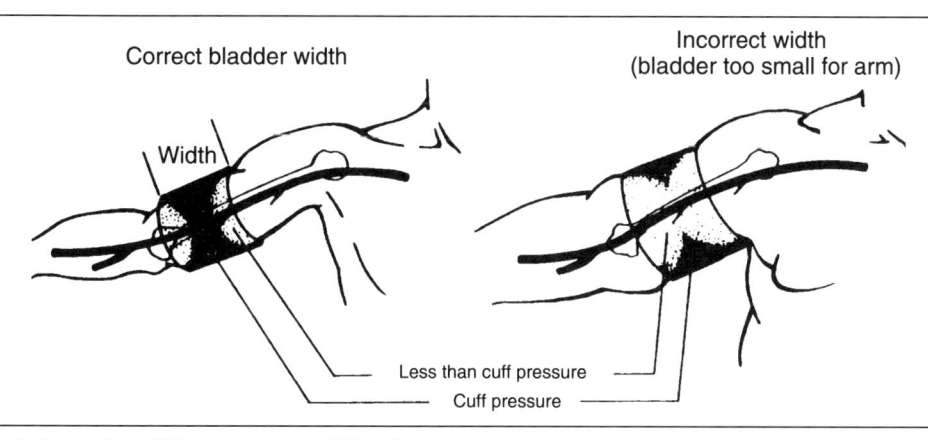

Fig. 16-6. Relationship of blood pressure cuff bladder to arm size. With correct bladder width (*left*), full cuff pressure is applied to the brachial artery. When the bladder width is too small (*right*), the artery has less than full pressure applied to it, resulting in an erroneously high pressure determination. (Reproduced with permission. From WM Kirkendall, M Feinleig, ED Freis, et al., *Recommendations for human blood pressure determination by sphygmomanometers*, 1987. Subcommittee on the American Heart Association Postgraduate Education Committee. *Circulation* 62:1145A, 1987. Copyright American Heart Association.)

flow creates a spectrum of audible sounds, which is classically divided into five phases, the last being silent. Correlating closely with systolic pressure is the appearance of the faint but progressively intense tapping sounds of phase I. Diastolic pressure determination is more difficult to determine and correlates with phase IV or V, depending on age and clinical conditions. Phase IV is marked by the abrupt muffling of the crisp, intense third-phase sounds to a distinct soft, blowing quality. Phase V is the point at which the sounds disappear. High flow rates in the brachial artery occur in conditions such as exercise and hyperthyroidism, but also in normal infants and children, and may be associated with a longer interval of phase IV muffled sounds. Diastolic pressure is thus underestimated by the fifth phase. Instead, the muffling that signals the onset of phase IV should be utilized for diastolic determination in children, recognizing that this may occur at a pressure slightly higher than one that is measured directly [43]. This is also relevant to patients of any age with a hyperkinetic state or aortic insufficiency. Both auscultatory and palpatory methods are of limited utility when limb perfusion is poor, such as in shock or other states of vasoconstriction, even though central arterial pressure may be normal [48].

Indirect measurement of pressure by transcutaneous Doppler, which detects arterial wall motion rather than auditory sound, is accurate when compared with direct measurement [49]. The ultrasound transducer, which is placed between the cuff and the artery, detects a change in the ultrasound field when the arterial wall moves during deflation of the cuff below systolic pressure. The first appearance of a signal caused by Doppler shift, converted to audible sound by the device, accurately indicates systolic pressure. Analogous to the Korotkov sounds, diastolic pressure correlates with a marked diminution in wall motion. Although often difficult to hear and therefore inherently inaccurate, the signal at this point changes to a muffled sound. The device can be used successfully in small infants, although a higher-frequency ultrasound field is required to accurately detect wall motion in the relatively small arteries of neonates, necessitating a transducer with 8 to 10 MHz output [50]. Ultrasound offers clear advantages in situations in which auscultation is difficult, including environmental noise, hearing loss, tiny arteries, obesity, and low-flow states [51]. Attention to cuff size is as important as in the auscultatory method [52].

The oscillometric principle offers the simplest

technique for fully automated indirect blood pressure monitoring. As the cuff is deflated below systolic pressure, the artery exerts pulsatile pressure to the surrounding tissue. The monitor senses the amplitude of the pulsations as they are transmitted to the cuff and uses a microprocessor to relate the degree of oscillation to pressure [53]. Systolic pressure is identified at the point at which oscillation rapidly begins to increase, while diastolic pressure correlates with the point at which oscillation amplitude suddenly decreases. Unlike other methods of indirect measurement, which derive mean blood pressure from measured systolic and diastolic values, oscillometry actually measures mean pressure by determining the point at which the oscillation reaches maximum amplitude.

Except in hypotensive, very low birthweight infants [54], oscillometrically determined blood pressure is reliable when compared to direct arterial and indirect Doppler methods, although systolic determination is more accurate than mean or diastolic [55–57]. Its superiority is based on the lack of observed variation inherent in other indirect methods, ease of cuff placement, independence from interference by sound or electrosurgical units, the ability to measure heart rate, automation, and alarm capability. Any oscillometric device used for children should be compatible with small cuffs and lower blood pressure, utilizing lower inflation pressures and maintaining adequately slow stepwise deflation.

Although indirect methods are noninvasive and thereby considered risk free, complications can occur. A cuff that is too tight or deflates improperly will cause venous congestion and possibly arterial occlusion in low-flow states. Heavy tubing that connects the cuff to the monitor should not rest on the child. Ulnar neuropathy has been associated with brachial cuffs in adult patients [58] and might be prevented by placing the cuff more proximally, away from the ulnar groove, and oriented so that the tubing exits proximally rather than distally. These maneuvers should not influence the accuracy of the device.

A new technique, using Penaz methodology in a finger cuff, provides continuous, real-time blood pressure measurement [59]. Its use in pediatrics has not been validated. While perhaps as accurate as the oscillometric technique in adults, the Penaz methodology can be inaccurate in states of vasoconstriction or poor perfusion [60], and it is not always possible to predict reliability when compared with direct measurement [61] (see Chap. 4).

Children with cardiac arrhythmias will have significant beat-to-beat fluctuation in systolic and diastolic pressure, which renders any indirect method of pressure measurement potentially inaccurate [62]. Pulsus paradoxus due to heart failure, obstructive pulmonary disease, or pericardial effusion will cause fluctuation of the arterial pressure with the respiratory cycle that will not be recognized by an automatic oscillometric technique [63].

Direct Invasive Arterial Pressure Measurement

Radial Artery Cannulation. Successful radial arterial cannulation is possible in all age groups, including premature infants [64–66]. Normally, there is extensive collateral circulation to the hand from radial and ulnar contribution to the palmar arterial arch. For cannulation the artery is immobilized by extending the wrist with the hand supinated and taped to a padded board in such a way that the fingers and thumb remain visible for signs of vascular insufficiency. Hyperextension of the wrist may cause occlusion of the radial artery in newborns and should be avoided. Locally injected 1 percent lidocaine can be used, with care taken to avoid inadvertent arterial puncture or obliteration of the small pulse. The point of maximal pulsation is located at the distal radius; alternatively, a cool fiberoptic light source directed laterally can be used to identify the artery by transillumination [67]. A small skin incision made carefully with a 20-gauge needle allows smooth percutaneous passage of the catheter assembly without shredding the plastic sheath. The needle should enter at 30 to 45 degrees. It is not always necessary to transfix the artery although this method is preferred by some, particularly in very small infants. Even with the stylet removed, blood return may not be obvious from small arteries and small catheters, necessitating slow withdrawal of the cannula. If arterial entry is achieved without transfixion, rotation of the bevel after puncture of the anterior wall as shown in Fig. 16-7 ensures that the stylet is completely within the vessel lumen and allows atraumatic threading of the catheter. Smaller sterile guide

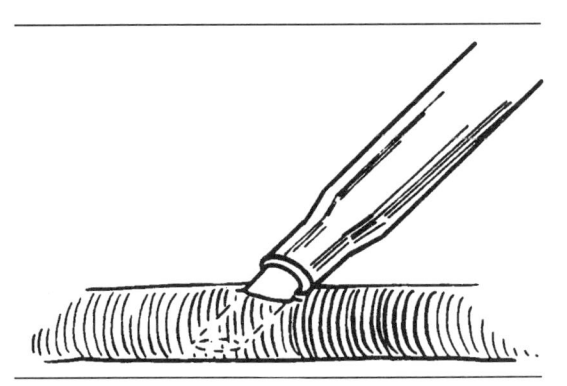

Fig. 16-7. A needle within the arterial lumen. After penetrating the artery, rotation of the bevel 180 degrees to the position shown places the needle completely within the small-vessel lumen and facilitates advancement of the catheter. (Reprinted with permission from GA Gregory, Monitoring During Surgery. In GA Gregory (ed), *Pediatric Anesthesia* (2nd ed). New York: Churchill Livingstone, 1989. Pp 477–500.)

wires and guide wire–catheter assemblies are available and may facilitate threading of the cannula for those familiar with their use; however, a wire or catheter should never be advanced against even slight resistance to avoid dissection or other damage to the vessel wall.

In infants the cannula should be connected to a stopcock by a short piece of tubing such as a T-connector, as shown in Fig. 16-8, and, after checking for blood return, flushed immediately with heparinized injections from a small syringe at 0.1 ml per second. The cannula should be secured with No. 3-0 or 4-0 sutures and covered with an occlusive adhesive dressing to allow minimal movement of the catheter within the artery. The T-connector allows withdrawal of blood samples through a 22- or 23-gauge needle inserted into the rubber injection port at the hub of the cannula while the tubing is clamped [64]. While this technique minimizes sampling dead space, the risk of exposure of personnel to contaminated needles should be considered. Any stopcock or injection port should be clearly labeled "arterial" to discourage the inadvertent infusion of hypertonic solution, vasoactive medication, or blood products. The system should be zeroed at the right atrium and continuously transduced, with alarms set to detect clinically significant blood pressure changes or technical complications, such as damping, occlusion, or disconnection and exsanguination.

The transducer and flush system should be completely free of bubbles. Flush solution should be isotonic, as hyperosmolar solution induces vessel spasm and endothelial damage that might increase the risk of thrombosis. Heparin solution of 1 to 2 units per milliliter should be continuously infused at 1 to 3 ml per hour. While normal saline diminishes the theoretic risk of bacterial colonization in dextrose solutions, the sodium load to a small infant (3 ml/hr = 11 mEq/day) must be considered.

Recommendations for catheter size vary, and although 23- or 24-gauge catheters are more appropriate for premature or small neonates most agree that 22-gauge is suitable for infants. Beyond the first several years of age, a 20-gauge catheter should suffice [1, 64].

In children with flow through the ductus arteriosus, a catheter on the right side allows preductal sampling. Vascular surgery may interfere with normal blood flow to an extremity and preclude a given site from monitoring, as in creation of a systemic-pulmonary shunt or any repair utilizing the subclavian artery. Prior catheterization, particularly by surgical cutdown, may render arterial access difficult. Because of the risk of vascular or neurologic damage, the nondominant hand should be selected for cannulation when available.

Fig. 16-8. Arterial catheter connection assembly showing pediatric T-connector tubing with injection port or stopcock available for sampling. The extremity is secured and the connectors are labeled clearly.

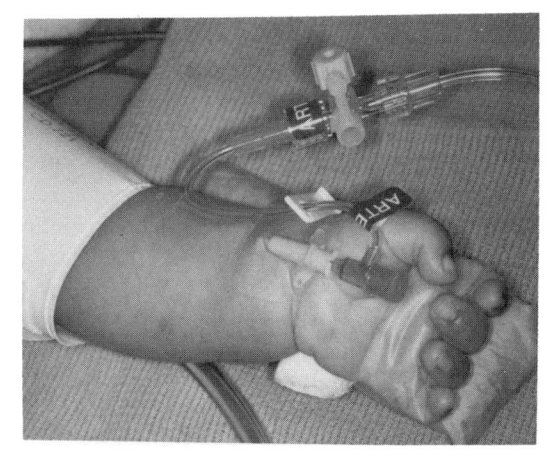

Temporary thrombosis following arterial cannulation is common but usually clinically inapparent [68]. Embolization can be observed in all major arteries of the arm, forearm, and hand but fortunately is usually asymptomatic and major complications are rare. Radial arteriography and Doppler flow studies in adults reveal the degree of thrombosis and the incidence of occlusion to correlate with the external diameter of the catheter in relation to the size of the vessel lumen [69–71] and possibly to the duration of cannulation [68]. Recanalization invariably occurs but may take weeks, with smaller vessels being the slowest [69]. Following removal of an arterial cannula, the pulse volume amplitude may increase gradually over 24 hours, indicating spasm at the time of decannulation [68]. There may be a more vasospastic tendency in pediatric patients [72].

The incidence of thrombosis and embolization has been minimized in adults by using smaller catheters and continuous heparinized flush systems rather than intermittent injection [73]. Although its safety is comparable to that seen with adult use, radial arterial catheterization in children is more frequently terminated prematurely due to malfunction. Endothelial damage may be enhanced by the catheter tip moving within a smaller vessel, thereby encouraging thrombus formation [74–76]. Nonetheless, vascular complications are similarly minor and usually transient. Blanching of the skin near the catheter occurs frequently, particularly during injection, probably related to increased local capillary pressure [64]. If skin blanching or signs of decreased distal perfusion persist, a catheter should be removed immediately. Likewise, if signs of clot formation interfere with either blood withdrawal or the pressure wave form a catheter should be removed. Attention to these details has been associated with the absence of major vascular complications in large series of infants and children [64–67, 74–76]. Although younger age and longer duration of cannulation may be associated with radial arterial occlusion, as in adults, all obstructed vessels eventually recanalize [75]. Isolated incidences of major vascular complications in children such as gangrene and digital necrosis typically occur in cases of preexisting vascular pathology or trauma, no preinsertion assessment of flow, injection of toxic solution, cannulas allowed to remain in situ despite signs of vascular compromise, and delays in treatment of occluded end arteries [77, 78]. When strict attention to technique has been followed, vascular complications have been associated with severe hypotension, vasopressor therapy, hypoxemia, and disseminated intravascular coagulation [78–80].

Later neurologic, vascular, or infectious sequelae may not be evident when clinical follow-up study beyond the perioperative period is not sought. Carpal tunnel syndrome from prior radial artery catheterization [65] and median nerve damage following brachial artery puncture or cannulation has been reported in newborns [81]. Osler's node formation has been reported following indwelling radial arterial cannulation in the adult [82]. Epiphyseal growth arrest can result from osteomyelitis, acute ischemia, or aseptic embolization, and has been observed following catheterization of radial, femoral, and umbilical arteries [83, 84]. Chronic reduction in blood supply from a damaged artery will decrease skeletal growth, but the discrepancy may be partially corrected following revascularization [85]. Finally, the risk of infection from any invasive catheterization demands strict adherence to sterile technique [86].

Manual flushing of arterial catheters must be done carefully to avoid cerebral embolization. As little as 3 ml injected into an adult radial artery can reach the subclavian-vertebral artery junction [87]. With neonatal catheters, flushed with 0.5 ml over one second, retrograde flow is seen from the radial artery to the aortic arch and left common carotid artery, and from the posterior tibial or umbilical artery to the descending aorta and superior mesenteric artery. Arterial injection is also associated with transient hypertension. These phenomena can be prevented by flushing at a rate not to exceed 0.5 ml over 5 seconds [88]. The volume to discard before obtaining blood for sampling should be equal to three times the dead space volume, and slightly more for coagulation studies [89]. The waste should never be reinjected into an artery.

Ulnar/Brachial Artery Cannulation. Alternative sites for arterial catheterization are available, although none is without risk. In the upper extremity the ulnar artery should be reserved for use when the radial is the dominant artery and has not been cannulated recently. The brachial artery, coursing from axillary to radial and ulnar arteries, should be avoided. Due to a lack of collateral circulation, its occlusion can result in loss of the distal arm [90]. In addition, the median nerve lies lateral to the artery in the antecubital fossa and can be damaged by either direct trauma or compression from a hematoma [81].

Axillary Artery Cannulation. The axillary artery is a continuation of the subclavian and is nearly as large as the femoral artery. It offers an acceptable alternative when other sides are unavailable or during circulatory insufficiency or peripheral vasoconstriction. Rich collateral circulation is supplied by the thyrocervical trunk of the subclavian artery. Complications are related to the presence of the neurovascular bundle in the axillary sheath. Vascular compromise is rare and has resolved following removal of the catheter [91, 92]. Injury to the cords of the brachial plexus by direct trauma or compression by hematoma occurs in adults. Neuropathy has not been evident in pediatric patients although more subtle neurologic deficit may have been overlooked in this age group [91, 93]. Careful location of the pulse and efforts to avoid large hematoma formation may be important factors.

With the arm supinated and abducted 90 degrees and while retracting redundant skin distally, the artery is palpated high in the axilla. The percutaneous introducer is inserted at a point distal to the humeral head and using the Seldinger technique the catheter is advanced until the tip is in the first portion of the subclavian artery [91]. In adults and most children, a 20-gauge catheter will suffice, although as small as 24-gauge has been used in neonates. For any blood gas or pressure measurement in the upper extremity, including the axillary artery, the same consideration to shunts or previous vascular surgery applies. Theoretically, it is preferable to use the left side in order to minimize embolization to the cerebral circulation, although it must be remembered that retrograde embolization has been observed from any site [87, 88].

Umbilical Artery Cannulation. Cannulation of the umbilical artery was common in neonates before the widespread use of percutaneous radial artery catheters. Constriction of the umbilical arteries is delayed in newborns with cardiorespiratory disease, although after the first few days it is usually no longer possible to cannulate the vessel [94]. In most infants a No. 3.0 or 3.5 French catheter can be inserted in the first day of life. Thrombosis does occur and, although usually asymptomatic, may result in significant occlusion or embolization. To minimize damage to vital arterial segments, the tip of the catheter should be placed above the aortic bifurcation but below the renal and inferior mesenteric arteries, corresponding to the third or fourth lumbar vertebral level. Nonetheless, the risk of vascular complications from thrombus, embolism (including air), and vasospasm cannot be eliminated. Despite prompt removal of the catheter, when evidence of ischemia exists major neurologic, gastrointestinal, renal, and lower-extremity sequelae can occur [94, 95].

Temporal Artery Cannulation. Temporal artery catheterization in newborns used to be thought of as a simple technique, relatively free from apparent short-term complications and with the advantage of a longer duration of catheter function [66, 96]. However, there have been reports of serious neurologic sequelae, including hemiplegia with computed tomography (CT) evidence of infarction in the distribution of the middle cerebral artery [97–99]. As a branch of the external carotid artery, the temporal artery is relatively contraindicated as the site of catheterization due to the risk of embolization to the nearby internal carotid artery.

Femoral Artery Cannulation. The largest artery accessible percutaneously is the femoral. Arising from the external iliac artery near the inguinal ligament and lying between the vein medially and nerve laterally, it can be cannulated easily using the Seldinger technique. Entry should never be superior to the inguinal ligament, where the external iliac artery courses posteriorly and uncontrollable bleeding can extend retroperitoneally. Hemorrhage can occur upon either insertion or removal of a catheter. Excessive local pressure to prevent hematoma is thought to be associated with increased risk of thrombus formation [100]. There are additional risk factors for thrombotic complications in children with heart disease, including polycythemia, low cardiac output, and relatively large catheter size. Prompt catheter removal and treatment with anticoagulation or thrombectomy are usually effective, although distal thrombosis or embolism carries a worse prognosis [100, 101]. Urinary and fecal contamination is of theoretic concern following isolated reports of septic arthritis of the hip in neonates after femoral venipuncture [102], but appears not to increase the risk of infection when the femoral artery is compared with other sites of cannulation [103].

Additional arteries are available in the lower extremity. The dorsalis pedis artery, superficially located parallel and lateral to the extensor hallucis longus, is the continuation of the anterior tibial artery. It is bilaterally nonpalpable in 5 percent of children and collateral circulation should be confirmed [104]. The plantar artery (the main arch of the foot analogous to the radioulnar communication in the hand) is supplied by the dorsalis pedis and the lateral plantar artery, a terminal branch of the posterior tibial artery. A modification of the Allen's test can be performed by occluding the dorsalis pedis artery, blanching the nail of the great toe, and then releasing the nail to assess reperfusion from lateral plantar flow. The patient must be supine with warm feet [105]. Both the dorsalis pedis and posterior tibial arteries have been cannulated in children and adults with relatively few complications. Thrombosis is reported, but when vessels were decannulated upon early evidence of occlusion no major complications occurred [105–107].

Technical Considerations. Interpretation of direct blood pressure measurement is dependent on the location of the catheter tip. During propagation of a pressure wave from the aorta to distal arteries, there is amplification of amplitude and contour (see Chap. 4). Primarily responsible are the reflection of pulse waves within the arterial system and a progressive increase in wall stiffness as arteries are followed distally. Amplification is highest in children and disappears progressively with age, associated with a decline in arterial distensibility and progressive arterial degenerative disease [108–110]. Nevertheless, with normal circulation direct measurement at radial, brachial, axillary, and femoral sites will reflect a systolic pressure only slightly higher than central aortic pressure. However, pedal

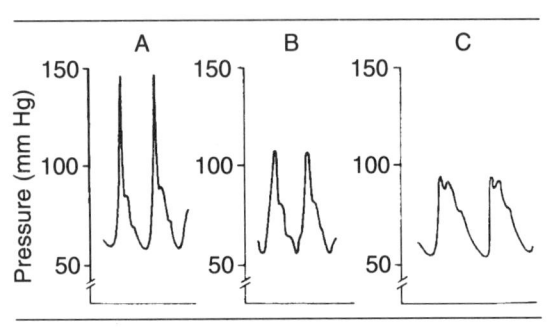

Fig. 16-9. Arterial pressure wave forms. Pedal artery pressure is compared in patients with marked (A) and minimal (B) systolic amplification. A typical radial artery pressure wave form without amplification of systolic pressure is represented in (C). (Reprinted with permission from MK Park, JI Robotham, and VF German. Systolic pressure amplification in pedal arteries in children. *Crit Care Med* 11:286, © by Williams & Wilkins, 1983.)

arterial pressure is variably and unpredictably amplified in children and therefore may lead to gross overestimation of systolic pressure [105, 106, 111], demonstrated in Fig. 16-9. Amplification may also be enhanced in conditions of increased vascular tone, such as hypovolemia, shock, hypothermia, and vasopressor therapy [108, 111].

Additional consideration should be given to the dynamic response of a system for direct pressure measurement [112, 113]. The catheter-transducer system must not only demonstrate accuracy for static calibration measurement, but also must be able to respond to the rapid and often hyperdynamic pressure wave forms in the pediatric patient. Natural frequency, defining how rapidly a system oscillates, is directly proportional to the radius and varies inversely with the square root of the length. A faster heart rate or rapid-pressure upstroke (dp/dt) as seen in children requires a higher natural frequency, usually greater than 10 Hz, for the best dynamic response [112]. High natural frequency will allow for a larger latitude in damping coefficient, which refers to how quickly a system comes to rest after a sudden change. Damping coefficient is inversely related to the third power of the radius and varies directly with the square root of the length of the catheter. With a damping coefficient that is too high (overdamped), a wave form is smoothed out, with loss of fine detail such as the dicrotic notch. With a low damping coefficient (underdamped), the wave form will overshoot and produce oscillation or ringing. Thus, underdamped systems overestimate systolic pressure, clinically by as much as 30 torr, and produce amplification of artifact [112, 114].

Although damping coefficients may be higher and resonant frequencies lower with small-gauge catheters, bench testing usually demonstrates no significant difference in accuracy within the clinical range [113]. Most error is introduced by the connection between the catheter and transducer. Connecting tubing that exceeds three feet in length can result in exaggerations of wave form and systolic pressure [114]. While catheters and transducer domes should be highly compliant, connecting tubing should be of low compliance [112]. Air is more compliant and elastic than fluid; small air bubbles reduce frequency response and cause underdamped distortion of wave forms. Experimentally, air amplifies systolic pressure significantly; diastolic and electronically averaged mean pressure are affected minimally, but mean derived from systolic and diastolic pressure is not reliable [114]. Abrupt diameter changes at tubing connectors tend to trap air bubbles. Distortion from air and long tubing are additive. On the other hand large amounts of air, unlike small bubbles, damp the response.

It is impractical to determine absolute indications for direct arterial monitoring. Venous or capillary blood samples can be used for routine laboratory determination of virtually everything but PaO_2 [115]. In clinical conditions in which noninvasive oxygen monitoring is unreliable, or if multiple blood samples are anticipated perioperatively, indwelling arterial access may be necessary. Except in severely diminished peripheral perfusion, noninvasive blood pressure measurement will usually suffice. In patients who will require further cardiac surgery, it is wise to avoid vascular cannulation whenever possible, as this may make things more difficult later on. However, if underlying cardiac disease, medical illness, or operative procedure is expected to result in circulatory instability in the perioperative period then the benefits of direct monitoring may clearly outweigh the risk.

Central Venous Access

Modification of the technique used for percutaneous access to central veins of adults allows successful cannulation in most children. However, the complications reported in adults have also occurred in children, and the pediatric cardiac patient may present additional risk because of anatomic and physiologic variation.

In children with normal anatomy, the subclavian vein courses behind the clavicle and is attached to this bone and first rib by loose connective tissue. The subclavian artery parallels the vein posteriorly and, medial to the clavicular midpoint, is separated from the vein by the scalenus anterior muscle. At this point over the first rib, the area is free of pleura and can be safely cannulated in infants and older children. Nonetheless, the risk of fatal arterial or pleural puncture always exists. Insertion of a needle either lateral to the clavicular midpoint or beyond the plane of the subclavian vein will direct it posteriorly into the pleura. The tangential direction of the needle increases the risk of a larger, linear tear. Unlike vessels in the neck or groin, the subclavian vessels are protected by the clavicle. Thus, bleeding may be profuse and difficult to control, with the inability to compress the vessel.

In infants the subclavian veins arch superiorly as they course centrally, particularly on the right [116]. As seen in Fig. 16-10, a catheter must change direction to traverse the high arch of the subclavian vein and the acute angle between the innominate vein and superior vena cava. Thus, inadvertent passage into the ipsilateral internal jugular or contralateral innominate vein may occur. The left side may be simpler due to the less acute angle [117] but proximity to the thoracic duct presents a theoretic disadvantage. After one year of age, the subclavian vein assumes the horizontal position characteristic of the adult [116].

Due to the life-threatening nature of its complications, the procedure should be carried out in a controlled, monitored setting with strict attention to technique. With the head extended slightly and arms adducted, a small roll under the thoracic spine should extend the shoulders symmetrically and open the small space between the clavicle and first rib. The Trendelenburg position may not be necessary [116, 118] and does not eliminate the risk of air embolism. A thin-walled needle attached to a syringe should enter below the midpoint of the clavicle and, once under the bone, should not exceed a 20-degree angle with the skin. With gentle negative pressure on the syringe, the needle is inserted and withdrawn slowly in a straight line, aiming just above the sternal notch until blood return occurs. When using a needle-catheter assembly in infants, care must be taken to advance sufficiently so that the tip of the plastic cannula lies within the vessel, while avoiding puncture of the posterior wall with the needle. Using the Seldinger technique a wire with the J-tip directed caudally will facilitate passage to the vena cava. Proper placement of the cannula must be confirmed by testing immediately for blood return and examining the chest x-ray for catheter tip location and evidence of pneumothorax. Complications include hemorrhage or arterial puncture; placement in extrathoracic veins, pericardium, or pleural space; and pneumothorax [57, 117, 119]. In patients with vascular anomalies, including repair or shunt procedures involving the subclavian or innominate vessels, cannulation by the infraclavicular approach may be hazardous.

The location and course of the internal jugular vein make it a somewhat safer alternative to the subclavian approach. It is usually as large or larger than the subclavian vein, and is more expansible, which enhances the utility of the Trendelenburg position [116]. While in infants the course from the right internal jugular vein follows a straight line through the right innominate vein to the superior vena cava (see Fig. 16-10), the course from the left is severely angulated at both the left innominate vein and the superior vena cava [118]. The longer, tortuous course to the right atrium, along with the higher location of apical pleura and the presence of the thoracic duct on the left, renders cannulation of the right side preferable. Unlike the subclavian vessel approach, the cervical approach allows direct compression when bleeding occurs.

The internal jugular approach is popular in both adults and children due to a high success rate and low incidence of complications [120–124]. Nonetheless, life-threatening complications do occur and additional skill is required for the more technically intricate catheterization in infants. Percu-

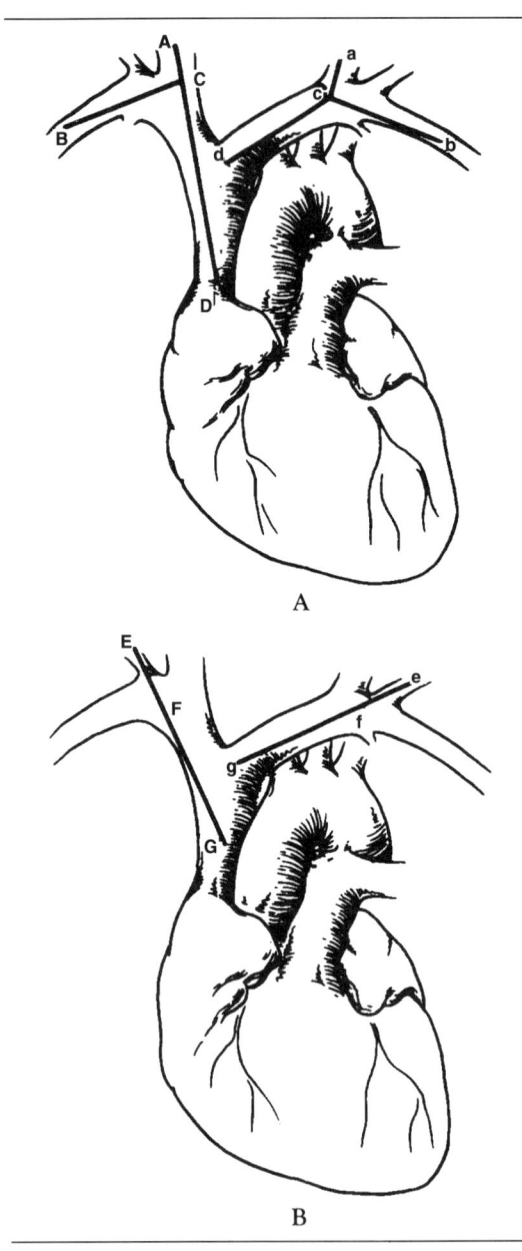

Fig. 16-10. Central venous anatomy in infants. A. The high arched course of the right and left subclavian veins is represented by angles BCD and bcd. The internal jugular veins course directly into the central venous circulation, as shown by angles ACD and acd. B. Likewise, the external jugular veins follow a nearly straight course represented by EFG and efg. (Reprinted with permission from LM Cobb, CD Vinocur, CW Wagner, et al., The central venous anatomy in infants. *Surg Gynecol Obstet* 165:230, 1987. By permission of *Surgery, Gynecology and Obstetrics*.)

taneous technique avoids the problems associated with surgical cutdown of neck veins, including scar formation and inability to use the vessel in the future [123]. While the procedure is essentially the same as in adults, the anatomic landmarks are less apparent in small children. In the 15- to 20-degree Trendelenburg position with the head turned to the contralateral side, a roll placed under the shoulders allows slight extension of the neck, unobtrusive placement of the infant's large occiput, tension of the sternocleidomastoid muscle, and optimal anatomic exposure. Location of the vessel can be accomplished with a small-gauge "finder" needle. At the apex of the triangle formed by the sternal and clavicular heads of the sternocleidomastoid muscle, the needle should enter the skin at an angle of 30 to 45 degrees, directed toward the ipsilateral nipple. If the landmarks of the triangle are not clear, as occurs with neuromuscular blockade, skin entry should be immediately lateral to the carotid artery at the midpoint of a line between the mastoid process and the suprasternal notch [120]. The needle should enter the vein within 1 to 2 cm of the skin surface. Excessively deep or caudal insertion increases the risk of damage to structures such as pleura or prevertebral sympathetic chain. If no blood return occurs during initial passage, the syringe and needle should be withdrawn very slowly with only gentle negative pressure. Inadvertent puncture of the carotid artery is often difficult to detect, as venous pressure may be very high or arterial saturation may be low in children with congenital heart disease. Determination of pressure with the transducer connected to the finder needle may be necessary. The catheter itself should advance easily and free blood return should be demonstrated before infusion.

A posterior approach, entering the skin at the midpoint of the posterior border of the clavicular head of the muscle and directing toward the suprasternal notch, can also be used [121, 123]. A low approach that uses as a landmark a notch near the sternal end of the clavicle, thereby avoiding the difficulty in identification of the sternocleidomastoid muscle in small children, has been described [125]. However, the technique may be associated with a greater risk of pneumothorax and intrapulmonary hemorrhage, the morbidity of which makes it difficult to justify this as a routine approach [126].

Due to the proximity of pleura and thoracic duct, the low approach is relatively contraindicated on the left, and is absolutely contraindicated in ipsilateral vascular anomalies such as a Blalock-Taussig shunt or a right-sided aortic arch [126, 127]. Complications of internal jugular vein cannulation include mediastinal extravasation, pneumothorax, tracheal puncture, carotid arterial puncture, superior vena caval obstruction, Horner's syndrome, and damage to the thoracic duct [121–123, 125, 126, 128–130]. Pneumothorax has also been reported following removal of an internal jugular sheath, presumably opening a pleural and parenchymal defect caused during insertion [131].

Alternatively, the external jugular vein can be used, offering an extremely safe site of entry away from other important structures. Although its valves and curved, nonfixed course through the neck may hinder initial advancement of a catheter or guide wire, the course to the innominate vein is nearly a straight line in infants [118] (see Fig. 16-10). Passage to the central circulation may be easier with the use of a J-wire if the radius of curvature of the J-tip is smaller than the diameter of the vein [132]. Although external jugular cannulation is considered safer, its success rate usually falls short of the internal approach [132–134].

The femoral vein allows access to the central circulation easily and without the risk of cerebrovascular or potentially fatal intrathoracic complications. The vein, which lies medial to the artery, should be entered caudal to the inguinal ligament to prevent uncontrollable retroperitoneal hematoma formation. The needle should be advanced at a 30-degree angle to the skin, and dropped to a more parallel position once inside the vein to facilitate passage of a J-wire through a small child's vessel. Contraindications include existing infection, ischemia, or thromboembolic disease involving the lower extremity, and trauma or major surgery of the abdomen or pelvis. When subsequent cardiac catheterization is anticipated in a child with heart disease, an alternative site should be considered. In the patient with congenital heart disease associated with interruption of the inferior vena cava, a superior approach is necessary [135]. Although there is no evidence that the incidence of thrombotic complications associated with femoral catheters is greater than with other vessels in either children or adults [135–137], deep venous thrombosis of the leg is potentially serious and concern is justified. Indeed, thrombosis should be considered a risk of central venous cannulation by any route. While thrombus formation may be clinically inapparent, prompt removal of the catheter on any sign of thrombotic obstruction such as leg swelling may reduce the risk of thromboembolic sequelae [135, 136]. Hypercoagulable states increase the risk of thrombosis at any site, and an alternative to the femoral approach might be considered in cyanotic children with polycythemia. While coagulopathy increases the risk of bleeding at any site, the femoral vessels can be easily compressed and therefore offer a safer alternative to thoracic or cervical vessels. A theoretic concern, bacterial contamination of the inguinal area, has not been shown to increase catheter-related infection [103].

A variety of smaller catheters are manufactured for pediatric use. Appropriate length is easily determined by visual estimation of the course from skin entry to central vena caval site. Appropriate diameter is determined not only by patient size but also by the intended use of the catheter. For children less than 2 years of age, the equivalent of No. 3 French (or 22 gauge) is usually appropriate, children 2 to 10 years of age can use No. 4 French (or 20 gauge), and older children and adolescents require No. 5 French or adult catheters [126]. While the minimum diameter is appropriate for simply monitoring central venous pressure, a larger size may be desirable for perioperative administration of fluid and blood products. Rapid infusion is possible peripherally through large-bore intravenous catheters but may be limited by the size, valves, and tortuosity of small veins [138]. Although the central circulation can accept extremely rapid flow rates, infusion may be limited by the length of some smaller-lumen pediatric catheters, following Poiseuille's law, which states that resistance to flow is inversely related to the fourth power of the radius but directly related to length. If fluid resuscitation is necessary, a lumen with greater cross-sectional area may be appropriate, but excessive length may negate the benefits of the larger lumen. Multiple-lumen catheters are also available for children. They allow administration of incompatible substances and accurate pressure monitoring simultaneously [139]. However, the variable distances between the ports of distal and proximal lumens may place the most proximal port outside the central circulation in infants, rendering it useless for pressure measurements [140] and dangerous for infusion of hyperosmolar, thrombogenic substances.

Although experience with smaller catheters has made possible percutaneous access to central veins in children, surgical cutdown may occasionally be necessary. In the arm the cephalic and basilic veins are available by cutdown, and central placement in infants is often more successful via the latter [141]. Turning the head to the ipsilateral side may prevent the catheter from coursing into the neck, and the semi-sitting position may also aid intrathoracic placement [142]. In the leg the distal saphenous vein is available but the distance to the central circulation precludes its use. Alternatively, the large and easily accessible proximal saphenous vein has been used but the risk of thrombosis should limit its use to emergency, short-term situations [143]. The umbilical vein is used occasionally in newborns, but likewise can cause thromboembolic complications and has been associated with hepatic necrosis following infusion of hyperosmolar substances [144].

The incidence of occult air embolism is unknown, but the potential morbidity in a child with an intracardiac shunt demands rigorous precautions, including the meticulous inspection of the entire length of tubing, injection ports, stopcocks, connection sites, needles, and syringes to avoid the potentially catastrophic consequences of air embolization in the systemic circulation. While documented right-to-left or bidirectional shunting places a patient at risk, the transient reversal of left-to-right shunt can occur during the cardiac cycle. Massive venous air embolism immediately following catheter removal has also been reported [145].

Except for the purpose of evacuating embolized air, a catheter tip in the right atrium is contraindicated due to the risk of cardiac perforation. A rare but lethal complication, perforation can occur during insertion or, more commonly, later. Rapid deterioration from pericardial tamponade will result, unless recognition is prompt and is followed by aspiration through the catheter, pericardiocentesis, and, if necessary, pericardiotomy. Perforation of the vena cava, resulting in hydrothorax [146, 147], and of the ventricle (frequently fatal) [148], can also occur. While most reports of cardiac perforation in children have been associated with the use of stiffer material such as polyethylene [149–151], perforation can occur with any pliable material as well, including Silastic [150].

Location of a central venous catheter is confirmed by x-ray or sonography, the latter offering greater sensitivity to catheter malposition in infants [152, 153]. Using the catheter tip as a properly grounded exploring ECG lead can also determine its position [154]. The catheter should be sutured in place near the entry site and immobilized to prevent kinking, accidental dislodgment, or distal migration. Nevertheless, movement of the neck, arm, or chest may advance the tip into the right atrium or ventricle, particularly when a long cannula is inserted through an arm vein. Placement in the external jugular vein has also been associated with excessive catheter movement in infants and the risk of perforation exists with central catheters inserted at any site [148–151, 155]. While most recommend placement of the catheter tip in the vena cava at the junction of the right atrium, others advocate the innominate–superior vena cava junction [155, 156]. Although inaccuracy may exist in the inferior vena cava [156], venous pressure measured in any of the intrathoracic central veins will reasonably reflect right atrial pressure [157].

Central venous pressure can be measured most accurately with a calibrated, recorded pressure curve using end expiratory mean pressure. Digital electronic measurements correlate closely, but because they usually average the signal over an interval of time the result is influenced by periodic fluctuations such as the respiratory cycle. Although currently available monitors use an algorithm that seeks end expiratory pressure as the long, stable portion of low-frequency variation, such a system may fail, with higher respiratory rates in children [158]. A digital value will be higher in patients with positive pressure ventilation and lower during spontaneous respiration. Measurement by water manometry is unreliable [159].

With certain limitations the central venous pressure tracing may reflect abnormal right ventricular physiology. Despite surgical correction of tetralogy of Fallot or a long-standing atrial septal defect, right ventricular dysfunction may persist. For example, in right ventricular failure, or with increased afterload in children with pulmonic stenosis or pulmonary hypertension, a prominent "a" wave is seen. Interpretation of ventricular function from central venous pressure requires intact function of the tricuspid valve, as atrial contraction through a stenotic valve will also produce a large a wave. With tricuspid regurgitation, whether congenital or acquired from right ventricular dilatation or intracardiac surgery, the pressure tracing will be dominated by a large "v" wave. Monitoring central venous pressure may be useful when right-sided function is critically dependent on preload, such as after the Fontan procedure. Avoidance of hypovolemia and maintenance of adequate systemic venous return are important in obstructive lesions such as valvular or infundibular pulmonary stenosis, including tetralogy of Fallot. Experience with adults and more recently with children has confirmed that in a variety of clinical situations central venous pressure is not a reliable indicator of left-sided filling or function, particularly when compliance is altered. In addition central venous blood does not accurately reflect mixed venous oxygen content.

Right Heart Catheterization

If direct measurement of pulmonary artery pressure, estimation of left ventricular filling pressure or function, measurement of mixed venous oxygen content, or determination of cardiac output is indicated, a central venous catheter is inadequate. Although right and left ventricular function curves are similar in shape, the relationship between atrial pressure and contralateral stroke work or cardiac output is not consistent. Differences in contractility and Frank-Starling forces exist between the ventricles. Clinically, this disparity is demonstrated by the inaccuracy of central venous pressure in assessment of biventricular function during left ventricular failure, myocardial ischemia or infarction, cor pulmonale, vasoactive drug infusion, inotropic therapy, and other critical or multisystem illness [160–164].

In the absence of mitral valve disease, left atrial pressure closely approximates left ventricular end diastolic pressure, the true left ventricular "filling pressure," and is estimated by pulmonary artery wedge pressure [165, 166]. With rapid heart rates and catheters of varying dynamic response, a wedge tracing may be difficult to interpret in children. An underdamped system will amplify artifact such as catheter whip in the pulmonary artery [112]. Children with mitral regurgitation will have wedge tracings dominated by giant v waves in which mean pulmonary artery wedge pressure may exceed pulmonary artery diastolic pressure. Care must be taken to avoid misinterpretation of a pulmonary wedge tracing that resembles a nonwedged pulmonary artery tracing due to underdamping or the presence of a large v wave in mitral regurgitation. Likewise, mitral stenosis will result in a prominent a wave and the pulmonary artery wedge pressure is no longer a reliable indicator of left ventricular preload. Wedge pressure will also be influenced by alveolar pressure unless the catheter tip rests in dependent lung below the left atrium (zone III of West) [167], where pulmonary venous pressure exceeds alveolar pressure. However, with proper placement pulmonary artery wedge pressure is an accurate reflection of left atrial pressure even during positive pressure ventilation with high levels of positive end-expiratory pressure [166, 168]. Pressure measurement is routinely performed at end expiration and the same limitations for central venous pressure measurement apply.

To avoid repeated balloon occlusion, pulmonary artery diastolic pressure is occasionally used to follow left ventricular end diastolic pressure. However, this relationship is unreliably altered in tachycardia, increased pulmonary blood flow from left-to-right shunt, increased pulmonary venous pressure from anomalous pulmonary venous systems, mitral valve disease or left ventricular dysfunction, and increased arteriolar resistance in children with true pulmonary hypertension [169–172]. In patients with left ventricular dysfunction, in whom an accentuated atrial systole contributes to left ventricular filling, true left ventricular end diastolic pressure is best reflected by the peak a wave in the wedge tracing [169]. Unfortunately, the a wave may be difficult to determine with rapid heart rates and smaller catheters.

Children with heart disease presenting for noncardiac surgery may occasionally require hemodynamic monitoring for coexisting cardiogenic shock, reactive pulmonary artery hypertension, critical valvular disease, septic shock, severe respiratory failure, or major surgery with significant third-space fluid loss. In these conditions appropriate treatment with volume expansion, inotropic agents, vasoactive drugs, or manipulation of ventilatory support depends on accurate hemodynamic assessment, and pulmonary artery catheterization is often justified. Other means of assessment, such as peripheral perfusion, oxygenation, acid-base status, and urine output, should never be ignored. However, the use of invasive hemodynamic monitoring is an important adjunct to patient management and can provide information that is not otherwise available [173].

The Swan-Ganz [174] flow-directed balloon-tipped pulmonary artery catheter with thermodilution cardiac output capability is available in sizes appropriate for infants and children. A No. 4 French catheter is ideal for most newborns and infants, a No. 5 French catheter will suffice for most children under 18 kg, and a No. 7 French can be used for older children and adolescents. The total length of the catheter and the distance from the central venous lumen to the tip vary according to catheter size and manufacturer. With the balloon tip wedged appropriately in the proximal pulmonary artery of a small infant, the standard central venous port at 15 cm from the tip would place the port in an extrathoracic vessel or inside the introducer sheath, resulting in inaccurate central venous pressure and cardiac output determination. Thus, smaller catheters are equipped with central venous pressure ports 7 to 10 cm from the tip. The appropriate distance can be estimated by measuring on the anterior surface of the patient or, more accurately, the chest radiograph. A nomogram is shown in Fig. 16-11; this most accurately predicts mid–right atrium to right pulmonary artery distance (MRA-to-RPA) using patient length, although a simpler derived equation.

$$\text{MRA-to-RPA} = 5.32 + 1.06 \times \text{square root of age}$$

can be used to predict MRA-to-RPA in most clinical situations [175]. A sheath introducer should be used with a protective sleeve to maintain sterility

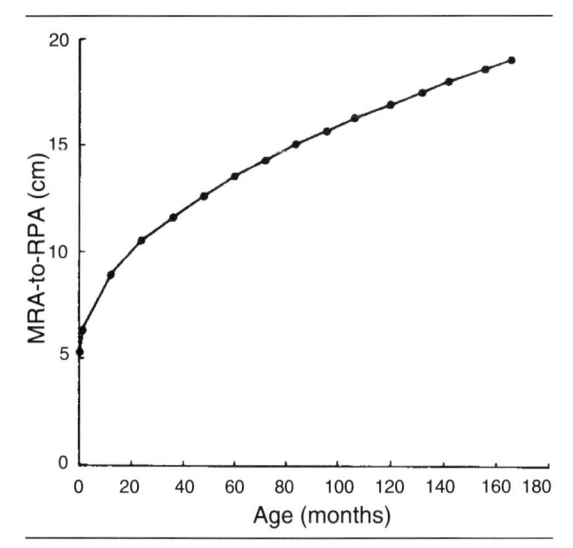

Fig. 16-11. MRA-to-RPA = 1.504 + 0.156 × length − 0.117 × SSSP. MRA-to-RPA = mean right atrial to right pulmonary artery distance; SSSP = suprasternal to suprapubic distance. (Reprinted with permission from LM Borland. Allometric determination of the distance from the central venous pressure port to wedge position of balloon-tip catheters in pediatric patients. *Crit Care Med* 14:974, © by Williams & Wilkins, 1986.)

and allow manipulation of the catheter after initial insertion [176]. The size of the introducer is usually one size French larger than the pulmonary artery catheter, but the sheath must not reach the right atrium. Likewise, a subclavian introducer in a small patient might reach the contralateral subclavian vein [177].

While essentially the same technique as in adults, pulmonary artery catheter placement in children is technically more difficult, even in the absence of cardiovascular anomalies. The relatively stiff catheter does not easily traverse the sharp curves of vessels and cardiac chambers, and difficulty in advancing beyond the right ventricle is common. Fluoroscopic guidance during manipulation of the catheter may assist in its placement. Two-dimensional echocardiography also allows visualization of the catheter and balloon location [178, 179]. The inflated balloon can cause transient obstruction to right atrial or ventricular outflow [128] and in the pulmonary artery can cause critical obstruction [129, 180]. Partial deflation of the balloon may facilitate its passage [128]. Inflation of the balloon in the pulmonary artery may increase right ventricular afterload and alter, or even reverse, a left-to-right shunt, as demonstrated by arterial oxygen desaturation and increased systemic arterial pressure in children with cardiac septal defects [129].

Additional difficulty arises when the catheter is passed through abnormal anatomy. With a $Q_P:Q_S$ ratio of 1 or greater, the catheter should pass into an intact pulmonary artery or surgical pulmonary artery conduit [134]. Atrial fibrillation, tricuspid stenosis, or regurgitant flow from severe tricuspid insufficiency may cause difficulty in advancing into the right ventricle [129, 181]. Subvalvular pulmonic stenosis or right ventricular dilatation may prevent the catheter from exiting the pulmonary outflow [180, 181]. Patients with unrepaired tetralogy of Fallot are at high risk for arrhythmia and pulmonary infundibular spasm, and a catheter in the pulmonary artery is relatively contraindicated [134]. In children with endocardial cushion or septal defects, it is possible to wedge the catheter in the pulmonary artery. Careful attention to the pressure tracing should alert one to entry into the systemic ventricle, as the inflated balloon may float the catheter into the left side and obstruct a major artery such as the carotid or descending aorta. Although in most infants the ductus arteriosus is functionally closed within the first 10 days of life [182], children with congenital heart disease have a higher incidence of persistent ductus arteriosus. A pulmonary artery catheter thus can be advanced inadvertently or migrate passively through the ductus, revealing systemic arterial pressure and oxygen tension [134, 183]. Transposition of the great arteries poses obvious difficulty, although it is possible to enter the pulmonary artery from the left or common ventricle [180].

Pulmonary artery pressure and reactivity are elevated at birth, particularly in term infants, and gradually fall to near adult levels within hours or days [182]. However, in children with elevated pulmonary vascular resistance due to congenital heart disease the pulmonary vasculature is highly reactive [129]. Prompt treatment of a pulmonary hypertensive crisis is necessary to prevent right ventricular failure and hypoxia from right-to-left shunt, particularly during acid-base or fluid imbalance, sepsis, respiratory insufficiency, or extubation. Thus, pulmonary artery monitoring may be justified in children with large left-to-right shunts or right ventricular dysfunction [184]. In any cardiac patient whose perioperative course might be complicated by increased pulmonary vascular resistance, low cardiac output, pulmonary venous congestion, or noncardiogenic pulmonary edema correct diagnosis, and subsequent intervention depends on accurate hemodynamic assessment.

Large series of pulmonary artery catheterization in children [128, 129, 134, 180] and adults [130, 164, 174, 177, 185–187] confirm its relative safety. Most significant complications are associated with obtaining central venous access. Choice of vein is subject to the same consideration as with central venous pressure monitoring, although in children the pulmonary artery catheter may be more difficult to place from the external jugular vein or distant sites such as femoral or arm veins. Arrhythmia is common, both supraventricular and ventricular, and as in adults, usually resolves spontaneously with advancement or withdrawal of the catheter. Although rarely seen in children, passage of the catheter may transiently disrupt right ventricular conduction [185]. In a child with left bundle branch block from a congenital or surgical lesion, progression to complete heart block is of theoretic concern [186, 188]. Placement of a transcutaneous cardiac pacing device before the procedure facilitates immediate treatment.

Pediatric balloon rupture is rare [128, 180], and possibly less frequent with newer catheters [129, 134], but can cause embolization of air and latex. Inflation volume ranges from 0.5 to 1.5 cc and strict attention to the manufacturer's specification is crucial. In any child with a right-to-left shunt, the balloon, including the dead space, should be inflated with sterile carbon dioxide, which minimizes the effects of gas embolism due to its high blood solubility. The inflated balloon will decrease in diameter by about 0.5 mm per minute as carbon dioxide diffuses through the latex wall [180].

Intracardiac knotting of the catheter has been reported in adults [189, 190] and children [80]. With the balloon deflated the catheter should be gently withdrawn under fluoroscopic guidance. Passage of a semiflexible guide wire can facilitate unknotting but great care should be taken to avoid perforation of the heart or vessels [189]. A tight knot will not allow the catheter to be drawn through the sheath introducer, and should never be pulled through an inaccessible vein such as the subclavian.

Pulmonary complications are rare if strict guidelines are followed. Rupture of the pulmonary artery is usually associated with a distally placed or permanently wedged catheter, and most commonly is associated with cardiac surgery or profound hypothermia [186, 191, 192]. Risk can be minimized by placement in a more proximal segment, prompt deflation of the balloon, and continuous monitoring of the pressure tracing for evidence of a permanent wedge position. Redundant intracardiac catheter length should be avoided, and catheter migration will frequently occur. Monitoring a right ventricular port, available on some catheters for migration to the pulmonary artery [193, 194], is unreliable due to the infinite variability in the size of pediatric patients. If a catheter wedges with only partial inflation of the balloon, the catheter should be withdrawn. The balloon should be allowed to deflate passively. Rupture of the pulmonary artery in adults is often associated with pulmonary hypertension, although the degree of causation or risk is not clear. Anticoagulation contributes to fatal outcome [191]. Any degree of hemoptysis during or following catheter insertion should be considered a warning sign of possible pulmonary artery rupture or dissection [193]. While hemorrhage may cease spontaneously or with the application of positive end expiratory pressure [195], the need for prompt endobronchial intubation or thoracotomy may arise. Pulmonary infarction can result from occlusion of an arterial segment by thrombus, embolism, a distally migrated catheter tip, or prolonged balloon inflation. Attention to catheter location, along with the use of heparin-bonded catheters and constant heparinized infusion through the lumen, should minimize the risk of infarction [185, 186, 196].

Cardiac Output

The thermodilution technique for measurement of cardiac output in infants and children is accurate by comparison with the Fick principle [197, 198] and dye dilution [199, 200] methods. It is much easier to perform and avoids the large amount of blood sampling required by dye dilution. A set of computation factors is supplied with each type of catheter. Earlier recommendations to prefill the catheter dead space with blood at body temperature are probably unnecessary [201]. The Stewart-Hamilton indicator dilution equation reveals the relationship of the variables:

$$Q = \frac{1.08(T_B - T_I)V_I C_T 60}{\int \Delta T_B(t)\, dt}$$

where Q = cardiac output (liters/min), $T_B - T_I$ = temperature of blood and injectate (°C), V_I = volume of injectate (liters), C_T = correction for heat gained by injectate during injection, 1.08 = empiric correction factor for specific heat and gravity of blood and injectate, 60 = factor for conversion of liters/sec to liters/min, and $\int \Delta T_B(t)\, dt$ = integral of the resultant temperature-time curve (°C/sec) [201].

In children a smaller injectate volume is necessary to avoid fluid overload, prolonged injection time through a narrower lumen, and distortion of the dilution curve due to recirculation of thermal indicator [197, 202]. Iced rather than room-temperature injectate improves the signal-to-noise ratio and allows greater accuracy at lower volume, which can range from 1 to 10 ml of either normal saline or dextrose 5 percent. While the specific gravity and specific heat of each solution are similar so that the computation factor need not change, the sodium load should be considered in smaller infants who require repeated determination. Using a smaller injectate volume in children, the cardiac output should be determined by averaging three consecutive, randomly timed determinations, which should be within 10 to 15 percent of each other. Variability will increase when stroke output varies, as in atrial fibrillation or heart block. Normal cardiac output indexed to surface area, along with derived hemodynamic variables, is presented in Table 16-3.

Although the computer calculates and displays the cardiac output, it is important to examine the thermodilution curve to detect distortion from artifact. The thermistor must be in the pulmonary artery, confirmed by an appropriate pressure tracing and an undistorted thermodilution curve with rapid return to thermal baseline [199]. Adequate mixing of the indicator in the blood and no loss of indicator before sampling are essential and the thermistor must sense mainstream flow [202]. Thus, with the tip of the catheter in the pulmonary artery the injectate port must be within the right atrium or a central vein. Likewise, loss of injectate retrograde through an introducer sheath will yield erroneous results. Injection from the right ventricle in the adult has produced reliable results [203] but adequate mixing has not been confirmed in children.

Like the Fick method thermodilution is unreliable when right and left heart output are unequal [204]. The presence of a left-to-right shunt causes recirculation of indicator, which adds an additional deflection to the thermodilution curve that either will overestimate systemic output or cannot be interpreted by the computer, but can be used to estimate Q_P/Q_S, as shown in Fig. 16-12 [205]. With a left-to-right shunt through a ductus arteriosus, the shunt flow will be included in the cardiac output determination when the thermistor is distal to the shunt. With a right-to-left shunt, systemic cardiac output is overestimated due to loss of indicator, bypassing the thermistor [198]. If a shunt in either direction is less than 10 percent, the error is usually insignificant [204]. Thermodilution is also less reliable during low-flow states, tending to overestimate cardiac output due to heat loss during the prolonged course to the pulmonary artery. In order for thermodilution to reflect total cardiac output, the catheter must be in a vessel through which all ve-

Table 16-3. Cardiac output and increasing age

Age	Cardiac output (liters/min)	Cardiac index (liters/min/m^2)
Term	0.4 ± 0.1	2.5 ± 0.6
6 mo	0.8 ± 0.2	2.0 ± 0.5
12 mo	1.1 ± 0.3	2.5 ± 0.6
2 yr	1.7 ± 1.4	3.1 ± 0.7
3 yr	2.1 ± 0.5	—
5 yr	2.7 ± 0.7	3.7 ± 0.9
12 yr	4.5 ± 1.0	4.3 ± 1.1
23 yr	6.5 ± 0.5	3.7 ± 0.3

Source: Reprinted with permission from GA Gregory, Pediatric Anesthesia. In RD Miller (ed), *Anesthesia* (2nd ed). New York: Churchill Livingstone, 1986.

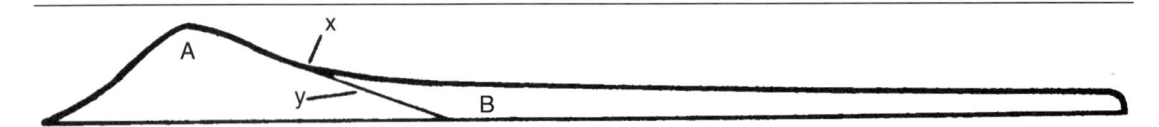

Fig. 16-12. Thermodilution curve obtained in a patient with atrial septal defect (ASD) and left-to-right shunt of 2.2:1.0. Early recirculation of indicator through the ASD results in a deflection at point x in the usual exponential portion of the downslope. Extrapolating the exponential downslope before x to the baseline allows transposition of line y to the original curve. The area under the curve is divided into A and B, and shunt ratio is calculated by the ratio of (A + B) to (A). (Reprinted with permission from F Morady, BH Brundage, and HJ Gelberg. Rapid method for determination of shunt ratio using a thermodilution technique. Am Heart J 106:369, 1983).

nous return flows. For example, in certain anomalous systemic venous connections, or following operations, such as Blalock-Taussig (subclavian to pulmonary artery), Waterston (ascending aorta to pulmonary artery), Potts (descending aorta to pulmonary artery), or Glenn (superior vena cava to right pulmonary artery) shunts, or a modified Fontan procedure where venous return is divided between the right and left pulmonary arteries, thermodilution cannot reliably determine cardiac output [134]. Congenital or surgically acquired pulmonary insufficiency changes the shape of the thermodilution curve to a shorter peak and a more gradual return to baseline, but the area under the curve is not significantly changed and allows determination of cardiac output. Severe tricuspid regurgitation usually overestimates cardiac output when measured by thermodilution. Low-flow states can magnify error caused by regurgitant flow [206, 207]. Infusion of cold intravenous fluid or blood should not interfere significantly if the infusion rate and temperature are not changed preceding or during thermodilution cardiac output determination [208]. Electrosurgical devices may interfere with the ability to interpret information from the thermistor.

Mixed Venous Oxygen Measurement

Mixed venous blood sampled from the pulmonary artery is a nonspecific indicator of tissue oxygenation. Mixed venous PO_2 (SvO_2) falls very predictably during severe impairment of intracellular oxygenation from either cardiac or respiratory etiology, correlating with hyperlactatemia [209]. It must be kept in mind that in the presence of intracardiac left-to-right shunt the pulmonary artery PO_2 does not reflect true PvO_2. A full discussion of SvO_2 measurement and interpretation is presented in Chap. 4.

Echocardiography

Limitations imposed by relying on central venous or pulmonary artery wedge pressure to determine left ventricular end diastolic pressure have been discussed. Interpretation of left ventricular end diastolic pressure also is limited, as it may not reliably reflect left ventricular diastolic volume and myocardial fiber length, especially when there is altered left ventricular compliance. Two-dimensional echocardiography offers a more direct method for assessment of ventricular function. Left ventricular diastolic volume represents true preload; contractility is reflected by ejection fraction, shortening fraction, mean velocity of circumferential fiber-shortening length, and systolic time intervals. Determination of wall stress more completely reflects afterload. Nonetheless, limitations to echocardiographic measurements exist, including the dependence of certain measurements on false geometric assumptions and the inability to hold certain parameters constant during clinical measurement.

Until recently transesophageal echocardiography was limited to children over 20 kg, in whom a biplane adult probe can be used safely [210]. The development of smaller probes has allowed the use of pulsed-wave Doppler and M-mode echocardiographic imaging with color-flow mapping in newborns with a device measuring only 6 to 7 mm in diameter at the tip [211, 212]. The advantages over precordial or epicardial acoustic windows are clear [210, 212–214]. Visualization of atrial situs, interatrial septum, and both systemic and pulmonary venous return is superior. Function of an interatrial baffle from a Mustard or Senning procedure or the circulation from a Fontan procedure can be assessed. Morphology and function of the atrioventricular valves are easily seen. Left ventricular volume and systolic function are easily assessed, and early left ventricular diastolic dysfunction from right ventricular dilation or hypertrophy, as in children with pulmonary hypertension, can be evaluated using pulsed Doppler [215]. The left ventricular outflow tract morphology is also clearly delineated. Although the central and right pulmonary arteries are easily seen, resolution of the left pulmonary artery and right ventricular outflow tract is difficult due to the distance from the esophageal probe. Likewise, the anteroapical portion of the interventricular septum may not be seen. Some of these problems may eventually be eliminated by the development of smaller biplane probes.

Quantitative Doppler measurements can be used to determine flow and thereby estimate cardiac output or shunt flows. A full discussion of pediatric Doppler and echocardiography is beyond the scope of this chapter.

THE FUTURE

Modification of technology developed for use in the adult has provided the ability to perform right-heart catheterization, thermodilution cardiac output, oximetry, and capnography safely and reliably in children. Pulse oximetry has radically changed the practice of anesthesia. Newer devices using reflectance spectrophotometry will allow continuous surface or intravascular monitoring of oxygenation in infants. Beat-to-beat blood pressure measurement might be possible noninvasively by refining existing techniques.

The field of echocardiography is rapidly developing and advances in miniaturization will allow greater resolution and measurement in pediatric patients. Transvascular applications will allow direct intravascular and intracardiac imaging. Simpler Doppler devices, such as transesophageal and transtracheal probes, might be ideal for routine practice. They require little expertise, but so far are subject to significant limitations imposed by errors in measurement of diameter and flow [216, 217]. A technique such as transthoracic bioimpedance allows totally noninvasive measurement in children, although its accuracy is questioned during various clinical conditions [218, 219].

With all monitoring modalities, new and old, the balance of risk against the benefit of information obtained must take into account the limitations of the device and method. All measurement is subject to error, and clinical correlation with all technologic data is essential.

REFERENCES

1. Gregory, GA. Monitoring During Surgery. In GA Gregory (ed), *Pediatric Anesthesia* (2nd ed). New York: Churchill Livingstone, 1989. Pp 477–500.
2. Wukitsch, MW, Petterson, MT, Tobler, DR, et al. Pulse oximetry: Analysis of theory, technology, and practice. *J Clin Monit* 4:290, 1988.
3. Yelderman, M, New, W. Evaluation of pulse oximetry. *Anesthesiology* 59:349, 1983.
4. Deckardt, TR, Steward, DJ. Noninvasive arterial hemoglobin oxygen saturation versus transcutaneous oxygen tension monitoring in the preterm infant. *Crit Care Med* 12:935, 1984.
5. Brown, M, Vender, JS. Noninvasive oxygen monitoring. *Crit Care Clin* 4:493, 1988.
6. Fanconi, S, Doherty, P, Edmonds, J, et al. Pulse oximetry in pediatric intensive care: Comparison with measured saturations and transcutaneous oxygen tension. *J Pediatr* 107:372, 1985.
7. Wasunna, A, Whitelaw, AGL. Pulse oximetry in preterm infants. *Arch Dis Child* 62:957, 1987.
8. Russel, RIR, Helms, PJ. Comparative accuracy of pulse oximetry and transcutaneous oxygen in assessing arterial saturation in pediatric intensive care. *Crit Care Med* 18:725, 1990.
9. Severinghaus, JW, Naifeh, KH. Accuracy of response of six pulse oximeters to profound hypoxia. *Anesthesiology* 67:551, 1987.
10. Fanconi, S. Reliability of pulse oximetry in hypoxic infants. *J Pediatr* 112:424, 1988.
11. Lucey, JF, Dongman, B. A reexamination of the role of oxygen in retrolental fibroplasia. *Pediatrics* 73:82, 1984.

12. Scheller, MS, Unger, RJ, Kelner, MJ. Effects of intravenously administered dyes on pulse oximetry readings. *Anesthesiology* 65:550, 1986.
13. Anderson, JV. The accuracy of pulse oximetry in neonates: Effects of fetal hemoglobin and bilirubin. *J Perinatol* 7:323, 1987.
14. Cote, CJ, Boldstein, EA, Cote, MA, et al. A single blind study of pulse oximetry in children. *Anesthesiology* 68:184, 1988.
15. Lubbers, D. Theoretical basis of the transcutaneous blood gas measurement. *Crit Care Med* 9:721, 1981.
16. Fenner, A, Muller, R, Busse, HG, et al. Transcutaneous determination of arterial oxygen tension. *Pediatrics* 55:244, 1975.
17. Swanstrom, S, Villa Elisaga, I, Cardona, L, et al. Transcutaneous PO_2 measurements in seriously ill newborn infants. *Arch Dis Child* 50:913, 1975.
18. Yahav, J, Mindorff, C, Levison, H. Validity of transcutaneous oxygen tension method in children with cardiorespiratory problems. *Am Rev Respir Dis* 124:586, 1981.
19. Tremper, KK, Shoemaker, WC. Transcutaneous oxygen monitoring of critically ill adults, with and without low flow shock. *Crit Care Med* 9:706, 1981.
20. Venus, B, Patel, KC, Pratap, KS, et al. Transcutaneous PO_2 monitoring during pediatric surgery. *Crit Care Med* 9:714, 1981.
21. Eberhard, P, Mindt, W. Interference of anesthetic gases at skin surface sensors for oxygen and carbon dioxide. *Crit Care Med* 9:717, 1981.
22. Monaco, F, McQuitty, J. Transcutaneous measurements of carbon dioxide partial pressures in sick neonates. *Crit Care Med* 9:756, 1981.
23. Hansen, TN, Tooley, WH. Surface carbon dioxide tension in sick infants. *Pediatrics* 64:942, 1979.
24. Laptook, A, Oh, W. Transcutaneous carbon dioxide monitoring in the newborn period,. *Crit Care Med* 9:759, 1981.
25. Bhat, R, Kim, WD, Shukla, A, et al. Simultaneous tissue pH and transcutaneous carbon dioxide monitoring in critically ill neonates. *Crit Care Med* 9:744, 1981.
26. Tremper, K, Shoemaker, W, Shippy, CR, et al. Transcutaneous PCO_2 monitoring on adult patients in the ICU and the operating room. *Crit Care Med* 9:752, 1981.
27. Tremper, K, Mentelos, RA, Shoemaker, W. Effect of hypercarbia and shock on transcutaneous carbon dioxide at different electrode temperatures. *Crit Care Med* 8:608, 1980.
28. Lee, HK, Broadhurst, E, Helms, P. Evaluation of two combined oxygen and carbon dioxide transcutaneous sensors. *Arch Dis Child* 64:279, 1989.
29. Whitesell, R, Asidaddao, C, Gollman, D, et al. Relationship between arterial and peak expired CO_2 during anesthesia and factors affecting the difference. *Anesth Analg* 60:508, 1981.
30. Raemer, DB, Francis, D, Philip, JH, et al. Variation in PCO_2 between arterial blood and peak expired gas during anesthesia. *Anesth Analg* 62:1065, 1983.
31. Fletcher, R. The relationship between the arterial to end-tidal PCO_2 difference and hemoglobin saturation in patients with congenital heart disease. *Anesthesiology* 75:210, 1991.
32. Badgwell, JM, Heavner, JE, May, WS, et al. End-tidal PCO_2 monitoring in infants and children ventilated with either a partial rebreathing or a nonrebreathing circuit. *Anesthesiology* 66:405, 1987.
33. Badgwell, JM, McLeod, ME, Lerman, J, et al. End-tital PCO_2 measurements sampled at the distal and proximal ends of the endotracheal tube in infants and children. *Anesth Analg* 66:959, 1987.
34. Weil, MH, Bisera, J, Trevino, RP, et al. Cardiac output and end-tidal carbon dioxide. *Crit Care Med* 13:907, 1985.
35. Barton, C, Callaham, M. Lack of correlation between end-tidal carbon dioxide concentrations and $PaCO_2$ in cardiac arrest. *Crit Care Med* 19:108, 1991.
36. Tanner, GE, Angers, DG, Barach, PG, et al. Effect of left-to-right, mixed right-to-left, and right-to-left shunts on inhalational anesthetic induction in children: A computer model. *Anesth Analg* 64:101, 1985.
37. London, MFG, Hollenberg, M, Wong, MG, et al. Intraoperative myocardial ischemia: Localization by continuous 12-lead electrocardiography. *Anesthesiology* 69:232, 1988.
38. Bell, C, Rimar, S, Barash, P. Intraoperative ST-segment changes consistent with myocardial ischemia in the neonate: A report of three cases. *Anesthesiology* 71:601, 1989.
39. Garson, A, Jr. Electrocardiography. In A Garson Jr, JT Brickner, DG McNamara (eds), *The Science and Practice of Pediatric Cardiology*. Philadelphia: Lea & Febiger, 1990. Pp 713–767.
40. Wong, RS, Baum, VC, Sangwan, S. Truncus arteriosus: Recognition and therapy of intraoperative cardiac ischemia. *Anesthesiology* 74:378, 1991.
41. Tawes, RL, Berry, CL, Aberdeen, E, et al. Myocardial ischemia in infants. *Ann Thorac Surg* 8:383, 1969.
42. Brownlee, JR, Serwer, GA, Dick, M, II, et al. Failure of electrocardiographic monitoring to detect cardiac arrest in patients with pacemakers. *Am J Dis Child* 143:105, 1989.
43. Kirkendall, WM, Feinleig, M, Freis, ED, et al.

Recommendation for human blood pressure determination by sphygmomanometers: Subcommittee on the American Heart Association Postgraduate Education Committee. *Circulation* 62:1145A, 1980.
44. Kirkendall, WM, Burton, AC, Epstein, FH, et al. Recommendations for human blood pressure determination by sphygmomanometers. *Circulation* 36:980, 1967.
45. Mitchell, PL, Parlin, RW, Blackburn, H. Effect of vertical displacement of the arm on indirect blood pressure measurement. *N Engl J Med* 271:72, 1964.
46. Sadove, MS, Schmidt, G, Wu, HH, et al. Indirect blood pressure measurement in infants: A comparison of four methods in four limbs. *Anesth Analg* 52:682, 1973.
47. Geddes, LA, Spencer, WA, Hoff, HE. Graphic recording of the Korotkov sounds. *Am Heart J* 57:361, 1959.
48. Cohn, JN. Blood pressure measurement in shock. Mechanism of inaccuracy in auscultatory and palpatory methods. *JAMA* 199:118, 1967.
49. Kirby, RR, Kemmerer, WT, Morgan, JL. Transcutaneous Doppler measurement of blood pressure. *Anesthesiology* 31:86, 1969.
50. Hochberg, HM, Saltzman, MB. Accuracy of an ultrasound blood pressure instrument in neonates, infants and children. *Curr Ther* 13:482, 1971.
51. Waltemath, CL, Preuss, DD. Determination of blood pressure in low-flow states by the Doppler technique. *Anesthesiology* 34:77, 1971.
52. Hill, GE, Machin, RH. Doppler determined blood pressure recordings: The effect of varying cuff sizes in children. *Can Anaesth Soc J* 23:323, 1976.
53. Yelderman, M, Ream, AK. Indirect measurement of mean blood pressure in the anesthetized patient. *Anesthesiology* 50:253, 1979.
54. Diprose, GK, Evans, DH, Archer, LNJ, et al. Dinamap fails to detect hypotension in very low birthweight infants. *Arch Dis Child* 61:771, 1986.
55. Friesen, RH, Lichtor, JL. Indirect measurement of blood pressure in neonates and infants utilizing an automated non-invasive oscillometric monitor. *Anesth Analg* 60:742, 1981.
56. Kimble, KJ. An automated oscillometric technique for estimating mean arterial blood pressure in critically ill newborns. *Anesthesiology* 54:423, 1981.
57. Groff, DB, Ahmed, N. Subclavian vein catheterization in the infant. *J Pediatr Surg* 9:171, 1974.
58. Sy, WP. Ulnar nerve palsy possibly related to use of automatically cycled blood pressure cuff. *Anesth Analg* 60:687, 1981.
59. Boehmer, RD. Continuous, real-time, non-invasive monitor of blood pressure; Penaz methodology applied to the finger. *J Clin Monit* 3:282, 1987.
60. Kurki, T, Smith, NT, Head, N, et al. Non-invasive continuous blood pressure measurement from the finger: Optimal measurement conditions and factors affecting reliability. *J Clin Monit* 3:6, 1987.
61. Gibbs, NM, Larach, DR, Derr, JA. The accuracy of Finapres noninvasive mean arterial pressure measurement in anesthetized patients. *Anesthesiology* 74:647, 1991.
62. Park, MK, Menard, SM. Accuracy of blood pressure measurement by the Dinamap monitor in infants and children. *Pediatrics* 79:907, 1987.
63. McGregor, M. Pulsus paradoxus. *N Engl J Med* 301:480, 1979.
64. Schleien, CL, Zahka, KG, Rogers, MC. Principles of Postoperative Management in the Pediatric Intensive Care Unit. In MC Rogers (ed), *Textbook of Pediatric Intensive Care*. Baltimore: Williams & Wilkins, 1986. Pp 411–458.
65. Koenigsberger, MR, Moessinger, AC. Iatrogenic carpal tunnel syndrome in the newborn infant. *J Pediatr* 91:441, 1977.
66. Zerella, JT, Trump, DS, Dorman, GW. Access for neonatal arterial monitoring. *J Pediatr Surg* 14:270, 1979.
67. Cole, FS, Todres, ID, Shannon, DC. Technique for percutaneous cannulation of the radial artery in the newborn infant. *J Pediatr* 92:105, 1978.
68. Bedford, RF, Wallman, H. Complications of percutaneous radial artery cannulation: An objective prospective study in man. *Anesthesiology* 38:228, 1973.
69. Bedford, RF. Radial arterial function following percutaneous cannulation with 18- and 20-gauge catheters. *Anesthesiology* 47:37, 1977.
70. Downs, JB, Rackstein, AD, Klein, EF, et al. Hazards of radial-artery catheterization. *Anesthesiology* 38:283, 1973.
71. Bedford, RF. Wrist circumference predicts the risk of radial-arterial occlusion after cannulation. *Anesthesiology* 48:377, 1978.
72. Ryan, JF, Raines, J, Daltohn, BC, et al. Arterial dynamics of radial artery cannulation. *Anesth Analg* 52:1017, 1973.
73. Downs, JB, Chapman, RL, Jr, Hawkins, IR. Prolonged radial-artery catheterization. An evaluation of heparinized catheters and continuous irrigation. *Arch Surg* 108:671, 1974.
74. Sellden, H, Nilsson, K, Larsson, LE, et al. Radial arterial catheters in children and neonates: A prospective study. *Crit Care Med* 15:1106, 1987.
75. Miyasaka, K, Edmonds, JF, Conn, AW. Complica-

tions of radial artery lines in the pediatric patient. *Can Anaesth Soc J* 23:9, 1976.
76. Randel, SN, Tsang, BHL, Wung, JT, et al. Experience with percutaneous indwelling peripheral arterial catheterization in neonates. *Am J Dis Child* 141: 848, 1987.
77. Mayer, T, Matlak, ME, Thompson, JA. Necrosis of the forearm following radial artery catheterization in a patient with Reye's syndrome. *Pediatrics* 65:141, 1980.
78. Johnson, FE, Sumner, DS, Strandness, DE. Extremity necrosis caused by indwelling arterial catheters. *Am J Surg* 131:375, 1976.
79. Cartwright, GW, Schreiner, RL. Major complication to percutaneous radial artery catheterization in the neonate. *Pediatrics* 65:139, 1980.
80. Smith-Wright, D, Green, T, Egar, M, et al. Complications of vascular catheterization in critically ill children. *Crit Care Med* 12:1015, 1984.
81. Pape, KE, Armstrong, DL, Fitzhardinge, PM. Peripheral median nerve damage secondary to brachial arterial blood gas sampling. *J Pediatr* 93:852, 1978.
82. Michaelson, ED, Walsh, RE. Osler's node—a complication of prolonged arterial cannulation. *N Engl J Med* 283:472, 1970.
83. Guy, RL, Holland, JP, Shaw, DG, et al. Limb shortening secondary to complications of vascular cannulae in the neonatal period. *Skeletal Radiol* 19:423, 1990.
84. Seibert, JJ, McCarthy, RE, Alexander, JE, et al. Acquired bone dysplasia secondary to catheter-related complications in the neonate. *Pediatr Radiol* 16:43, 1986.
85. Rubinstein, RA, Jr, Taylor, LM, Jr, Porter, JM, et al. Limb growth after late bypass graft for occlusion of the femoral artery. *J Bone Joint Surg* 72-A:935, 1990.
86. Band, JD, Maki, DG. Infections caused by arterial catheters used for hemodynamic monitoring. *Am J Med* 67:735, 1979.
87. Lowenstein, E, Little, JW, Lo, HH. Prevention of cerebral embolization from flushing radial artery cannulas. *N Engl J Med* 285:1414, 1971.
88. Butt, WW, Gow, R, Whyte, H, et al. Complications resulting from use of arterial catheters: Retrograde flow and rapid elevation in blood pressure. *Pediatrics* 76:250, 1985.
89. Merenstein, GB. Heparinized catheters and coagulation studies. *J Pediatr* 79:117, 1971.
90. Bjork, L, Enghoff, E, et al. Local circulatory changes following brachial artery catheterization. *Vasc Dis* 2: 283, 1965.
91. Cantwell, GP, Holzman, BH, Caceres, MJ. Percutaneous catheterization of the axillary artery in the pediatric patient. *Crit Care Med* 18:880, 1990.
92. De Angelis, J. Axillary arterial monitoring. *Crit Care Med* 4:205, 1976.
93. Lawless, S, Orr, R. Axillary arterial monitoring of pediatric patients. *Pediatrics* 84:273, 1989.
94. Kitterman, JA, Phibbs, RH, Tooley, WH. Catheterization of umbilical vessels in newborn infants. *Pediatr Clin North Am* 17:895, 1970.
95. Krishnamoorthy, KS, Fernandez, RJ, Todres, ID, et al. Paraplegia associated with umbilical artery catheterization in the newborn. *Pediatrics* 58:443, 1976.
96. Prian, GW. Temporal artery catheterization for arterial access in the high-risk newborn. *Surgery* 82: 734, 1977.
97. Bull, MJ, Schreiner, RL, Garg, BP, et al. Neurologic complications following temporal artery catheterization. *J Pediatr* 96:1071, 1980.
98. Simmons, MA, Levine, RL, Lubchenco, LO. Warning: Serious sequelae of temporal artery catheterization. *J Pediatr* 92:284, 1978.
99. Prian, GW, Wright, GB, Rumack, CM, et al. Apparent cerebral embolization after temporal artery catheterization. *J Pediatr* 93:115, 1978.
100. Morris, TR, Bouhoutsos, J. The dangers of femoral artery puncture and catheterization. *Am Heart J* 89:260, 1975.
101. Shah, A, Gnoj, J, Fisher, VJ. Complications of selective coronary arteriography by the Judkins technique and their prevention. *Am Heart J* 90:353, 1975.
102. Asnes, RS, Arendar, GM. Septic arthritis of the hip: A complication of femoral venipuncture. *Pediatrics* 38:837, 1966.
103. Russell, JA, Joel, M, Hudson, RJ, et al. Prospective evaluation of radial and femoral artery catheterization sites in critically ill patients. *Crit Care Med* 11: 936, 1983.
104. Barnhorst, DA, Barner, HB. Prevalence of congenitally absent pedal pulses. *N Engl J Med* 278: 264, 1968.
105. Johnstone, RE, Greenhow, DE. Catheterization of the dorsalis pedis artery. *Anesthesiology* 39:654, 1973.
106. Youngberg, JA, Miller, ED. Evaluation of percutaneous cannulations of the dorsalis pedis artery. *Anesthesiology* 44:80, 1976.
107. Spahr, RC, MacDonald, HM, Holzman, IR. Catheterization of the posterior tibial artery in the neonate. *Am J Dis Child* 133:945, 1979.
108. O'Rourke, MF, Blazek, JV, Morreels, CL, Jr, et al. Pressure wave transmission along the human aorta: Changes with age and in arterial degenerative disease. *Circ Res* 23:567, 1968.
109. Kroeker, EJ, Wood, EH. Comparison of simultane-

ously recorded central and peripheral arterial pressure pulse during test, exercise and tilted position in man. *Circ Res* 3:623, 1955.
110. Park, MK, Guntheroth, WG. Direct blood pressure measurements in brachial and femoral arteries in children. *Circulation* 41:231, 1970.
111. Park, MK, Robotham, JI, German, VF. Systolic pressure amplification in pedal arteries in children. *Crit Care Med* 11:286, 1983.
112. Gardner, RM. Direct blood pressure measurement—dynamic response requirements. *Anesthesiology* 54:227, 1981.
113. Fiser, DH, Graves, SA, van der AA, J. Catheters for arterial pressure monitoring in pediatrics. *Crit Care Med* 13:580, 1985.
114. Shinozaki, T, Deane, RS, Mazuzan, JE. The dynamic responses of liquid-filled catheter systems for direct measurement of blood pressure. *Anesthesiology* 53:498, 1980.
115. Jung, RC, Galchum, OJ, Massey, FJ. The accuracy of venous and capillary blood for the prediction of arterial pH, PCO_2, and PO_2 measurements. *Am J Clin Pathol* 45:129, 1966.
116. Cobb, LM, Vinocur, CD, Wagner, CW, et al. The central venous anatomy in infants. *Surg Gynecol Obstet* 165:230, 1987.
117. Morgan, WW, Harkins, GA. Percutaneous introduction of long-term indwelling vascular catheters in infants. *J Pediatr Surg* 7:538, 1972.
118. Pietsch, JB, Nagaraj, HS, Groff, DB. Simplified insertion of central venous catheter in infants. *Surg Gynecol Obstet* 158:91, 1984.
119. Filston, HC, Grant, JP. A safer system for percutaneous subclavian venous catheterization in newborn infants. *J Pediatr Surg* 14:564, 1979.
120. English, ICW, Frew, RM, Pigott, JF. Percutaneous catheterization of the internal jugular vein. *Anaesthesia* 24:521, 1969.
121. Prince, S, Sullivan, L, Hackel, A. Percutaneous catheterization of the internal jugular vein in infants and children. *Anesthesiology* 44:170, 1976.
122. Hall, DMB, Geefhuysen, J. Percutaneous catheterization of the internal jugular vein in infants and children. *J Pediatr Surg* 12:719, 1977.
123. Krausz, MM, Berlatsky, Y, Ayalon, A, et al. Percutaneous cannulation of the internal jugular vein in infants and children. *Surg Gynecol Obstet* 148:591, 1979.
124. Schulman, RJ, Pokorny, WJ, Martin, CG, et al. Comparison of percutaneous and surgical placement of central venous catheters in neonates. *J Pediatr Surg* 21:348, 1986.
125. Rao, TLD, Wong, AY, Salem, MR. A new approach to percutaneous catheterization of the internal jugular vein. *Anesthesiology* 46:362, 1977.
126. Cote, CJ, Jobes, DR, Schwartz, AJ, et al. Two approaches to cannulation of the child's internal jugular vein. *Anesthesiology* 50:371, 1979.
127. Schwartz, AJ. Percutaneous aortic catheterization—hazard of supraclavicular internal jugular vein catheterization. *Anesthesiology* 46:77, 1977.
128. Pollack, MM, Red, TP, Holbrook, PR, et al. Bedside pulmonary artery catheterization in pediatrics. *J Pediatr* 96:274, 1980.
129. Damen, J, Wever, JEAT. The use of balloon-tipped pulmonary artery catheters in children undergoing cardiac surgery. *Intensive Care Med* 13:266, 1987.
130. Damen, J, Bolton, D. A prospective analysis of 1400 pulmonary artery catheterizations in patients undergoing cardiac surgery. *Acta Anaesthesiol Scand* 30:386, 1986.
131. Dauber, M. Delayed onset of pneumothorax following internal jugular vein cannulation. *Anesthesiology* 74:201, 1991.
132. Humphrey, MJ, Blitt, CD. Central venous access in children via the external jugular vein. *Anesthesiology* 57:50, 1982.
133. Nicolson, SC, Sweeney, MF, Moore, RA, et al. Comparison of internal and external jugular cannulation of the central circulation in the pediatric patient. *Crit Care Med* 13:747, 1985.
134. Introna, RPS, Martin, DC, Pruett, JK, et al. Percutaneous pulmonary artery catheterization in pediatric cardiovascular anesthesia: Insertion techniques and use. *Anesth Analg* 7C:562, 1990.
135. Kanter, RK, Zimmerman, JJ, Strauss, RH, et al. Central venous catheter insertion by femoral vein: Safety and effectiveness for the pediatric patient. *Pediatrics* 77:842, 1986.
136. Williams, JF, Seneff, MG, Friedman, BC, et al. Use of femoral venous catheters in critically ill adults: Prospective study. *Crit Care Med* 19:550, 1991.
137. Newman, BM, Jewett, TC, Jr, Karp, MP, et al. Percutaneous central venous catheterization in children: First line choice for venous access. *J Pediatr Surg* 21:685, 1986.
138. Hodge, D, Delgado-Paredes, C, Sleisher, G. Central and peripheral catheter flow rates in "pediatric" dogs. *Ann Emerg Med* 15:1151, 1986.
139. Ikeda, S, Schweiss, JF. Maximum infusion rates and CVP accuracy during high-flow delivery through multilumen catheters. *Crit Care Med* 13:586, 1985.
140. Briscoe, CE. A comparison of jugular and central venous pressure measurements during anesthesia. *Br J Anaesth* 45:173, 1973.
141. Gilhooly, J, Lindenberg, J, Reynolds, JW. Central

venous silicone elastomer catheter placement by basilic vein cutdown in neonates. *Pediatrics* 78:636, 1986.
142. Bridges, BB, Carden, E, Takacs, FA. Introduction of central pressure catheters through arm veins with a high success rate. *Can Anaesth Soc J* 26:128, 1979.
143. Dronen, SC, Yee, AS, Tomlanovich, MC. Proximal saphenous vein cutdown. *Ann Emerg Med* 10:328, 1981.
144. Wigger, HJ, Bransilver, BR, Blanc, WA. Thomboses due to catheterization in infants and children. *J Pediatr* 76:1, 1970.
145. Turnage, WS, Harper, JV. Venous air embolism occurring after removal of a central venous catheter. *Anesth Analg* 72:559, 1991.
146. Ross, P, Jr, Seashore, JH. Bilateral hydrothorax complicating central venous catheterization in a child: Case report. *J Pediatr Surg* 24:263, 1989.
147. Henderson, AM, Sumner, E. Late perforation by central venous cannulae. *Arch Dis Child* 59:776, 1984.
148. Aldridge, HE, Jay, AWL. Central venous catheters and heart perforation. *Can Med Assoc J* 135:1082, 1986.
149. Fischer, GW, Scherz, RG. Neck vein catheters and pericardial tamponade. *Pediatrics* 52:868, 1978.
150. Opitz, JC, Toyama, W. Cardiac tamponade from central venous catheterization: Two cases in premature infants with survival. *Pediatrics* 70:139, 1982.
151. Agarwal, KC, Ali Khan, MA, Falla, A, et al. Cardiac perforation from central venous catheters: Survival after cardiac tamponade in an infant. *Pediatrics* 73:333, 1984.
152. Stark, DD, Brasch, RC, Gooding, CA. Radiographic assessment of venous catheter position in children: Value of the lateral view. *Pediatr Radiol* 14:76, 1984.
153. Diemer, A. Central venous Silastic catheters in newborns: Localization by sonography and radiology. *Pediatr Radiol* 17:15, 1987.
154. Michenfelder, JD, Terry, HR, Jr, Daw, EF, et al. Air embolism during neurosurgery: A new method of treatment. *Anesth Analg* 45:390, 1966.
155. Maschke, SP, Rogove, HJ. Cardiac tamponade associated with a multilumen central venous catheter. *Crit Care Med* 12:611, 1984.
156. Wilson, JN, Brow, JB, Demong, CV, et al. Central venous pressure in optimal blood volume maintenance. *Arch Surg* 85:563, 1962.
157. Guyton, AC, Jones, CE. Central venous pressure: Physiological significance and clinical implications. *Am Heart J* 86:431, 1973.
158. Ellis, DM. Interpretation of beat-to-beat blood pressure values in the presence of ventilatory changes. *J Clin Monit* 1:65, 1985.
159. Verweij, J, Kester, A, Stroes, W, et al. Comparison of three methods for measuring central venous pressure. *Crit Care Med* 14:288, 1986.
160. Cohn, JN, Tristani, FE, Khatri, IM. Studies in clinical shock and hypotension. VI. Relationship between left and right ventricular function. *J Clin Invest* 48:2008, 1969.
161. Civetta, JM, Gabel, JC, Laver, MB. Disparate ventricular function in surgical patients. *Surg Forum* 22:131, 1971.
162. Forrester, JS, Diamond, G, McHugh, TJ, et al. Filling pressures in the right and left sides of the heart in acute myocardial infarction. *N Engl J Med* 285:190, 1971.
163. Toussaint, GPM, Burgess, JJH, Hampson, LG. Central venous pressure and pulmonary wedge pressure in critical surgical illness. *Arch Surg* 109:265, 1974.
164. Archer, G, Cobb, LA. Long term pulmonary artery pressure monitoring in the management of the critically ill. *Ann Surg* 180:747, 1974.
165. Lappas, D, Lell, WA, Gabel, JC, et al. Indirect measurement of left atrial pressure in surgical patients: Pulmonary-capillary wedge and pulmonary-artery diastolic pressures compared with left-atrial pressure. *Anesthesiology* 38:394, 1973.
166. Roy, R, Powers, SR, Feustel, PJ, et al. Pulmonary wedge catheterization during positive end-expiratory pressure ventilation in the dog. *Anesthesiology* 46:385, 1977.
167. West, JB, Dollery, CT, Naimark, A. Distribution of blood flow in isolated lung: Relations to vascular and alveolar pressures. *J Appl Physiol* 19:713, 1964.
168. Tooker, J, Huseby, J, Butler, J. The effect of Swan-Ganz catheter height on the wedge pressure–left atrial pressure relationship in edema during positive-pressure ventilation. *Am Rev Respir Dis* 117:721, 1978.
169. Fisher, ML, DeFelice, CE, Parigi, AF. Assessing left ventricular pressure with flow-directed (Swan-Ganz) catheters: Detection of sudden changes in patients with left ventricular dysfunction. *Chest* 68:542, 1975.
170. Bouchard, RJ, Gault, JH, Ross, J, Jr. Evaluation of pulmonary arterial end-diastolic pressure as an estimate of left ventricular end-diastolic pressure in patients with normal and abnormal left ventricular performance. *Circulation* 44:1072, 1971.
171. Scheinman, M, Evans, GT, Weiss, A, et al. Relationship between pulmonary artery end-diastolic

pressure and left ventricular filling pressure in patients in shock. *Circulation* 47:317, 1973.
172. Jenkins, BS, Bradley, RD, Branthwaite, MA. Evaluation of pulmonary arterial end-diastolic as an indirect estimate of left atrial mean pressure. *Circulation* 42:75, 1970.
173. Eisenberg, PR, Jaffe, AS, Shuster, DP. Clinical evaluation compared to pulmonary artery catheterization in the hemodynamic assessment of critically ill patients. *Crit Care Med* 12:549, 1984.
174. Swan, HJ, Ganz, W, Forrester, J, et al. Catheterization of the heart in man with use of a flow-directed balloon-tipped catheter. *N Engl J Med* 283:447, 1970.
175. Borland, LM. Allometric determination of the distance from the central venous pressure port to wedge position of balloon-tip catheters in pediatric patients. *Crit Care Med* 14:974, 1986.
176. Bilen, Z, Weinberg, PF, Gowani, Y, et al. Clinical utility and cost-effectiveness of protective sleeve pulmonary artery catheters. *Crit Care Med* 19:491, 1991.
177. Sise, MJ, Hollingsworth, P, Brimm, JE, et al. Complications of the flow-directed pulmonary-artery catheter: A prospective analysis in 219 patients. *Crit Care Med* 9:315, 1981.
178. Tuggle, DW, Pryor, R, Ward, K, et al. Real-time echocardiography: A new technique to facilitate Swan-Ganz catheter insertion. *J Pediatr Surg* 22:1169, 1987.
179. Xin-fang, Wang, Jia-en, Wang, Lin-sheng Cao, et al. Application of two-dimensional echocardiography in location of balloon of the Swan-Ganz catheter. *Chin Med J* 103:117, 1990.
180. Stanger, P, Heymann, MA, Hoffman, JL, et al. Use of the Swan-Ganz catheter in cardiac catheterization of infants and children. *Am Heart J* 83:749, 1972.
181. Baraka, A, Nawfal, M, Dahdah, S. Difficult pulmonary artery catheterization in the pediatric patient with tricuspid regurgitation. *Anesthesiology* 74:393, 1991.
182. Rudolph, AM, Drorbaugh, JE, Auld, PAM, et al. Studies on the circulation in the neonatal period: The circulation in the respiratory distress syndrome. *Pediatrics* 27:551, 1961.
183. Moore, RA, McNicholas, K, Gallagher, JD, et al. Migration of pediatric pulmonary artery catheters. *Anesthesiology* 58:102, 1983.
184. Jones, ODH, Shore, DF, Rigby, ML, et al. The use of tolazoline hydrochloride as a pulmonary vasodilator in potentially fatal episodes of pulmonary vasoconstriction after cardiac surgery in children. *Circulation* 64 (Suppl II):134, 1981.

185. Elliott, CG, Zimmerman, GA, Clemmer, TP. Complications of pulmonary artery catheterization in the care of critically ill patients. *Chest* 76:647, 1979.
186. Shah, KB, Rao, T, Laughlin, S, et al. A review of pulmonary artery catheterization in 6245 patients. *Anesthesiology* 61:271, 1984.
187. Katz, JD, Cronau, LH, Barash, PG, et al. Pulmonary artery flow-guided catheters in the perioperative period: Indications and complications. *JAMA* 237:2832, 1977.
188. Abernathy, WS. Complete heart block caused by the Swan-Ganz catheter. *Chest* 65:349, 1974.
189. Mond, HG, Clark, DW, Nesbitt, SJ. Technique for unknotting an intracardiac flow-directed balloon catheter. *Chest* 67:731, 1975.
190. Lipp, H, O'Donoghue, D, Resnekov, L. Intracardiac knotting of a flow-directed balloon catheter. *N Engl J Med* 284:220, 1971.
191. Pape, LA, Haffajee, CL, Markis, JE, et al. Fatal pulmonary hemorrhage after use of the flow-directed balloon-tipped catheter. *Ann Intern Med* 90:344, 1979.
192. Golden, MS, Pinder, T, Jr, Anderson, WT, et al. Fatal pulmonary hemorrhage complicating the use of a flow-directed balloon-tipped catheter in a patient receiving anticoagulant therapy. *Am J Cardiol* 32:865, 1973.
193. Santora, T, Ganz, W, Gold, J, et al. New method for monitoring pulmonary artery catheter location. *Crit Care Med* 19:422, 1991.
194. Robertie, PG, Johnston, WE, Williamson, MK, et al. Clinical utility of a position-monitoring catheter in the pulmonary artery. *Anesthesiology* 74:440, 1991.
195. Scuderi, PE, Prough, DS, Price, JD, et al. Cessation of pulmonary artery catheter induced endobronchial hemorrhage associated with the use of PEEP. *Anesth Analg* 62:236, 1983.
196. Foote, GA, Schabel, SI, Hodges, M. Pulmonary complications of the flow-directed balloon-tipped catheter. *N Engl J Med* 290:927, 1974.
197. Wyse, SD, Pfitzner, J, et al. Measurement of cardiac output by thermodilution in infants and children. *Thorax* 30:262, 1975.
198. Freed, MD, Keane, JF. Cardiac output measured by thermodilution in infants and children. *J Pediatr* 92:39, 1978.
199. Mathur, J, Harris, EA, Barratt-Boyes, BG. Measurement of cardiac output by thermodilution in infants and children after open-heart operations. *J Thorac Cardiovasc Surg* 72:221, 1976.
200. Colgan, FJ, Stewart, S. An assessment of cardiac output by thermodilution in infants and children

following cardiac surgery. *Crit Care Med* 5:220, 1977.
201. Maruschak, GF, Potter, AM, Schauble, JF, et al. Overestimation of pediatric cardiac output by thermal indicator loss. *Circulation* 65:380, 1982.
202. Callaghan, ML, Weintraub, WH, Coran, AH. Assessment of the thermodilution cardiac output in small subjects. *J Pediatr Surg* 11:629, 1976.
203. Pesola, GR, Carlon, GC. Thermodilution cardiac output: Proximal lumen versus right ventricular port. *Crit Care Med* 19:563, 1991.
204. Vargo, TA. Cardiac Catheterization—Hemodynamic Measurements. In A Garson, Jr, JT Brickner, DG McNamara (eds), *The Science and Practice of Pediatric Cardiology*. Philadelphia: Lea & Febiger, 1990. Pp 913–945.
205. Morady, F, Brundage, BH, Gelberg, HJ. Rapid method for determination of shunt ratio using a thermodilution technique. *Am Heart J* 106:369, 1983.
206. Goldenberg, IF, Ochi, RP, Emery, RW, et al. Overestimation of Fick cardiac output by thermodilution method in patients with severe tricuspid regurgitation. *Crit Care Med* 16:428, 1988.
207. Nadeau, S, Noble, WH. Limitations of cardiac output measurements by thermodilution. *Can Anaesth Soc J* 33:780, 1986.
208. Wetzel, RC, Latson, TW. Major errors in thermodilution cardiac output measurement during rapid volume infusion. *Anesthesiology* 62:684, 1985.
209. Simmons, DH, Alpas, AP, Tashkin, DP, et al. Hyperlactatemia due to arterial hypoxemia or reduced cardiac output or both. *J Appl Physiol* 45:195, 1978.
210. Dan, M, Bonato, R, Mazzucco, A, et al. Value of transesophageal echocardiography during repair of congenital heart defects. *Ann Thorac Surg* 50:637, 1990.
211. Ritter, SB. Transesophageal echocardiography in children: New peephole to the heart. *J Am Coll Cardiol* 16:447, 1990.
212. Stumper, OFW, Elzenga, NJ, Hess, J, et al. Transesophageal echocardiography in children with congenital heart disease: An initial experience. *J Am Coll Cardiol* 16:433, 1990.
213. Cryan, SE, Kimball, TR, Meyer, RA, et al. Efficacy of intraoperative transesophageal echocardiography in children with congenital heart disease. *Am J Cardiol* 63:594, 1989.
214. Muhiudeen, IA, Roberson, DA, Silverman, NH, et al. Intraoperative echocardiography in infants and children with congenital cardiac shunt lesions: Transesophageal versus epicardial echocardiography. *J Am Coll Cardiol* 16:1687, 1990.
215. Louie, EK, Rich, S, Brundage, BH. Doppler echocardiographic assessment of impaired left ventricular filling in patients with right ventricular pressure overload due to primary pulmonary hypertension. *J Am Coll Cardiol* 8:1298, 1986.
216. Siegel, LC, Fitzgerald, DC, Engstrom, RH. Simultaneous intraoperative measurement of cardiac output by thermodilution and transtracheal Doppler. *Anesthesiology* 74:664, 1991.
217. Wong, DH, Watson, T, Gordon, I, et al. Comparison of changes in transit time ultrasound, esophageal Doppler, and thermodilution cardiac output after changes in preload, afterload, and contractility in pigs. *Anesth Analg* 72:584, 1991.
218. Introna, RPS, Pruett, JK, Crumrine, RC, et al. Use of transthoracic bioimpedance to determine cardiac output in pediatric patients. *Crit Care Med* 16:1101, 1988.
219. Mickell, JJ, Lucking, SE, Chaten, FC, et al. Trending of impedance-monitoring cardiac variables: Method and statistical power analysis of 100 control studies in a pediatric intensive care unit. *Crit Care Med* 18:645, 1990.

17
Noncyanotic Heart Disease

GERALD A. SCHIFF

Most anesthesiologists are faced on a daily basis with patients who have adult-type cardiovascular disease such as ischemic or valvular heart disease, and, therefore, are well versed with the preoperative assessment and anesthetic implications of these lesions. However, the pediatric patient with coexisting congenital heart disease (CHD) presents a special challenge for the anesthesiologist. CHD is represented by a wide range of anatomic lesions that are infrequently encountered in daily anesthetic practice. Each year in the United States, there are approximately 3.75 million live births, and about 0.8 percent of these infants manifest some form of CHD [1–3]. Some of these children will require palliative or corrective surgery early in life. These lifesaving procedures, however, are only performed in a limited number of institutions. These children may present for noncardiac surgery either before cardiac surgery or between one of several cardiac operations staged to treat CHD. Other children, with benign asymptomatic lesions, will not require surgical intervention at an early age, and in some situations, a child may even present for noncardiac surgery with a previously unrecognized cardiac lesion. These children are frequently seen at the community hospital for common surgical procedures, such as myringotomy, tonsillectomy, dental restorations, or herniorrhaphy. It is crucial, therefore, that all anesthesiologists understand and be familiar with the pathophysiologic changes that are produced by anatomic cardiac defects. This chapter does not focus on the management of these children for cardiac surgery, but instead clarifies the basic pathophysiologic principles and reviews the basic perioperative guidelines pertaining to children with noncyanotic congenital heart disease.

PATHOPHYSIOLOGY OF CONGENITAL HEART DISEASE

Although more than 100 different congenital heart lesions are known [4–10], nearly 90 percent of all cardiac defects are accounted for by the 10 most common lesions (Table 17-1). One can further classify congenital heart disease by asking questions about the flow characteristics of the various lesions [11]. First, is there an abnormal shunt pathway for blood flow through an intracardiac, extracardiac, or combined defect? Second, is there an increase or decrease in pulmonary or systemic blood flow? Finally, is there an obstruction to or reduction in blood flow due to a supravalvular, subvalvular, or primary valvular abnormality?

The major alterations in blood flow in lesions that have shunts, occur in the pulmonary circulation. Pulmonary blood flow will either be in-

Table 17-1. Common congenital heart defects

Heart defect	% of total defects
Ventricular septal defect	28
Secundum atrial septal defect	10
Patent ductus arteriosus	10
Tetralogy of Fallot	10
Pulmonic stenosis	10
Aortic stenosis	7
Coarctation of the aorta	5
Transposition of the great arteries	5
Primum atrial septal defect	3
Total anomalous pulmonary venous return	1

Source: Reprinted with permission from RK Stoelting and SF Dierdorf, *Anesthesia and Coexisting Disease*. New York: Churchill Livingstone, 1983. P 48.

creased, resulting in a volume and/or pressure overload to the pulmonary circulation, or decreased, secondary to an abnormal shunt pathway and obstruction to pulmonary blood flow, resulting in a relative inability to oxygenate the blood. In the third group of congenital heart lesions, there is no shunting of blood. The primary problem in this group of patients is obstruction to blood flow (for example, aortic stenosis or coarctation of the aorta). The major pathophysiologic consequence of obstruction to blood flow is the increased myocardial work needed to overcome the obstruction. The increased work required to pump blood in the presence of an obstruction to flow causes ventricular hypertrophy, decreased chamber compliance, and elevated myocardial oxygen consumption (Table 17-2).

To further illustrate the effect of shunting, one can apply the cardiovascular equivalent of Ohm's law,

$$Q = \frac{P}{R}$$

where Q = blood flow (cardiac output), P = blood pressure (generated within a cardiac chamber), and R = vascular resistance (offered by the pulmonary or systemic vascular bed). Examples of this application will aid in understanding the pathophysiology and management of shunt lesions (Fig. 17-1).

Ventricular septal defect is an example of a shunting lesion with increased pulmonary blood flow. Blood is shunted into the lung because left ventricular pressure is greater than right ventricular pressure, and right ventricular outflow (i.e., pulmonary vascular resistance) offers less impedance to flow than left ventricular outflow (the systemic vascular resistance in the aorta). The resistance, and consequently the degree, of shunting is determined by the size of the ventricular septal defect itself. The larger the ventricular septal defect, the less resistance it offers, and the greater the flow

Table 17-2. Flow characteristics of various congenital cardiac lesions

Increased pulmonary blood flow lesions
Atrial septal defect
Ventricular septal defect
Patent ductus arteriosus
Endocardial cushion defect (atrioventricular canal abnormality)
Transposition of the great arteries*
Anomalous pulmonary venous return*
Truncus arteriosus*
Single ventricle*

Decreased pulmonary blood flow lesions
Tetralogy of Fallot
Pulmonic atresia
Tricuspid atresia
Ebstein's anomaly
Truncus arteriosus*
Transposition of the great arteries*
Single ventricle*

Obstructive lesions
Aortic stenosis
Pulmonic stenosis
Coarctation of the aorta
Asymmetric septal hypertrophy

*Systemic hypoxemia occurs as a result of the mixing of systemic and pulmonary venous returns. Classification as an increased or decreased pulmonary blood flow lesion depends on the absence or presence within the anatomic variation of obstruction to pulmonary blood flow.
Source: Reprinted and modified with permission from AS Schwartz and DR Jobes, Congenital Heart Disease—Special Anesthetic Considerations. In TJ Conahan (ed), *Cardiac Anesthesia*. Menlo Park: Addison-Wesley, 1982.

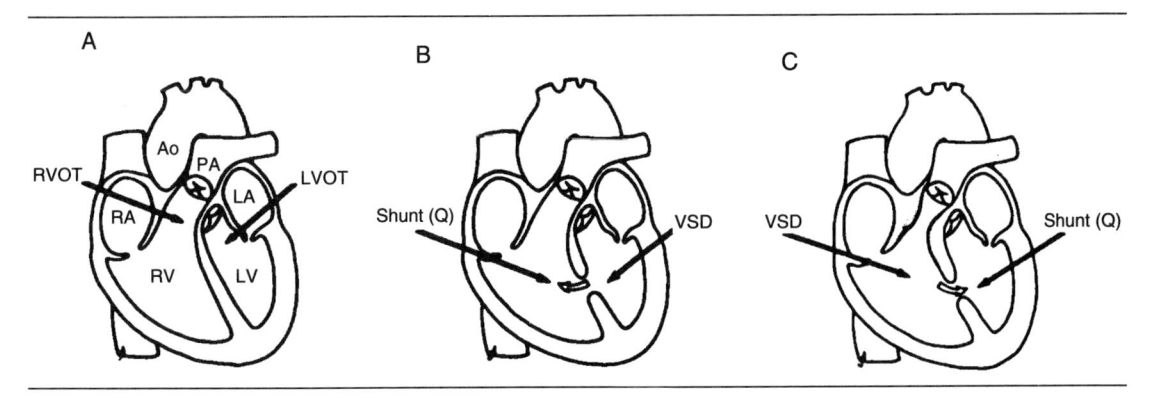

Fig. 17-1. Diagrammatic representation of a normal heart and congenital heart lesions in which there is a pathophysiologic alteration in pulmonary blood flow (PBF). Ao = aorta; LA = left atrium; LV = left ventricle; LVOT = left ventricular outflow tract; PA = pulmonary artery; Q = shunt blood flow; RA = right atrium; RV = right ventricle; RVOT = right ventricular outflow tract; VSD = ventricular septal defect. A. A normal heart showing the anatomic relationships between the cardiac chambers and the outflow tracts of the ventricles. B. An increased PBF lesion is exemplified by a VSD. When (1) the VSD is large diameter offering low resistance to blood flow (R) and (2) RVOT and PA offer low R, then (3) LV pressure > RV pressure and Q, indicated by the open arrow, is left-to-right increasing PBF. C. A decreased PBF lesion is exemplified by tetralogy of Fallot. When (1) the VSD is large diameter offering low R, (2) RVOT is obstructed (subpulmonic muscular hypertrophy), (3) RVOT R > LVOT R, then (4) RV pressure > LV pressure and Q, indicated by the open arrow, is right-to-left decreasing PBF. (Reprinted with permission from CL Lake, *Pediatric Cardiac Anesthesia*. Norwalk: Appleton & Lange, 1988. P 11.)

across it from the left ventricle to the right ventricle and pulmonary vascular bed (Fig. 17-2).

Tetralogy of Fallot is an example of a shunting lesion with decreased pulmonary blood flow. Blood is shunted away from the lungs because the right ventricular outflow tract is obstructed (subpulmonic muscular hypertrophy and/or valvular or supravalvular stenosis) and offers more resistance to blood flow than the interventricular communication (ventricular septal defect) that is present. The ventricular septal defect acts to decompress the right ventricle, which cannot empty normally because of its obstructed outflow tract. Right ventricular pressure, which commonly equals or exceeds left ventricular pressure in tetralogy of Fallot, is elevated in an attempt to overcome the resistance to normal right ventricular outflow. As long as the systemic vascular resistance is relatively low and there is no impedance to left ventricular emptying, blood flows from the right ventricle through the ventricular septal defect, carrying deoxygenated blood to the left ventricle and out to the systemic circulation (Fig. 17-3).

In complex shunting lesions, mixing of the systemic and pulmonary venous return occurs as a result of abnormal circulatory pathways (for example, transposition of the great arteries) or common vascular chambers to both the systemic and pulmonary circulations (for example, truncus arteriosus or single ventricle). Since there is continuous mixing of blood, bidirectional shunting occurs, right-to-left as well as left-to-right. One or the other shunt may predominate, depending on the presence or absence of anatomic variations that produce obstructions to pulmonary or systemic blood flow. In the absence of pulmonary outflow obstruction, pulmonary blood flow is increased since the pulmonary bed offers less resistance to ventricular outflow than does the systemic circulation. However, despite the increased pulmonary blood flow, these patients are usually hypoxemic since the right-to-left shunt component transfers deoxygenated blood to the systemic arterial circulation. When an obstruction to pulmonary blood flow is superimposed, the resistance to flow into the pulmonary circuit increases relative to that of the systemic circulation. Therefore, pulmonary blood flow is quantitatively as well as functionally de-

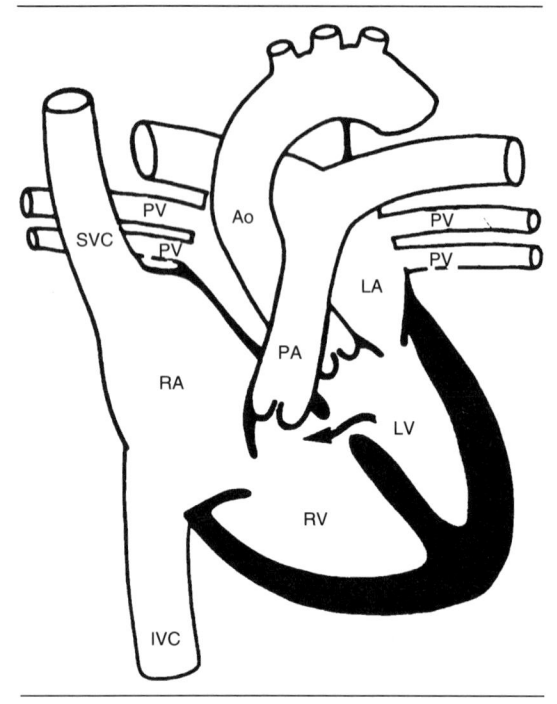

Fig. 17-2. Schematic diagram of a ventricular septal defect located just below the muscular ridge that separates the body of the right ventricle (RV) from the pulmonary artery (PA) outflow tract. Blood flow is along a pressure gradient from the left ventricle (LV) to the RV. The resulting left-to-right intracardiac shunt is associated with a pulmonary blood flow that exceeds the volume of LV ejection into the aorta (Ao). Decreases in systemic vascular resistance decrease the pressure gradient across the defect and reduce the magnitude of the shunt. PV = pulmonary vein; RA = right atrium; LA = left atrium; SVC = superior vena cava; IVC = inferior vena cava. (Reprinted with permission from RK Stoelting and SF Dierdorf, *Anesthesia and Coexisting Disease*. New York: Churchill Livingstone, 1983. P 50.)

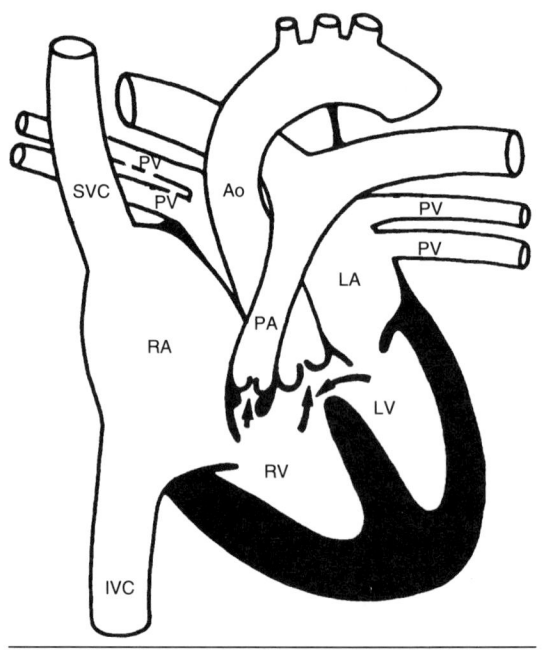

Fig. 17-3. Schematic diagram of the anatomic cardiac defects associated with tetralogy of Fallot. Defects include (1) a ventricular septal defect, (2) an aorta (Ao) that overrides the septum and pulmonary artery (PA) outflow tract, (3) obstruction to blood flow through a narrowed PA or stenotic pulmonary valve, and (4) right ventricular hypertrophy. The resistance to PA outflow results in a pressure gradient that favors blood flow across the ventricular septal defect from the right ventricle (RV) to the left ventricle (LV). The resulting right-to-left intracardiac shunt combined with the obstruction to ejection of the right ventricular stroke volume leads to a marked reduction in pulmonary blood flow and the development of arterial hypoxemia. Events that increase pulmonary vascular resistance or decrease systemic vascular resistance will increase the magnitude of the shunt and accentuate arterial hypoxemia. PV = pulmonary vein; RA = right atrium; LA = left atrium; SVC = superior vena cava; IVC = inferior vena cava. (Reprinted with permission from RK Stoelting, SF Dierdorf, *Anesthesia and Coexisting Disease*. New York: Churchill Livingstone, 1983. P 54.)

creased and the degree of right-to-left shunting is increased. Further detailed analysis of these complex lesions can be found in Chapter 18.

Anesthesia and perioperative hemodynamic manipulations can alter the pathophysiologic expression of CHD. The effects of various anesthetics and other medications have the potential to alter several components of the flow-pressure-resistance relationship. The cardiac depressant effects of volatile anesthetic agents may decrease the cardiac output, thereby limiting the ability of each ventricle to produce flow. Furthermore, with the increased myocardial depression, the ventricle may no longer be able to generate effective intracardiac pressures, which may alter the pressure differential between chambers and its effect on shunting. In certain circumstances, however, a decrease in contractility may produce a desirable effect; for example, in the patient with tetralogy of Fallot and subpulmonic infundibular hypertrophy, there is a dynamic obstruction to the right ventricular outflow tract. This can be exacerbated by tachycardia and hypovolemia, which reduces ventricular size, and by excessive contractility, which increases the degree of muscular contraction and obstruction. Halothane will decrease contractility and heart rate, decrease the right ventricular outflow obstruction, improve pulmonary blood flow, and lessen the degree of hypoxemia. One can use the side effects of many medications in this way to alter shunting hemodynamics.

PREOPERATIVE ASSESSMENT

Preoperative assessment of the child with CHD is necessary to plan a safe anesthetic course. Routine evaluation should include a detailed history and physical examination; chest x-ray; electrocardiogram; laboratory tests, including hematocrit, electrolytes, glucose, blood urea nitrogen (BUN), and creatinine; echocardiography; and, if necessary, cardiac catheterization. As many as 20 percent of children with CHD will have extracardiac anomalies as part of a variety of systemic congenital syndromes, which may complicate the anesthetic management. For example, children with Down's, Treacher Collins, and Pierre Robin syndromes may also have significant airway abnormalities in addition to their cardiac lesions [12] (Table 17-3).

History

Children with CHD may be asymptomatic or may have signs of cyanosis or congestive heart failure. The frequency and duration of cyanotic spells are important to note. Cyanosis may be present at rest, may be induced by crying or exercise, and may be relieved by squatting or compressing the femoral arteries. These latter two maneuvers work by increasing the systemic vascular resistance and improve oxygenation by decreasing the amount of right-to-left shunt. These maneuvers mimic the pharmacologic basis for treating acute desaturation with α-adrenergic agonists [13].

Manifestations of congestive heart failure include tachypnea and dyspnea. Children with increased pulmonary blood flow are prone to frequent lung infections, and it is sometimes difficult to distinguish respiratory distress stemming from a lung infection from that caused by congestive heart failure. Older children sometimes describe bouts of chest pain and palpitations and may tire more easily than their peers. These patients may be receiving multiple medications, including digoxin, diuretics, antiarrhythmics, β-blockers, prostaglandins, and inotropic agents.

Physical Examination

Physical examination is used to correlate significant findings with the patient's history. It should be determined whether the child's growth and development are age appropriate. Failure to thrive may be a sign of congestive heart failure unless hypoxemia is present.

Blood pressure in the upper and lower extremities should be checked in patients with aortic arch abnormalities. If the subclavian artery had previously been used for a Blalock-Taussig shunt, an erroneous blood pressure may be present in that arm, and a different extremity should be used to measure and monitor blood pressure. The cardiac examination should include inspection of precordial activity as well as auscultation for heart sounds, murmurs, and clicks. The respiratory system should be assessed for active infection, bronchospasm, and possible associated airway abnormalities. One should also note the presence of scars from previous surgical cutdowns that may limit the choice of venous or arterial catheterization sites. Knowledge of the patient's current weight is mandatory before any pediatric anesthetic can be given.

Cyanotic patients frequently become polycythemic in the body's attempt to improve oxygen-carrying capacity. Children taking diuretics may be hypokalemic, may have elevated BUN and creatinine levels, or have a hypochloremic metabolic alkalosis. Persistent severe hypoxemia or inadequate cardiac output may result in metabolic acidosis. Calcium and glucose should always be measured in neonates and critically ill children.

Chest X-ray and ECG

The chest x-ray should be reviewed for evidence of cardiomegaly, pulmonary vascular congestion, and

Table 17-3. Syndromes with congenital cardiac defects

Syndrome	Cardiac lesions	Syndrome	Cardiac lesions
Trisomy 21 (Down)	ECD, VSD, ASD, TOF, PDA	Forney (deafness, freckles)	MI
Trisomy 18	VSD, PDA, ASD, bicuspid PV, CoA, bicuspid AV	Leopard (deafness, lentigines)	PS
		Neurofibromatosis	PS, renal artery stenosis
		Tuberous sclerosis	Rhabdomyoma
5p-(cri du chat)	VSD, PDA, ASD, PS	Kartagener (bronchiectasis)	Dextrocardia
4p-(Wolf)	VSD, ASD, PDA, PS		
XO (Turner)	CoA, AS, VSD, ASD	Ivemark asplenia or polysplenia	Complex cyanotic heart disease
Ellis–van Creveld	Single atrium, ECD, PDA	Marfan	Dilation of proximal aorta (AI, aneurysm), MVP, cystic medial necrosis
Laurence-Moon-Biedl	TOF, VSD		
Carpenter	PDA, VSD		
Holt-Oram	ASD, VSD, TOF, PS, PDA	Ehlers-Danlos	MVP, arterial rupture
Fanconi	PDA, VSD	Cutis laxa	Peripheral PS
Thrombocytopenia, absent radius	ASD, TOF	Osteogenesis imperfecta	MVP, AI
		Pseudoxanthoma elasticum	Coronary artery disease
Rubinstein-Taybi	CAV, ASD	Glycogen storage disease II (Pompe)	Massive cardiac enlargement due to glycogen deposition
Vater	Variable		
Noonan	PS (dysplastic PV), ASD		
Di George	Interrupted aortic arch type B, aberrant right subclavian, right aortic arch, truncus arteriosus, TOF	Homocystinuria	Thrombosis of arteries
		Mucopolysaccharidoses Type I, Hurler	Pseudoatherosclerosis, AI, MI
		Type II, Hunter	AI
		Types IV, V, VI, Hunter	AI
Smith-Lemli-Opitz	VSD, PDA	Friedreich ataxia	Cardiomyopathy
Facial dysmorphism	PDA	Myotonic dystrophy	MVP, cardiomyopathy
de Lange	VSD, PDA, ASD, TOF	Muscular dystrophy	Cardiomyopathy
Goldenhar	TOF, VSD, PDA, CoA	Jervell and Lange-Nielsen (deafness)	Prolonged QT and RT intervals, VF
Williams' elfin face	Supravalvular AS, peripheral AS, peripheral PS, interrupted arch	Romano Ward (no deafness)	Prolonged QT interval, VF
		Refsum (polyneuritis)	Arrhythmia, heart block
Asymmetric crying facies	Variable	Familial periodic paralysis	Hypokalemia, SVT

ECD = endocardial cushion defect; VSD = ventricular septal defect; ASD = atrial septal defect; TOF = tetralogy of Fallot; PDA = patent ductus arteriosus; PV = pulmonary valve; CoA = coarctation of aorta; AV = aortic valve; PS = pulmonic stenosis; AS = aortic stenosis; TGA = transposition of great arteries; LH = left heart; CAV = canalis atrioventricularis; MI = mitral insufficiency; AI = aortic insufficiency; MVP = mitral valve prolapse; VF = ventricular fibrillation; SVT = supraventricular tachycardia.
Source: Modified from J Katz and DJ Steward (eds), *Anesthesia and Uncommon Pediatric Diseases*. Philadelphia: Saunders, 1987.

areas of consolidation or atelectasis. To assess heart size accurately, the chest film should ideally be taken with the patient in the upright position. Patients with left-to-right shunt ratios greater than 2:1 will have evidence of increased pulmonary vascular markings. A small pulmonary artery and pulmonary vessels that extend only to the midlung are indicative of a right-to-left shunt. The chest x-ray may also show airway compression from an anomalous vessel. One should remember that the presence of a "normal" chest x-ray does not rule out CHD. The electrocardiogram, although not diagnostic of any one specific lesion, provides useful information about heart rate and rhythm. It also should be evaluated for ventricular strain patterns (ST and T-wave changes) characteristic of excessive pressure or volume load on the ventricles.

Echocardiography

Advances in echocardiographic imaging of the heart have significantly improved the diagnosis and evaluation of CHD [14]. In some patients, for example, those with atrial septal defect, patent ductus arteriosus, or coarctation of the aorta, this noninvasive technique can replace cardiac catheterization and provide an accurate anatomic diagnosis [15, 16]. Echocardiography has also been shown to be a valuable adjunct in assessing patients who have undergone prior corrective cardiac procedures. One can measure cardiovascular reserve by measuring left ventricular systolic function and ejection fraction. These two-dimensional studies have been shown to compare favorably with volumes recorded at cardiac catheterization [17]. Doppler measurements of pressure gradients across semilunar valves and other obstructions often are accurate. Pressure gradients can be calculated by measuring the velocity of flow at the obstructed site and converting that into a gradient that can be used to predict the severity of valvular stenosis [18]. Noninvasive Doppler estimates of pulmonary and systemic blood flow correlate well with measurements of these flows at the time of cardiac catheterization. Despite the value of echocardiography in the diagnosis of anatomic defects and ventricular function, cardiac catheterization remains the gold standard for the ultimate assessment of cardiac anatomy and physiologic function.

ANTIBIOTIC PROPHYLAXIS

The prevention of bacterial endocarditis is a major preoperative concern in the management of the patient with CHD. In general, all individuals known to have intracardiac lesions should be considered candidates for antibiotic prophylaxis, with the exception of those patients with an isolated secundum atrial septal defect, a secundum atrial septal defect repaired without a patch more than 6 months ago, and a patent ductus arteriosus ligated and divided more than 6 months earlier [19, 20]. In addition, prophylaxis is indicated in acquired lesions, such as rheumatic, atherosclerotic, or calcific disease; prolapsing mitral valve with regurgitation; hypertrophic obstructive cardiomyopathy; or calcified mitral annulus. Prophylaxis is also required in those patients with an intracardiac prosthesis or patch, such as prosthetic valves or surgically created systemic to pulmonary shunts, and in those with a previous history of bacterial endocarditis (Tables 17-4 and 17-5). These intracardiac or vascular abnormalities cause an alteration in blood flow, producing local areas of turbulence that increase the risk of endocardial or arterial endothelial infection in the face of transient bacteremia. Antibiotics may prevent the development of bacterial endocarditis, and prophylaxis is therefore recommended. The standardized antibiotic protocols of the American Academy of Pediatrics and the American Heart Association are listed in Table 17-6.

Table 17-4. Criteria for institution of prophylaxis for bacterial endocarditis

---

Endocarditis prophylaxis recommended
Prosthetic cardiac valves (including biosynthetic valves)
Most congenital cardiac malformations
Surgically constructed systemic-pulmonary shunts
Rheumatic and other acquired valvular dysfunction
Asymmetric septal hypertrophy (idiopathic hypertrophic subaortic stenosis)
Previous history of bacterial endocarditis
Mitral valve prolapse with insufficiency*

Endocarditis prophylaxis not recommended
Isolated secundum atrial septal defect
Secundum atrial septal defect repaired without a patch 6 or more months earlier
Postoperative coronary artery bypass graft (CABG) surgery

---

*Definitive data to provide guidance in management of patients with mitral valve prolapse are particularly limited. It is clear that, in general, such patients are at low risk of developing endocarditis, but the risk-benefit ratio of prophylaxis in mitral valve prolapse is uncertain.

Source: Reproduced and modified by permission of *Pediatrics*. From Committee on Rheumatic Fever and Bacterial Endocarditis, Prevention of bacterial endocarditis. *Pediatrics* 75:603, 1985.

Table 17-5. Procedures for which endocarditis prophylaxis is indicated[a]

All dental procedures likely to induce gingival bleeding (not simple adjustment of orthodontic appliances or shedding of deciduous teeth)
Tonsillectomy and/or adenoidectomy
Surgical procedures or biopsy involving the respiratory mucosa
Bronchoscopy, especially with a rigid bronchoscope[b]
Incision and drainage of infected tissue
Genitourinary and gastrointestinal procedures

[a] This table lists common procedures, but is not meant to be all inclusive.
[b] The risk with flexible bronchoscopy is low, but the necessity for prophylaxis is not yet defined.
Source: Reproduced and modified by permission of *Pediatrics*. From Committee on Rheumatic Fever and Bacterial Endocarditis, Prevention of bacterial endocarditis. *Pediatrics* 75:603, 1985.

PREMEDICATION

The selection and timing of preoperative medication are important in the anesthetic management of patients with CHD. One should aim to have the patient arrive in the operating room calm and sedated without causing respiratory depression. This will smooth the induction of anesthesia considerably and allow smaller amounts of anesthetic agents to be used during induction, thereby reducing the risk of hypotension [21]. Additionally, in a patient with a right-to-left shunt, premedication will help to avoid crying and struggling during induction, which could increase the magnitude of the right-to-left shunt and worsen hypoxemia.

Age and physical condition of the patient determine the amount of premedication warranted. Neonates and young infants in general do not require sedation, but should receive an anticholiner-

Table 17-6. Prophylaxis regimens for bacterial endocarditis

Type of regimen	Antibiotic protocol	Type of regimen	Antibiotic protocol
For dental/respiratory procedures		Parenteral regimen for penicillin-allergic patients	Vancomycin, 1 gm IV slowly over 1 hr starting 1 hr before; no repeat dose is necessary
Standard regimen for dental procedures that cause gingival bleeding, and oral respiratory tract surgery	Penicillin V, 2 gm orally 1 hr before, then 1 gm 6 hr later for patients unable to take oral medications; 2 million units aqueous penicillin G IV or IM 30–60 min before a procedure and 1 million units 6 hr later		
		For gastrointestinal/genitourinary procedures *	
		Standard regimen	Ampicillin, 2 gm IM or IV plus gentamicin, 1.5 mg/kg IM or IV ½ to 1 hr before procedure; one follow-up dose can be given 8 hr later
Special regimens			
Parenteral regimens for use when maximal protection is desired, i.e., patients with prosthetic heart valves	Ampicillin, 1–2 gm IM or IV, plus gentamicin, 1.5 mg/kg IM or IV ½ hr before procedure, followed by 1 gm oral penicillin V 6 hr later; alternatively, parenteral regimen can be repeated once 8 hr later	Special regimens	
		Oral regimen for minor or repetitive procedures in low-risk patients	Amoxicillin, 3 gm orally 1 hr before procedure and 1.5 gm 6 hr later
		Penicillin-allergic patients	Vancomycin, 1 gm IV slowly over 1 hr, plus gentamicin, 1.5 mg/kg IM or IV given 1 hr before procedure; can be repeated once 8–12 hr later
Oral regimen for penicillin-allergic patients	Erythromycin, 1 gm orally 1 hr before, then 500 mg 6 hr later		

*Pediatric doses: amoxicillin, 50 mg/kg per dose; ampicillin, 50 mg/kg per dose; erythromycin, 20 mg/kg first dose, then 10 mg/kg; gentamicin, 2 mg/kg per dose; penicillin V, full adult dose if greater than 27 kg, half adult dose if less than 27 kg; aqueous penicillin G, 50,000 units/kg (25,000 units/kg for follow-up); vancomycin, 20 mg/kg per dose. The intervals between doses are the same as for adults. Total doses should not exceed adult doses.
Source: Reproduced and modified by permission of *Pediatrics*. From Committee on Rheumatic Fever and Bacterial Endocarditis, Prevention of bacterial endocarditis. *Pediatrics* 75:603, 1985.

gic drug, either atropine, 0.01 mg/kg, or glycopyrrolate, 0.005 mg/kg. Since small children are unable to increase their stroke volume, cardiac output is more rate dependent and the anticholinergic premedication will help avoid bradycardia. For the older child, a combination of a barbiturate such as pentobarbital, a narcotic such as morphine, and an anticholinergic is very effective. An adolescent could be given oral diazepam after a proper preoperative evaluation. Once a child is premedicated, he or she must be under constant observation with oxygen and resuscitative equipment readily available [22].

In general, withholding food and fluids preoperatively conforms to the general guidelines for pediatric patients. For the infant receiving around-the-clock feedings, giving the child the last oral intake, consisting of 5 percent dextrose or apple juice, 2 to 3 hours preoperatively is sufficient. For older children, the time limit should be extended appropriately. If a child is not scheduled for early-morning surgery, strong consideration should be given to starting an intravenous line preoperatively to avoid dehydration.

INDUCTION OF ANESTHESIA

The choice of anesthetic induction technique depends on the age of the child, the degree of cooperation that can be expected, the presence or absence of adequate premedication, the presence of intravenous access, the child's lesion and cardiovascular status, and the anticipated responses to the various anesthetic agents. If the child arrives in the operating room with a functioning intravenous catheter, then, depending on the lesion, a slow or rapid intravenous induction can proceed safely. The older child with a noncyanotic lesion such as an atrial septal defect, without evidence of congestive heart failure would certainly tolerate an induction consisting of barbiturates, narcotics, benzodiazepines, or an inhalation induction with a potent agent without any expected complications (see Appendix). Certainly, a young child without an IV line and without significant hemodynamic compromise would tolerate an inhalation induction.

The anesthetic challenge surrounds the cyanotic patient, the child in congestive heart failure with increased right-sided pressures, and the neonate who presents without IV access. An educated assessment of the situation must be made by the anesthesiologist as to whether he or she anticipates any airway difficulties, the ease with which intravenous access can be established after induction, and the degree of shunting and pulmonary blood flow present. One should not hastily give a potent agent to a child who has limited ventricular reserve. This will rapidly lead to a decreased cardiac output, decreased perfusion, metabolic acidosis, increased pulmonary vascular resistance and decreased systemic vascular resistance, hypoxemia, and cardiovascular collapse. The child's safety must predominate over the momentary discomfort of an intramuscular injection. Ketamine is a useful drug for this purpose in this patient population. It will support the circulation by increasing heart rate and blood pressure, while inducing anesthesia, provided that the sympathetic nervous system is functioning appropriately. In the cyanotic patient with a right-to-left shunt, it will tend to maintain pulmonary blood flow and oxygen saturation by its effect on maintaining systemic vascular resistance. Although there has been some concern that ketamine could similarly also increase pulmonary vascular resistance, Hickey and associates [23] have shown that this does not occur in children, provided that ventilation and oxygenation are maintained.

Historically, narcotics have been viewed as the mainstay of cardiac anesthesia pharmacology. In patients ranging from the severely compromised premature neonate to the octogenarian with acquired valvular and atherosclerotic heart disease, narcotics have proven attractive as the primary anesthetic for their lack of myocardial depression, relative vascular stability, potency, and duration of action. There are patients who would not tolerate potent inhalation agents, benzodiazepines, barbiturates, or even nitrous oxide; however, assuming normal volume status, they will tolerate narcotics that can provide a stress-free anesthetic [24, 25].

Most of the patients with noncyanotic CHD will tolerate a standard inhalation induction with oxygen, nitrous oxide, and halothane. The speed of induction of an inhalation agent is determined by the rate of increasing the partial pressure of the agent within the alveoli and the distribution and transfer of anesthetic from the blood to the brain. Anesthetic equilibration is usually relatively rapid between the alveoli, arterial blood, and brain, with the limiting factor being the rate of rise of the alveolar partial pressure of anesthetic [26]. In patients with CHD who have decreased pulmonary blood flow, anesthetic transfer from the alveoli to the arterial blood is slowed. The right-to-left shunting of systemic venous blood into the arterial circulation further lowers the arterial partial pressure and therefore delays the rate of rise of the partial pressure of anesthetic in the brain; consequently, the rate of anesthetic induction is slowed [27, 28]. Clinically, this can be overcome by using higher concentrations, by the use of a soluble anesthetic agent, and by increasing the minute ventilation.

In the case of left-to-right shunting, the speed of inhalation induction is unchanged. The patient with increased pulmonary blood flow maintains a normal systemic cardiac output by compensatory increases in blood volume and right heart output. Assuming a constant inspired anesthetic concentration and a rapid initial rise in alveolar partial pressure and full anesthetic equilibration between the alveoli and the pulmonary blood after the first pass through the lung, there will be no increased partial pressure of anesthetic in the blood during the subsequent recirculation through the lungs; therefore, the rate of rise of anesthetic delivery to the brain cannot be increased.

The speed of induction of intravenous agents may also be affected by shunting of blood in CHD. In patients with left-to-right shunts and increased pulmonary blood flow, the appearance of the drug in the systemic circulation is not delayed. However, because of the dilution by the increased pulmonary blood flow and recirculation through the lungs, the initial peak concentration is lower and its effect is prolonged. In cyanotic lesions with right-to-left shunting, the onset time is shortened since the systemic venous blood bypasses the pulmonary circulation and the bolus is shunted directly into the systemic circulation.

Monitoring during the anesthetic induction will depend on the general health and cooperation of the patient. A squirming uncooperative 2-year-old may only allow placement of a precordial stethoscope and pulse oximeter before induction; however, once induction is accomplished, electrocardiography and blood pressure cuff should be rapidly applied and intravenous access obtained as quickly as possible. An indwelling arterial catheter is strongly recommended for children with a history of congestive heart failure who are undergoing noncardiac surgery, for closer hemodynamic monitoring and for frequent arterial blood gas sampling. One should remember that acidosis, hypoxia, hypercarbia, and hypothermia are the most easily preventable causes of increased pulmonary vascular resistance and decreased pulmonary blood flow; therefore, care should be taken to maintain adequate ventilation, oxygenation, and body temperature.

Special vigilance must be taken when starting and manipulating intravenous lines in any patient with a shunt lesion. Air bubbles floating in the venous system may be shunted to the systemic arterial circulation through any communication between the pulmonary and systemic circulations, for example, atrial septal defect, ventricular septal defect, patent ductus arteriosus, and so forth. Children with right-to-left shunts are at the greatest risk; however, even lesions in which the predominant direction is left-to-right can have episodes of bidirectional shunting or frank right-to-left shunting. Some of the most feared complications arising in these patients are found in the heart and in the central nervous system, resulting in embolic strokes or abscess formation and coronary embolism leading to myocardial infarction.

Meticulous insertion and use of these catheters can prevent many complications. Intravenous tubing, connection sites, injection ports, and stopcocks must be flushed free of all air before connection to a patient. Blood should back-bleed to fill the catheter before its attachment to the intravenous tubing. Small amounts of solution should be ejected from the syringe to clear air from the needle and hub before intravenous injection. All stopcock ports should be filled with fluid before a syringe is inserted; then the syringe should be held upright so that any remaining air bubble will rise to the plunger end. One should avoid injecting the last milliliter from a syringe into the intravenous tubing, as this area frequently conceals hidden bubbles. Central lines should be placed with the patient in the Trendelenburg position during positive pressure ventilation to reduce the chance of negative pressure aspiration or air [29]. Many anesthesiologists are wary of using nitrous oxide after induction in children with right-to-left shunts, in

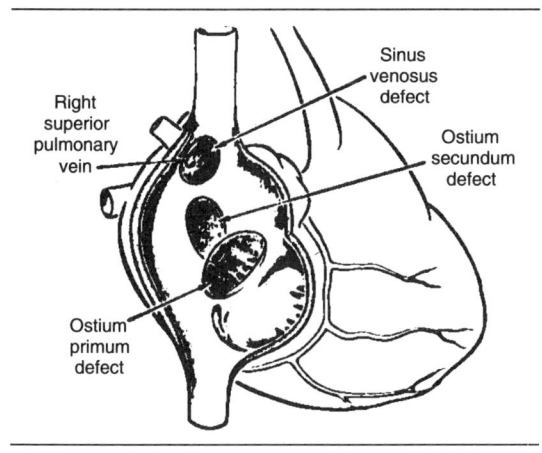

Fig. 17-4. View of the atrial septum illustrating the location of the various atrial septal defects. (Reprinted with permission from AK Ream and RP Fogdall (eds), *Acute Cardiovascular Management: Anesthesia and Intensive Care.* Philadelphia: Lippincott, 1982.)

order to avoid the possibility of unintentionally increasing the size of intravenous air bubbles [30, 31].

SPECIFIC NONCYANOTIC LESIONS

Atrial Septal Defect

Atrial septal defects (ASD) can be divided into three distinct categories: ostium primum, ostium secundum, and sinus venosus types (Fig. 17-4). Ostium primum defects or partial atrioventricular canal defects are located low in the atrial wall. They frequently are associated with a cleft in the anterior leaflet of the mitral and tricuspid valves, causing prolapse and regurgitation directly into the atria, which may predispose to the early development of cardiac failure. The ostium secundum type is the most common form of ASD, occurring in 80 percent of cases [32]. It frequently involves the area of the foramen ovale, is variable in size, and is usually found as an isolated cardiac lesion. The sinus venosus type of atrial septal defect is much rarer and is frequently associated with partial anomalous pulmonary venous return of the right pulmonary veins.

The pathophysiology of atrial septal defect is a

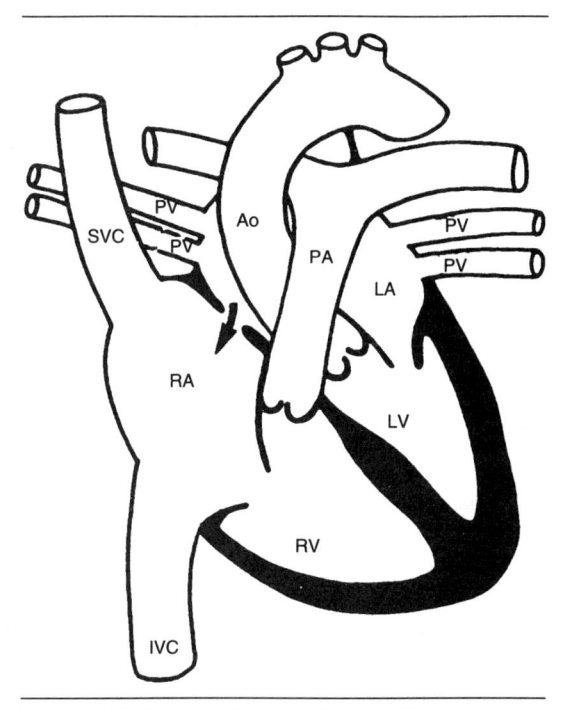

Fig. 17-5. Schematic diagram of a secundum atrial septal defect located in the center of the interatrial septum. Blood flows along a pressure gradient from the left atrium (LA) to the right atrium (RA). The resulting left-to-right intracardiac shunt is associated with increased flow through the pulmonary artery (PA). Surgical closure of the defect is indicated when the pulmonary artery blood flow is double the flow into the aorta (Ao). Decreases in systemic vascular resistance or increases in pulmonary vascular resistance will decrease the pressure gradient across the defect, leading to a reduction in the magnitude of the shunt. RV = right ventricle; LV = left ventricle; SVC = superior vena cava; IVC = inferior vena cava; PV = pulmonary vein. (Reprinted with permission from RK Stoelting and SF Dierdorf, *Anesthesia and Coexisting Disease.* New York: Churchill Livingstone, 1983. P 48.)

shunt that depends on the pressure gradient between the right and left atria generated by their respective ventricles during diastole (Fig. 17-5). In the neonatal period, the compliance and thickness of both ventricles are comparable, so that minimal shunting exists. However, as the left ventricle increases in thickness, and the pulmonary vascular resistance decreases, left-to-right shunting occurs. The left-to-right shunt causes an increase in pulmonary blood flow, although the pulmonary vascular resistance usually stays within normal limits until the end of the second decade [33]. Symptoms of fatigue and dyspnea usually develop with a pulmonary to systemic flow ratio above three, and at that level pulmonary vascular resistance tends to become elevated. Once fixed pulmonary hypertension develops, its course is usually progressive, with severe dyspnea on exertion, decrease in the left-to-right shunt, shunt reversal, and cyanosis. This is known as Eisenmenger's syndrome with pulmonary hypertension and fixed reversal of shunt. Surgery is usually recommended in the presence of an increased pulmonary blood flow ratio greater than 1.5 before the development of severe pulmonary vascular disease.

The patient with normal growth and development, and no history of dyspnea or cyanosis, would be expected to have an uncomplicated asymptomatic ASD. Anesthesia could proceed in any fashion that the anesthesiologist believes would be comfortable, with the following guidelines. Neither intravenous nor inhalational general anesthesia is contraindicated. Vigilance should be exercised to protect against air bubbles in the intravenous tubing. Air bubble traps are recommended. Unless a definitive confirmation of isolated ostium secundum atrial septal defect is known, bacterial prophylaxis should be given for procedures that have been associated with an increased risk for endocarditis (See Table 17-5). Invasive hemodynamic monitoring should not be necessary, assuming no other medical indication.

Ventricular Septal Defect

Ventricular septal defects (VSD) (see Fig. 17-2; Fig. 17-6) are the most common type of congenital heart defect, occurring both as isolated abnormalities or as a component of a systemic congenital syndrome. The ventricular septum consists of a fibrous component, the membranous septum, and a muscular portion. One can classify these lesions based on their anatomic location [34]. Type I, or supracristal, defects are located above the crista supraventricularis just under the annulus of the aorta. The incidence of this lesion is 5 percent. Type II, or infracristal, defects are the most common type of VSD (incidence of about 80%) and are found

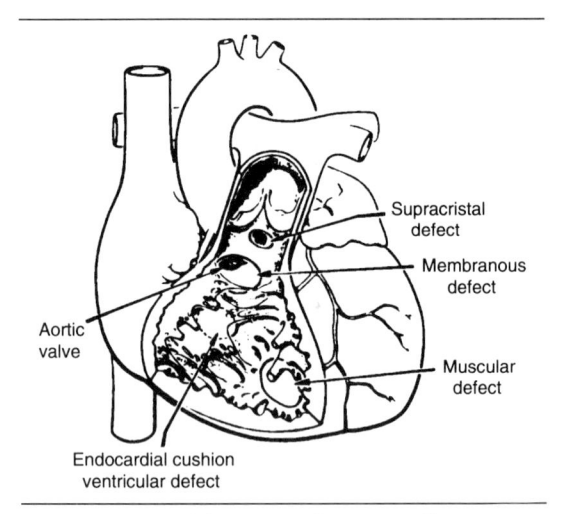

Fig. 17-6. View of the ventricular septum illustrating the location of the various ventricular septal defects. (Reprinted with permission from AK Ream and RP Fogdall (eds), *Acute Cardiovascular Management: Anesthesia and Intensive Care*. Philadelphia: Lippincott, 1982.)

lower in the membranous septum beneath the crista supraventricularis. Type III, or canal type, defects are the septal defects accompanying complete atrioventricular canal and result from incomplete fusion of the endocardial cushions. Type IV (incidence of 3–8%) may be single or multiple (Swiss cheese defect) and may be located anywhere within the muscular septum [35].

The physiologic circulatory alteration caused by a VSD depends primarily on its size and the status of the pulmonary vascular system. A small VSD with high resistance to flow permits only a small left-to-right shunt. A large interventricular communication allows a large left-to-right shunt only if there is no pulmonic stenosis or high pulmonary vascular resistance since these factors determine shunt flow. Resistance to left ventricular emptying also affects shunt flow because it is an important factor in determining left ventricular pressure. Large defects allow both ventricles to function hemodynamically as a single pumping chamber with two outlets, equalizing the pressure in the systemic and pulmonary circulations. In such patients the magnitude of the left-to-right shunt varies inversely with pulmonary vascular resistance.

A wide spectrum exists in the natural history of

VSD, ranging from spontaneous closure to congestive heart failure and death in infancy. Within this spectrum are the possible development of pulmonary vascular obstruction, right ventricular outflow tract obstruction, aortic regurgitation, and infective endocarditis [36, 37]. It is unusual for a VSD to cause difficulties in the immediate postnatal period, although congestive heart failure during the first 6 months of life is a frequent occurrence. Spontaneous closure occurs by age 3 years in approximately 40 percent of patients; however, occasionally, VSDs do not close until the child is 8 to 10 years old. Closure is more common in patients born with a small VSD; nonetheless, in 7 percent of patients with a large defect and congestive failure spontaneous closure may occur. A persistent tiny VSD is not life threatening unless bacterial endocarditis develops; however, with proper precautions the incidence of this complication is less than 1 percent. If a moderate to large defect maintains its size after birth, the net left-to-right shunt tends to increase during the first month of life as pulmonary vascular resistance falls. Children with large shunts tend to develop recurrent upper and lower respiratory tract infections, failure to gain weight, and congestive heart failure. These children usually benefit from primary intracardiac closure with full cardiopulmonary bypass early in childhood [38]. It is of the utmost importance to identify patients in whom irreversible pulmonary hypertension (Eisenmenger's syndrome) may develop to offer them surgical correction at an early age.

The electrocardiogram in the child with a VSD may be essentially normal or may show left or biventricular hypertrophy. Chest x-ray may be normal or may reveal cardiomegaly, left atrial enlargement, and pulmonary vascular engorgement in those patients with a history of congestive heart failure.

The anesthetic plan for these patients as well as the necessity for invasive monitoring should be tailored to the severity of the cardiac pathophysiology and the complexity of the surgery planned. Neither inhalation nor intravenous general anesthesia is contraindicated, except in the infant in congestive heart failure who is presenting for emergency surgery. It may be prudent in this case to choose a narcotic or ketamine-based anesthetic instead of a potent myocardial depressant. Vigilance should be exercised to protect against air bubbles in the intravenous tubing. Air bubble traps are suggested. The recommended guidelines previously discussed for antibiotic prophylaxis should be followed. There are no specific contraindications to regional anesthesia in a child with a ventricular septal defect. One should note that a patient with a surgically corrected type II VSD may have postoperative right bundle branch block and left anterior hemiblock and has a high incidence of progression to complete heart block. However, prophylactic use of permanent pacemakers in the asymptomatic patient is not currently recommended [39, 40].

The postoperative care of these patients should be tailored to the severity of the patient's illness. An asymptomatic patient presenting for routine ambulatory surgery can be discharged home in the usual fashion. The symptomatic patient, however, may not only benefit from hospitalization, but may also require intensive care monitoring postoperatively. These details should be addressed preoperatively in conjunction with the patient's cardiologist and surgeon.

Atrioventricular Canal

Complete atrioventricular (AV) canal is caused by failure of the endocardial cushions to fuse with the septum primum (Figs. 17-7 and 17-8). This produces defects of the atrial septum, and the ventricular septum, a cleft in the mitral valve, and an abnormal tricuspid valve. The four chambers communicate, yielding systemic pressures in both ventricles and a large left-to-right shunt. Occasionally, these lesions are associated with pulmonary stenosis and a concomitant right-to-left shunt, but in the absence of pulmonary stenosis, an AV canal leads to markedly increased pulmonary blood flow, causing pulmonary hypertension and heart failure at an early age. Complete surgical repair is usually required by age 2. These children frequently have their pulmonary arteries banded in early infancy to decrease pulmonary blood flow; however, because of the high mortality associated with this approach, many centers are now finding improved results with primary repair in infancy [41–43]. The urgency for corrective surgery depends on the degree of shunting, the extent of valvular incompetence, and the onset of pulmonary changes.

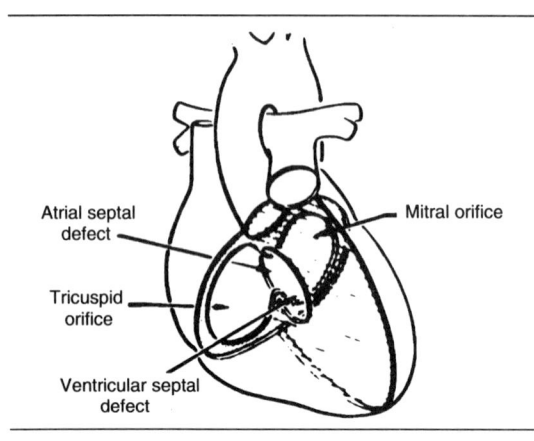

Fig. 17-7. Diagrammatic view of endocardial cushion defect illustrating relative positions of atrioventricular valves. (Reprinted with permission from AK Ream and RP Fogdall (eds), *Acute Cardiovascular Management: Anesthesia and Intensive Care.* Philadelphia: Lippincott, 1982.)

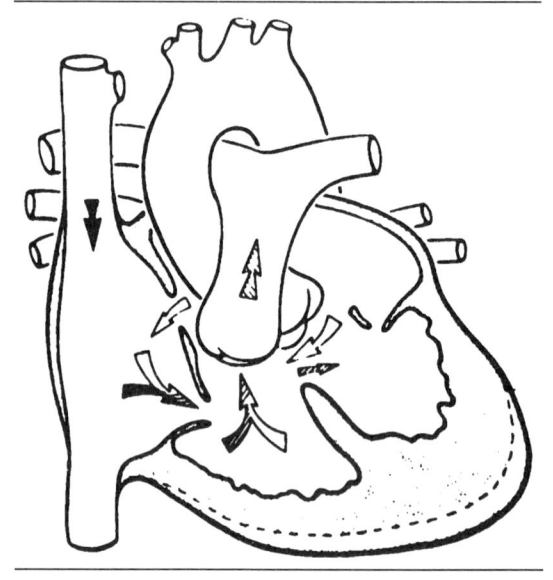

Fig. 17-8. Flow diagram of endocardial cushion defect illustrating mixing at atrial and ventricular levels and biventricular hypertrophy. (Reprinted with permission from AK Ream and RP Fogdall (eds), *Acute Cardiovascular Management: Anesthesia and Intensive Care.* Philadelphia: Lippincott, 1982.)

On physical examination, both right and left ventricular impulses are prominent. Systolic and diastolic murmurs may be present and the heart is enlarged on chest x-ray. Right atrial and ventricular enlargement are present on the electrocardiogram, and dysrhythmias, such as atrial fibrillation, nodal bradycardia, paroxysmal ventricular tachycardia, and complete heart block, occur in approximately 20 percent of patients [44].

In addition to the utilization of the standard anesthetic monitors, including pulse oximetry, strong consideration should be given to invasive arterial blood pressure monitoring with frequent arterial blood gas sampling. Any induction technique is acceptable provided that ventilation is maintained, as this lesion primarily causes a left-to-right shunt. In patients with more advanced disease in the presence of pulmonary hypertension with right heart failure, intramuscular ketamine may be preferable to potent inhalation agents. These children should be admitted for postoperative observation in a monitored unit following surgery, as the added stresses in the postoperative period could exacerbate pulmonary hypertension with increased congestive heart failure. One must remember that the patient recovering from general anesthesia may be prone to hypoventilation and rises in the arterial carbon dioxide tension ($PaCO_2$), which could acutely increase the pulmonary vascular resistance and cause reversal of the left-to-right shunt.

Patent Ductus Arteriosus

The ductus arteriosus allows continuous blood flow between the pulmonary and systemic circulations (Fig. 17-9). In the fetus, in the presence of high pulmonary vascular resistance, elevated circulating prostaglandins, and a low arterial oxygen tension (PaO_2), the ductus remains relatively dilated, allowing the majority of the right ventricular cardiac output to bypass the unexpanded lungs and flow directly to the descending aorta [45, 46]. The diameter of the ductus arteriosus in the fetus can approach that of the aorta and the main pulmonary trunk. Immediately after birth, with the expansion of the lungs and the cessation of placental blood flow, the pulmonary vascular resistance drops, the arterial PaO_2 rises, and the level of circulating prostaglandin falls, allowing for the constriction of the ductus arteriosus. Physiologic closure of the ductus occurs in the first 10 to 15 hours of life [47]. Full

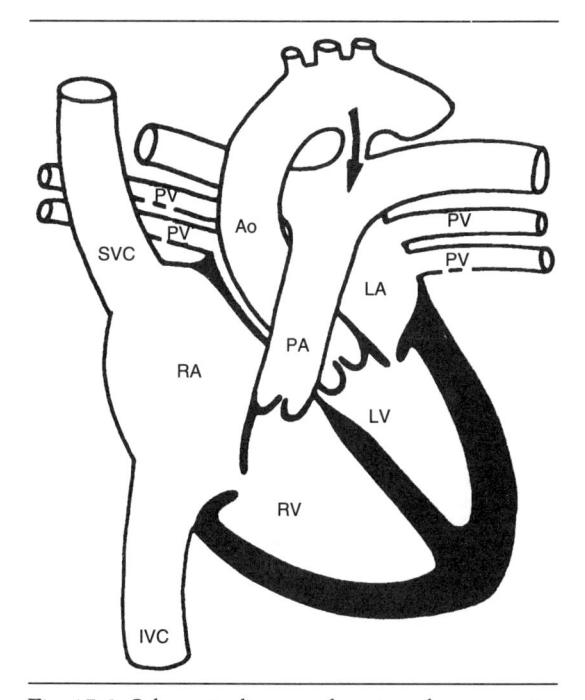

Fig. 17-9. Schematic diagram of a patent ductus arteriosus connecting the arch of the aorta (Ao) with the pulmonary artery (PA). Blood flow is from the high-pressure Ao into the PA. The resulting systemic to pulmonary shunt (left-to-right shunt) leads to increased pulmonary blood flow. Reductions in systemic vascular resistance or increases in pulmonary vascular resistance will decrease the magnitude of the shunt through the ductus arteriosus. SVC = superior vena cava; RA = right atrium; IVC = inferior vena cava; PV = pulmonary vein; RV = right ventricle; LA = left atrium; LV = left ventricle. (Reprinted with permission from RK Stoelting and SF Dierdorf, *Anesthesia and Coexisting Disease.* New York: Churchill Livingstone, 1983. P 52.)

anatomic closure of the ductus as a result of muscular constriction and thrombosis occurs by the end of the third month [48]. If the ductus fails to close shortly after birth, a functional left-to-right shunt usually develops.

Infants with a large patent ductus arteriosus (PDA) usually show signs and symptoms of left ventricular failure, that is, failure to thrive, tachypnea, and tachycardia. These children are usually corrected early in life. Occasionally, the older child or adult presents with a systolic heart murmur and upon evaluation is found to have a PDA. These patients are at an increased risk to develop bacterial endocarditis, aneurysmal dilatation of the aorta, and progressive heart failure. Extended studies describing the course of long-standing PDA suggest that the life expectancy is decreased by one half [49].

The anesthetic management of a patient with an isolated coexisting PDA should follow the general guidelines for those patients with a simple left-to-right shunt. Invasive arterial monitoring is not specifically required for a patient with a PDA. Myocardial function is usually preserved and these patients would tolerate any inhalation, intravenous, or regional anesthetic. They are at risk for bacterial endocarditis, and antibiotic prophylaxis is recommended. These patients are also at risk for air emboli, and bubble traps are also recommended.

The premature infant in congestive heart failure because of a ductus that has not yet closed occasionally needs emergency surgery, for example, exploratory laparotomy for necrotizing enterocolitis. These children are critically ill, demand minimal anesthesia, and frequently require full cardiovascular and metabolic resuscitation. They should receive a carefully titrated anesthetic, free of any myocardial depressants, with full invasive monitoring as indicated.

One should note that these patients differ from neonates with complex congenital heart disease and obstruction to pulmonary blood flow at some level, who rely on the PDA as a life-preserving conduit to maintain some degree of pulmonary blood flow. In general, these patients should receive a permanent shunting procedure to reliably maintain pulmonary blood flow before definitive corrective cardiac surgery. It is unlikely that this type of PDA would present as coexisting cardiac disease for noncardiac surgery before placement of a shunt. This is discussed further in Chap. 18.

Coarctation of the Aorta

Coarctation of the aorta is a congenital narrowing of the descending aorta at the aortic isthmus that occurs either just before or opposite the ductus arteriosus. One must review fetal blood flow to understand the development of coarctation of the aorta. Fetal cardiac output is divided equally between the aorta and the pulmonary artery. Aortic blood flows predominantly to the coronary arteries and to the cerebral vessels. Pulmonary blood flow is shunted predominantly across the ductus arteriosus to the descending aorta. The aortic isthmus, the segment between the brachiocephalic artery and the ductus arteriosus, is narrower than any other aortic segment, since it carries the least amount of blood during fetal development. At birth, the flow pattern changes, allowing increased blood flow across the aortic isthmus, therefore allowing for the rapid growth of this section of the aorta. A decrease in left ventricular outflow in the fetal and postnatal period will reduce flow across the isthmus and result in a preductal coarctation [50]. The most common lesions associated with coarctation are VSD, hypoplastic left heart syndrome, patent ductus arteriosus, and malformations of the aortic and mitral valves [51]. Closure of the ductus and the invagination of the posterior aortic wall can lead to postductal coarctation. In fact, coarctation of the aorta is the most common cause of congestive heart failure diagnosed between the first and third weeks of life, the normal time of ductal closure.

Patients with coarctation who survive infancy are usually asymptomatic during the first two decades of life. They rarely present in congestive failure; instead, they are usually identified on routine physical examination with different blood pressures in the upper and lower extremities, a systolic cardiac murmur, and hypertension. Since the renal arteries lie distal to the coarctation, the renal vascular bed is perfused at a lower pressure. This may explain the involvement of the renin-angiotensin-aldosterone system in the etiology of hypertension in patients with coarctation [52]. Adults with coarctation may present with left ventricular hypertrophy, or left bundle branch block on the electrocardiogram. The chest x-ray universally shows rib notching secondary to the development of enlarged intercostal artery collateral blood flow, as well as signs of left ventricular hypertrophy.

The anesthetic management of these patients depends on the location of the coarctation, preductal or postductal; coexisting cardiac anomalies; and/or congestive heart failure. Patients with a coexisting preductal coarctation frequently are neonates who are receiving prostaglandin infusion to maintain patency of the ductus arteriosus. The right-to-left shunt from the pulmonary artery to the descending aorta facilitates some perfusion to the lower half of the body to protect against severe metabolic acidosis. The prostaglandin infusion should remain in a dedicated intravenous line until the coarctation is repaired, and one must be careful to avoid flushing this line, as an inadvertent bolus of prostaglandin could result in a marked decrease in blood pressure. One should remember to place a blood pressure monitor on the right upper extremity to provide accurate information about cerebral blood flow. These patients commonly have some degree of left ventricular dysfunction and may not tolerate potent myocardial depressants.

Patients with postductal coarctation are frequently asymptomatic for many years. Anesthesia can be maintained with either intravenous or inhalation agents. Drugs that can significantly raise arterial blood pressure such as ketamine and pancuronium should be avoided. Monitoring should be tailored to the patient's proposed surgery and medical condition. One should recognize that bleeding might present as a significant complication in these patients during abdominal or thoracic surgery secondary to the presence of massively dilated arteries to supply collateral blood flow to the lower half of the body.

Aortic Stenosis

Congenital aortic stenosis accounts for approximately 5 to 10 percent of all congenital cardiac lesions. The classification is based on their specific anatomic obstruction: valvular, subvalvular, or supravalvular. Valvular aortic stenosis, which occurs in approximately 85 percent of cases, is an obstruction at the level of the valve. It is frequently associated with a bicuspid valve whose leaflets become stiff, thickened, and fused. Subvalvular stenosis develops either because of the presence of a discrete membranous obstruction below the true aortic valve or because of a muscular band that impinges on the left ventricular outflow tract and obstructs blood flow. Supravalvular stenosis is rare; when it does occur, it is often associated with supravalvular pulmonic stenosis and mental retardation (Williams' syndrome). The obstruction to flow appears just above the sinuses of Valsalva, which can subject the coronary arteries to high systolic blood pressures, causing abnormal dilatation and premature atherosclerotic changes.

Critical aortic stenosis presents in the newborn

period with severe congestive heart failure, reduced left ventricular volumes, and left ventricular hypertrophy. These children require emergent valvuloplasty or surgery. Mortality from surgery is 50 percent; however, the number approaches 100 percent without surgical intervention [53]. Since these children rarely require noncardiac surgery before correction, this subject is not discussed further in this chapter.

In contrast to the newborn with critical aortic stenosis, the older patient typically presents for evaluation of an asymptomatic systolic murmur. Development of symptoms of dyspnea, syncope, or chest pain usually indicates severe aortic stenosis, and corrective surgery is recommended [54]. The risk of sudden death may be as high as 7.5 percent of patients with aortic stenosis [55].

The anesthetic management of patients with aortic stenosis is the same whether the obstruction is valvular, subvalvular, or supravalvular. The obstruction to left ventricular emptying increases left ventricular pressure, which causes left ventricular hypertrophy and increased myocardial work. The increased myocardial mass requires increased oxygen delivery, which may be compromised by tachycardia since this increases oxygen consumption while decreasing diastolic perfusion time of the coronary arteries. Tachycardia also results in inadequate left ventricular filling and decreased cardiac output to further decrease coronary perfusion. Similarly, bradycardia may reduce cardiac output because stroke volume is limited by the flow rate across the stenotic lesion. Induction and maintenance of anesthesia with either intravenous or inhalational agents are acceptable, with the understanding that one should avoid significant tachycardia and reduction of diastolic blood pressure. Systemic vascular resistance should be maintained to prevent subendocardial ischemia. These patients may have an increased risk of ischemia-induced arrhythmias, especially with the use of halothane anesthesia. Spinal anesthesia is relatively contraindicated in the patient with aortic stenosis. Invasive hemodynamic monitoring should be considered based on the patient's medical condition. The recommended guidelines concerning antibiotic prophylaxis should be followed. See Chap. 6 for a more complete discussion of aortic stenosis.

Partial Anomalous Pulmonary Venous Return

Partial anomalous pulmonary venous return (PAPVR) is a congenital lesion in which one or more of the pulmonary veins, but not all, are connected to the right atrium or to one or more of its venous tributaries. An atrial septal defect, usually one of the sinus venosus type, commonly accompanies this anomaly, frequently involving the veins of the right upper and middle lobe and the superior vena cava. There is therefore an inherent left-to-right shunt. Excluding atrial septal defects, other major cardiac malformations, including VSD and tetralogy of Fallot, occur in approximately 20 percent of patients with PAPVR. In the usual patient with isolated PAPVR, the hemodynamic state and physical findings are similar to those found in an atrial septal defect. Any type of inhalation, intravenous, or regional anesthetic is well tolerated. Invasive monitoring is not specifically indicated. The recommended guidelines for antibiotic prophylaxis should be followed. A discussion of total anomalous pulmonary venous return can be found in Chap. 18.

In general, the basic principles outlined in this chapter governing the anesthetic management of noncyanotic heart disease can be applied to all such lesions. A thorough understanding of the patient's anatomy and pathophysiology must be present before any anesthetic is started, and appropriate support should be available in the hospital, at least for consultation, before a child is accepted for elective surgery. Recently, there have been reports of children with hypoplastic left heart syndrome who received anesthesia for elective noncardiac surgery [56]. However, for the present these cases remain the domain of the specialized tertiary care center.

REFERENCES

1. Wegman, ME. Annual summary of vital statistics—1985. *Pediatrics* 78:983, 1986.
2. Smith, RM. *Anesthesia for Infants and Children* (4th ed). St. Louis: Mosby, 1980.
3. Keith, JD. Prevalence, Incidence and Epidemiology.

In JD Keith, RD Rowe, P Vlad (eds), *Heart Disease in Infancy and Childhood* (3rd ed). New York: Macmillan, 1978.
4. Perloff, JK. *The Clinical Recognition of Congenital Heart Disease* (3rd ed). Philadelphia: Saunders, 1987.
5. Stevenson, JG. Acyanotic lesions with normal pulmonary blood flow. *Pediatr Clin North Am* 25:725, 1978.
6. Stevenson, JG. Acyanotic lesions with increased pulmonary blood flow. *Pediatr Clin North Am* 25:743, 1978.
7. Kawabori, I. Cyanotic congenital heart defects with decreased pulmonary blood flow. *Pediatr Clin North Am* 25:759, 1978.
8. Kawabori, I. Cyanotic congenital heart defects with increased pulmonary blood flow. *Pediatr Clin North Am* 25:777, 1978.
9. Young, D. Pathophysiology of congenital heart disease. *Int Anesthesiol Clin* 18:5, 1980.
10. Fink, BW. *Congenital Heart Disease: A Deductive Approach to its Diagnosis* (2nd ed). Chicago: Year Book, 1985.
11. Schwartz, AJ, Jobes, DR. Congenital Heart Disease—Special Anesthetic Considerations. In TJ Conahan (ed), *Cardiac Anesthesia*. Menlo Park: Addison-Wesley, 1982.
12. Greenwood, RD. Cardiovascular malformations associated with extracardiac anomalies and malformation syndromes. *Clin Pediatr* 23:145, 1984.
13. Nudel, DB, Berman, MA, Talner, NS. Effects of acutely increasing systemic vascular resistance on oxygen tension on tetralogy of Fallot. *Pediatrics* 58:248, 1976.
14. Sanders, S. Echocardiography and related techniques in the diagnosis of congenital heart defects. *Echocardiography* 1:185, 1984.
15. Huhta, JC, Glasow, P. Surgery without catheterization for congenital heart defects: Management of 100 patients. *J Am Coll Cardiol* 9:823, 1987.
16. Gutgesell, HP. Accuracy of two dimensional echocardiography in the diagnosis of congenital heart disease. *Am J Cardiol* 55:514, 1985.
17. Silverman, N, Ports, T, Snider, A, et al. Determination of left ventricular volume in children. Echocardiographic and angiographic comparisons. *Circulation* 62:548, 1980.
18. Stamm, R, Martin, R. Quantification of pressure gradients across stenotic valves by Doppler ultrasound. *J Am Coll Cardiol* 2:707, 1983.
19. Committee on Rheumatic Fever and Bacterial Endocarditis: Prevention of bacterial endocarditis. *Pediatrics* 75:603, 1985.
20. Chadwick, EG, Shulman, ST. Prevention of infective endocarditis. *Modern Concepts Cardiovasc Dis* 55:11, 1986.
21. Saidman, LJ, Eger, EI, II. Effect of nitrous oxide and of narcotic premedication on the alveolar concentration of halothane required for anesthesia. *Anesthesiology* 25:302, 1964.
22. DeBock, TL, Davis, PJ, Tome, J, et al. Effect of premedication on arterial oxygen saturation in children with congenital heart disease. *J Cardiothoracic Anesth* 4:425, 1990.
23. Hickey, PR, Hansen, DD, Cramolini, GM, et al. Pulmonary and systemic responses to ketamine in infants with normal and elevated pulmonary vascular resistance. *Anesthesiology* 62:287, 1985.
24. Stanley, TH, Webster, LR. Anesthetic requirements and cardiovascular effects of fentanyl-oxygen and fentanyl-diazepam-oxygen anesthesia in man. *Anesth Analg* 57:411, 1978.
25. Hickey, PR, Hansen, DD, Wessel, DL, et al. Blunting of stress responses in the pulmonary circulation of infants by fentanyl. *Anesth Analg* 64:1137, 1985.
26. Eger, EI, II. Uptake and Distribution of Inhaled Anesthetics. In RD Miller (ed), *Anesthesia* (2nd ed). New York: Churchill Livingstone, 1986.
27. Stoelting, RK, Longnecker, DE. Effect of right-to-left shunt on the rate of increase in arterial anesthetic concentration. *Anesthesiology* 36:352, 1972.
28. Tanner, GE, Angers, DG, Barash, PG, et al. Effect of left-to-right, mixed left-to-right, and right-to-left shunts on inhalational anesthetic induction in children: A computer model. *Anesth Analg* 64:101, 1985.
29. Campbell, FW, Schwartz, AJ. Anesthesia for noncardiac surgery in the pediatric patient with congenital heart disease. *Refresher Courses in Anesthesiology* 14:75, 1986.
30. Munson, ES. Transfer of nitrous oxide into body air cavities. *Br J Anesth* 46:202, 1974.
31. Mehta, M, Sokoll, MD, Gergis, SD. Effects of venous air embolism on the cardiovascular system and acid base balance in the presence and absence of nitrous oxide. *Acta Anaesthesiol Scand* 28:266, 1984.
32. Behrendt, DM. Atrial Septal Defect. In E Arciniegas (ed), *Pediatric Cardiac Surgery*. Chicago: Year Book, 1985.
33. Cohn, LH, Morrow, AG, Braunwald, E. Operative treatment of atrial septal defect: Clinical and hemodynamic assessments in 175 patients. *Br Heart J* 29:725, 1967.
34. Becu, LM, Fontana, RS, Dushave, JW, et al. Anatomic and pathologic studies in ventricular septal defect. *Circulation* 14:649, 1956.

35. Friedman, WF, et al. Multiple muscular ventricular septal defects. *Circulation* 32:35, 1965.
36. Herth, JD, Rose, V, Collins, G, Kidd, VSL. Ventricular septal defect. Incidence, morbidity and mortality in various age groups. *Br Heart J* 33:81, 1971.
37. Dickinson, DF, Arnold, R, Wilkinson, JJ. Ventricular septal defects in children born in Liverpool. Evaluation of natural course and surgical implications in selected population. *Br Heart J* 46:47, 1981.
38. Sade, RM, Williams, RG, Castenada, AR. Corrective surgery for congenital cardiovascular defects in early infancy. *Am Heart J* 90:656, 1975.
39. Godman, MJ, Roberts, NK, Izuhawa, T. Late postoperative conduction disturbances after repair of ventricular septal defect in tetralogy of Fallot. *Circulation* 49:214, 1974.
40. Okarama, EO, Guller, B, Molohy, JD, Weidman, WH. Etiology of right bundle branch block pattern after surgical closure of ventricular septal defects. *Am Heart J* 90:14, 1975.
41. Berger, TJ, Kirklin, JW, Blackstone, EH, et al. Primary repair of complete atrioventricular canal in patients less than 2 years old. *Am J Cardiol* 41:906, 1978.
42. Silverman, N, Levitsky, S, Fisher, E, et al. Efficacy of pulmonary artery banding in infants with complete atrioventricular canal. *Circulation* 68:148, 1983.
43. Castenada, A, Mayer, JE, Jones, RA. Repair of complete atrioventricular canal in infancy. *World J Surg* 9:590, 1985.
44. Somerville, J. Ostium primum defect: Factors causing deterioration in the natural history. *Br Heart J* 27:413, 1965.
45. McMurphy, DM, Heymann, MA, Rudolph, AM, Melman, KL. Developmental change in constriction of the ductus arteriosus: Response to oxygen and vasoactive substances in the isolated ductus arteriosus of the fetal lamb. *Pediatr Res* 6:231, 1972.
46. Coceani, F, Olley, PM. The response of the ductus arteriosus to prostaglandins. *Can J Physiol Pharmacol* 51:220, 1973.
47. Moss, AJ, Emmanouilides, G, Duffie, ER. Closure of the ductus arteriosus in the newborn infant. *Pediatrics* 32:25, 1963.
48. Christie, A. Normal closing time of the foramen ovale and the ductus arteriosus: An anatomic and statistical study. *Am J Dis Child* 40:323, 1930.
49. Campbell, M. Natural history of persistent ductus arteriosus. *Br Heart J* 30:4, 1968.
50. Campbell, M. Natural history of coarctation of the aorta. *Br Heart J* 32:633, 1970.
51. Rudolph, AM, Heymann, MA, Spitznas, U. Hemodynamic considerations in the development of narrowing of the aorta. *Am J Cardiol* 30:514, 1972.
52. Alpert, BS, Bain, HH, Balfe, JW, et al. Role of the renin-angiotensin-aldosterone system in hypertensive children with coarctation of the aorta. *Am J Cardiol* 43:828, 1979.
53. Sandor, GGS, Olley, PM, Trusler, GA, et al. Long term follow-up of patients after valvotomy for congenital valvular aortic stenosis in children. *J Thorac Cardiovasc Surg* 80:171, 1980.
54. Friedman, WF, Pappelbaum, SJ. Indications for hemodynamic evaluation and surgery in congenital aortic stenosis. *Pediatr Clin North Am* 18:1207, 1971.
55. Lambert, EC, Menon, VA, Wagner, HR, Vlad, P. Sudden unexpected death from cardiovascular disease in children. *Am J Cardiol* 34:89, 1974.
56. Karl, HW, Hensley, FA, Jr, Cyran, SE, et al. Hypoplastic left heart syndrome: Anesthesia for elective noncardiac surgery. *Anesthesiology* 72:753, 1990.

Appendix: Drugs and Dosages in Patients with Congenital Heart Disease

Drug	Dose	Drug	Dose
Inotropes and vasopressors		*Diuretics*	
Epinephrine	1–10 µg/kg	Furosemide	0.5–1.0 mg/kg
Isoproterenol	Infusion, 0.01–0.1 µg/kg/min	Mannitol	0.5 gm/kg
		Anesthetics	
Dopamine	Infusion, 2–20 µg/kg/min	Thiopental	2–5 mg/kg
Dobutamine	Infusion, 5–15 µg/kg/min	Diazepam	0.1–0.2 mg/kg
Amrinone	Load dose, 1–2 mg/kg	Midazolam	5–10 µg/kg and titrate up
	Infusion, 5–15 µg/kg/min	Ketamine	1–2 mg/kg IV
Norepinephrine	Infusion, 0.1–1.0 µg/kg/min		3–7 mg/kg IM
Ephedrine	0.1–0.5 mg/kg	Morphine	0.1–0.2 mg/kg and titrate up
Phenylephrine	0.5–1.0 µg/kg	Meperidine	0.5–2.0 mg/kg and titrate up
	Infusion, 0.1 µg/kg/min	Fentanyl	2–50 µg/kg and titrate up
Calcium chloride	10–15 mg/kg	Sufentanil	Induction, 0.5–10.0 µg/kg
Calcium gluconate	100–200 mg/kg	Droperidol	0.05–0.1 mg/kg
Vasodilators		Naloxone	5–10 µg/kg
Nitroglycerin	Start 0.2 µg/kg/min	*Miscellaneous*	
Sodium nitroprusside	Start 0.2 µg/kg/min	Sodium bicarbonate	⅓ × body wt (kg) × base excess; give ½ calculated dose, then check arterial blood gas
Trimethaphan	Start 5 µg/kg/min		
Hydralazine	0.1 mg/kg, repeat after 30 min if needed		
Tolazoline	0.5–2.0 mg/kg bolus	Potassium chloride	Maximum 0.5 mEq/kg over 60 min with continuous ECG monitoring
	Infusion, 1–2 mg/kg/hr		
Prostaglandin E1	0.05–0.1 µg/kg/min		
		Dantrolene	3 mg/kg up to 10 mg/kg
Antiarrhythmics		Diphenhydramine	0.5–1.5 mg/kg
Lidocaine	1 mg/kg	Glucose	250–500 mg/kg
	Infusion, 10–30 µg/kg/min	Heparin	3 mg/kg
Procainamide	1–2 mg/kg slowly over 10 min	*Muscle relaxants and reversals*	
Verapamil	0.1–0.2 mg/kg	Pancuronium	0.04–0.1 mg/kg
Adenosine	0.05–0.1 mg/kg	d-Tubocurarine	0.25–0.5 mg/kg
Edrophonium	0.1–0.2 mg/kg	Atracurium	0.3–0.5 mg/kg
Phenytoin	5 mg/kg	Vecuronium	0.05–0.1 mg/kg
Bretylium	5–10 mg/kg	Succinylcholine	1.0–2.0 mg/kg
Anticholinergics		Neostigmine	0.06 mg/kg
Atropine	0.01–0.03 mg/kg	Pyridostigmine	0.2 mg/kg
Scopolamine	0.006–0.01 mg/kg		
Glycopyrrolate	0.005–0.01 mg/kg		

18
Cyanotic Congenital Heart Disease

Corey S. Scher

The anesthetic implications for the child with cyanotic congenital heart disease who is undergoing noncardiac surgery have changed dramatically within the last decade. At the same time, our growing understanding of pediatric cardiopulmonary physiology continues to evolve. In years past, the child with tetralogy of Fallot presented to the operating room with one of many possible palliative shunts to relieve right ventricular hypertension and systemic desaturation. In those children without shunts, the anesthetic plan employed agents that would improve pulmonary blood flow to correct systemic saturation. The understanding that normal postnatal changes of myocardial hyperplasia, coronary and pulmonary angiogenesis, and alveologenesis are determined by a normal physiologic relationship between the heart and lungs has influenced cardiologists and surgeons to reevaluate their approach to these children [1, 2]. Therefore, in the last decade there has been a movement to perform a complete primary repair early in infancy in the child with cyanotic heart disease [3], since the problems associated with shunts and bands are thus avoided. It is hoped that providing a normal anatomic and physiologic relationship between the heart and the lungs early in the postnatal period will prevent irreversible end-organ damage and foster normal cardiopulmonary development.

Although initial clinical outcome studies of primary repair of children with cyanotic heart disease are favorable [4, 5], many problems remain for this subset of patients. Due to anatomic variations, not all children are candidates for primary repair and some must receive a palliative procedure. In those patients who have been repaired, many are not "cured" [6]. For some forms of cyanotic heart disease, an operation to approximate normal anatomic and physiologic relationship has yet to be established.

The child with cyanotic heart disease who presents for noncardiac surgery may be different than in years past. While the anatomic lesions have not changed, the anesthetic implications have. They are dependent on whether the patient has had a complete primary repair, primary repair with residual desaturation, palliative surgery, or medical treatment only. Because of the great diversity of cyanotic heart disease, emphasis here is placed on physiology of the immature cardiopulmonary system and the pathophysiology that results when lesions resulting in cyanosis are superimposed on the immature cardiopulmonary system. Understanding the patient's pathophysiology and previous attempts at management will enable the clinician to formulate and implement a sound anesthetic plan and deliver care with minimal morbidity.

TRANSITION FROM THE FETAL TO THE ADULT CIRCULATION

The child with cyanotic heart disease has an immature cardiopulmonary physiology, intracardiac shunting, and alterations in pulmonary blood flow. These lesions prevent the normal transition from the fetal circulation to the adult circulation. Understanding of normal transition is essential to the clinician when faced with the child who has cyanotic heart disease, so that management principles can be targeted toward helping the child approximate an adult-type circulation.

The fetal circulation has been classically described as parallel in nature. This is in contrast with the adult series type circulation (Fig. 18-1). The fetal right ventricle plays the same role as in postnatal life by delivering the majority of its output for oxygen uptake at the placenta. The fetal left ventricle delivers the majority of its output to the heart, brain, and upper body for oxygen consumption. Fetal circulatory anatomy is such that the right ventricle receives blood that is less saturated with oxygen and the left ventricle receives blood that is more saturated with oxygen.

A nonuniform flow of blood in the heart is accomplished by the anatomic structure of the right atrium and fetal venous channels [7]. Poorly saturated blood from the superior vena cava and coronary sinus constitutes one quarter of the venous return and flows across the tricuspid valve and into the right ventricle. One half of the venous return receives oxygen from the placenta and travels in the umbilical vein. The umbilical venous return splits in the liver. One half of this blood is used to deliver oxygen to most of the liver and the other half passes through to the ductus venosus. These two sources of well-saturated blood meet up again along the medial aspect of the inferior vena cava and cross the foramen ovale into the left atrium and left ventricle. This blood becomes desaturated to a small degree by 10 percent of the venous return stemming from the lungs (Fig. 18-2).

At birth, many physiologic changes occur to replace the relatively inefficient fetal oxygen delivery and uptake system. Umbilical cord occlusion, ventilation, oxygenation, myocardial function, and vasoactive metabolites each play a role in the elimination of intra- and extracardiac shunts and lowering the pulmonary vascular resistance (Fig. 18-3).

Umbilical cord occlusion simply eliminates the placenta as the source of oxygen and causes an elevation of the systemic vascular resistance (SVR). Ventilation alone has been demonstrated to dramatically affect the distribution of blood volumes

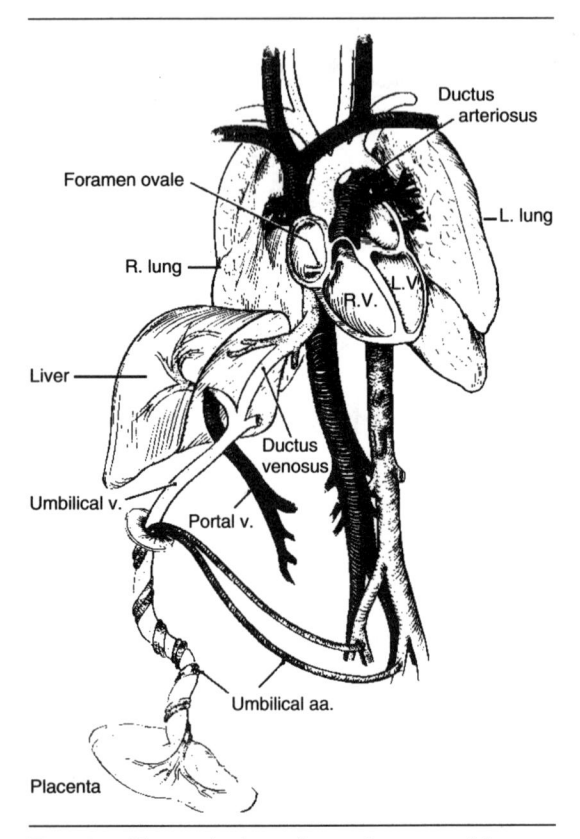

Fig. 18-1. Human fetal circulation. Intensity of dots within vessels indicates degree of oxygen desaturation of hemoglobin. Note possible course of blood from the placenta through the liver or through the ductus venosus to the inferior vena cava, and then to the heart. Also note major sites of mixing of blood of varying oxygen content: portal vein, hepatic vein, inferior vena cava, foramen ovale, and ductus arteriosus. (Reprinted with permission from FH Adams, Fetal and Neonatal Circulation. In FH Adams, et al. (eds), *Moss' Heart Disease in Infants, Children and Adolescents* (3rd ed). Baltimore: Williams & Wilkins Co., 1983. © 1983, the Williams & Wilkins Co., Baltimore.)

18. Cyanotic Congenital Heart Disease   443

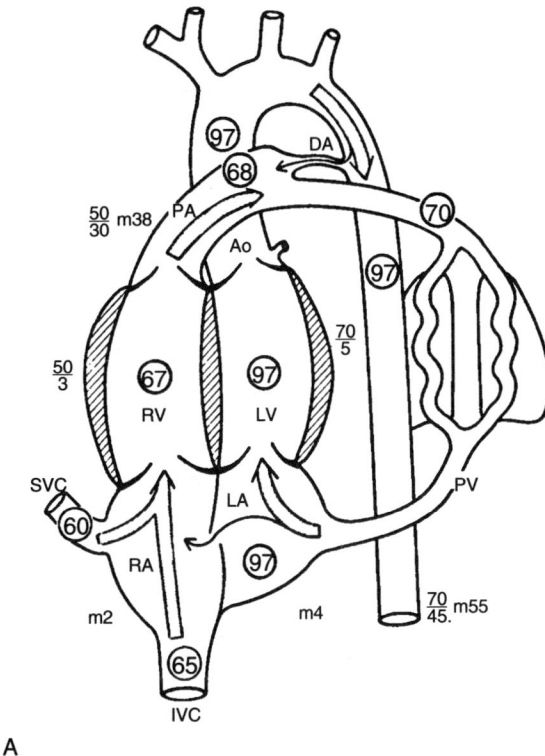

Fig. 18-2. A. Transitional circulation. B. Mature circulation. Ao = aorta; LV = left ventricle; RV = right ventricle; RA = right atrium; LA = left atrium; PA = pulmonary artery; PV = pulmonary vein; SVC = superior vena cava; IVC = inferior vena cava; m = mean pressure; DA = ductus arteriosus. Circled numbers represent oxygen saturation. (Reprinted with permission from AM Rudolph, *Congenital Diseases of the Heart*. Chicago: Year Book, 1974. P 19.)

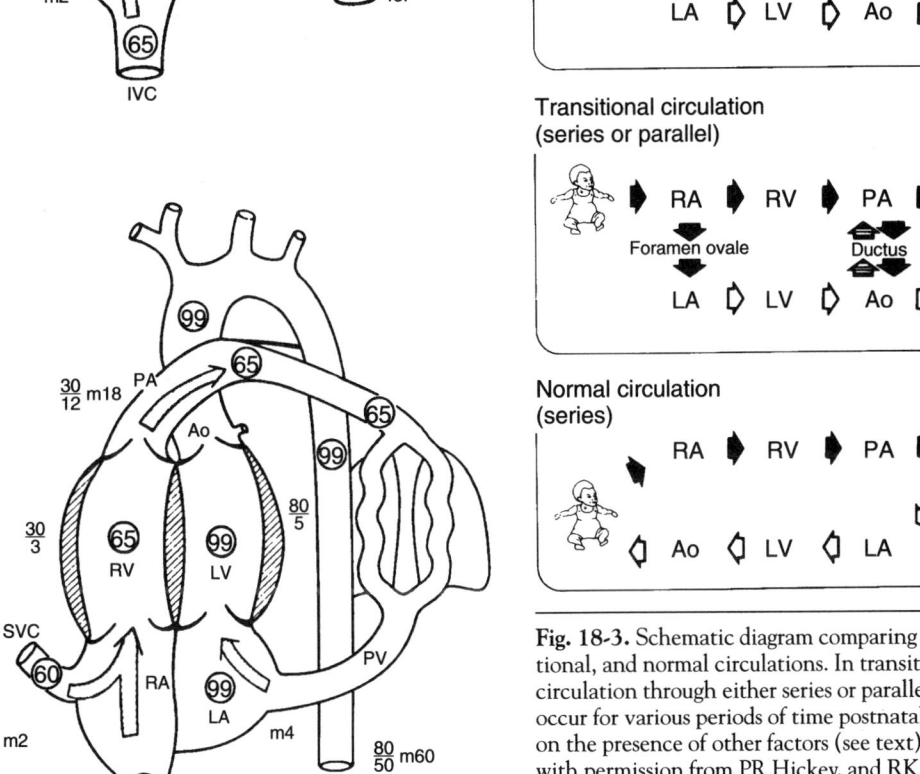

Fig. 18-3. Schematic diagram comparing fetal, transitional, and normal circulations. In transitional stage, circulation through either series or parallel circuits can occur for various periods of time postnatally, depending on the presence of other factors (see text). (Reprinted with permission from PR Hickey, and RK Crone. Cardiovascular Physiology and Pharmacology in Children. In J Ryan, D Todres, C Cote, et al., *A Practice of Anesthesia for Infants and Children*. Orlando, FL: Grune & Stratton, 1986.)

Fig. 18-4. Normal solid line and abnormal changes in pulmonary arterial tree during the first year of life. Pulmonary vascular resistance, arterial smooth-muscle percentage, and pressure normally fall within the first year of life. A large, unrestrictive ventricular septal defect (*dotted line*) with a large LR shunt results in an initial increase in flow and a later increase in vascular resistance. (Reprinted with permission from AM Rudolph, *Congenital Diseases of the Heart*. Chicago: Year Book, 1974. Pp. 79–87.)

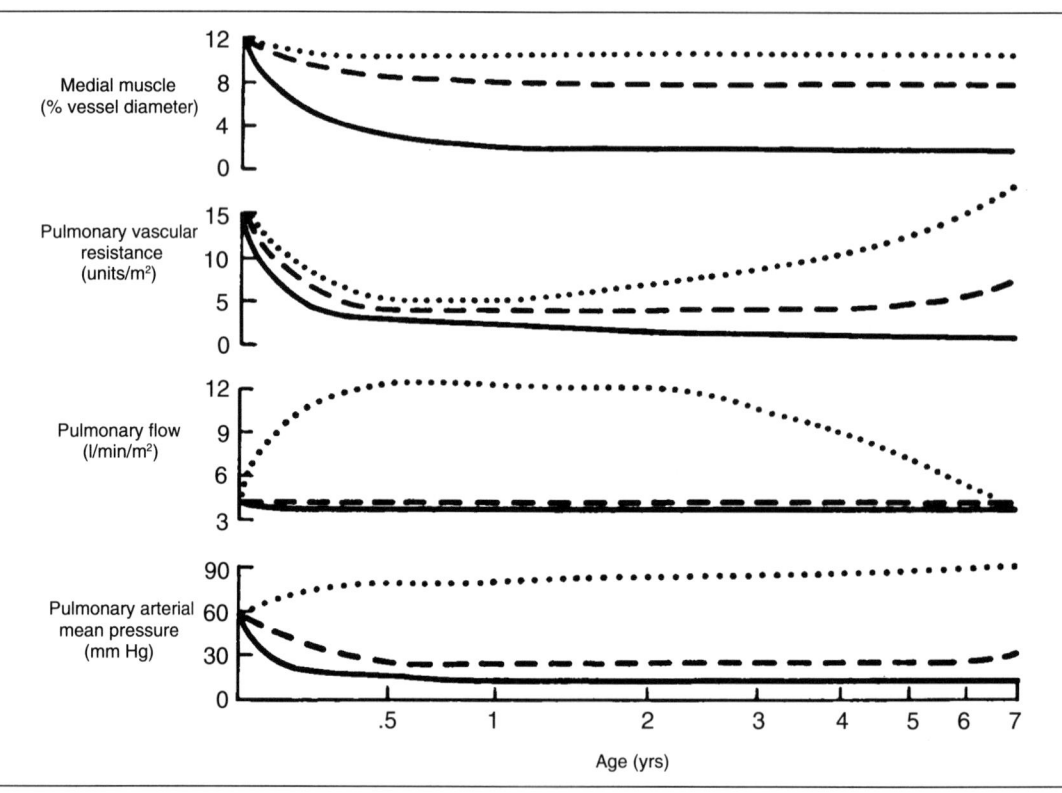

[8]. Ventilation initiates the reabsorption of lung water and lowers pulmonary vascular resistance (PVR), with an associated large increase in pulmonary blood flow. Oxygenation plays a dual role by lowering PVR further and participating in the mechanisms that effect closure of the ductus arteriosus [9].

It has been demonstrated that the initiation of ventilation causes the production of massive amounts of endogenous prostacyclins [10]. These vasoactive metabolites of the cyclooxygenase system are powerful vasodilators and are major contributors to the lowering of the elevated fetal PVR in the first few hours of life [11]. Recently, elevated leukotrienes have been documented when pulmonary resistance does not fall in the first few hours of life [12].

The myocardium acts in synchrony with cord clamping, ventilation, oxygenation, and prostacyclin release to pump blood in a direction that is optimal for oxygen delivery and uptake. As the PVR is falling in the first few days of life, right ventricular compliance improves and filling pressures decrease (Fig. 18-4). There is little tendency for the right ventricular (RV) septum to bulge into the left ventricle (LV) and impair LV filling when RV pressures are low. The right ventricle can now pump (with little resistance) blood through the lungs and increase LV preload. As LV preload and pulmonary flows increase, the foramen ovale will functionally close. With a rise in blood oxygen content and a postnatal decrease in circulating prostaglandins of placental origin, the ductus arteriosus will close functionally within 24 to 48 hours after birth. With a low PVR and closed foramen ovale and ductus arteriosus, blood ejected from the left ventricle will be well saturated and destined for the systemic circulation.

Normal development of the pulmonary vascular bed and myocardium are interdependent. The PVR continues to drop over the first few years of life as a result of extensive remodeling of the pulmonary arterial tree [13]. Normal arborization of the pulmonary vascular tree will not occur if the pulmonary vascular bed is exposed to abnormal stress (Fig. 18-5). Acidosis, hypoxemia, and abnormal pulmonary blood flows that are inherent to congenital heart disease are factors that modulate pulmonary vascular and parenchymal development [14]. Sustained increases in pulmonary blood flow and pressures will cause structural alterations in the pulmonary arteries [15]. These changes may be irreversible in spite of treatments that lower these flows and pressures. Decrease in pulmonary blood flow in the poorly arborized but well muscularized neonatal arterial tree leads to a hypoxic vasoconstrictive response that far exceeds an adult response [16]. Anatomic investigations on neonates who have pulmonary hypertension show both hypertrophy of the pulmonary arterial musculature and extension of the muscular development of the pulmonary arterioles closer to the alveolar-capillary unit when compared to normal development [17]. Similar to patients who have excessive pulmonary flow, patients with low pulmonary blood flow may have pulmonary vascular changes that persist despite repair of their lesions [18].

Those patients with low pulmonary blood flow resulting in cyanosis frequently have the adaptive response of polycythemia to increase oxygen delivery. The increase in hematocrits of these patients increases blood viscosity and ventricular afterload. This effect has been demonstrated to be of greater significance in the pulmonary than in the systemic circulation [19].

Developing neonatal hearts are less compliant than adult hearts. Noncontractile elements involved with protein synthesis occupy most of the immature myofibril (Fig. 18-6). The contractile

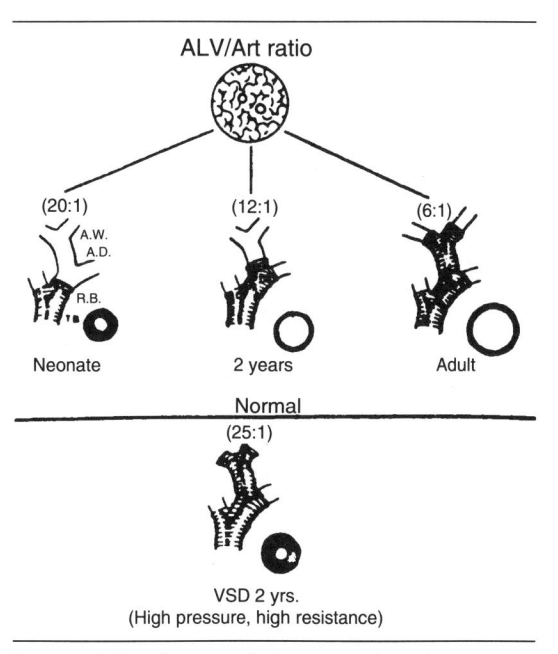

Fig. 18-5. Developmental changes in the pulmonary arterial tree in normal patients and in the presence of a ventricular septal defect (VSD) with a large LR shunt. Alveolar to arteriolar (ALV/art) ratio decreases with age because of extensive arborization of the arterial tree as the arteriolar lumen increases and the muscle layer thins and spreads distally. Pulmonary hypertension and high flow from a left-to-right shunt in a VSD cause pulmonary vascular obstructive disease marked by decreased numbers of pulmonary arterioles (ALV/art of 25:1), decrease in vessel lumen, increase in muscle thickness, and more distal spread of muscle. Letters indicate arterioles from level of terminal bronchiolus (TB) to the alveolar wall (AW). RB = respiratory bronchiole; AD = alveolar duct. (Reprinted with permission from MB Rabinovitch, SG Haworth, AR Castenada, et al., Lung biopsy in congenital heart disease: A morphometric approach to pulmonary vascular disease. *Circulation* 58:1107–1119, 1978.)

mass accounts for 30 percent of the myofibril in the infant compared to 60 percent in the adult [20]. Since right and left ventricles are equal in size, ventricular interaction via septal displacement is much more common than in adults. An increase in filling pressure in one ventricle quickly leads to septal shift and an increase in filling pressure in the other ventricle. The result may be biventricular failure, an event uncommon in adults. The Starling curve

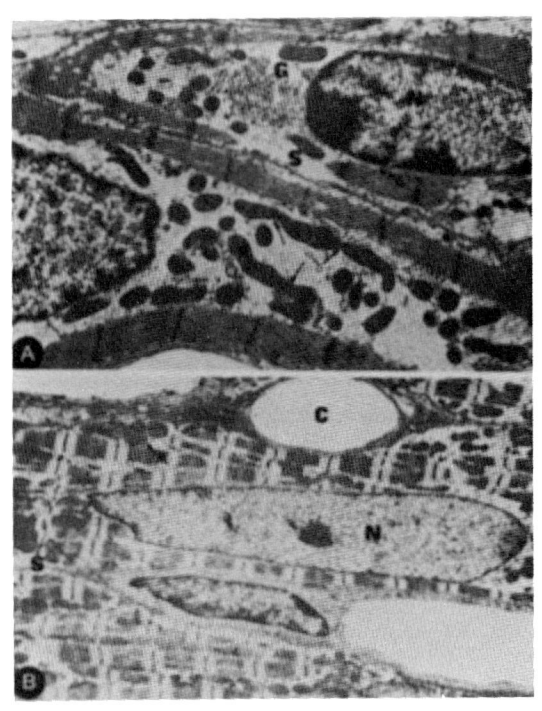

Fig. 18-6. Transmission electron micrographs of myocardial cells from fetal (A) and 36-day postnatal (B) lambs. The fetal cells have myofibrils located below the sarcolemma (S). The mitochondria (M) are long and appear to be budding in certain areas (*arrows*). Nucleus (N) and Golgi apparatus (G) are identified. The neonatal myocardial cell has a larger amount of contractile tissue extending into the interior of the cell. A capillary (C) is seen in this specimen. (Reprinted with permission from CA Sheldon, WF Friedman, and HD Sybers, Scanning electron microscopy of fetal and neonatal lamb cardiac cells. *J Mol Cell Cardiol* 8:853, 1976.)

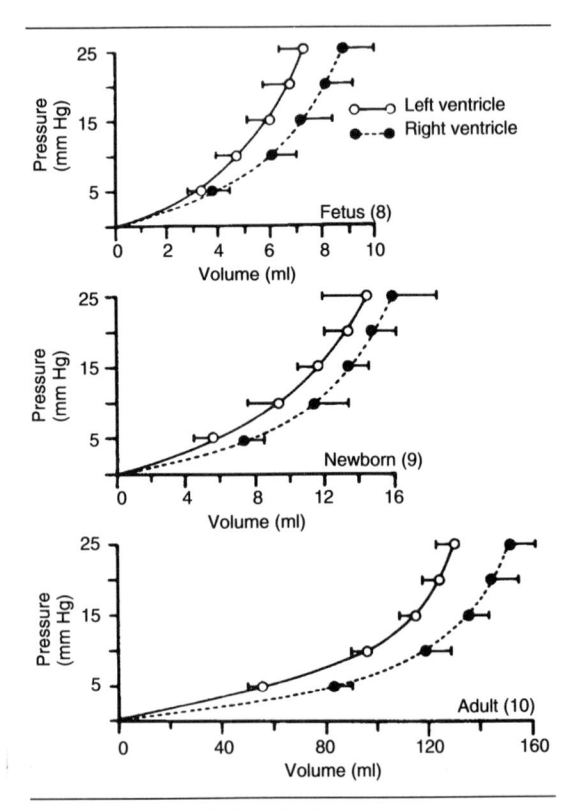

Fig. 18-7. Average left and right ventricular pressure-volume curves for each age group. Numbers in parentheses are numbers of animals studied. Each point and horizontal bars are mean values ± SE. No significant differences were observed between the two ventricles in the fetus. In the newborn, the left ventricular pressure-volume curve was significantly shifted to the left of the right ventricular curve at 15 and 20 mm Hg ($p < .05$). In the adult significantly greater left ventricular pressures existed at every volume when compared to those for the right ventricle ($p < .001$). (Reprinted with permission from T Romero, J Covell, and W Friedman, A comparison of pressure-volume relations of the fetal, newborn and the adult heart. *Am J Physiol* 222:1285, 1972.)

for the infant demonstrates that stroke volume changes only over a narrow range of filling pressures (Fig. 18-7). Additional intravascular volume will bring the patient to the plateau of the Starling function curve, where stroke volume is fixed and cardiac output is rate dependent. Further increases will lead to congestive heart failure. The neonatal myocardium is very sensitive to pressure and volume shifts.

After the placenta is removed at birth, abnormal blood flows created by an arrangement of shunts and obstructions cause major developmental alteration on the tenuous neonatal myocardium and lung. The abnormally developing heart and lungs act on each other by pressure, flow, and volume alterations to exacerbate the effects of fixed anatomic cardiac lesions.

PREOPERATIVE EVALUATION OF THE CHILD WITH CYANOTIC HEART DISEASE

Systemic Effects of the Cyanotic State

Although an understanding of the course of blood flow through the heart and lungs is the essence of preoperative evaluation when preparing an anesthetic plan, the state of cyanosis does affect other systems, which require careful consideration.

In the previous section we referred to the effects of polycythemia and increased blood viscosity on ventricular afterload. Recently, investigators have looked to see if the response to chronic hypoxemia is maladaptive or adequately physiologic. A regression equation has been generated by one group relating hemoglobin concentration to oxygen saturation in patients with adequate iron stores. Children who are less than 8 years of age with an oxygen saturation of greater than 80 percent generally have low serum erythropoietin titers and compensate for chronic hypoxemia at levels of hemoglobin that do not produce a state of hyperviscosity [21]. These patients generally have hemoglobins of 18.1 gm/dl or less. Patients with oxygen saturations of less than 75 percent generally have high serum erythropoietin titers, elevated red cell 2,3–diphosphoglyceric acid (2,3-DPG) concentrations, and hyperviscosity. This latter group of patients are at risk for the hyperviscosity syndrome, and meticulous attention must be paid to their state of hydration, as they are at significant risk for cerebral and renal thrombosis [22].

Poorly defined coagulopathies with hypofibrinogenemia and thrombocytopenia correlating with the degree of hypoxemia have been described [23]. Poor platelet function is well known in these patients [24], and these hematologic abnormalities may preclude the use of regional anesthetics in these patients.

With the current trend toward early intervention, it is more likely that the child with cyanotic congenital heart disease has had palliative surgery or a definitive repair. These patients may have been exposed to moderate to deep hypothermia and cardiopulmonary bypass with or without deep hypothermic circulatory arrest. Neurologic sequelae of these procedures, including strokes, diffuse hypoxic ischemic injury, intracranial hemorrhages, delayed choreoathetoid syndrome, and spinal cord lesions, have been reported [25–27]. Cases of diffuse cortical atrophy on magnetic resonance imaging scan after cardiac surgery in children have also been reported [28]. A recent survey of six pediatric cardiac surgery units in North America reported a small but definite incidence of neurologic symptoms following open heart surgery in children [29]. Although the incidence of these injuries is small and part of the "cost of doing business," intensive investigations continue to define the pathophysiology of neuronal injury during open heart surgery in children. A careful neurologic examination should be performed on this subset of patients before they undergo their noncardiac procedure.

It is well recognized that patients with cyanotic heart disease who have not had a palliative procedure or primary repair are at risk for neurologic injury from cerebrovascular accidents, cerebral abscesses, and hypercyanotic spells [30]. In patients with severe right-to-left shunts, the phagocytic filtering action of the pulmonary capillary bed is bypassed and bacteria may colonize tissue. Poorly perfused, hypoxic brain tissue can serve as a site of abscess formation. Any child with a severe right-to-left shunt who presents with focal neurologic signs must be evaluated for a brain abscess. This may be a disastrous sequela of a bacteremic state in the perioperative period, which is not uncommon after emergency surgery.

Several combined congenital syndromes, such as Möbius' syndrome (transposition of the great vessels, bilateral facial weakness with unilateral or bilateral abducens palsy), Klippel-Feil defect, and Poland syndrome, are associated with cyanotic heart disease [31]. The association of neurologic and congenital heart disease may support the unifying hypothesis proposed by Bavinck and Weaver [32] that an intrapartum insult occurs during the fourth to seventh week of gestation, consistent with the vascular theory of embryopathogenesis. These authors have suggested that the development of the subclavian, basilar, vertebral, and internal thoracic arteries is interrupted during the sixth intrauterine week. Brain and myocardial development would subsequently be affected [32].

Extensive preoperative neurologic surveys have not been reported for children with uncorrected cyanotic heart disease. A prospective investigation of electroencephalographic abnormalities in children with congenital heart disease found a 20 percent incidence of abnormalities that were mostly focal in nature [33]. This finding is somewhat unexpected because one would think that the incidence would be higher, that abnormalities would be diffuse, and that chronic anoxia would be the etiology. A postmortem investigation of 100 children with congenital heart disease found that in addition to the changes of acute and chronic anoxia, 11 percent had telangiectasia of the cerebral vasculature with calcifications [34]. This derangement of cerebral vasculature may explain the EEG findings.

The child who has had a palliative procedure (e.g., a Blalock-Taussig [BT] shunt) is also at risk for neurologic injury. Hand grip strength should be assessed if the patient had a shunt involving the subclavian artery. Hand grip strength tested many years post–BT shunt may be reduced on the side of the shunt [35]. A shunt that improves oxygenation, thus lessening potential neuronal injury, may be too large and create a new set of neurologic problems. Shunts that create torrential pulmonary blood flow will severely restrict the child's activity and normal neurodevelopment [36]. Therefore, neurologic assessment of all patients with cyanotic heart disease presenting for noncardiac surgery is an essential component of the preoperative evaluation.

Because of the dynamic relationship of the cardiac and pulmonary systems, the preoperative pulmonary evaluation must be individualized to each patient's lesion and previous treatment plan. The child who has had an early primary repair of tetralogy of Fallot will have different respiratory function than a child who has had a BT shunt. There have been attempts to elucidate the relationship between pulmonary mechanics and pulmonary hemodynamics in children [37]. It has been demonstrated that although lung volumes are basically unchanged in patients with congenital heart disease, a significant reduction in compliance occurs in patients with left-to-right shunts [38]. A recent study employing the multiple occlusion technique and echocardiography demonstrated a significant negative relationship between total respiratory system compliance and the right pulmonary artery to aortic ratio. This ratio reflects pulmonary vascular engorgement [39]. Chest x-ray scores had poor relationship to total respiratory compliance. It has been proposed that pulmonary vascular engorgement resulting from a combination of elevated pulmonary blood flow and pulmonary arterial pressure rather than either factor alone is responsible for the reduction in lung compliance [39]. In patients with reduced pulmonary blood flow secondary to right-to-left shunts, an extensive network of collateral vessels develops to optimize oxygen uptake in the lungs. The variability of this neovascularization in patients with right-to-left shunts accounts for the small amount of data available on lung compliance in this subset of patients.

In children who have normal histories and physical examinations, many centers have eliminated tests of hepatic function. However, recently the effect of heart failure or cyanotic heart disease, or both, on the liver has been examined. Hepatic dysfunction measured by laboratory data and histologic liver studies was compared to three areas of cardiac dysfunction: hypoxemia, systemic venous congestion, and low cardiac output. These investigators found that patients with both hypoxemia and systemic venous congestion had significant hepatic dysfunction, and patients with low cardiac output had the most deranged liver function tests. Prothrombin times as a reflection of liver dysfunction were also abnormal [40]. We can conclude from their work that preoperative liver function testing should not be excluded from children with cyanotic heart disease.

Frequently, the preoperative urine analysis is waived by the anesthesiologist due to the inability to keep a urine collecting bag on a small infant. We are reluctant to order a suprapubic tap in order to obtain a urine specimen. However, it is known that glomerular lesions can occur in patients with cyanotic heart disease. Spear and Vitsky [41] described glomerular enlargement, congestion, and capillary dilatation. Mesangial hypercellularity, focal glomerular sclerosis, and diffuse thickening of the glomerular basement membrane have also been described. These morphologic changes translate into the functional abnormalities of a reduced glomerular filtration rate and effective renal plasma flow.

Proteinuria accompanies these morphologic and functional changes. It has also been demonstrated that the proteinuria may be reversed by lowering the hematocrit in the polycythemic patient [42]. In select patients this may be an important consideration in "tuning up" the patient before elective noncardiac surgery.

General Preoperative Cardiovascular Considerations

Patients with congenital cyanotic heart disease have the common denominator of having a communication between the systemic and pulmonary circulation. This communication is usually located in the heart and is referred to as a central cardiac shunt. The direction of blood flow through the shunt varies within the cardiac cycle and over time (Fig. 18-8). The presence of a central cardiac shunt will alter the developing heart and lungs through significant pressure and volume overloads on the pulmonary vasculature and chambers of the heart.

The most important aspect of the preoperative evaluation for the patient with cyanotic heart disease is an understanding of each patient's central shunt and the factors that control the magnitude and direction of the shunt. Patients who share the diagnosis of tetralogy of Fallot may not have shunts of similar direction, magnitude, or ability to be controlled by therapeutic manipulation.

For simple shunts, outflow resistance is determined by the pulmonary vascular resistance on the right and systemic vascular resistance on the left. A shunt is termed "restrictive" if it is fixed in magnitude by a small shunt orifice. A large shunt is termed "nonrestrictive" or "dependent" when shunt direction and magnitude are determined by the balance between the resistances of the pulmo-

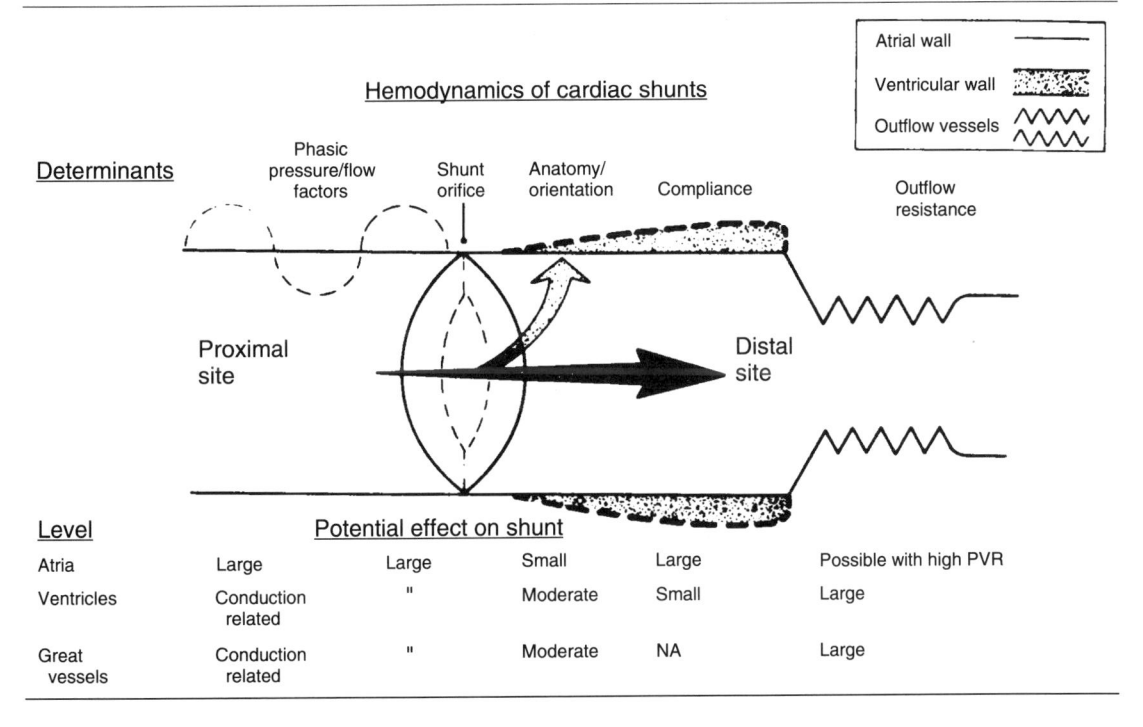

Fig. 18-8. Effects of the many determinants on central cardiac shunting at various levels. PVR = pulmonary vascular resistance. (Reprinted with permission from W Berman, Jr., The Hemodynamics of Shunts in Congenital Heart Disease. In K Johansen and WW Burggran (eds), *Cardiovascular Shunts: Phylogenic, Ontogenic, and Clinical Aspects*. Vol. 21. Copenhagen, Denmark: Alfred Benzon Foundation, 1985.)

Level	Phasic pressure/flow factors	Shunt orifice	Anatomy/ orientation	Compliance	Outflow resistance
Atria	Large	Large	Small	Large	Possible with high PVR
Ventricles	Conduction related	"	Moderate	Small	Large
Great vessels	Conduction related	"	Moderate	NA	Large

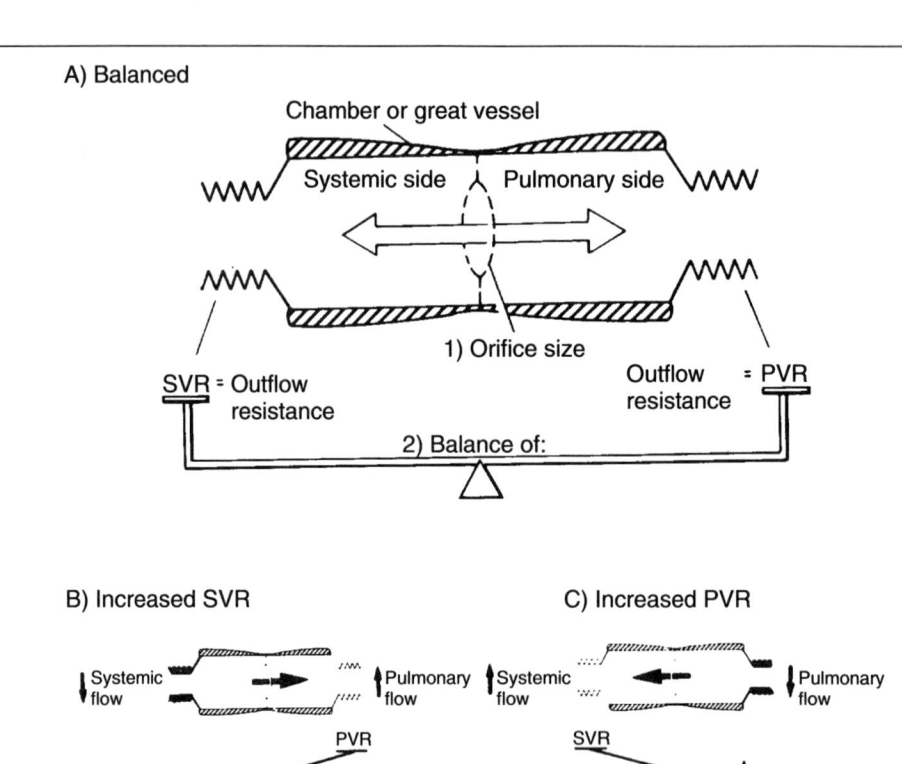

nary and systemic vascular beds. A shunt is termed "bidirectional" when a communication between two chambers is large enough that the two chambers function as one common chamber and complete mixing occurs [43]. In the absence of an obstructive lesion, patients with bidirectional central shunts have a tendency toward pulmonary overcirculation, since the pulmonary vascular resistance is much lower than the systemic vascular resistance (Fig. 18-9). The larger the orifice of a simple central shunt, the greater potential impact the SVR and PVR may have on the direction of blood through the shunt.

A shunt is designated as being complex if a fixed outflow obstruction is present on either the right or left side of the circulation. The obstructive lesion may be in the heart or in a great vessel. The shunts may be partial or total and may be dynamic or fixed. Blood flow tends to be away from the obstruction,

Fig. 18-9. The determinants of magnitude and direction of simple shunts. Orifice size is important in determining magnitude of shunting and pressure gradient across shunt, and is generally fixed. Balanced PVR and SVR are dynamic and determine the direction of shunt and variations of magnitude around limits fixed by orifice size. A. Balanced PVR/SVR. B. Increased pulmonary blood flow with increased SVR. C. Increased systemic flow with increased PVR. (Reprinted with permission from W Berman, Jr., The Hemodynamics of Shunts in Congenital Heart Disease. In K Johansen, and WW Burggran (eds), *Cardiovascular Shunts: Phylogenic, Ontogenic and Clinical Aspects*. Vol. 21. Copenhagen, Denmark: Alfred Benzon Foundation, 1985.)

as outflow resistance is the result of the resistance of a vascular bed and the resistance of the obstructive lesion. There will be less impact on shunt fraction with manipulation of SVR or PVR when the patient has a complex shunt. Some patients present with more than one obstructive lesion. The direction of the shunt in these patients will be determined by the nature of each obstructive lesion and

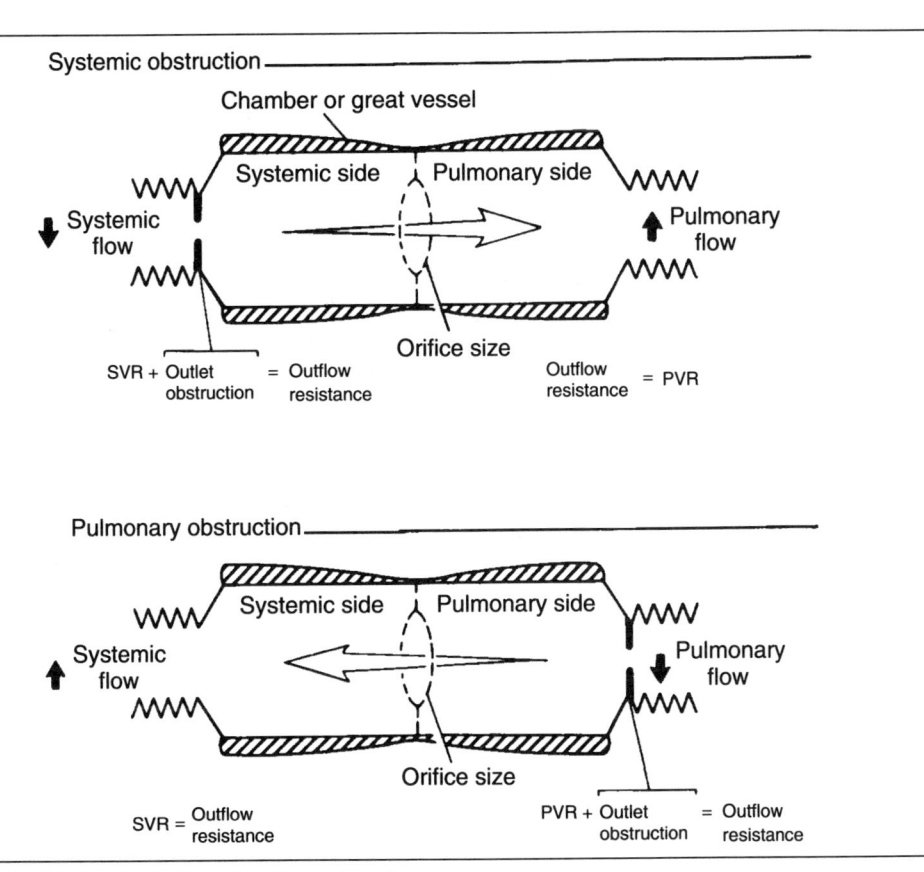

Fig. 18-10. The determinants of complex shunting with systemic or pulmonary outflow obstruction. Orifice size again limits magnitude, but the balance of outflow resistances includes outlet obstruction on either side of the circulation in addition to SVR or PVR. The addition of outflow obstruction increases flow on the opposite side and decreases flow on the same side. (Reprinted with permission from W Berman, Jr., The Hemodynamics of Shunts in Congenital Heart Disease. In K Johansen and WW Burggran (eds), *Cardiovascular Shunts: Phylogenic, Ontogenic, and Clinical Aspects.* Vol. 21. Copenhagen, Denmark: Alfred Benzon Foundation, 1985.)

the balance of the PVR and SVR (Fig. 18-10). Cardiac catheterization data, echocardiography, and previous operative reports will help define shunt direction. They also define variables in the patient's cardiovascular status that are subject to therapeutic manipulation to improve oxygen-carrying capacity (Fig. 18-11).

With the trend toward early total operative repair, the anesthesiologist must have an understanding of the cardiovascular status (myocardial, valvular, and electrical) of the "corrected patient." Residual shunts may exist. Cardiac chambers that are now designated to pump blood systemically may not be up to the task when stressed. Operative procedures may have altered normal cardiac conduction. Each specific corrective surgery carries a different spectrum of myocardial, valvular, and electrical disturbances.

With this background, individual cases representing the most common cyanotic heart diseases are presented for discussion to highlight management principles. Many principles highlighted in the tetralogy of Fallot presentation can be applied to the anesthetic management of other cyanotic heart diseases.

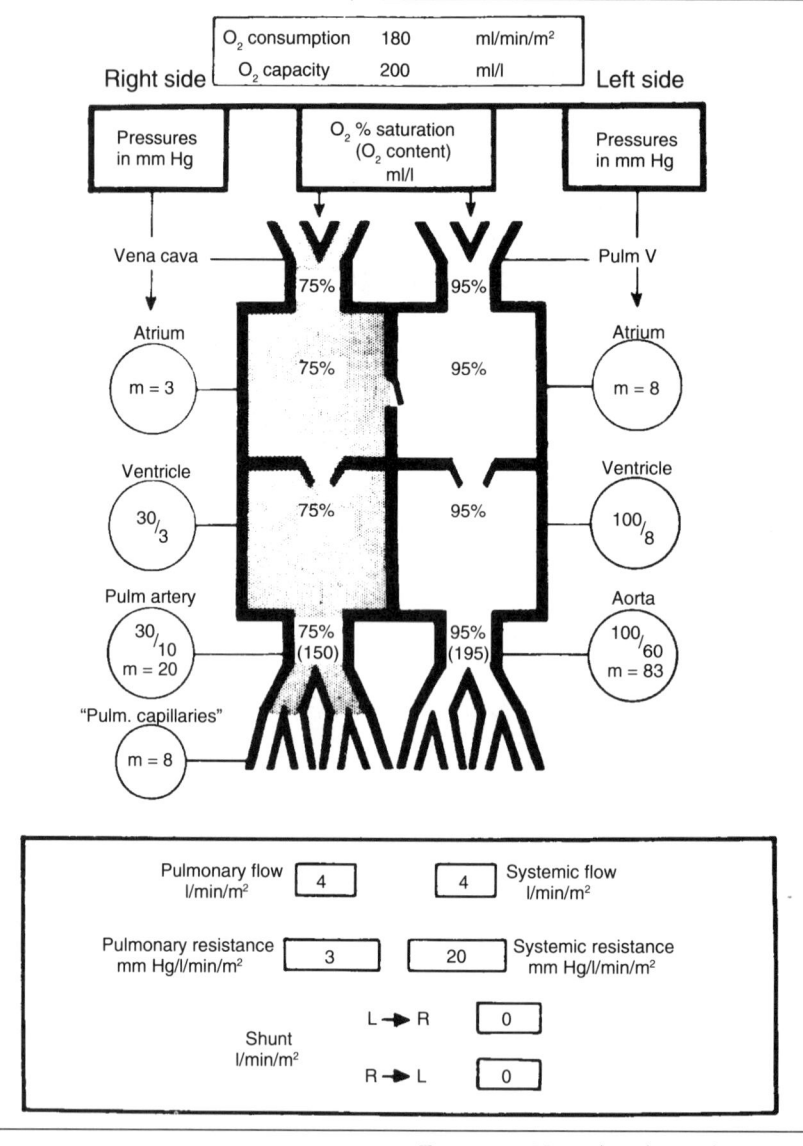

Fig. 18-11. Normal cardiac catheterization findings in a child. Numbers in chambers are oxygen saturations (%) and numbers in parentheses are oxygen content. Pressures in chambers are shown in circles. Note probe patent foramen ovale. (Reprinted with permission from AS Nadas, and DC Fyler, *Pediatric Cardiology*. Philadelphia: Saunders, 1972.)

SPECIFIC CYANOTIC LESIONS

Tetralogy of Fallot

A 2-month-old boy with a history of tetralogy of Fallot presents to the hospital with a 2-day history of vomiting with each feeding. Physical examination reveals an incarcerated inguinal hernia. The cardiologists following the baby have determined that the child has adequate pulmonary blood flow and that systemic to pulmonary shunting would compromise the adequacy of subsequent complete repair. Oxygen saturation by pulse oximetry is 82 percent (Fig. 18-12).

The diagnosis of tetralogy of Fallot in this patient was made in the newborn nursery when he

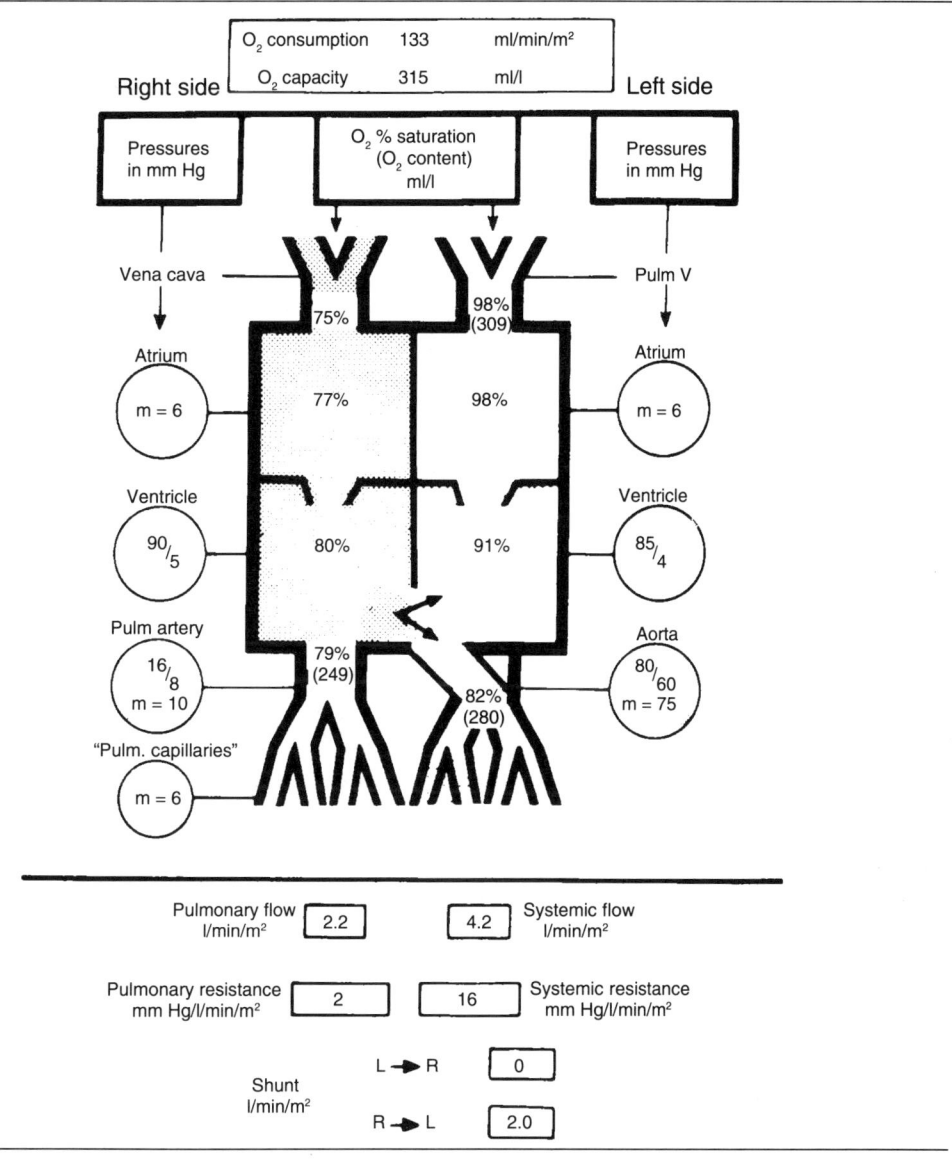

Fig. 18-12. Catheterization findings in a patient with tetralogy of Fallot. For key, see legend for Fig. 18-11. (Reprinted with permission from AS Nadas, and DC Fyler, *Pediatric Cardiology*. Philadelphia: Saunders, 1972.)

presented with cyanosis that was unresponsive to oxygen. The classic anatomic features of tetralogy include a ventricular septal defect (VSD), right ventricular outflow tract obstruction, overriding of the aorta, and right ventricular hypertrophy. The VSD and right ventricular outflow tract obstruction are due to the anterior displacement of a part of the infundibular septum into the outflow area of the right ventricle. The aorta is directed anteriorly and overrides both right and left ventricles. Anatomic concerns about the future repair of patients with tetralogy include (1) the location of the right ventricular outflow tract obstruction, (2) 25 percent of these patients have a right-sided aortic arch, and (3) 8 percent of these patients have abnormalities in the origin and distribution of the coronary arteries [44].

This patient's complex shunt is defined by the ventricular septal defect and the obstruction in the pulmonary outflow tract. Blood that enters the right ventricle will take the path of least resistance and cross over to the left ventricle without participating in pulmonary oxygenation. In the patient described above, some blood must be entering the pulmonary vasculature to account for the systemic arterial saturation of 82 percent. An extensive network of systemic to pulmonary collateral vessels may develop in response to chronic hypoxemia to improve oxygenation. In addition, the pulmonary outflow tract obstruction is often not fixed and may be at the infundibular level. Although the exact mechanisms that regulate the resistance of a dynamic right-sided obstruction are not well defined, management principles are well established to relieve the hypercyanotic state that develops if the infundibular orifice becomes critically narrowed. The administration of 100 percent oxygen, morphine sulfate, or β-blockers are useful in relieving infundibular spasm. Phenylephrine can be given to drive the SVR up to force blood over from the left ventricle to the right ventricle and out the pulmonary outflow tract [45]. Although the patient presented has made some physiologic adjustment to give him a systemic oxygen saturation of 82 percent, his condition must be viewed as tenuous and always subject to the stresses that create a life-threatening hypercyanotic state.

The multisystem derangement that results from the cyanotic state is described in the preoperative assessment section. Patients with cyanotic heart disease presenting for noncardiac surgery must be considered medical as well as surgical emergencies. The anesthesiologist can get a feel for the patient by asking the parents how often and what are the predisposing factors that cause hypercyanotic spells in their baby. A baseline neurologic history should be taken from the parents. Fluid resuscitation must begin in this patient at the time of surgical diagnosis to reduce the hyperviscosity state. Assessment of dehydration and fluid resuscitation should follow standard guidelines of pediatric fluid and electrolyte balance [46]. It has been the experience of most pediatricians that the physical examination of the patient will be more revealing after rehydration has begun. Additionally, the lethargic baby will become more alert with fluid therapy and a more accurate preoperative neurologic assessment can be made.

Oxygen delivery should begin at once. Face mask oxygen is effective, but its application may be the source of further excitement to the baby, thus predisposing him or her to a hypercyanotic spell. The rejection rate of a face mask has been shown to be 80 percent in infants. The compliance and effectiveness of oxygenation using the blow-by method employing anesthesia tubing connected to a 3-in. tape roll placed near the child's face is 100 percent [47].

Preoperative laboratory data should be collected and based on the present history and physical examination. Preoperative chest x-ray and electrocardiogram will reveal changes typical for tetralogy of Fallot, but are unlikely to add additional information that would alter anesthetic management. However, a complete blood count, coagulation profile, and serum chemistries including liver function tests would be helpful in assessing the effect of the present illness on the preexisting cyanotic state. Urine for specific gravity would also be helpful but is sometimes difficult to obtain.

No formal "recipe" can be given for this patient when formulating an anesthetic management plan. Any number of techniques and agents can be employed in the attempt to maintain or improve systemic saturation by decreasing PVR and maintaining or increasing SVR. An attempt must be made to maintain a stress-free state in the postoperative period, with adequate pain relief to prevent hypercyanotic spells. The patient presented can be summarized as a 2-month-old with a full stomach, predisposed to hypercyanotic spells, going for a procedure that is likely to last less than one hour, who will need excellent pain relief and intensive observation in the postoperative period. In this short procedure with minimal expected blood loss, noninvasive monitors would provide all necessary data to conduct a safe anesthetic. A rapid-sequence induction consisting of atropine or glycopyrrolate, ketamine and succinylcholine or a short-acting, nondepolarizing muscle relaxant should approach induction goals. Maintenance of anesthesia with an inhalational agent, nitrous oxide narcotic technique, or a combination of narcotics and inhalational agents would all be acceptable, keeping in mind that intraoperative hypercyanotic spells may occur at any time. Halothane will be better tolerated than isoflurane, sevoflurane, or desflurane, because of its minimal effect on SVR. If the patient desaturates in the operating room, the endotracheal tube and airway should be checked in the usual fashion; however, a hypercyanotic spell is now high on the list of possible causes.

During a hypercyanotic spell, sympathetic tone of the patient should be lowered by increasing the depth of anesthesia. Phenylephrine, 5 to 10 μg/kg IV or 2 to 5 μg/kg/min, and propranolol, 0.01 μg/kg, have been shown, by color-flow Doppler echocardiography, to reverse the increased right-to-left flow and improve pulmonary outflow tract obstruction, respectively, during intraoperative hypoxemic spells [48]. The volatile inhalational anesthetic agents with their negative inotropic properties may also be useful in that they may decrease the infundibular obstruction. The inspired concentration of oxygen should also be increased to lower the PVR [49]. If the spell persists, arterial blood gases should be analyzed to determine acid-base status. Supervening metabolic acidosis will increase PVR and perpetuate the hypercyanotic spell.

A postoperative plan that provides analgesia in an attempt to give comfort and prevent a hypercyanotic spell must be formulated. Validated instruments of pain measurement for infants are available but require training and experience before they can be used [50]. At this time, we must use our clinical judgment to determine the severity of pain in these patients.

The attempt at pain relief and surveillance for hypercyanotic or "tet" spells mandate that the patient spend at least the first 24 hours in an intensive care setting. Ilioinguinal nerve blocks, continuous intravenous narcotic infusions, or intermittent narcotic boluses have been used with success for years by clinicians. The intensive care postoperative setting allows consideration for continuous epidural (caudal) or intrathecal narcotic analgesia.

In the section on general considerations for patients with chronic hypercyanosis, it is noted that these patients are at risk for coagulopathies. If the patient does not have a coagulopathy, a caudal epidural catheter, L3-L4 epidural catheter (for children older than 2 years of age), or single-shot caudals or epidurals (narcotics) will provide excellent analgesia without the systemic effects of intravenous narcotics. Recently, it has been appreciated that the lung is an important organ involved in the disposition of local anesthetics [51]. The lung acts as a sponge after an intravenous injection of local anesthetics and there is a large concentration gradient between the venous and arterial side of the circulation. If the lung is taken out of the loop in the biodisposition of local anesthetics, as in a patient with tetralogy of Fallot, blood concentration of local anesthetic may be extremely high in patients with significant right-to-left shunts. Therefore, anesthetic techniques and agents used for a regional block should be selected to offset the adverse effects of possible high blood levels of local anesthetic that may be seen in patients with right-to-left shunts.

Transposition of the Great Vessels

A 5-year-old boy with transposition is hit by an automobile while crossing the street. A thorough evaluation by the trauma team reveals that the child only has a fracture of the left leg with significant blood loss into the leg. The rest of his workup is entirely normal. He is alert and stable but frightened. His past medical history is that he was born with transposition of the great vessels. An atrial septostomy was performed in the first week of life and the mother states that the child had a Mustard procedure at 1 year of age as a corrective operation. He has limited exercise tolerance and is in the 20th percentile for height and weight (Fig. 18-13).

The child born with transposition of the great vessels (TOGV) has an aorta originating from the right ventricle and a pulmonary artery originating from the left ventricle. This anatomic arrangement defines the *d*-transposition, whereby systemic venous blood returns to the right side of the heart but is ejected out through the aorta. With this arrangement, the systemic and pulmonary circulations function in parallel and the net result is that only a small proportion of blood will reach appropriate vascular beds via intercirculatory shunts. Intracardiac mixing occurs through a VSD in half of the cases and subpulmonic stenosis is frequently associated with the VSD. If a VSD is not present, mixing must occur at some level to maintain adequate saturation. The intercirculatory mixing volume is

456 The Pediatric Patient

Fig. 18-13. Catheterization findings in a patient with d-transposition of the great arteries with ventricular and atrial septal defects. For key, see legend for Fig. 18-11. (Reprinted with permission from AS Nadas, and DC Fyler, *Pediatric Cardiology*. Philadelphia: Saunders, 1972.)

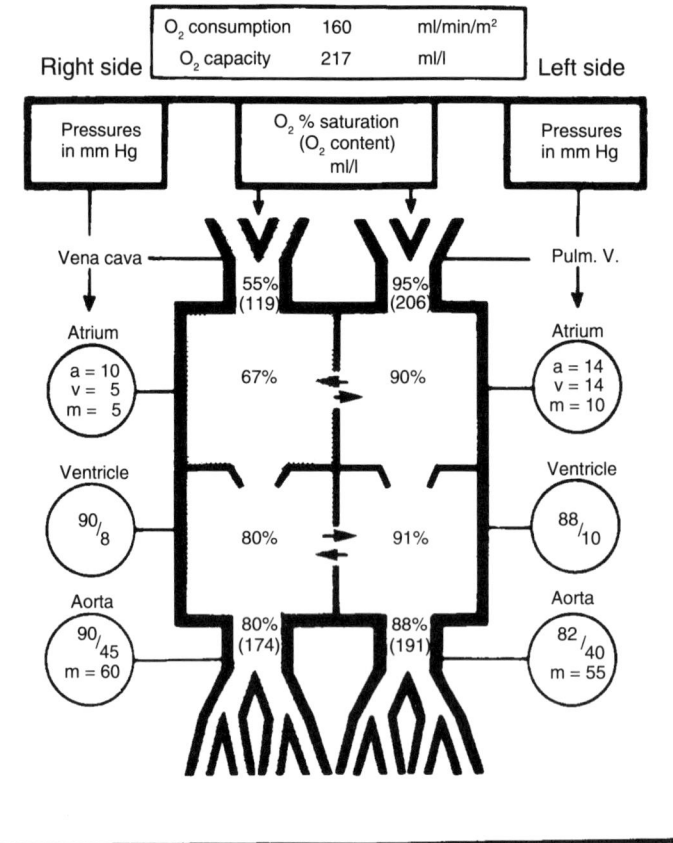

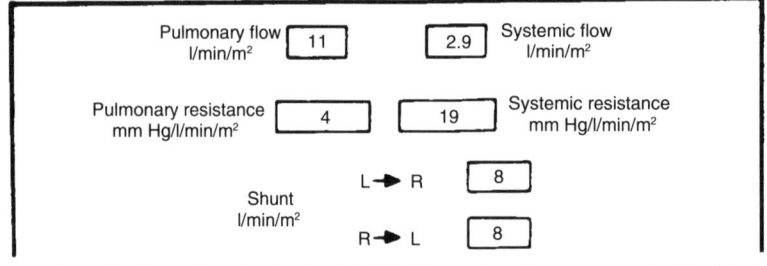

equal to the effective pulmonary blood flow, effective systemic blood flow, and net right-to-left and net left-to-right anatomic shunts. The volumes of right-to-left and left-to-right shunted blood that participate in gas exchange at the pulmonary and systemic capillary levels are small in comparison to large portions of blood recirculating within each circulation [52].

In the patient presented here, an atrial shunt was created by balloon septostomy to increase pulmonary blood flow. When the interatrial or intraventricular communications are of adequate size, the level of arterial oxygen saturation is the result of the pulmonary to systemic blood flow ratio. If the PVR increases or if the left ventricle fails, arterial oxygen saturation will be lowered [53]. The flow patterns through the balloon-created interatrial shunt vary during the cardiac cycle. In the absence of a VSD, the interatrial shunt is from right to left during ventricular diastole as the result of a lower resistance to filling in the left ventricle compared to the right ventricle. The shunt is from the left to right atrium during ventricular systole because the left atrium is less distensible and thus less compliant than the right atrium. Flow patterns are not as well defined in the presence of a large VSD [54] (Fig. 18-14). In sum, the interchange between the parallel systemic and pulmonary circulations in the patient with TOGV is controlled by local pressure gradients that are determined by (1) respiratory cycle phase, (2) local pathology, (3) the compliance of the cardiac chambers, (4) the volume of blood flow, and (5) the resistance of pulmonary and systemic circulations.

The various surgical approaches used in the past to correct TOGV have exchanged problems of systemic desaturation and pulmonary overcirculation with dysrhythmias, right and left ventricular dysfunction, tricuspid valve insufficiency, caval and pulmonary venous obstruction, and residual interatrial shunts [55]. Intraatrial corrective surgery (Mustard or Senning) utilizes surgical techniques to form a new systemic venous atrium, which extends from the superior (SVC) and inferior (IVC) vena cava to the mitral valve and effectively separates and redirects the two circulations. The atria are essentially converted from pumping chambers that have an important contribution to cardiac output to tenuous pathways that lead desaturated blood to be pumped out by the left ventricle for pulmonary oxygenation and saturated blood to be pumped by the right ventricle destined for the systemic vascular bed.

For optimal blood flow through surgically created atrial baffles, the patient's volume status must be normal. Ventilation should be controlled to prevent hypercapnia and an increase in both PVR and SVR. Poor baffle flow may be the result of caval or pulmonary venous obstruction. The patient with caval obstruction may present with the SVC syndrome and the patient with pulmonary venous obstruction may be in respiratory distress. This respiratory distress may be manifested by copious amounts of bloody secretions in the endotracheal

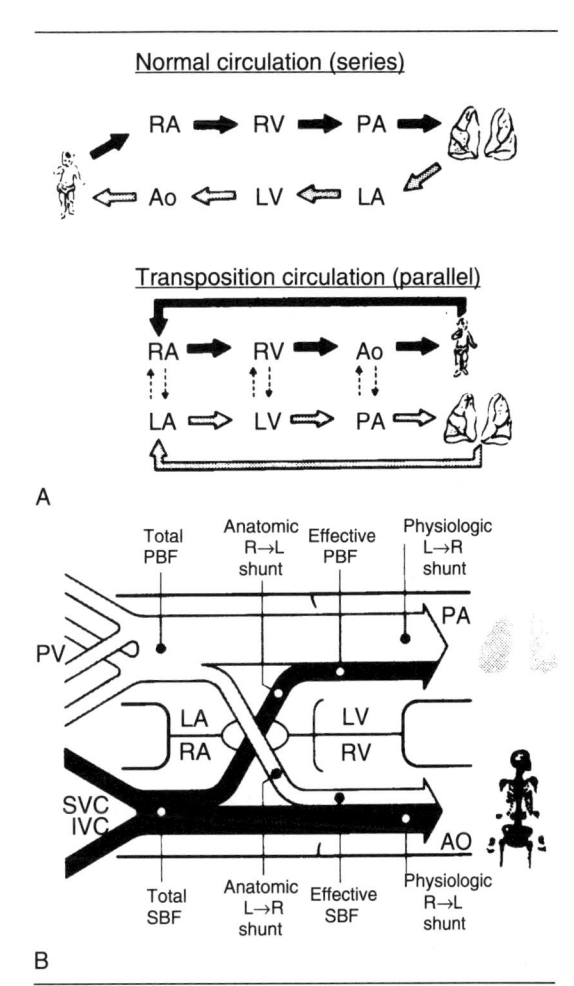

Fig. 18-14. The circulatory pathways in complete transposition. A. Systemic and pulmonary circulation pathways: in series, with normally related great arteries; in parallel, with TOGV. Solid arrows = relatively unoxygenated blood; stippled arrows = oxygenated blood; dashed arrows = intercirculatory shunts. B. Circulation schema demonstrating flows and shunts in infants with TOGV and intact ventricular septum. PV = pulmonary veins; SVC, IVC = superior and inferior vena cava; LA, RA = left and right atrium; LV, RV = left and right ventricle; PA = pulmonary artery; Ao = aorta; PBF, SBF = pulmonary and systemic blood flow. (Reprinted with permission from MH Paul, Transposition of the Great Arteries. In FH Adams, et al. (eds), *Moss' Heart Disease in Infants, Children and Adolescents* (3rd ed). Baltimore: Williams & Wilkins Co., 1983. © 1983, the Williams & Wilkins Co., Baltimore.)

tube, inadequate oxygenation, and low cardiac output. The right ventricle becomes the systemic pumping ventricle for life. Depressed right ventricular function and tricuspid valve insufficiency have been demonstrated in these patients while at rest [56]. This contrasts with a remarkable clinical performance of these children at play [57].

A history of the child's activity level should give the clinician an adequate data base concerning the performance of the systemically pumping right ventricle. Simply stated, an anesthetic plan is formulated that does not have negative impact on baffle flow, right ventricular ejection, or tricuspid valve function. As cardiac arrhythmias are not uncommon after baffle surgery, antiarrhythmic medications should be readily available and one should provide for pacing capability.

Although the patient presented above had intraatrial corrective surgery, more and more patients with transposition of the great vessels will have earlier corrective surgery with more "physiologically sound" operations. In 1954, complete anatomic correction of TOGV by direct contraposition of the transposed vessels was attempted, but clinical success was not obtained until the late 1970s. This arterial switch procedure is technically difficult due to the transfer of the coronary ostia and reconstruction of the right ventricular outflow tract. Patients who have had this anatomic correction have perioperative problems related to the anatomic correction.

The left ventricle becomes the systemic pumping chamber and, if it is not adequately prepared, left ventricular failure will ensue. Inadequate coronary arterial flow that results in myocardial ischemia may be the result of the reimplantation of the coronary arteries. Stenosis of either great vessel anastomosis is a possible late complication of the surgery. The anesthetic implications for the child who has had a successful hemodynamic correction are associated with any persisting morbidity related to the definitive correction, that is, neurologic, renal insufficiency, persistent myocardial ischemia, and antimicrobial prophylaxis.

The patient presented in this section must be viewed as a medical emergency. Restoration of normal systemic venous pressures with volume must be complete before the induction of anesthesia. Although it is reported that young children show little tendency to lower systemic venous pressure with epidural or spinal anesthesia employing local anesthetics, these techniques have not been used in this tenuous population. The epidural or subarachnoid space in these patients should probably be reserved only for the deposition of narcotics for postoperative pain relief. After volume restoration, the choice of agents for general anesthesia is secondary to the adherence to the principles that maintain atrial baffle flow (i.e., normocapnia, euvolemia, normal acid-base status, and avoidance of heat loss).

A child with TOGV with adequate mixing (large VSD or patent ductus arteriosus) may present to the operating room for a noncardiac operation before a definitive cardiac procedure. This scenario is becoming increasingly less common as every effort at early correction is made with long-term end-organ development in mind. If such a patient does present for noncardiac surgery, every attempt to define the anatomic features that support adequate mixing must be made. PVR and SVR can then be modified to maintain adequate oxygenation.

Tricuspid Atresia

A 5-year-old boy presents to the operating room with a diagnosis of acute appendicitis. A Blalock-Taussig shunt was placed at 1 month of age to relieve severe cyanosis secondary to tricuspid atresia. One year ago a Fontan procedure was performed for an increasing cyanotic state. The patient's cardiac status has been stable and he has made dramatic improvements on the growth curve (Fig. 18-15).

Tricuspid atresia is the common term applied to numerous congenital cardiac disorders that have an associated atresia of the tricuspid valve. Patients with tricuspid atresia may have associated cardiac anomalies that confer decreased, normal, or increased pulmonary blood flow, which determines symptomatology and treatment. The variability and severity of the various types of tricuspid atresia have led to the development of many classification systems to aid the clinician [58]. Tricuspid atresia is postulated to be the result of a misalignment between the ventricular loop and the atria during organogenesis [59].

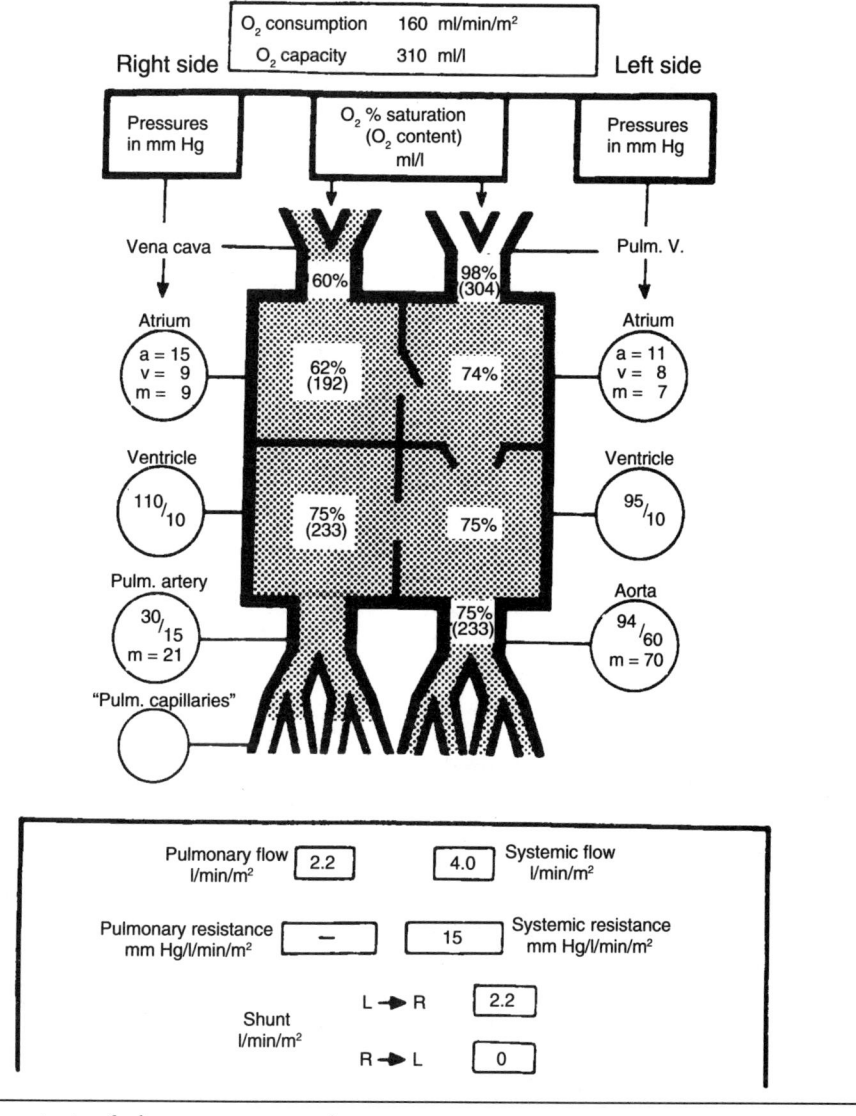

Fig. 18-15. Catheterization findings in a patient with tricuspid atresia. Note the necessary atrial septal defect and ventricular septal defect. For key, see legend for Fig. 18-11. (Reprinted with permission from AS Nadas, and DC Fyler, *Pediatric Cardiology*. Philadelphia: Saunders, 1972.)

In general patients with tricuspid atresia have diminished pulmonary blood flow with cyanosis and they present within the first few days of life. Those patients with excessive pulmonary blood flow present later in infancy with congestive heart failure that is characteristic of an associated d-transposition. The more commonly observed central cyanosis is the result of an obligatory right-to-left shunt through an atrial septal defect. Cyanosis is worse in those patients with an intact ventricular septum or pulmonic stenosis and least severe when a large VSD exists.

Hypercyanotic spells are common in patients with tricuspid atresia, usually in infants less than 6 months of age [60]. The etiology of the spells is believed to be related to either closure of a VSD or severe progressive narrowing of the pulmonary outflow tract. The physiology is not unlike that of patients having "tet" spells and their appearance is indicative of critically low pulmonary blood flow. These patients have end-organ changes that are typical of the cyanotic state.

The case presented represents a common scenario for the patient with the diagnosis of tricuspid atresia. Systemic venous blood enters the right atrium and cannot enter the pumping right ventricle (RV) due to an atretic tricuspid valve. The embryologically poorly developed RV continues to lose potential as an effective pumping chamber by never facing the stimulation of the volume load necessary for normal geometric growth. Blood is shunted through an atrial septal defect (ASD) and mixing occurs via a patent ductus arteriosus (PDA) or through an extensive network of large, collateral aortopulmonary vessels. In our patient the closure of the PDA required an infusion of prostaglandin E_1 (PGE_1; 0.05–0.1 mg/kg/min) on the third day of life to maintain ductal patency. Prostaglandin E_1 is most effective in children less than 4 days of age with an arterial oxygen tension (PaO_2) of less than 40 [61].

The clinical course of the patient presented here is similar to that of infants in the New England Regional Infant Cardiac Program. In the infants with a diagnosis of tricuspid atresia, 57 percent were hospitalized by the age of 1 month and all but one were hospitalized by 6 months [62]. The patient met the criteria for a Fontan procedure at age 4, whereby the right atria provide the pulsatile force for venous blood to enter the lungs for oxygenation. The original Fontan operation has had many modifications. Commonly, the ASD is closed and the right atrium is anastomosed to the right or main pulmonary artery. The success of the operation requires that there be essentially no pressure gradient between the left atrium and the "pumping" right atrium.

To ensure that there is no gradient between the left and right atrium in the postoperative period, patients selected for the Fontan procedure must have normal left ventricular function, be in sinus rhythm, and have no evidence of pulmonary vascular disease. Long-term postoperative catheterization studies have demonstrated that these patients have systemic venous hypertension with mean right atrial pressures between 12 and 16 [63]. In exchange for correction of chronic hypoxemia, the Fontan places the patient's cardiovascular function in a tenuous state. Minor degrees of obstruction to right atrial emptying due to rhythms other than sinus, anatomic obstruction, or increases in left atrial pressure will cause major circulatory compromise. A procedure that was once thought of as possibly curative is now recognized as being only palliative [64].

The anesthetic implications of the case presented surround optimal right atrial emptying. The PVR of the patient must be minimized to improve pulmonary blood flow through the lungs, and left ventricular function must be optimal to maintain the flow between the right and left atrium. In the preoperative period these goals can be accomplished by keeping the patient warm, well hydrated, and comfortable with analgesics as needed. Any anesthetic technique that does not compromise right atrial emptying is acceptable. However, large amounts of negative inotropy may cause elevation of left atrial and pulmonary pressures. Elevated airway pressure from mechanical ventilation will increase PVR and may have deleterious effects [65]. The anesthetic plan should allow for the resumption of spontaneous ventilation at the end of the procedure and extubation as early as possible. The anesthetic plan does not end when the patient is transported to the recovery room. Almost all of the common problems encountered in the recovery room (i.e., pain, full bladder, inadequate ventilation, hypothermia, and an elevated SVR) will confer negative effects on right atrial emptying.

Eisenmenger's Syndrome

A 7-year-old girl with a diagnosis of Eisenmenger's syndrome sustained a compound fracture of the left tibia after a fall. A cardiac catheterization at age 6 revealed a PDA with equalization of pulmonary and systemic pressures. The cardiac lesion was considered inoperable because of severe pulmonary hypertension. An intravenous line is started in the emergency room and pain medication is held because she appears blue. After lower-extremity x-rays are taken, she is transported to the operating room for open reduction and internal fixation.

Pulmonary hypertension resulting from congenital heart disease was first described by Eisenmenger

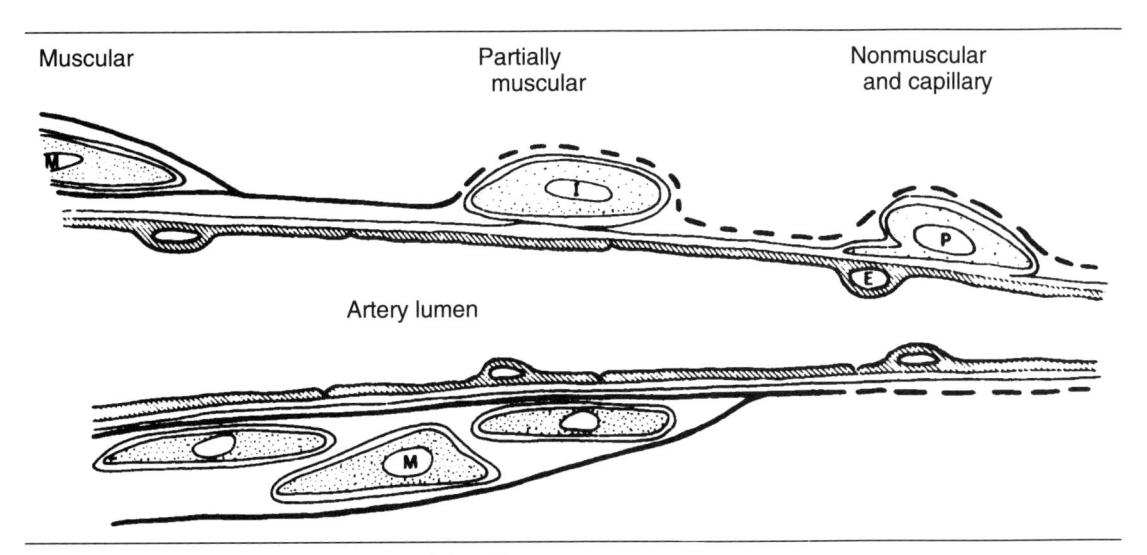

Fig. 18-16. Diagrammatic representation of the cells in the wall of the distal part of the pulmonary artery. The smooth-muscle cells (M) of the medial muscular coat are surrounded by a discrete basement membrane and are situated between both an internal and external elastic lamina (*thick black lines*). In the nonmuscular region of this partially muscular artery, the intermediate cell (I) is seen. This cell is surrounded by a basement membrane that fuses with that of the endothelial cell (E) and is situated internal to the single fragmented elastic lamina (*broken dashed lines*). In the wall of the nonmuscular artery and alveolar capillary, the pericyte (P) is found. This cell is ensheathed by a basement membrane, which is continuous with and thereby shares the basement membrane of the associated artery; like the "intermediate" cell, it is situated internal to the elastic lamina. (Reprinted with permission from B. Meyrick and L. Reid, Ultrastructural features of the distended pulmonary arteries of the normal rat. *Anat. Rec.* 193:71, 1979. Copyright John Wiley and Sons. Reprinted by permission of Wiley-Liss, a division of John Wiley and Sons, Inc.)

in 1897 [66]. A variety of congenital heart lesions characterized by left-to-right shunting (atrial septal defect, ventricular septal defect, PDA, etc.) will cause a progressive elevation of pulmonary vascular resistance, eventually resulting in the reversal of the shunt and cyanosis [67].

The normal growth and development of the pulmonary vascular bed are linked to normal hemodynamics. Lung biopsy evaluations have demonstrated that the severity of altered development and remodeling of the pulmonary vascular bed correlate with the hemodynamic state [68] (Fig. 18-16). A grading system that links pulmonary vasculature histology and degrees of pulmonary hypertension has been developed [69]. The exact etiology of the cellular morphologic changes is speculative, but probably relates to trauma from a widened pulmonary pulse pressure or vasoactive mediators.

The preoperative evaluation of the child who has congenital heart disease with pulmonary overcirculation includes cardiac catheterization and analysis of lung biopsy tissue to determine if the patient should receive a palliative or corrective procedure. As was mentioned in the discussion of the patient with tricuspid atresia, the success of the Fontan procedure is dependent on a low PVR.

In our patient a neglected PDA has led to irreversible pulmonary vascular changes and a high pulmonary vascular resistance. Table 18-1 lists some of the factors that cause this fixed elevated PVR. The histopathology of the pulmonary vasculature in our patient progressed through three grades to make her lesion inoperable. When she had grade A disease, there was an abnormal extension of muscle into small peripheral arteries with a mild increase in the wall thickness of the normally

Table 18-1. Factors determining the development of pulmonary vascular disease in patients with common varieties of congenital heart disease

	Major factors			Minor factors				
	↑P_{pa}	↑P_{pv}	↑QPA	↑PO_{2PA}	↓PO_{2SA}	↓PH_{SA}	Hematocrit↑	PVD
ASD, secundum	−	−	+	+	−	−	−	Unlikely
ASD, primum	−	±	+	+	−	−	−	Possible
TAVC	+	+	+	+	±	±	±	Highly probable
Large VSD	+	±	+	+	−	−	−	Probable
with mitral disease	+	+	+	+	−	−	−	Virtually certain
TF	−	−	−	−	+	+	+	Unlikely until late
with Potts	+	±	+	+	±	−	±	Probable
TGA	±	±	+	+	+	±	+	Virtually certain
with VSD	+	+	+	+	+	±	+	Certain

PVD = pulmonary vascular disease; P_{pa} = mean pulmonary arterial pressure; P_{pv} = mean pulmonary venous pressure; PO_{2PA} = oxygen pressure in pulmonary artery; PO_{2SA} = oxygen pressure systemic artery; PH_{SA} = PH in systemic artery; QPA = flow in pulmonary artery; ASD = atrial septal defect; VSD = ventricular septal defect; TF = tetralogy of Fallot; TAVC = total anomalous venous connection; TGA = transposition of the great arteries; − = absent; + = present; ± = sometimes absent/sometimes present; PH = pH.
Source: Reprinted and adapted with permission from AS Nadas and DC Fyler, *Pediatric Cardiology.* Philadelphia: Saunders, 1972. P 684.

muscular arteries. With increasing age, the patient developed grade B pulmonary vascular disease characterized by increased extension of muscle with more severe medial hypertrophy of normally muscular arteries. Now, with grade C disease, the patient's pulmonary vascular bed has all of the characteristics of grade B disease, with a reduced arterial concentration and reduced arterial size [70]. Although patients with grade C pulmonary vascular disease may have only a mildly elevated resting PVR, stress or hypoxia, or both, may cause severe elevations of PVR.

The anesthetic management of the patient with Eisenmenger's syndrome must incorporate an understanding of the patient's underlying congenital heart and secondary pulmonary vascular disease. It is important to determine if the PVR of the patient will improve with the administration of oxygen [71]. In our patient with a PDA, blood in the left extremity will be postductal, that is, a mixture of saturated and shunted blood. Blood in the right hand will be preductal and have improved oxygen saturation. By placing a pulse oximeter probe on the right hand (SaO$_2$ = 94%) and left hand (82%), an oxygen challenge test will determine the reactivity of the pulmonary vascular bed. Patients with marked improvement in the postductal saturation will have dilated their pulmonary vascular bed in response to oxygen. Blood that previously could not enter the pulmonary vascular bed facing a high resistance can now take part in oxygen exchange. If the postductal saturation has no appreciable change after the oxygen challenge test, drugs and anesthetic techniques that lower SVR greater than PVR are more likely to have a negative impact on the patient. Therefore, regional anesthesia employing local anesthetics would increase the right-to-left shunt and worsen cyanosis [72].

Information concerning the specific nature of the patient's intracardiac or aortopulmonary communication should not be difficult to obtain, as most of these patients have had extensive cardiac workups. It is likely that the true incidence of this syndrome will decline in areas of the world where the capability of an extensive early cardiac investigation exists.

The anesthetic plan should be aimed at manipulating all variables that can affect the SVR:PVR ratio to improve oxygenation. In the emergency phase, simple measures, such as warming blankets, analgesics, hydration, and supplemental oxygen, can lower PVR. In the operating room and during the postoperative period, meticulous attention must be given to patients receiving mechanical ventilation. Hyperinflation can increase PVR, and hypoventilation may result in postoperative atelectasis, with concomitant hypoxia, hypercarbia, and a resulting elevated PVR. The focus of the management of the case is not in the selection of the muscle relaxants, narcotics, inhalational agent, and sedative hypnotics (although agents that decrease SVR may be contraindicated), but in oxygenation, acid-base balance, temperature control, and a postoperative analgesic plan. A patient with a full bladder, who is nauseated, cold, and in pain, will have a PVR:SVR ratio that will confer hypoxia.

Total and Partial Anomalous Pulmonary Venous Connections

The incidence of abnormal pulmonary venous connections is low and the likelihood of a child with this anomaly presenting for noncardiac surgery is even more unusual. A brief discussion is presented here to familiarize the anesthesiologist with this entity that incorporates many management principles inherent to the child with cyanotic heart disease who is presenting for noncardiac surgery.

Under normal conditions, the two right and two left pulmonary veins carry oxygenated blood to the left atrium. Patients with abnormalities of the pulmonary venous system may have anomalous connections, stenotic connections, and abnormal numbers of pulmonary veins. This entity can become complicated when a patient has an abnormal number of connections that are hooked up in one of many locations other than the left atrium and one or more of these connections are stenotic. A classification system based on embryologic principles of pulmonary venous development is used to explain these anatomically and physiologically abnormal conditions [73].

If all of the pulmonary veins connect anomalously to the right atrium or to one of its venous tributaries, the condition is termed *total anomalous pulmonary venous connection (TAPVC)*. If one or more but not all of the veins have anomalous connections, the condition is termed *partial anomalous pulmonary venous connection (PAPVC)*.

There is a wide clinical spectrum to match almost every conceivable connection between pulmonary veins and various systemic tributaries in patients with PAPVC. Right pulmonary veins can anomalously connect with the right atrium, superior vena cava, or inferior vena cava. The left-sided pulmonary veins can connect anomalously with the coronary sinus and left innominate vein [74]. Connections to the azygos vein have also been described. If all but one of the pulmonary veins connect anomalously, the clinical picture will not be unlike that of a patient with TAPVC. More commonly, the veins of one lung connect anomalously and the clinical picture is not cyanosis but rather symptoms that occur in late childhood due to pulmonary overcirculation. Pulmonary overcirculation leads to increases in the PVR, which in turn leads to a progressive right-to-left shunt (Fig. 18-17).

Most patients with PAPVC have an atrial septal defect and it is the evaluation of the ASD that leads to the finding of anomalous pulmonary venous connections (Fig. 18-18). At surgery, the atrial septal defect is closed and all anomalous venous connections are repaired. Because of all the possible anomalous connections, with their respective impact on the pulmonary vascular bed, no formal prognostic data have been presented for these patients. Presumably, it is the state of the pulmonary vascular bed after surgical repair that will determine functional outcome.

Patients with TAPVC have all of their pulmonary veins connected to the right atrium or a systemic venous tributary. Interatrial communication is necessary for survival. One third of the patients have a concomitant major cardiac malformation (i.e., TOGV, pulmonary atresia, single ventricle, truncus arteriosus, etc.).

The distribution of the mixed venous blood will depend on the size of the intracardiac communication and the relative resistances of the pulmonary and systemic vascular beds. A major variable in these patients is the condition of the pulmonary vascular bed, which depends on the presence or absence of obstruction in the anomalous pulmonary veins. As the patient's PVR falls after birth, an increasing proportion of mixed venous blood enters the pulmonary circulation. Pulmonary blood flow may be three to five times systemic flow. With adequate mixing and no anomalous pulmonary venous obstruction, the oxygen saturation in the right atrium and left atrium should be greater than 90 percent. Within the first few months of life, the right ventricle will demonstrate that it is not up to the task of pumping the excessive blood that must traverse the pulmonary circuit. Right heart failure is common in these infants by 6 months of age.

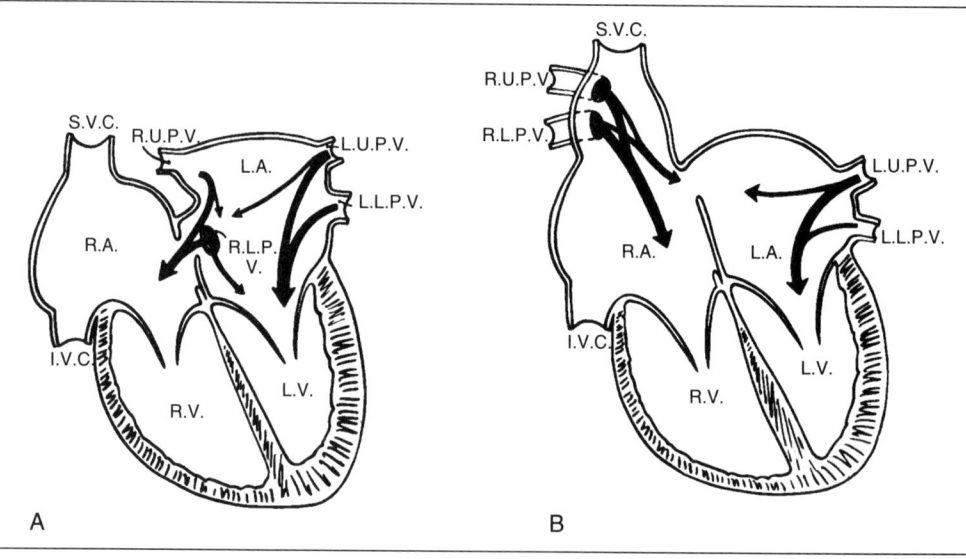

The clinical picture for the baby with TAPVC with concomitant pulmonary venous obstruction is the same irrespective of the site of obstruction. Cyanosis presents within the first few days of life. Obstruction in the anomalous pulmonary vessels leads to elevated hydrostatic pressure in the pulmonary veins and a tendency toward pulmonary edema. Reflex mechanisms characterized by reflex pulmonary arteriolar constriction, increased pulmonary lymphatic flow, and alternative pulmonary venous bypass channels come into action, with the net result of decreased pulmonary blood flow, cyanosis, pulmonary hypertension, and right heart failure [72]. Although the oxygen saturation in the right and left atrium is similar, a smaller percentage of mixed venous blood enters the mixed venous sample and the net result is significant desaturation. Clinically, these cyanotic patients are also tachypneic. Early surgical repair has replaced procrastination with improving results. The prognosis for each patient is linked to the preoperative state

Fig. 18-17. Partial anomalous pulmonary venous drainage: A. In atrial septal defect. The right pulmonary vein orifices are closer than the left to the atrial septal defect, and thus more of the right pulmonary vein blood drains anomalously to the right atrium. B. The major portion of blood from the right pulmonary veins drains anomalously while a small amount shunts right to left, and thus drains normally to the left atrium. A small portion of systemic venous blood from the SVC also reaches the left atrium. The majority of blood from the normally connected left pulmonary veins reaches the left ventricle, but some shunts left to right. RUPV and LUPV = right and left upper pulmonary vein; RLPV and LLPV = right and left lower pulmonary vein. (Reprinted with permission from RV Lucas, Anomalous Venous Connections, Pulmonary and Systemic. In FH Adams and GC Emmanouilides (eds), *Moss' Heart Disease in Infants, Children and Adolescents*. Baltimore: Williams & Wilkins Co., 1983. © 1983, the Williams & Wilkins Co., Baltimore.)

of the pulmonary vascular bed and the adequacy of the new venous–left atrial anastomosis. More data are needed on the outcome of the initial surgical repair before anesthetic implications can be defined.

Pulmonary Atresia with Intact Ventricular Septum

Although the name of this lesion appears to describe this rare cardiac abnormality, actually tremendous variability is found in the pathophysiol-

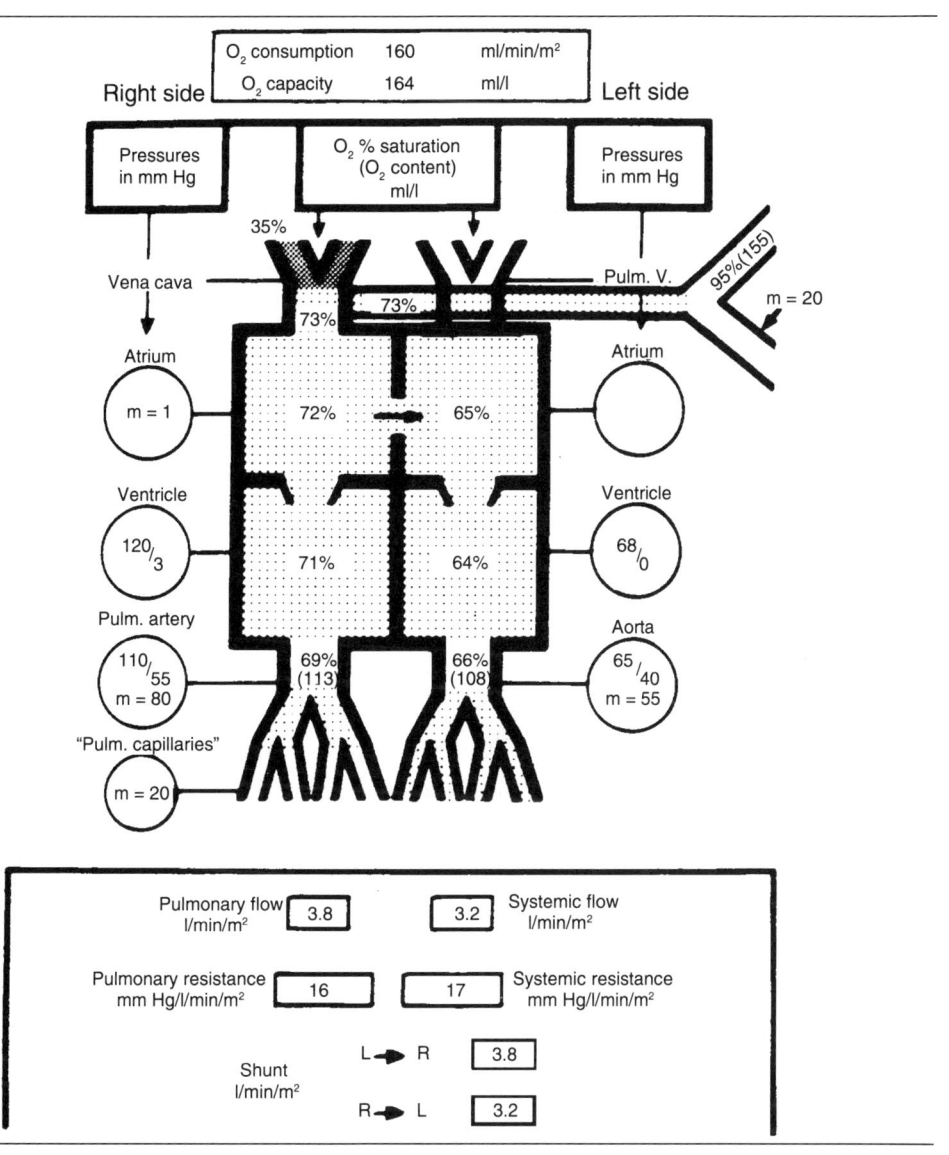

Fig. 18-18. Catheterization findings in a patient with total anomalous pulmonary venous connection with obstruction of pulmonary venous inflow. For key, see legend for Fig. 18-11. (Reprinted with permission from AS Nadas, and DC Fyler, *Pediatric Cardiology* (3rd ed). Philadelphia: Saunders, 1972.)

ogy among patients with pulmonary atresia with an intact VSD. In 80 percent of these patients, the pulmonary cusps are fused and in the remaining 20 percent, obstruction is due to a combination of infundibular and valvular atresia (Fig. 18-19).

There is great variation in the size and function of the right ventricle, ranging at one extreme from hypoplasia to marked dilatation at the other [75]. The right atrium is consistently dilated and the level of dilatation depends on the adequacy of the tricuspid valve. An atrial septal defect or a patent foramen ovale must exist to allow for mixing of desaturated and saturated blood. The newborn will tolerate this arrangement as long as left atrial pressures remain low and the ductus arteriosus remains

Fig. 18-19. Catheterization findings in a patient with pulmonary atresia and intact ventricular septum. For key, see legend for Fig. 18-11. (Reprinted with permission from AS Nadas, and DC Fyler, *Pediatric Cardiology*. Philadelphia: Saunders, 1972.)

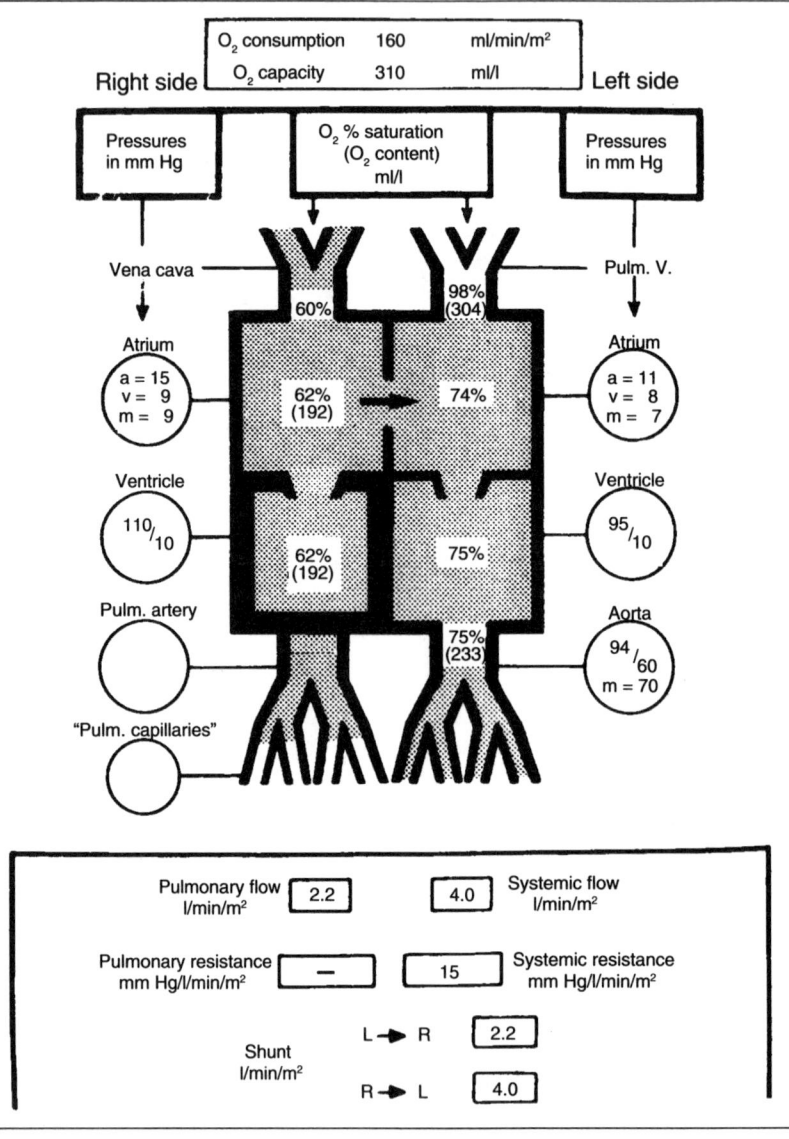

patent. Shortly after birth, left atrial pressure increases and the ductus that was transporting pulmonary blood flow closes. The net result is systemic hypoxemia.

Angiography will reveal detailed information concerning the size of the right ventricle and pulmonary arteries along with the diagnosis of pulmonary atresia. Immediate improvement in the precarious condition of the patient will depend on medical or surgical maneuvers, or both, to improve pulmonary blood flow. Prostaglandin infusions, acid-base correction, and respiratory support will be followed by either palliative or corrective surgery. If the patient has a hypoplastic right ventricle, an aortopulmonary shunt is created. If the right ventricle appears normal, a pulmonary valvotomy is performed. Obviously, alterations of PVR/SVR will have a profound effect on the degree of hypoxemia.

Like patients with TAPVC, these patients rarely present to the operating room for noncardiac surgery. The prognosis for these patients, like all patients with congenital cyanotic heart disease, lies in the potential of restoring a normal anatomic and physiologic relationship between the cardiac chambers and the pulmonary vascular bed.

Plans for the anesthetic management of children with cyanotic heart disease who need noncardiac surgery can be formulated by understanding the path of blood flow through cardiac chambers, valves, and great vessels that results in systemic oxygenation. These patients can be categorized into three groups: (1) patients who have had no cardiac surgery to improve systemic saturation, (2) patients who have had shunting procedures to improve pulmonary blood flow and thus systemic saturation, and (3) patients who have had cardiac surgery to increase pulmonary blood flow and foster normal cardiopulmonary growth. The anesthetic considerations for each method of increasing systemic saturation are different.

The condition of children who have had no previous surgical procedure may be quite tenuous. Variables that have negative impact on pulmonary blood flow (i.e., acid-base status, temperature, mode of ventilation, level of analgesia, etc.) may have the most pronounced effects on this set of patients. For example, the patient with tetralogy of Fallot may have severe desaturation with crying. Additionally, the multisystem effects of the cyanotic state need to be incorporated into perioperative management.

The anesthetic implications for children who have had a noncardiac surgical procedure to improve pulmonary blood flow (e.g., Blalock-Taussig shunt) not only include the above factors that affect shunt flow but relate to the size of the shunt as well. Shunts may be too small, with a resulting systemic desaturation, or too large, with irreparable changes in the pulmonary vascular bed.

Some children have had cardiac surgery to improve systemic saturation and foster normal cardiopulmonary development by establishing a more normal cardiac chamber relationship. These patients may be left with electrical disturbances, myocardial dysfunction, residual shunts, and multisystemic effects of the bypass process. The child with a surgically repaired transposition of the great vessels is not "cured."

Sound clinical anesthetic management principles come from appreciation of each defined disease in relation to the cardiac treatment initiated to date. Each cardiac treatment plan will influence the cyanotic state and organ development. Each anesthetic plan becomes highly individualized and targeted toward adhering to the principles of the cyanotic state, shunting, and postoperative pain relief.

REFERENCES

1. Rabinovitch, M, Herrera-DeLeon, V, Castenaeda, AR, et al. Growth and development of the pulmonary vascular bed in patients with tetralogy of Fallot with or without pulmonary atresia. *Circulation* 64: 1234–1249, 1981.
2. Flanagan, MF, Fujii, AM, Colan, SD, et al. Inhibitory effects on myocardial perfusion in pressure overload hypertrophy in immature lambs. *Pediatr Res* 23: 218A, 1988.
3. Castenaeda, A, Mayer, JE, Jonas, RA, et al. The neonate with critical congenital heart disease: Repair-A surgical challenge. *J Thorac Cardiovasc Surg* 98: 869–875, 1989.
4. Castenaeda, A, Freed, M, Williams, R, et al. Repair of tetalogy of Fallot in infancy, early and late results. *J Thorac Cardiovasc Surg* 74:372–381, 1977.
5. Kirklin, J, Blacksone, E, Pacifico, A, et al. Routine primary repair vs two-stage repair of tetralogy of Fallot. *Circulation* 60:373–386, 1979.
6. Perrault, H, Drblik, S, Montigny, M, et al. Comparison of cardiovascular adjustments to exercise in adolescents 8–15 years of age after correction of tetralogy of Fallot, ventricular septal defect or atrial septal defect. *Am J Cardiol* 64:213–217, 1989.
7. Teitel, DF. Circulatory adjustments to postnatal life. *Semin Perinatol* 12:96–103, 1988.
8. Iwamoto, HS, Teitel, D, Rudolph, AM. Effects of birth related events on blood flow distribution. *Pediatr Res* 22:634–640, 1987.
9. Moss, AJ, Emmanouilides, GC, Adams, FH, et al. Response of the ductus arteriosus and pulmonary and systemic arterial pressure to changes in oxygen environment in newborn infants. *Pediatrics* 33: 937–941, 1964.

10. Leffler, CW, Hessler, JR, Green, RS. The onset of breathing at birth stimulates pulmonary vascular prostacyclin synthesis. Pediatr Res 18:938, 1984.
11. Spitzer, AR, Davis, J, Clarke, WT, et al. Pulmonary hypertension and persistent fetal circulation in the newborn. Clin Perinatol 15:389–413, 1988.
12. Cassin, S. Role of prostaglandins, thromboxane and leukotrienes in control of the pulmonary circulation in the fetus and newborn. Semin Perinatol 11:53, 1987.
13. Hislop, A, Reid, L. Pulmonary arterial development during childhood: Branching pattern and structure. Thorax 28:129–135, 1973.
14. Davies, G, Reid, L. Growth of the alveoli and pulmonary arteries in childhood. Thorax 25:669–681, 1970.
15. Heath, D, Edwards, JE. The pathology of hypertensive pulmonary vascular disease. Circulation 18:533–547, 1958.
16. James, LS, Rowe, RD. The pattern of response of pulmonary and systemic arterial pressures in newborn and older infants to short periods of hypoxia. J Pediatr 51:5–11, 1957.
17. Murphy, JD, Rabinovitch, M, Goldstein, JD, et al. The structural basis of persistent pulmonary hypertension of the newborn infant. J Pediatr 98:962, 1981.
18. Hoffman, JIE, Rudolph, AM, Heyman, MA. Pulmonary vascular disease with congenital heart lesions. Pathologic features and causes. Circulation 64:874–877, 1981.
19. Lister, G, Hellenbrand, WE, Kleinman, CS. Physiologic effects of increasing hemoglobin concentration in left-to-right shunting in infants with ventricular septal defects. N Engl J Med 306:502–506, 1982.
20. Friedman, WF. Intrinsic physiological properties of the developing heart. Prog Cardiovasc Dis 15:87–111, 1972.
21. Gidding, SS, Stockman, JA, III. Erythropoietin in cyanotic heart disease. Am Heart J 116:128–132, 1988.
22. Phornohutkul, C, Rosenthal, A, Nadas, A. Cerebrovascular accidents in infants and children with cyanotic congenital heart disease. Am J Cardiol 32:329–334, 1973.
23. Paul, MH, Currinblay, Z, Miller, RA, et al. Thrombocytopenia in cyanotic congenital heart disease. Circulation 24:1013–1017, 1961.
24. Ekert, H, Sheers, M. Preoperative and postoperative platelet function in cyanotic congenital heart disease. J Thorac Cardiovasc Surg 67:184–190, 1974.
25. Greely, WJ, Ungerleider, RM, Smith, LR, et al. The effects of deep hypothermic cardiopulmonary bypass and total circulatory arrest on cerebral blood flow in infants and children. J Thorac Cardiovasc Surg 97:737–745, 1989.
26. Ferry, PC. Neurologic sequelae of cardiac surgery in children. Am J Dis Child 141:309–312, 1987.
27. Robinson, R, Samuels, M, Pohl, K. Choreic syndrome after cardiac surgery. Arch Dis Child 63:1466–1469, 1988.
28. McConnell, JR, Fleming, WH, Chu, W-K, et al. Magnetic resonance imaging of the brains in infants and children before and after cardiac surgery: A prospective study. Am J Dis Child 144:374–378, 1990.
29. Ferry, PC. Neurologic sequelae of open heart surgery in children. Am J Dis Child 144:369–373, 1990.
30. Cottril, CM, Kaplan, S. Cerebrovascular accidents in cyanotic congenital heart disease. Am J Dis Child 125:484–487, 1973.
31. Raroque, HG, Hershewe, GL, Snyder, RD. Mobius syndrome and transposition of the great vessels. Neurology 38:1894–1895, 1988.
32. Bavinck, JN, Weaver, DD. Subclavian artery supply disruption sequence: Hypothesis of a vascular etiology for Poland, Klipper-Feil, and Möbius anomalies. Am J Med Genet 23:903–918, 1986.
33. John, K, Bachman, DS, Cooper, RF, et al. Electroencephalographic abnormalities in children with congenital heart disease. Arch Neurol 42:794–796, 1985.
34. Cohen, MM. The central nervous system in congenital heart disease. Neurology 10:452–456, 1960.
35. Zahka, KG, Manolio, TA, Rykiel, MJ, et al. Handgrip strength after the Blalock-Taussig shunt: 14 to 34 year follow-up. Clin Cardiol 11:627–629, 1988.
36. Hesz, N, Clark, EB. Cognitive development in transposition of the great vessels. Arch Dis Child 63:198–200, 1988.
37. Howlett, G. Lung mechanics in normal infants and infants with congenital heart disease. Arch Dis Child 47:707–715, 1972.
38. Bancalari, E, Jesse, MJ, Gelband, H, et al. Lung mechanics in congenital heart disease with increased and decreased pulmonary blood flow. J Pediatr 90:192–195, 1977.
39. Davies, CJ, Cooper, SG, Fletcher, ME, et al. Total respiratory compliance in infants and young children with congenital heart disease. Pediatr Pulmonol 8:155–161, 1990.
40. Mace, S, Borkat, MD, Liebman, J. Hepatic dysfunction and cardiovascular abnormalities. Am J Dis Child 139:60–65, 1985.
41. Spear, GS, Vitsky, BH. Hyalinization of afferent and efferent glomerular arterioles in cyanotic congenital heart disease. Am J Med 41:309–315, 1966.

42. de Jong, PE, Weening, JJ, Donker, AJM, et al. The effect of phlebotomy on renal function and proteinuria in a patient with congenital cyanotic heart disease. Nephron 33:225–226, 1983.
43. Hickey, PR, Wessel, DL. Anesthesia for Treatment of Congenital Heart Disease. In JA Kaplan (ed), Cardiac Anesthesia (2nd ed.) New York: Grune & Stratton, 1987. Pp 635–715.
44. Dabizzi, RP, Caprioli, G, Aiazzi, L, et al. Distribution and anomalies of coronary arteries in tetralogy of Fallot. Circulation 61:95–102, 1980.
45. Nudel, D, Berman, N, Talner, N. Effects of acutely increasing systemic vascular resistance on arterial oxygen tension in tetralogy of Fallot. Pediatrics 58:248–251, 1976.
46. Graef, JW (ed). Manual of Pediatric Therapeutics. Boston: Little, Brown, 1988.
47. Amar, D, Brodman, E, Winikoff, SA, et al. An alternative oxygen delivery system for infants and children in the post-anesthesia care unit. Can J Anaesth 38:49–53, 1990.
48. Greeley, WJ, Stanley, TE, III, Ungerleider, RM, et al. Intraoperative hypoxemic spells in tetralogy of Fallot. Anesth Analg 68:815–819, 1989.
49. Clarke, WR, Gause, G, Marshall, BE, et al. The role of lung perfusate PO_2 in the control of the pulmonary vascular resistance in exteriorized fetal lambs. Respir Physiol 79:19–31, 1990.
50. McGrath, PA. Pain in Children: Nature, Assessment and Treatment. New York: Guilford Press, 1990.
51. Rothstein, P, Cole, JS, Pitt, BR. Pulmonary extraction of (3H) bupivacaine: Modification by dose, propranolol and interaction with (14C)-5-hydroxytryptamine. J Pharmacol Exp Ther 240:410–414, 1987.
52. Paul, MH. Transposition of the Great Arteries. In FH Adams and GC Emmanouilides (eds), Moss' Heart Disease in Infants, Children and Adolescents (3rd ed). Baltimore: Williams & Wilkins, 1983. Pp 296–332.
53. Mair, D, Ritter, DG. Factors influencing intercirculatory mixing in patients with complete transposition of the great arteries. Am J Cardiol 30:6–53, 1972.
54. Rashkind, WJ. Shunting at the ventricular level in transposition of the great vessels. Circulation 44 (Suppl II): 11–71, 1971.
55. Trusler, GA, Williams, WG, Izukawa, T, et al. Current results with the Mustard operation in isolated transposition of the great arteries. J Thorac Cardiovasc Surg 80:381, 1980.
56. Hagler, DJ, Ritter, DG, Mair, DD, et al. Long-term follow-up of Mustard operation survivors. Circulation 50:46–53, 1974.
57. Parrish, MD, Grahm, TO, Bender, HW, et al. Radionuclide angiographic evaluation of right and left ventricular function during exercise after repair of transposition of the great arteries: Comparison with normal subjects and patients with congenitally corrected transposition. Circulation 67:178–183, 1983.
58. Godman, MJ, Friedli, B, Pasternac, A, et al. Hemodynamic studies in children four to ten years after the Mustard operation for transposition of the great arteries. Circulation 53:532, 1976.
59. Barrit, DW, Urich, H. Congenital tricuspid incompetence. Br Heart J 18:133, 1956.
60. Ando, M, Satomi, G, Takao, A. Atresia of Tricuspid or Mitral Valve Orifice: Anatomic Spectrum and Morphogenetic Hypothesis. In R Van Praagh, A Takao (eds), Etiology and Morphogenesis of Congenital Heart Disease. Mount Kisco, NY: Futura Publishing Co., 1980.
61. Dick, M, Fyler, DC, Nadas, AS. Tricuspid atresia: The clinical course of 101 patients. Am J Cardiol 36(3): 327–337, 1975.
62. Freed, MD, Heymann, MA, Lewis, AB. Prostaglandin E_1 in infants with ductus arteriosus–dependent congenital heart disease. Circulation 64:899, 1981.
63. Report of the New England Regional Infant Cardiac Program. Pediatrics 65 (No. 2, Suppl): 388, 392–403, 1980.
64. Stanton, RE, Lurie, PR, Lindensmith, G. The Fontan procedure for tricuspid atresia. Circulation 64 (Suppl II): 140, 1981.
65. Fontan, F, Kirklin, JW, Fernandez, G, et al. Outcome after a "perfect" Fontan operation. Circulation 81:1521–1536, 1990.
66. Williams, DB, Kiernan, PD, Metke, MP. Hemodynamic response to positive end-expiratory pressure following right atrium–pulmonary artery bypass (Fontan procedure). J Thorac Cardiovasc Surg 87:856–861, 1984.
67. Eisenmenger, V. Die angeborenen Defecte der Kammerscheidewand des Herzen. Z Klin Med Suppl 132:1, 1897.
68. Bond, VF. Eisenmenger's complex. Report of two cases and review of cases with autopsy study. Am Heart J 42:424, 1951.
69. Rabinovitch, M, Haworth, SG, Castaneda, AR, et al. Lung biopsy in congenital heart disease. A morphometric approach to pulmonary vascular disease. Circulation 58:1107, 1978.
70. Meyrick, B, Reid, L. Ultrastructural findings in lung biopsy material from children with congenital heart defects. Am J Pathol 101:527, 1980.
71. Swan, HJC, Burchell, HB, Wood, EH. Effect of oxygen on pulmonary vascular resistance in patients

with pulmonary hypertension associated with atrial septal defect. *Circulation* 20:66–73, 1959.
72. Pollack, KL, Chestnut, DH, Wenstrom, KD. Anesthetic management of a parturient with Eisenmenger's syndrome. *Anesth Analg* 70:212–215, 1990.
73. Lucas, RV, Jr, Anderson, RC, Aplatz, K, et al. Congenital causes of pulmonary venous obstruction. *Pediatr Clin North Am* 10:781, 1963.
74. Lucas, RV. Anomalous Venous Connections, Pulmonary and Systemic. In FH Adams, GC Emmanouilides (eds), *Moss' Heart Disease in Infants, Children and Adolescents* (3rd ed). Baltimore: Williams & Wilkins, 1983. Pp 458–489.
75. Dhanavaravibul, S, Nora, J, McNamara, DG. Pulmonary valvular atresia with intact ventricular septum: Problems in diagnosis and results of treatment. *J Pediatr* 77:1010, 1970.

Index

Index

Abdominal complications after cardiac surgery, 292–295
Accelerated junctional rhythm, 228
Acebutolol in arrhythmias, 222
Acidosis
  diabetic ketoacidosis, 350
  in pericardial tamponade, 181
Action potentials, 215–216
Adamkiewicz artery in spinal cord ischemia, 255–256
Adenosine
  in arrhythmias, 223
  dosage in congenital heart disease, 440
Adrenal disorders, perioperative glucocorticoids in, 337
β-Adrenergic blockers
  in alcoholic heart disease, 364
  in aortic dissection, 249
  in arrhythmias, 222
  in atrial fibrillation, 226
  in hyperthyroidism, 371, 373
  in hypertrophic cardiomyopathy, 207
  intraoperative, in ischemic heart disease, 100
  in ischemia in aortic stenosis, 117
  in mitral prolapse, 162
  in mitral stenosis, 143
  perioperative use of, 94
    in blood pressure management, 344
  postoperative, in hypertension, 102
  in pregnancy, affecting fetus, 308–309, 325
  in supraventricular tachycardia, 225, 226
β-Adrenergic receptors in failing heart, 194–195
  down-regulation by beta agonists, 195
Afterload, 12
  in aortic regurgitation, 124
  in aortic stenosis, 113, 117
  in ischemic cardiomyopathy, 196
  in mitral regurgitation, 149, 155
  in mitral stenosis, 133, 134
Age
  and blood pressure changes, 396
  and cardiac output changes, 411
AIDS, 376–378
  anesthetic management in, 377
  cardiovascular effects of, 376–377
  epidemiology of, 376
  opportunistic infections in, 377
  pathophysiology of, 376
Alcoholic heart disease, 361–364
  anesthetic management in, 364
  clinical features of, 363–364
  electrocardiography in, 362–363
  malnutrition in, 363
  pathophysiology of, 362
Alfentanil
  cardiovascular effects of, 42–43
  chemical structure of, 40
  in ischemic heart disease, 98
  in pericardial tamponade, 182–183
  pharmacokinetics of, 41
Allen test, modification of, 402
Aminophylline in asthma, 360
Amiodarone
  in arrhythmias, 221
  in hypertrophic cardiomyopathy, 207
  in Wolff-Parkinson-White syndrome, 232
Amoxicillin in endocarditis prophylaxis, 428
Ampicillin in endocarditis prophylaxis, 428
Amrinone
  dosage in congenital heart disease, 440
  in ischemic cardiomyopathy, 195, 198
  preoperative use of, 101
  in pulmonary hypertension in mitral stenosis, 143
Amyloidosis
  cardiomyopathy in, 199
  hypothyroidism with, 369
Analgesic pumps, patient-controlled, 102, 164–165
Anatomy
  of aorta, 241–242
  of heart
    aortic valve, 5, 109
    chambers, 4–5
    conduction system, 9–12

473

Anatomy, of heart—Continued
  coronary arteries, 3, 6
  external, 3
  mitral valve, 5–6, 129–130
  skeletal framework, 4
  venous system, 6
  of pericardium, 6, 175–176
Anemia in renal failure, 354–356
Aneurysm of thoracic aorta, 242–243
  in ascending aorta, 249–250
  in descending aorta, 253–259
Angina
  in aortic regurgitation, 120
  in aortic stenosis, 111
  in cardiomyopathy
    hypertrophic, 205
    ischemic, 195
    restrictive, 200
  chronic stable, 83
  in mitral prolapse, 159, 160
  in mitral regurgitation, 154
  in mitral stenosis, 136
  Prinzmetal's, 84
  in pulmonary hypertension, 328
  unstable, 84
Angiography
  in aortic dissection, 246
  in cardiomyopathy
    hypertrophic, 206
    restrictive, 201
  coronary, in ischemic heart disease, 89
  in diabetes mellitus, 348
  in ischemic heart disease, 88–89
  in mitral prolapse, 161
  in mitral regurgitation, 150–151
  in mitral stenosis, 136, 139–140
  predictive value of, 91
  in pregnancy, affecting fetus, 324
Angioplasty, percutaneous transluminal, 92–93
Angiotensin-converting enzyme inhibitors, perioperative use of, 94
Antecubital vein
  as access for transvenous pacemaker, 272
  cannulation of, 71
Antiarrhythmic agents, 216–223
  adenosine, 223
  β-adrenergic blockers, 222
  amiodarone, 221
  bretylium, 221–222
  classification of, 216–217
  disopyramide, 220
  lidocaine, 220
  phenytoin, 220–221

in pregnancy, affecting fetus, 307–308
  procainamide, 219–220
  quinidine, 217–219
  sites of action of, 217, 218
  verapamil, 222–223
Antibiotic prophylaxis
  for cesarean section in atrial septal defect, 317
  in congenital heart disease, 427–428
  in mitral valve prolapse, 165
    for vaginal or cesarean delivery, 314
  in pregnancy
    in corrected cardiac disease, 329
    in ventricular septal defect, 318
Anticholinergics, dosage in congenital heart disease, 440
Anticoagulants in pregnancy, affecting fetus, 307
Antihypertensive agents
  considerations in selection of, 345
  perioperative, 344–345
Anxiety attacks in mitral prolapse, 160
Aorta
  anatomy of, 241–242
  ascending aortic surgery, 249–250
    interpositional tubular graft in, 250
  coarctation of, 435–436
  crossclamping of
    in ascending thoracic aorta, 251
    in descending thoracic aorta, 254, 256–258
  cystic medial necrosis, 243
  descending aortic surgery
    atrial-to-femoral artery bypass in, 258
    Gott shunt in, 258
    monitoring with somatosensory evoked potentials, 258–259
    one-lung ventilation in, 253–254
    spinal cord ischemia in, 255–259
  dissection of
    in Marfan syndrome in pregnancy, 328
    in thoracic aorta, 243–249
  in tetralogy of Fallot, 453

thoracic, disorders of, 241–260.
  See also Thoracic aortic disorders
  in transposition of great vessels, 455
Aortic arch, 241
  repair of, 250–253
    cerebral protection in, 251–253
Aortic valve disease, 109–126
  anatomic considerations in, 5, 109
  in pregnancy, 299
  regurgitation, 119–128
    acute, 120, 121
    anesthetic management in, 125–126
    in aortic dissection, 245
    chest films in, 123
    diastolic function in, 120–121
    echocardiography in, 123–124
    electrocardiography in, 122–123
    epidemiology of, 119
    hemodynamic goals in, 124–125
    myocardial ischmia in, 121
    natural history of, 120
    pathophysiology of, 120
    physical examination in, 121–122
    in pregnancy, 314–315
    preoperative evaluation in, 124
    systolic function in, 120
  stenosis, 109–119, 157
    anesthetic management in, 117–119
    causes of, 111
    chest films in, 116
    congenital, 436–437
    diastolic function in, 112–113
    echocardiography in, 116
    electrocardiography in, 116
    epidemiology of, 109
    hemodynamic goals in, 117
    myocardial ischemia in, 113–115
    natural history of, 111
    pathophysiology of, 111–115
    physical examination in, 115
    in pregnancy, 315–316
    preoperative evaluation in, 116
    symptoms of, 115
    systolic function in, 112
Arrhythmias, 215–237
  accelerated junctional rhythm, 228
  after cardiac surgery, 290–291, 329

in alcoholic heart disease, 362–363
antiarrhythmic agents in, 216–223. *See also* Antiarrhythmic agents
in aortic regurgitation, 124
in aortic stenosis, 117
atrial fibrillation, 226–227. *See also* Fibrillation, atrial
atrial flutter, 227–228
atrial tachycardia
multifocal, 228
paroxysmal, 225
bradycardia, 224–225
and effects of volatile anesthetic agents, 21
electrolyte management in, 236
in hypertension, 342
in hypertrophic cardiomyopathy, 206
implantable cardioverter defibrillators in, 281
impulse generation in, 216
intraoperative
causes of, 223–224, 237
control of, 100
in lupus erythematosus, 375
mechanisms of, 216
in mitral prolapse, 159, 162–163
in mitral stenosis, 141–142
in pregnancy, 311
from nitrous oxide, 16
pacing in. *See* Pacing
in pericarditis, 185
perioperative prognosis in, 93–94
premature ventricular contractions, 232–233, 336, 364
preoperative evaluation of, 336
reentry in, 216
in renal failure, 354, 355
risk factors for, 342
sick sinus syndrome, 225, 276, 369
sinus tachycardia, 225
supraventricular tachycardia, 225–226, 229
ventricular fibrillation, 233
ventricular tachycardia, 206, 233
in Wolff-Parkinson-White syndrome, 228–232
Arterial cannulation for blood pressure monitoring, 65–69
in childhood, 398–403
Arteriography. *See also* Angiography
coronary, in ischemic heart disease, 89
Arthritis, rheumatoid, 366–368

Asthma, 357, 359–361
anesthetic management in, 360–361
cardiac effects of, 360
clinical features of, 360
epidemiology of, 359
pathophysiology of, 359
Atherosclerosis
aneurysms of thoracic aorta in, 242
in diabetes mellitus, 347
in lupus erythematosus, 374
myocardial ischemia in, 82
Atracurium
in aortic regurgitation, 126
in cardiomyopathy
hypertrophic, 208
ischemic, 197
dosage in congenital heart disease, 440
in ischemic heart disease, 100
in mitral stenosis, 145
in pericardial tamponade, 183
in pericarditis, 187
Atria, 4, 5
Atrial fibrillation, 226–227. *See also* Fibrillation, atrial
Atrial flutter, 227–228
in Wolff-Parkinson-White syndrome, 229
Atrial kick, 5, 130
in aortic regurgitation, 121
in aortic stenosis, 112
in mitral stenosis, 133
Atrial pacing, transesophageal, 270
Atrial septal defect, 431–432
in partial anomalous pulmonary venous connection, 463
in pregnancy, 316–317
in tricuspid atresia, 460
Atrial tachycardia
multifocal, 228
paroxysmal, 225
Atrial-to-femoral artery bypass, in surgery of descending aorta, 258
Atrioventricular block, 233–234
first-degree, 234
second-degree, 234
third-degree, 234
Atrioventricular canal, 433–434
Atrioventricular node, 9, 215
Atrioventricular sulcus, 3
Atropine
in bradycardia, 225
dosage in congenital heart disease, 440
in hypertrophic cardiomyopathy, 208

in pericardial tamponade, 182
for premedication in childhood, 429
Autonomic neuropathy
in AIDS, 377
in diabetes mellitus, 348, 349
Autoregulation of blood flow, 8
volatile anesthetic agents affecting, 20
Axillary artery cannulation, 67
in children, 401

Bachmann's bundle, 9
Balloon counterpulsation, intraaortic
after pericardiectomy, 187
complications of, 288–289, 295
in ischemic cardiomyopathy, 195
in mitral regurgitation, 155, 156
Barbiturates, 27–29
in aortic regurgitation, 126
in aortic stenosis, 119
central nervous system effects of, 27
for cesarean section
in mitral prolapse, 314
in mitral stenosis, 311
in hypertrophic cardiomyopathy, 208
in ischemic heart disease, 98
methohexital, 29
in mitral regurgitation, 157–158
in mitral stenosis, 145, 311
in pericardial tamponade, 182
for premedication in childhood, 429
respiratory effects of, 27–28
thiopental and thiamylal, 28–29
Barlow syndrome. *See* Mitral valve disease, prolapse
Benzodiazepines, 29–34
in alcoholic heart disease, 364
in aortic regurgitation, 126
in aortic stenosis, 118–119
in cardiomyopathy
hypertrophic, 208
ischemic, 197
diazepam, 29–31
in hypertension, 345
in ischemic heart disease, 98
midazolam, 31–34
in mitral regurgitation, 157
in mitral stenosis, 145
opioids with, 43
in pericardial tamponade, 181, 182
in pericarditis, 187
in renal failure, 356
respiratory effects of, 29

Bicarbonate dosage in congenital heart disease, 440
Biliary tract, opioids affecting, 39
Biopsy, transvenous endomyocardial, in restrictive cardiomyopathy, 201
Bleeding, gastrointestinal, after cardiac surgery, 292–293
Blood flow
  fetal, transition to adult circulation, 442–446
  myocardial, 7–8
    and oxygen demand, 82
    volatile anesthetic agents affecting, 18–19, 20
  pulmonary
    effects of lesions in, 421–425
    nitrous oxide affecting, 16
Blood pressure. *See also* Hypertension; Hypotension
  changes with age, 396
  etomidate affecting, 35
  invasive monitoring of, 65–69
    axillary artery cannulation in, 67
    in children, 398–403
    complications from, 68–69
    femoral artery catheterization in, 67
    inaccuracies in, 67
    in ischemic heart disease, 96
    radial artery cannulation in, 66–67
  monitoring in children, 396–403
    axillary artery cannulation in, 401
    brachial artery cannulation in, 401
    dorsalis pedis artery cannulation in, 402
    femoral artery cannulation in, 401–402
    interpretation of direct measurements in, 402–403
    invasive, 398–403
    noninvasive, 396–398
    oscillometry in, 397–398
    Penaz methodology in, 398
    plantar artery cannulation in, 402
    radial artery cannulation in, 398–400
    sphygmomanometer in, 396–397
    temporal artery cannulation in, 401
    transcutaneous Doppler in, 397–398

  ulnar artery cannulation in, 398–400
  umbilical artery cannulation in, 401
  noninvasive monitoring of, 58–59
    automatic intermittent, 59
    in children, 396–398
    continuous, 59
    inaccuracies in, 58
    Riva-Rocci technique in, 58–59, 396
  opioids affecting, 41
  propofol affecting, 37
  systolic, and changes in myocardial oxygen consumption, 7
Blood volume
  in anemia with renal failure, 356
  and pericardial pressure, 179
  in pregnancy, 301
Bowel obstruction after cardiac surgery, 294
Brachial artery cannulation in children, 401
Bradycardia, 224–225
  from amiodarone, 221
Bretylium
  in arrhythmias, 221–222
  dosage in congenital heart disease, 440
  in pregnancy, affecting fetus, 308
  in premature ventricular contractions, 232–233
  in ventricular tachycardia, 233
Bronchitis, chronic, 357
Bronchospasm in asthma, 360
  anesthetic management in, 361
Bundle branch block, 234–236
  bifascicular, 234
  hemiblock
    left anterior, 234
    left posterior, 234, 236
  left, 234, 235
  from pulmonary artery catheter, 77
  right, 234, 235
Bundle of His, 9, 215
Bupivacaine, for labor and delivery in tetralogy of Fallot, 319
Bypass grafting, coronary artery, 92

Calcifications
  mitral valve, 131, 147
  myocardial, in renal failure, 354
Calcium channel blockers. *See also* Nifedipine; Verapamil
  in hypertrophic cardiomyopathy, 207

  perioperative use of, 94
  in blood pressure management, 344
  in pregnancy, affecting fetus, 325
Calcium chloride dosage in congenital heart disease, 440
Calcium gluconate dosage in congenital heart disease, 440
Cancer, pericardial tamponade in, 174, 182
  example of emergency operation in, 183–184
Capillary network in ischemic cardiomyopathy, 192–193
Capnography, 390–391
Captopril, in hypertension in renal failure, 353
Carbon dioxide
  capnography, 390–391
  transcutaneous monitoring, 390
Cardiac output, 10
  in anemia with renal failure, 355
  changes with age, 411
  determination in children, 410–412
  in pregnancy, 301–303
Cardiac Risk Index, 89, 91
Cardiomyopathy, 191–209
  alcoholic, 362
  classification of, 192
  congestive or dilated, 191–198
    in AIDS, 376
  hypertrophic, 202–209
    anesthetic management in, 207–209
    angiography in, 206
    chest films in, 206
    in childhood, 205
    diastolic dysfunction in, 203–204
    echocardiography in, 206
    electrocardiography in, 206
    gross morphology of, 202–203
    histopathology of, 203
    medical therapy in, 207
    mitral regurgitation in, 202
    myocardial ischemia in, 203, 204, 205
    natural history of, 204–205
    outflow tract obstruction in, 203
    pathophysiology of, 202–204
    symptoms of, 205–206
    systolic function in, 204, 205
    in idiopathic hypertrophic subaortic stenosis, 203
    in pregnancy, 323–324
  ischemic, 86, 191–198

β-adrenergic receptors in, 194–195
afterload sensitivity in, 196
anesthetic management in, 195–198
capillary changes in, 192–193
clinical features of, 195
in diabetes mellitus, 348
down-regulation of β-adrenergic receptors in, 195, 197
effects of β-adrenergic agonists in, 195
monitoring in, 197
myocardial changes in, 193–194
pathogenesis of, 191–194
preload dependence in, 196
in lupus erythematosus, 375
in pregnancy, 321–324
in idiopathic hypertrophic subaortic stenosis, 323–324
peripartum, 321–323
in renal failure, 354
restrictive, 198–202
anesthetic management in, 201–202
clinical features of, 200–201
compared to constrictive pericarditis, 200, 201
etiology of, 199
pathophysiology of, 199–200
Cardiovascular system in pregnancy, 300–303
Cardioversion
in atrial fibrillation, 226, 227
in atrial flutter, 228
direct-current, affecting pacemaker function, 280
in supraventricular tachycardia, 226
in ventricular tachycardia, 233
Cardioverter defibrillators, implantable, 281
Carotid artery puncture, in pulmonary artery catheterization, 76
Carotid sinus, hypersensitive, permanent pacing in, 276
Carpenter syndrome, cardiac lesions in, 426
Catecholamine depletion, effects of ketamine in, 288, 290
Catheterization
arterial, for blood pressure monitoring, 65–69
in children, 398–403
cardiac
in ischemic heart disease, 89

in restrictive cardiomyopathy, 201
in central venous pressure monitoring, 69–71
in children, 403–407
pulmonary artery, 71–78
in children, 407–410
Cellular ultrastructure, myocardial, 17
Central nervous system, drugs affecting. See Neurologic conditions, drug-induced
Central venous pressure monitoring, 69–71
antecubital vein approach in, 71
in children, 403–407
complications from, 71
femoral vein approach in, 71
internal jugular vein cannulation in, 70
in pericardial tamponade, 178–179
subclavian vein cannulation in, 70–71
Cerebral protection in aortic arch repair, 251–253
Cerebrospinal fluid drainage, before crossclamping of descending aorta, 256, 257
Cesarean section
in aortic insufficiency, 315
in aortic stenosis, 316
in atrial septal defect, 317
in coronary artery disease, 325
in Eisenmenger syndrome, 320
hemodynamic effects of, 303
in idiopathic hypertrophic subaortic stenosis, 323–324
in Marfan syndrome, 329
in mitral prolapse, 314
in mitral regurgitation, 313
in mitral stenosis, 311–312
in peripartum cardiomyopathy, 323
in primary pulmonary hypertension, 327
in tetralogy of Fallot, 319
in ventricular septal defect, 318
Chambers of heart, 4–5
Chest films
in aortic dissection, 246
in aortic regurgitation, 123
in aortic stenosis, 116
in congenital heart disease, 425–426
in emphysema, 357
in hypertension, 341
in hypertrophic cardiomyopathy, 206

in hypothyroidism, 369
in ischemic heart disease, 87
in lupus erythematosus, 375
in mitral prolapse, 161
in mitral regurgitation, 150–151
in mitral stenosis, 136
in pericardial tamponade, 174
in pericarditis, 185
in restrictive cardiomyopathy, 201
Chest pain. See Angina
Cholecystitis, acute, after cardiac surgery, 294–295
Chordae tendineae
in mitral stenosis, 131
rupture of, 147
mitral prolapse in, 160
Chronotropic reserve, 12
Cimetidine interaction with procainamide, 219–220
Clonidine, perioperative use of, 94
in blood pressure management, 344
Clotting factor deficiencies after cardiac surgery, 291
Coagulopathies
after cardiac surgery, 291, 329
in cyanotic heart disease, 447
Coarctation of aorta, 435–436
Cocaine
arrhythmias from, 223
sinus tachycardia from, 225
Coma
hyperosmolar, in diabetes mellitus, 350
myxedema, 369
Computed tomography in aortic dissection, 246
Conduction system, 9–12, 215
abnormalities of, 216
in children, 395
heart block in, 233–236
in rheumatoid arthritis, 367–368
Congenital heart disease. See also Pediatric patients
antibiotic prophylaxis in, 427–428
aortic stenosis, 436–437
atrial septal defect, 431–432
atrioventricular canal, 433–434
blood flow characteristics in, 422
chest films in, 425–426
coarctation of aorta, 435–436
common defects in, 422
cyanotic, 441–467. See also Cyanotic congenital heart disease

Congenital heart disease—
    Continued
  drugs and dosages in, 440
  echocardiography in, 427
  electrocardiography in, 426–427
  induction of anesthesia in, 429–431
  monitoring in, 387–413
  noncyanotic, 421–437
  partial anomalous pulmonary venous return, 437, 463
  patent ductus arteriosus, 434–435
  pathophysiology of, 421–425
  physical examination in, 425
  in pregnancy, 299, 316–321
  premedication in, 428–429
  preoperative assessment in, 425–427
    in cyanotic disease, 449–452
  syndromes with, 426
  ventricular septal defect, 432–433
Contractility, myocardial
  echocardiography of, 62
  in mitral regurgitation, 149, 154
  in mitral stenosis, 134
  nitrous oxide affecting, 13–14
  preoperative evaluation of, 335
  volatile agents affecting, 16–17
Conus ligament, 4
Cor pulmonale, 358
  anesthetic management in, 361
  in mitral stenosis, 135, 140
  in obesity hypoventilation syndrome, 365
Coronary arteries, 3, 6
  arteriography in ischemic heart disease, 89
  blood flow regulation in, 7–8
  bypass grafting, 92
  collateral vessels, 8
  disease of. See Ischemic heart disease
  intermediate vessels, 6
Coronary blood flow. See Blood flow, myocardial
Coronary steal
  in aortic stenosis, 118
  from nitroprusside, 100
  volatile anesthetic agents affecting, 19–21
Coronary sulcus, 3
Corticosteroids
  in pericarditis, 367
  perioperative
    dosage of, 337
    in hypothyroidism, 370

potency of, 338
  for spinal cord protection in surgery of descending aorta, 257
Cortisol levels, etomidate affecting, 35
Cough
  in asthma, 360
  in chronic bronchitis, 357
Creatinine levels in renal failure, 353
Cri du chat syndrome, cardiac lesions in, 426
Crying facies, asymmetric, cardiac lesions in, 426
Curare in ischemic heart disease, 100
Cutis laxa, cardiac lesions in, 426
Cyanosis
  in congenital heart disease. See Cyanotic congenital heart disease
  maneuvers for relief of, 425
  in pulmonary hypertension, 328
Cyanotic congenital heart disease, 441–467
  Eisenmenger syndrome, 320, 460–463
  induction of anesthesia in, 429
  preoperative evaluation in, 449–452
  pulmonary atresia with intact ventricular septum, 464–467
  pulmonary venous connection anomalies, 463–464
  systemic effects of, 447–449
  tetralogy of Fallot, 318, 452–455
  and transition from fetal to adult circulation, 442–446
  transposition of great vessels, 455–458
  tricuspid atresia, 458–460
Cystic medial necrosis, aortic, 243

Dantrolene, dosage in congenital heart disease, 440
Death, sudden
  in hypertrophic cardiomyopathy, 205
  in mitral prolapse, 159, 160
  in mitral stenosis, postpartum, 311
Defibrillators, cardioverter, implantable, 281
de Lange syndrome, cardiac lesions in, 426

Delirium, emergence, ketamine-induced, 34
Depolarization, 215
Desflurane, 16–22
  in aortic regurgitation, 125
  molecular structure of, 14
Dexamethasone, for cerebral protection in aortic arch repair, 252
Dextrocardia, 392
Diabetes mellitus, 346–352
  anesthetic management in, 351–352
  autonomic neuropathy in, 348, 349
  clinical features of, 347
  coronary artery disease in, 347–348
  epidemiology of, 346–347
  in hemochromatosis, 352
  hyperosmolar coma in, 350
  ketoacidosis in, 350
  metabolic effects on cardiovascular function, 349–350
  pathophysiology of, 347
  perioperative hyperglycemia management in, 350–351
  renal failure in, 352
  small-vessel disease in, 348
  ventricular function abnormalities in, 348–349
Dialysis in renal failure, 353
Diastole, 10
  end diastolic volume, 10
  filling phases of, 10
  pressure time index, 8
Diastolic function, 130
  in aortic regurgitation, 120–121
  in aortic stenosis, 112–113
  in cardiomyopathy
    hypertrophic, 203–204
    restrictive, 199
  in diabetes mellitus, 348
  in hypertension, 340
  in mitral regurgitation, 148–149
  in mitral stenosis, 132, 133
Diazepam, 29–31
  in aortic regurgitation, 126
  cardiovascular effects of, 30–31
  dosage in congenital heart disease, 440
  in ischemic cardiomyopathy, 197
  in mitral stenosis, 143
  nitrous oxide with, 31
  opioids with, 31
  for premedication in childhood, 429

Di George syndrome, cardiac lesions in, 426
Digoxin
  in atrial fibrillation, 227
  interaction with quinidine, 218
  perioperative use of, 94
  in pregnancy, placental transfer of, 306–307
  in Wolff-Parkinson-White syndrome, 232
Diphenhydramine dosage in congenital heart disease, 440
Dipyridamole thallium imaging, 88, 335
  predictive value of, 91–92
Disopyramide
  in arrhythmias, 220
  in hypertrophic cardiomyopathy, 207
Dissociative state, ketamine-induced, 34
Diuretics
  dosage in congenital heart disease, 440
  in hypertension, 340, 342–343
Dobutamine
  dosage in congenital heart disease, 440
  in ischemic cardiomyopathy, 195, 198
  in mitral regurgitation, 156
  in pericardial tamponade, 180
  preoperative use of, 101
Dopamine
  dosage in congenital heart disease, 440
  in ischemic cardiomyopathy, 195, 198
  in pregnancy, affecting uterine blood flow, 305
Dorsalis pedis artery cannulation, 402
Double product, and changes in myocardial oxygen consumption, 7
Down syndrome, cardiac lesions in, 426
Doxacurium
  in aortic regurgitation, 126
  in aortic stenosis, 119
  in ischemic cardiomyopathy, 197
  in mitral stenosis, 145
Dressler syndrome, pericarditis in, 185
Droperidol
  in alcoholic heart disease, 364
  in aortic regurgitation, 126

in aortic stenosis, 119
in diabetes mellitus, 352
dosage in congenital heart disease, 440
in hypertension, 345
in hyperthyroidism, 373
in mitral regurgitation, 157
in mitral stenosis, 145
Ductus arteriosus patency, 433–434
  closure with prostaglandin E_1, 460
  in Eisenmenger syndrome, 461
  in tricuspid atresia, 460
Dyspnea
  in aortic regurgitation, 120
  in aortic stenosis, 115
  in asthma, 360
  in cardiomyopathy
    hypertrophic, 205
    ischemic, 195
    restrictive, 200
  in chronic bronchitis, 357
  in emphysema, 357
  in hypertension, 340
  in mitral regurgitation, 150, 153
  in mitral stenosis, 131, 134, 135
  in pulmonary hypertension, 328

Echocardiography, 61–65
  in aortic dissection, 246–247
  in aortic regurgitation, 123–124
  in aortic stenosis, 116
  in cardiomyopathy
    hypertrophic, 206
    restrictive, 201
  in children, 412–413
  in congenital heart disease, 427
  in hypertension, 342
  in ischemic heart disease, 64–65, 89
  in mitral prolapse, 158, 161
  in mitral regurgitation, 151
  in mitral stenosis, 137–139
  in pericardial tamponade, 175
  in pericarditis, 186
  technical aspects of, 62–64
  transesophageal, 61, 62, 339
    in ischemic heart disease, 96–97
Ectopy, ventricular, 232–233
  preoperative evaluation of, 336
Edema, pulmonary
  in aortic regurgitation, 123
  in aortic stenosis, 113
  in ischemic cardiomyopathy, 195
  in mitral regurgitation, 150
  in mitral stenosis, 131, 132–133, 134, 135, 140

from pericardiocentesis, 181
in renal failure, 353
Edrophonium
  bradycardia from, 224
  dosage in congenital heart disease, 440
Effusions, pericardial, and cardiac tamponade, 173. See also Tamponade, pericardial
Ehlers-Danlos syndrome
  aortic dissection in, 243
  aortic regurgitation in, 119
  cardiac lesions in, 426
  mitral valve prolapse in, 313
Eisenmenger syndrome, 432, 460–463
  in pregnancy, 317, 319–321
Ejection fraction, 10
  in aortic stenosis, 112
  in diabetes mellitus, 348
  in ischemic cardiomyopathy, 194
  in mitral regurgitation, 149, 154
  in mitral stenosis, 133, 134, 140
  and perioperative risk, 336
Electrocardiography, 59–61
  in alcoholic heart disease, 362–363
  ambulatory, 87–88, 336, 344
  in aortic dissection, 246
  in aortic regurgitation, 122–123
  in aortic stenosis, 116
  in cardiomyopathy
    hypertrophic, 206
    restrictive, 201
  in children, 391–396
  computer ST segment analysis in, 60–61
    in ischemic heart disease, 96
  in congenital heart disease, 426–427
  delta wave in Wolff-Parkinson-White syndrome, 228
  in hypertension, 341–342
  in hyperthyroidism, 372
  in hypothyroidism, 369
  in ischemic heart disease, 60–61, 87–88, 96
    postoperative, 101
  in lupus erythematosus, 375
  in mitral prolapse, 161
  in mitral regurgitation, 151
  in mitral stenosis, 137
  in pericardial tamponade, 175
  in pericarditis, 185, 353–354, 355
  predictive value of, 90–91
  in pregnancy, 301
  stress testing in, 88

Electrocautery, affecting pacemaker function, 278-280
Ellis-van Creveld syndrome, cardiac lesions in, 426
Embolism, pulmonary, after cardiac surgery, 295-296
Emergence reactions, ketamine-induced, 34
Emergency surgery in ischemic heart disease, 102
Emphysema, 357
Enalapril
    in hypertension in renal failure, 353
    intraoperative use of, 94, 95
Encainide in Wolff-Parkinson-White syndrome, 232
End-organ dysfunction
    in diabetes mellitus, 346
    in hypertension, 339, 340
Endocarditis
    in AIDS, 376
    antibiotic prophylaxis for, 427-428
    in lupus erythematosus, 375
Endocrine system, etomidate affecting, 35
Enflurane, 16-22
    in AIDS, 377
    in aortic regurgitation, 125
    in cardiomyopathy
        hypertrophic, 208
        ischemic, 198
    in hypertension, 345
    in hyperthyroidism, 373
    in ischemic heart disease, 99
    in lupus erythematosus, 375
    in mitral prolapse, 164
    in mitral regurgitation, 157
    in mitral stenosis, 144
    molecular structure of, 14
Ephedrine
    dosage in congenital heart disease, 440
    in pregnancy, affecting uterine blood flow, 304-305
Epicardial pacing, 275
Epidural anesthesia
    in aortic regurgitation, 126
    in aortic stenosis, 119
    bradycardia from, 225
    in diabetes mellitus, 352
    in hypertension, 346
    in ischemic heart disease, 97
    for labor and delivery
        in aortic insufficiency, 315
        in aortic stenosis, 316
        in atrial septal defect, 317

in coronary artery disease, 325
in Eisenmenger syndrome, 320
in idiopathic hypertrophic subaortic stenosis, 323-324
in Marfan syndrome, 328-329
in mitral prolapse, 314
in mitral regurgitation, 312-313
in mitral stenosis, 311
in tetralogy of Fallot, 319
in ventricular septal defect, 318
in mitral prolapse, 164
in mitral stenosis, 145-146
in obesity, 366
in pericardial tamponade, 183
in pregnancy, affecting fetus, 304-305
in renal failure, 356
in tetralogy of Fallot, 455
Epinephrine
    in bronchospasm, 361
    dosage in congenital heart disease, 440
    in ischemic cardiomyopathy, 195, 198
    in pregnancy, affecting uterine blood flow, 305
    sinus tachycardia from, 225
Ergonovine test in variant angina, 89
Erythromycin in endocarditis prophylaxis, 428
Erythropoietin therapy, in anemia with renal failure, 354-355
Esmolol
    in aortic dissection, 249
    in arrhythmias, 222
    in asthma, 360
    in atrial fibrillation, 226
    in perioperative blood pressure management, 344-345
    in pregnancy, affecting fetus, 309
    in sinus tachycardia, 225
Etomidate, 35-36
    in cardiomyopathy
        hypertrophic, 208
        ischemic, 198
        restrictive, 202
    cardiovascular effects of, 35-36
    central nervous system effects of, 35
    for cesarean section in coronary artery disease, 325-326
    endocrine effects of, 35
    in ischemic heart disease, 98
    in mitral prolapse, 164

in mitral regurgitation, 157
in mitral stenosis, 145
nitrous oxide with, 36
in pericardial tamponade, 182
Evoked potentials, somatosensory, in monitoring for spinal cord ischemia, 258-259
Exercise stress tests, 335

Facial dysmorphism syndrome, cardiac lesions in, 426
Fallot tetralogy. See Tetralogy of Fallot
Fanconi syndrome, cardiac lesions in, 426
Femoral artery
    cannulation of, 67
        in children, 401-402
    obstruction after intraaortic balloon counterpulsation, 288-289
Femoral vein
    as access for transvenous pacemaker, 272
    cannulation of, 71
        in children, 405-406
Fentanyl
    in aortic regurgitation, 126
    in aortic stenosis, 118
    bradycardia from, 224
    in cardiomyopathy, ischemic, 197, 198
    cardiovascular effects of, 42
    for cesarean section
        in coronary artery disease, 325-326
        in Eisenmenger syndrome, 320
    chemical structure of, 40
    diazepam with, 31
    dosage in congenital heart disease, 440
    in ischemic heart disease, 98
    midazolam with, 33
    in pericardial tamponade, 181, 182
    pharmacokinetics of, 39
Fetal blood flow, transition to adult circulation, 442-446
Fibrillation
    atrial, 226-227
        in hypertrophic cardiomyopathy, 206
        in mitral prolapse, 162
        in mitral stenosis, 131, 133, 142
        in Wolff-Parkinson-White syndrome, 229
    ventricular, 233

Fibrosis, endomyocardial, 199
Fibrous trigones, 4
Fick equation, 10
Finapres device, 59
Floppy-valve syndrome. *See* Mitral valve disease, prolapse
Fluid retention in renal failure, 353
Fluid therapy
 in pericardial tamponade, 180
 in surgery of descending thoracic aorta, 253
Flumazenil as benzodiazepine antagonist, 29
Flutter, atrial, 227–228
 in Wolff-Parkinson-White syndrome, 229
Fontan procedure in tricuspid atresia, 460
Forney syndrome, cardiac lesions in, 426
Friedreich ataxia, cardiac lesions in, 426
Furosemide
 for cerebral protection in aortic arch repair, 252
 dosage in congenital heart disease, 440

Gastrointestinal system
 intestinal ischemia and infarction after cardiac surgery, 295
 opioids affecting, 39
 in pregnancy, 303–304
 ulcers after cardiac surgery, 292–293
Glomerular filtration rate, and serum creatinine levels, 353
Glucocorticoids, potency of, 338. *See also* Corticosteroids
Glucose
 dosage in congenital heart disease, 440
 serum levels
  in cerebral ischemia, 252
  in diabetes mellitus, 346, 350–351
  perioperative glucocorticoids affecting, 337
  in spinal cord ischemia, 257
Glycopyrrolate
 dosage in congenital heart disease, 440
 for premedication in childhood, 429
Goiter, and hyperthyroidism, 370, 371
Goldenhar syndrome, cardiac lesions in, 426

Gorlin's formula, 132
Gott shunt in protection against spinal cord ischemia, 258
Graves' disease, 370–373. *See also* Hyperthyroidism
Halothane, 16–22
 in alcoholic heart disease, 364
 in aortic regurgitation, 125
 in aortic stenosis, 118
 arrhythmias from, 223
 in cardiomyopathy
  hypertrophic, 208
  ischemic, 198
 for cesarean section
  in mitral prolapse, 314
  in mitral stenosis, 312
 in congenital heart disease, 429
 in hypertension, 345
 in ischemic heart disease, 98, 99
 for labor and delivery, in idiopathic hypertrophic subaortic stenosis, 324
 in mitral prolapse, 164
 in mitral regurgitation, 156, 157
 in mitral stenosis, 144
 molecular structure of, 14
 in tetralogy of Fallot, 455
Heart block
 from amiodarone, 221
 atrioventricular, 233–234
 bundle branch, 234–236
 in children, 395
 permanent pacing in, 276
 in rheumatoid arthritis, 367
 temporary pacing in, 267–269
Heart failure
 β-adrenergic receptors in, 194–195
 in alcoholism, 364
 in aortic dissection, 245
 in aortic regurgitation, 120
 in aortic stenosis, 111
 in cardiomyopathy
  ischemic, 194
  restrictive, 201
 in congenital heart disease, 425
 in crossclamping of descending aorta, 257
 in hypertension, 340, 341, 343
 in ischemic heart disease, anesthetic choice in, 97
 in lupus erythematosus, 374
 in mitral regurgitation, 149, 156
 in mitral stenosis, 131, 134, 135, 140
 in renal failure, 354
 right-sided

 in chronic obstructive pulmonary disease, 357, 359
 in obesity hypoventilation syndrome, 365
 signs and symptoms of, 336
 in ventricular septal defect, 317
Heart rate
 in aortic regurgitation, 124
 in aortic stenosis, 113, 115, 117
 and changes in myocardial oxygen consumption, 7
 in mitral regurgitation, 155
 in mitral stenosis, 141–142
 nitrous oxide affecting, 16
 opioids affecting, 43
 volatile anesthetic agents affecting, 21
Heart sounds, 10
 in anemia, 356
 in aortic regurgitation, 122
 in aortic stenosis, 115
 in hypertension, 340
 in hyperthyroidism, 372
 in mitral regurgitation, 150
 in mitral stenosis, 135–136
Hematoma from pulmonary artery catheterization, 77
Hemochromatosis, 352
 restrictive cardiomyopathy in, 199, 201
Hemoptysis in mitral stenosis, 135
Heparin
 dosage in congenital heart disease, 440
 in pregnancy, affecting fetus, 307
 rebound after cardiac surgery, 291
Hibernating myocardium, 86
His bundle, 9, 215
 bundle branch block, 234–236
Histamine levels, morphine affecting, 41
HIV infection. *See* AIDS
Holt-Oram syndrome, cardiac lesions in, 426
Holter monitoring, 87–88
 preoperative, 336
 silent ischemia detection in, 336, 344
Homocystinuria, cardiac lesions in, 426
Hunter syndrome, cardiac lesions in, 426
Hurler syndrome, cardiac lesions in, 426
Hydralazine
 dosage in congenital heart disease, 440
 in mitral regurgitation, 155

Hydralazine—Continued
  in pericardial tamponade, 181
  in perioperative blood pressure management, 344–345
  in pregnancy, affecting uterine blood flow, 306
Hypercyanotic spells
  in tetralogy of Fallot, 318, 454, 455
  in tricuspid atresia, 459–460
Hypereosinophilic syndrome, 199
Hyperglycemia
  in diabetes mellitus, 346
    perioperative management of, 350–351
  from perioperative glucocorticoids, 337
Hyperosmolar coma in diabetes mellitus, 350
Hypertension, 339–346
  after cardiac surgery, 290
  in alcoholism, 362
  anesthetic management in, 343, 345–346
  and autonomic neuropathy in diabetics, 349
  blood pressure management in, 343–345
  clinical features of, 340–343
  in diabetes mellitus, 347
  epidemiology of, 339
  intraoperative, control of, 100
  in lupus erythematosus, 374
  in obesity, 365
  pathophysiology of, 339–340
  physical examination in, 341–342
  postoperative, in ischemic heart disease, 102
  pulmonary. See Pulmonary hypertension
  in renal failure, 353
Hyperthyroidism, 370–373
  anesthetic management in, 373
  clinical features of, 372
  electrocardiography in, 372
  epidemiology of, 370–371
  laboratory evaluation of, 371–372
  pathophysiology of, 371
  treatment of, 372–373
Hypertrophic subaortic stenosis, idiopathic, 203
  in pregnancy, 323–324
Hypertrophy of heart
  in cardiomyopathy, 202–209. See also Cardiomyopathy, hypertrophic

  in hyperthyroidism, 371
  left ventricular
    in aortic regurgitation, 120
    in aortic stenosis, 111
    in hypertension, 339–340
  right ventricular, in pulmonary hypertension, 326
Hypotension
  after cardiac surgery, 287
  anesthetic-induced, 101
  with atrial fibrillation, 226
  in ischemic heart disease
    postoperative, 102
    treatment of, 97
  in mitral stenosis, 144
  in pericardial tamponade, 174
Hypothermia
  bradycardia from, 224
  for cerebral protection in aortic arch repair, 251–252
  for protection against spinal cord ischemia, 257
Hypothyroidism, 368–370
  anesthetic management in, 370
  cardiovascular effects of, 369
  clinical features of, 369
  epidemiology of, 368
  laboratory evaluation of, 368
  pathophysiology of, 368
  preoperative preparation in, 369–370
Hypoventilation syndrome in obesity, 365

Ileus, adynamic, after cardiac surgery, 294
Immune system
  in AIDS, 376
  in hypothyroidism, 368
  in lupus erythematosus, 373, 374
  in rheumatoid arthritis, 367
Immunodeficiency syndrome, acquired, 376–378. See also AIDS
Infarction
  intestinal, after cardiac surgery, 295
  myocardial, 85
    compared to acute pericarditis, 354
    in diabetes mellitus, 347–348
    pericarditis after, 185
    and perioperative morbidity, 90
    and postinfarction permanent pacing, 276
    and postoperative reinfarction, 93, 101
    in pregnancy, 324

    right heart, 85
    subendocardial, 85
    transmural, 85
    ventricular dysfunction in, 85–86
Infundibulum of heart, 5
Inhalation anesthetic agents, 13–22. See also Nitrous oxide; Volatile anesthetic agents
Inotropes, dosage in congenital heart disease, 440
Inotropic reserve, 12
Insulin, effects in diabetes mellitus, 347, 350
Interventricular sulcus, 3
Intestinal ischemia and infarction, after cardiac surgery, 295
Intravenous anesthetic agents, 27–44. See also specific agents
  barbiturates, 27–29
  benzodiazepines, 29–34
  etomidate, 35–36
  ketamine, 34–35
  opioids, 37–44
  propofol, 36–37
Iodine, radioactive, in hyperthyroidism, 372
Ischemia
  cerebral, and protection in aortic arch repair, 251–253
  intestinal, after cardiac surgery, 295
  of leg, after intraaortic balloon counterpulsation, 288–289, 295
  myocardial. See Ischemic heart disease
  of papillary muscles, and mitral regurgitation, 147–148
  spinal cord
    and monitoring with somatosensory evoked potentials, 258–259
    in surgery of descending thoracic aorta, 255–257
Ischemic heart disease, 7, 81–102
  anesthetic management in, 96–101
  in aortic regurgitation, 121, 125
  in aortic stenosis, 113–115
    management of, 117
  cardiac catheterization in, 89
  cardiomyopathy in, 86, 191–198
  causes of, 8
  chest films in, 87
  choice of anesthetic in, 97–98
  in chronic obstructive pulmonary disease, 357–358

chronic stable angina in, 83
in diabetes mellitus, 347–348
diagnosis of, 86–89
echocardiography in, 64–65, 89
electrocardiography in, 60–61, 87–88
emergency surgery in, 102
epidemiology of, 81
epidural anesthesia in, 97
etiology and pathophysiology of, 82–83
in hypertension, 340
in hypertrophic cardiomyopathy, 203, 204, 205
in hypothyroidism, 369
infarction in, 85. *See also* Infarction, myocardial
left main coronary artery disease in, 84
mitral prolapse in, 159
mitral regurgitation in, 154
in mitral stenosis, 136
myocardial protection in, 99–101
nitrous oxide affecting, 14–16
nuclear imaging in, 88–89
in obesity, 365
in pericardial tamponade, 176
perioperative morbidity in, 89–92
pharmacologic strategy in, 98–100
physical examination in, 86–87
postoperative management in, 101–102
in pregnancy, 299, 324–326
preoperative evaluation of, 336
preoperative management in, 93–96
Prinzmetal's angina in, 84
risk factors for, 324
silent ischemia in, 84–85
detection in preoperative Holter monitoring, 336, 344
in diabetes mellitus, 348
spinal anesthesia in, 97
strategy evaluation in, 92–93
stress testing in, 88
subendocardial, 82–83
in aortic stenosis, 112
unstable angina in, 84
ventricular dysfunction in, 85–86
ventricular tachycardia in, 233
Isoflurane, 16–22
in AIDS, 377
in alcoholic heart disease, 364
in aortic regurgitation, 125
in aortic stenosis, 118
in cardiomyopathy

hypertrophic, 208
ischemic, 198
restrictive, 202
in coronary steal, 19–21
in hypertension, 345
in hyperthyroidism, 373
in ischemic heart disease, 98–99
in lupus erythematosus, 375
in mitral prolapse, 164
in mitral regurgitation, 156
in mitral stenosis, 144
molecular structure of, 14
in pericardial tamponade, 182
Isoproterenol
in bradycardia, 225
dosage in congenital heart disease, 440
in pericardial tamponade, 180, 181
in pericarditis, 187
in pregnancy, affecting uterine blood flow, 305–306
Ivemark asplenia, cardiac lesions in, 426

Jervell and Lange-Nielsen syndrome, cardiac lesions in, 426
Jod-Basedow phenomenon, 371
Jugular vein
external, cannulation in children, 405
internal
as access for transvenous pacemaker, 272
cannulation of, 70
in children, 404–405
in pulmonary artery catheterization, 72
Junctional rhythm, accelerated, 228

Kaposi's sarcoma of heart, in AIDS, 376
Kartagener syndrome, cardiac lesions in, 426
Kent fibers in Wolff-Parkinson-White syndrome, 228
Ketamine, 34–35
in AIDS, 377
in alcoholic heart disease, 364
in aortic regurgitation, 126
in aortic stenosis, 119
arrhythmias from, 223
in cardiomyopathy
hypertrophic, 208
ischemic, 198
restrictive, 202
cardiovascular effects of, 34–35

central nervous system effects of, 34
for cesarean section
in Eisenmenger syndrome, 320
in tetralogy of Fallot, 319
in congenital heart disease, 429
dosage in, 440
in diabetes mellitus, 352
effects in catecholamine depletion, 288, 290
in hypertension, 345
in ischemic heart disease, 98
in lupus erythematosus, 375
in mitral prolapse, 164
in mitral regurgitation, 157
in mitral stenosis, 145
in obesity, 366
in pericardial tamponade, 181, 182
in pericarditis, 187
in pulmonary disease, 361
in renal failure, 356
respiratory effects of, 34
Ketoacidosis, diabetic, 350
Kidneys
in cyanotic heart disease, 448–449
failure of, 352–356
after cardiac surgery, 291
anemia in, 354–356
anesthetic management in, 356
arrhythmias in, 354, 355
cardiomyopathy in, 354
epidemiology of, 352
fluid retention and pulmonary edema in, 353
hypertension in, 353
pathophysiology of, 352–353
pericarditis in, 353–354
Korotkov sounds, 58, 396–397
Kussmaul sign
in pericardial tamponade, 175
in pericarditis, 186

Labetalol
in aortic dissection, 249
in perioperative blood pressure management, 344
in pregnancy, affecting fetus, 309
Labor and delivery. *See also* Pregnancy
cardiac output in, 303
cesarean section in. *See* Cesarean section
Laurence-Moon-Biedl syndrome, cardiac lesions in, 426
Leg ischemia, after intraaortic balloon counterpulsation, 288–289, 295

Leopard syndrome, cardiac lesions in, 426
Levocardia, 392
Libman-Sacks endocarditis in lupus erythematosus, 375
Lidocaine
 in arrhythmias, 220
 dosage in congenital heart disease, 440
 for labor and delivery in idiopathic hypertrophic subaortic stenosis, 324
 in pregnancy
  affecting fetus, 308
  in mitral regurgitation, 313
  in premature ventricular contractions, 232
  in Wolff-Parkinson-White syndrome, 229
Lithotripsy, affecting pacemaker function, 280
Liver
 in cyanotic heart disease, 448
 opioids affecting, 39
Loeffler's hypereosinophilic syndrome, 199
Lorazepam in ischemic cardiomyopathy, 197
Lown-Ganong-Levine syndrome, 228
Lupus erythematosus, 373–376
 anesthetic management in, 375–376
 cardiovascular effects of, 374–375
 electrocardiography in, 375
 epidemiology of, 373–374
 laboratory evaluation of, 374
 pathophysiology of, 374
Lupus-like syndrome, drug-induced, 219, 374

Magnesium levels, in arrhythmias, 236
Magnetic resonance imaging
 affecting pacemaker function, 280
 in aortic dissection, 247
Mahaim fibers in preexcitation syndrome, 228
Malnutrition in alcoholism, 363
Mannitol
 for cerebral protection in aortic arch repair, 252
 dosage in congenital heart disease, 440
Marfan's syndrome
 aortic dissection in, 243, 244

 aortic regurgitation in, 119
 cardiac lesions in, 426
 mitral valve prolapse in, 313
 pregnancy in, 328–329
Means-Lerman scratch in hyperthyroidism, 372
Meperidine
 cardiovascular effects of, 42
 chemical structure of, 40
 dosage in congenital heart disease, 440
 pharmacokinetics of, 39
Metaraminol in pregnancy, affecting uterine blood flow, 304
Methimazole in hyperthyroidism, 372
Methohexital, cardiovascular effects of, 29
Methoxamine in pregnancy, affecting uterine blood flow, 304
Methoxyflurane, molecular structure of, 14
Methylprednisolone, for cerebral protection in aortic arch repair, 252
Metocurine
 in ischemic heart disease, 100
 in pericardial tamponade, 183
 in pericarditis, 187
Metoprolol
 in aortic dissection, 249
 in arrhythmias, 222
 in pregnancy, affecting fetus, 309
Midazolam, 31–34
 in aortic regurgitation, 126
 in aortic stenosis, 118
 in cardiomyopathy, ischemic, 197, 198
 cardiovascular effects of, 32–34
 for cerebral protection in aortic arch repair, 252
 dosage in congenital heart disease, 440
 fentanyl with, 33
 in ischemic heart disease, 98
 in mitral stenosis, 143
Mineralocorticoids, potency of, 338
Minoxidil, in hypertension in renal failure, 353
Mitral valve disease, 129–165
 anatomic considerations in, 5–6, 129–130
 physiologic aspects of, 130–131
 in pregnancy, 299
 prolapse, 158–165
  anatomic considerations in, 160
  anesthetic management in, 164
  angiography in, 161

  antibiotic prophylaxis in, 165
  arrhythmias in, 159, 162–163
  causes of, 159
  chest films in, 161
  echocardiography in, 158, 161
  electrocardiography in, 161
  epidemiology of, 158
  hemodynamic goals in, 163
  in hyperthyroidism, 372
  monitoring in, 163–164
  natural history of, 159
  physical examination in, 160
  postoperative concerns in, 164–165
  in pregnancy, 313–314
  preoperative evaluation in, 161–162
  regurgitation in, 147
  symptoms in, 160
 regurgitation, 146–158
  anesthetic management in, 156–158
  angiography in, 151–153
  atrial compliance in, 149
  in cardiomyopathy
   dilated, 194
   hypertrophic, 202, 203
  causes of, 147
  chest films in, 150–151
  echocardiography in, 151
  electrocardiography in, 151
  epidemiology of, 146–148
  hemodynamic goals in, 155
  in mitral prolapse, 159, 160
  monitoring in, 154–155
  natural history of, 148
  pathophysiology of, 148–150
  pharmacologic agents in, 155–156
  physical examination in, 150
  postoperative concerns in, 158
  in pregnancy, 312–313
  preoperative evaluation in, 153–154
  with prosthetic valves, 151
  symptoms of, 150
 stenosis, 131–146
  anesthetic management in, 143–146
  angiography in, 139–140
  chest films in, 136
  chest pain in, 136
  congenital, 131
  echocardiography in, 137–139
  electrocardiography in, 137
  epidemiology of, 131
  hemodynamic goals in, 141–142
  left atrium in, 133

left ventricle in, 133–134
monitoring in, 141
natural history of, 131–132
pathophysiology of, 132–135
pharmacologic therapy in, 142–143
physical examination in, 135–136
in pregnancy, 299, 310–312
preoperative evaluation in, 140–141
pulmonary and right ventricular function in, 134–135
symptoms of, 135
Mivacurium, in aortic regurgitation, 126
Mobitz atrioventricular block, 234
Moderator band, 4
Monitoring of patients, 57–78, 338–339
in alcoholic heart disease, 364
in aortic dissection, 249
in aortic regurgitation, 125
in aortic stenosis, 118
in pregnancy, 315, 316
arterial cannulation in, 65–69
blood pressure in, 58–59
in cardiomyopathy
hypertrophic, 208
ischemic, 197
restrictive, 202
central venous pressure in, 69–71
in diabetes mellitus, 351
echocardiography in, 61–65
in Eisenmenger syndrome in pregnancy, 320
electrocardiography in, 59–61
in hypothyroidism, 370
invasive, 65–78
in ischemic heart disease, 96–97
in Marfan's syndrome in pregnancy, 328
in mitral prolapse, 163–164
in mitral regurgitation, 154–155
in mitral stenosis, 141
in pregnancy, 311
noninvasive, 58–65
in obesity, 366
pediatric, 387–413, 430
capnography in, 390–391
cardiac output in, 410–412
central vascular access in, 403–407
echocardiography in, 412–413
electrocardiography in, 391–396
hemodynamic, 391–413
mixed venous oxygen measurement in, 412

pulmonary artery catheterization in, 407–410
pulse oximetry in, 387–389
respiratory, 387–391
systemic blood pressure in, 396–403
transcutaneous measurements in
carbon dioxide, 390
oxygen, 389–390
in pericardial tamponade, 179–180
in pericarditis, 187
postpartum, in coronary artery disease, 326
in primary pulmonary hypertension
postpartum, 328
in pregnancy, 327
pulmonary artery catheterization in, 71–78
somatosensory evoked potentials in, for spinal cord integrity, 258–259
in tetralogy of Fallot, in pregnancy, 319
in ventricular septal defect, in pregnancy, 318
Monoamine oxidase inhibitors, interaction with opioids, 43–44
Morphine
in aortic dissection, 249
bradycardia from, 224
cardiovascular effects of, 41–42
chemical structure of, 40
dosage in congenital heart disease, 440
in ischemic heart disease, 98
in mitral stenosis, 143
pharmacokinetics of, 39
Mucopolysaccharidoses, cardiac lesions in, 426
Multiorgan failure after cardiac surgery, 296
Murmurs
in aortic regurgitation, 122
in aortic stenosis, 115, 157
in mitral prolapse, 160–161
in mitral regurgitation, 150
in mitral stenosis, 135, 136
Muscle relaxants
in aortic regurgitation, 126
in aortic stenosis, 119
bradycardia from, 224
in cardiomyopathy
hypertrophic, 208
ischemic, 197

in diabetes mellitus, 352
dosage in congenital heart disease, 440
in hypertension, 345
in ischemic heart disease, 99–100
in mitral regurgitation, 158
in mitral stenosis, 145
in pericardial tamponade, 181
in pericarditis, 187
Muscles
dystrophy of, cardiac lesions in, 426
opioids affecting, 39
Myocarditis
in AIDS, 376
in lupus erythematosus, 374
Myotonic dystrophy, cardiac lesions in, 426
Myxedema coma, 369
Myxoma, atrial, mitral valve in, 131

Naloxone dosage in congenital heart disease, 440
Narcotics. See Opioids
Neostigmine
bradycardia from, 224
dosage in congenital heart disease, 440
Neurofibromatosis, cardiac lesions in, 426
Neurologic conditions
after cardiac surgery, 292
in cyanotic heart disease, 447–448
drug-induced
from barbiturates, 27
from etomidate, 35
from ketamine, 34
from opioids, 38
from propofol, 36
Neuromuscular junctions, opioids affecting, 39
Neuropathy, autonomic
in AIDS, 377
in diabetes mellitus, 348, 349
Nifedipine
in hypertension in renal failure, 353
in hypertrophic cardiomyopathy, 207
in perioperative blood pressure management, 344
Nimodipine, for cerebral protection in aortic arch repair, 252
Nitrates in pregnancy, affecting fetus, 325
Nitric oxide in mitral stenosis, 144

Nitroglycerin
  dosage in congenital heart disease, 440
  in hypertension in renal failure, 353
  intracoronary infusion of, 100
  in ischemia in aortic stenosis, 117
  in mitral regurgitation, 155, 156
    in pregnancy, 313
  in mitral stenosis in pregnancy, 312
  in perioperative blood pressure management, 344
  in pregnancy, affecting uterine blood flow, 306
Nitroprusside
  in aortic dissection, 249
  dosage in congenital heart disease, 440
  in hypertension in renal failure, 353
  in mitral regurgitation, 155
  in pericardial tamponade, 180, 181
  in perioperative blood pressure management, 344
  in pregnancy, affecting uterine blood flow, 306
  in pulmonary hypertension in mitral stenosis, 143
  untoward effects of, 100
Nitrous oxide, 13–16
  in aortic regurgitation, 125–126
  in aortic stenosis, 118
  in congenital heart disease, 429
  diazepam with, 31
  effects on myocardial ischemia, 14–16, 99
  etomidate with, 36
  and heart rate, 16
  hemodynamic effects of, 22
  in hypertension, 345
  in ischemic cardiomyopathy, 198
  in mitral regurgitation, 156
  in mitral stenosis, 144
  molecular structure of, 14
  and myocardial contractility, 13–14
  in obesity, 366
  opioids with, 43, 182
  in pericardial tamponade, 181, 182
  in pericarditis, 187
  and pulmonary circulation, 16
  in pulmonary disease, 361
Nodulus Arantii, 5
Noonan syndrome, cardiac lesions in, 426

Norepinephrine
  dosage in congenital heart disease, 440
  in pregnancy, affecting uterine blood flow, 305
Normeperidine, 39

Obesity, 364–366
  anesthetic management in, 366
  epidemiology of, 364–365
  hemodynamic concerns in, 365–366
  hypoventilation syndrome in, 365
  pathophysiology of, 365
  Pickwickian syndrome in, 365
Ogilvie syndrome after cardiac surgery, 294
Opioids, 37–44
  in AIDS, 377
  in alcoholic heart disease, 364
  in aortic regurgitation, 126
  in aortic stenosis, 118–119
  benzodiazepines with, 43
  bradycardia from, 224
  in cardiomyopathy
    ischemic, 197
    restrictive, 202
  cardiovascular effects of, 41–43
  central nervous system effects of, 38
  for cesarean section
    in mitral stenosis, 312
    in tetralogy of Fallot, 319
  in congenital heart disease, 429
  diazepam with, 31
  hepatorenal and gastrointestinal effects of, 39
  in hypertension, 345
  interactions with other drugs, 43–44
  in ischemic heart disease, 98, 99
  in lupus erythematosus, 375
  midazolam with, 33
  in mitral regurgitation, 156, 157
  in mitral stenosis, 144–145
  neuromuscular junction effects of, 39
  nitrous oxide with, 43, 182
  pharmacodynamics of, 39–41
  for premedication in childhood, 429
  propofol with, 37
  receptors for, 38
  in renal failure, 356
  respiratory effects of, 38–39
Opportunistic infections in AIDS, 377

Oscillometry in blood pressure measurements, 397–398
Osteogenesis imperfecta, cardiac lesions in, 426
Outflow tract obstruction
  in idiopathic hypertrophic subaortic stenosis, 323
  in tetralogy of Fallot, 453
Oximetry, pulse, 387–389
Oxygen
  mixed venous measurements in children, 412
  saturation determination, 74–76
  myocardial supply and demand, 7
    in aortic regurgitation, 121, 125
    in aortic stenosis, 113, 315
    and coronary blood flow, 82
    etomidate affecting, 35–36
    in hyperthyroidism, 371
    left ventricular hypertrophy affecting, 339–340
    postoperative events affecting, 102
  in pregnancy, 303
  volatile anesthetic agents affecting, 18
  therapy with
    in bronchospasm, 361
    in obesity hypoventilation syndrome, 365
    in tetralogy of Fallot, 454
  transcutaneous monitoring, 389–390
  transport of, 74–75
Oxyhemoglobin dissociation curve, 75

Pacemaker syndrome, 277
Pacing
  codes for modes used in, 276, 284
  epicardial, 275
  manufacturers of units for, 285
  overdrive
    in atrial flutter, 228
    in premature ventricular contractions, 232
    in tachycardias, 267
  permanent, 275–281
    atrial inhibited, 277
    and cardioverter defibrillators, 281
    in children, 396
    direct-current cardioversion affecting, 280
    dual-chamber, 276, 277

electrocautery affecting, 278–280
indications for, 275–276
lithotripsy affecting, 280
magnetic resonance imaging affecting, 280
modes used in, 276–277
perioperative management of, 280–281
preoperative evaluation in, 277–278
rate-modulated, 276–277, 281
ventricular inhibited, 277
pulmonary artery catheters in, 268–269, 274
temporary, 267–275
indications for, 267–269
transvenous, 270–275
transcutaneous, noninvasive, 268, 269–270
transesophageal atrial, 270
transvenous, temporary, 270–275
in bradycardia, 225
catheter placement in, 270–272
complications of, 275
post-insertion care in, 274–275
technique of, 272–274
Pain. *See also* Angina
analgesic pumps in, patient-controlled, 102, 164–165
in aneurysms of thoracic aorta, 242
in aortic dissection, 244–245
in pericarditis, 185
postoperative control in mitral prolapse, 164–165
Palpitations
in hypertrophic cardiomyopathy, 206
in pulmonary hypertension, 328
Pancreatitis after cardiac surgery, 293–294
Pancuronium
in aortic regurgitation, 126
in aortic stenosis, 119
in cardiomyopathy
hypertrophic, 208
ischemic, 197
dosage in congenital heart disease, 440
in ischemic heart disease, 100
in lupus erythematosus, 375
in mitral regurgitation, 158
in mitral stenosis, 145
in pericardial tamponade, 183
in pericarditis, 187

Papillary muscles, 6
dysfunction in ischemic heart disease, 86
ischemia of, and mitral regurgitation, 147–148
in mitral valve disease, 129–130
rupture of, 149–150
Patent ductus arteriosus, 433–434
and prostaglandin E$_1$, 460
in Eisenmenger syndrome, 461
in tricuspid atresia, 460
Pectinate muscles, 4
Pediatric patients
asthma in, 359
bradycardia in hypoxia, 225
congenital disorders in. *See* Congenital heart disease
cyanotic heart disease in, 441–467
hypertrophic cardiomyopathy in, 205
ketamine affecting, 34
monitoring of, 387–413, 430. *See also* Monitoring of patients, pediatric
noncyanotic heart disease in, 421–437
Penaz methodology in blood pressure measurements, 398
Penicillin in endocarditis prophylaxis, 428
Pericardial disease, 173–187
pericarditis, 184–187. *See also* Pericarditis
tamponade, 173–184. *See also* Tamponade, pericardial
Pericardial fluid, 176
Pericardiectomy, 186–187
Pericardiocentesis, 173–174, 181
Pericarditis, 184–187
in AIDS, 376
anesthetic management in, 186–187
causes of, 184
clinical features of, 354
compared to acute infarction, 354
constrictive, 184
compared to restrictive cardiomyopathy, 200, 201
diagnosis of, 185–186
in hypothyroidism, 369
in lupus erythematosus, 374–375
pathophysiology of, 185
in renal failure, 353–354, 356
in rheumatoid arthritis, 367
tamponade in, 186
Pericardium, 6, 175–176
Periodic paralysis, familial, cardiac lesions in, 426

Perioperative medications in ischemic heart disease, 94–96
Phenylephrine
in anesthetic-induced hypotension, 101
dosage in congenital heart disease, 440
in mitral stenosis, 144
in pregnancy, 311
for perfusion pressure in aortic stenosis, 117
in pregnancy, affecting uterine blood flow, 304–305
in tetralogy of Fallot, 454, 455
Phenytoin
in arrhythmias, 220–221
for cerebral protection in aortic arch repair, 252
dosage in congenital heart disease, 440
in pregnancy, affecting fetus, 308
in premature ventricular contractions, 233
Phosphate therapy in diabetes mellitus, 351
Physical examination
in aortic regurgitation, 121–122
in aortic stenosis, 115
in congenital heart disease, 425
in hypertension, 341–342
in ischemic heart disease, 86–87
in mitral stenosis, 135–136
Physostigmine, bradycardia from, 224
Pickwickian syndrome in obesity, 365
Pipecuronium
in aortic regurgitation, 126
in aortic stenosis, 119
in ischemic cardiomyopathy, 197
in mitral regurgitation, 158
in mitral stenosis, 145
Plantar artery cannulation, 402
Platelet count after cardiac surgery, 291
Pneumothorax from central venous pressure monitoring, 71
Pompe disease, cardiac lesions in, 426
Porphyria, barbiturates contraindicated in, 27–28
Postcardiac surgical patients, 287–296
arrhythmias in, 290–291
coagulopathies in, 291
gastrointestinal complications in, 292–295
hemodynamic problems in, 287–290

Postcardiac surgical patients—Continued
  hypertension in, 290
  hypotension in, 287
  neurologic complications in, 292
  pregnancy in, 329–330
  renal failure in, 291
  respiratory pathology in, 290
  vascular complications in, 295–296
  vasodilatation in, 288
  ventricular dysfunction in, 288–290
Postcardiotomy syndrome, pericarditis in, 185
Postpartum period
  in aortic stenosis, 316
  cardiac output in, 303
  cardiomyopathy in, 321
  in Eisenmenger syndrome, 320–321
  in primary pulmonary hypertension, 328
Potassium therapy
  in diabetes mellitus, 351
  dosage of potassium chloride in congenital heart disease, 440
  in premature ventricular contractions, 232
  preoperative, in hypertension, 342–343
Preeclampsia, and peripartum cardiomyopathy, 322
Preexcitation syndrome, 228
Pregnancy, 299–330
  after cardiac surgery, 329–330
  aortic dissection in, 244
  ascending aortic aneurysm in, 260
  atrial septal defect in, 316–317
  cardiac medications in, affecting fetus, 304–309
  cardiomyopathies in, 321–324
  cardiovascular system in, 300–303
  congenital heart disease in, 316–321
    left-to-right shunts, 316–318
    right-to-left shunts, 318–321
  coronary artery disease in, 324–326
  Eisenmenger syndrome in, 317, 319–321
  epidemiology of cardiac disease in, 299–300
  gastrointestinal system in, 303–304
  management of cardiac disease in, 310–311
  in Marfan's syndrome, 328–329
  physiologic changes in, 300–304
  pulmonary hypertension in, primary, 326–328
  respiratory system in, 303
  tetralogy of Fallot in, 318–319
  valvular heart disease in, 310–316
    aortic, 314–316
    mitral, 310–314
  ventricular septal defect in, 317–318
Preload, 12
  in aortic regurgitation, 120–121, 124
  in aortic stenosis, 113, 117
  in ischemic cardiomyopathy, 196–197
  in mitral regurgitation, 149, 155
  in mitral stenosis, 132, 133, 134
Premature ventricular contractions, 232–233
  in alcoholic heart disease, 363, 364
  preoperative evaluation of, 336
Premedication in ischemic heart disease, 96
Procainamide
  in arrhythmias, 219
  dosage in congenital heart disease, 440
  interaction with cimetidine, 219
  in pregnancy, affecting fetus, 308
  in premature ventricular contractions, 232
  in ventricular tachycardia, 233
  in Wolff-Parkinson-White syndrome, 229
Propofol, 36–37
  in aortic regurgitation, 126
  in aortic stenosis, 119
  cardiovascular effects of, 37
  central nervous system effects of, 36
  in ischemic heart disease, 98
  in mitral prolapse, 164
  in mitral regurgitation, 156, 157
  in mitral stenosis, 145
  opioids with, 37
  in pericardial tamponade, 182
  respiratory effects of, 37
Propranolol
  in aortic dissection, 249
  in arrhythmias, 222
  bradycardia from, 224
  in hyperthyroidism, 373
  in hypertrophic cardiomyopathy, 208
  in mitral prolapse, 163
  in pregnancy, affecting fetus, 308–309
  in sinus tachycardia, 225
  in tetralogy of Fallot, 455
  verapamil with, 223
Propylthiouracil in hyperthyroidism, 372
Prostaglandin E$_1$
  in patent ductus arteriosus, 460
  dosage in congenital heart disease, 440
Pseudoxanthoma, cardiac lesions in, 426
Pulmonary artery
  catheterization of, 71–78, 336–337
    catheter insertion technique in, 72–74
    in children, 407–410
    in chronic obstructive pulmonary disease, 359
    complications from, 76–78
    determination of mixed venous oxygen saturation in, 74–76
    indications for, 72
    in ischemic heart disease, 96
    pacing with, 268–269, 274
    rupture from artery in, 77
    in transposition of great vessels, 455
Pulmonary atresia with intact ventricular septum, 464–467
Pulmonary blood flow
  effects of lesions in, 421–425
  nitrous oxide affecting, 16
Pulmonary disease, chronic obstructive, 356–359
  anesthetic management in, 360–361
  cardiac effects of, 357–359
  clinical features of, 359
  multifocal atrial tachycardia in, 228
Pulmonary edema. See Edema, pulmonary
Pulmonary embolism after cardiac surgery, 295–296
Pulmonary hypertension
  in asthma, 360
  causes of, 326
  in Eisenmenger syndrome, 319–320, 432, 460–461
  in mitral regurgitation, 149
  in mitral stenosis, 131, 134, 140
    management of, 143
  in obesity hypoventilation syndrome, 365

primary
   in pregnancy, 326–328
   vasospasm in, 327
Pulmonary venous return anomaly
   partial, 437, 463
   total, 463–464
Pulmonic valve, 5
Pulse, 10
   in anemia, 356
   in aortic regurgitation, 121
   in aortic stenosis, 115
   in pericardial tamponade, 174
Pulse oximetry, 387–389
Pulsus paradoxus in pericardial tamponade, 174, 177
Purkinje fibers, 215
Pyridostigmine dosage in congenital heart disease, 440

Quinidine
   in arrhythmias, 217–219
   interaction with digoxin, 218
   in pregnancy, affecting fetus, 308

Radial artery cannulation, 66–67
   in children, 398–400
Radiography. See Chest films
Reentry mechanism in arrhythmias, 216
Refsum's syndrome, cardiac lesions in, 426
Regional anesthesia. See Epidural anesthesia; Spinal anesthesia
Renal failure. See Kidneys, failure of
Repolarization, 215
Respiratory system
   in asthma, 357, 359–361
   barbiturates affecting, 27
   benzodiazepines affecting, 29
   cardiac surgery affecting, 290
   in chronic obstructive pulmonary disease, 356–359
   etomidate affecting, 35
   ketamine affecting, 34
   monitoring in pediatric disorders, 387–391
   in obesity, 365
   opioids affecting, 38–39
   in pregnancy, 303
   propofol affecting, 37
Revascularization, prophylactic, indications for, 92
Rheumatic heart disease
   mitral regurgitation in, 146–147
   mitral stenosis in, 131
   in pregnancy, 299
Rheumatoid arthritis, 366–368

cardiac disease in, 367–368
   anesthetic management in, 368
   clinical features of, 367
   epidemiology of, 366–367
   pathophysiology of, 367
Romano Ward syndrome, cardiac lesions in, 426
Rubinstein-Taybi syndrome, cardiac lesions in, 426

Scopolamine
   dosage in congenital heart disease, 440
   in mitral stenosis, 143, 145
Semilunar valves, 5
Septal defects
   atrial, 431–432
   ventricular, 432–433
Sevoflurane, 16–22
   in aortic regurgitation, 125
   molecular structure of, 14
Shunting lesions
   effects of, 421–425
   preoperative evaluation of, 449–451
Sick sinus syndrome, 225
   bradycardia in, 224
   in hypothyroidism, 369
   permanent pacing in, 276
Silent myocardial ischemia, 84–85
   detection in preoperative Holter monitoring, 336, 344
   in diabetes mellitus, 348
Sinoatrial node, 9, 215
Sinus node dysfunction, permanent pacing in, 276
Sinus tachycardia, 225
Skeletal framework of heart, 4
Smith-Lemli-Opitz syndrome, cardiac lesions in, 426
Sodium levels in arrhythmias, 236
Somatosensory evoked potentials, in monitoring for spinal cord ischemia, 258–259
Sphygmomanometry, 58–59
   in children, 396–397
Spinal anesthesia
   in aortic regurgitation, 126
   in aortic stenosis, 119
   for labor and delivery, 316
   bradycardia from, 225
   in ischemic heart disease, 97
   in mitral stenosis, 145
   in pericardial tamponade, 183
   in pregnancy, affecting fetus, 304–305
Spinal cord ischemia
   and monitoring with somato-

sensory evoked potentials, 258–259
   in surgery of descending thoracic aorta, 255–257
Starling's effect, 12
Stress reduction, perioperative, 93
Stress testing, 335
   in diabetes mellitus, 348
   in ischemic heart disease, 88
   in mitral prolapse, 162
Stress ulcers after cardiac surgery, 292–293
Stroke volume, 10
Stunned myocardium, 86, 288
Subclavian vein
   as access for transvenous pacemaker, 272
   cannulation of, 70–71
   in children, 403–404
Succinylcholine
   in aortic regurgitation, 126
   in aortic stenosis, 119
   bradycardia from, 224
   for cesarean section
      in mitral prolapse, 314
      in mitral stenosis, 311
   dosage in congenital heart disease, 440
   in mitral stenosis, 145
Sufentanil
   in aortic regurgitation, 126
   in aortic stenosis, 118
   bradycardia from, 224
   in cardiomyopathy, ischemic, 197, 198
   cardiovascular effects of, 42
   chemical structure of, 40
   dosage in congenital heart disease, 440
   in ischemic heart disease, 98
   in mitral stenosis, 144–145
   pharmacokinetics of, 39–41
Superoxide dismutase, for spinal cord protection in surgery of descending aorta, 257
Swan-Ganz catheter. See Pulmonary artery, catheterization of
Syncope
   in aortic stenosis, 111, 115
   in hypersensitive carotid sinus syndrome, 276
   in hypertrophic cardiomyopathy, 205–206
   in mitral prolapse, 160
Systemic diseases, 335–378
   AIDS, 376–378
   alcoholism, 361–364
   asthma, 359–361

Systemic diseases—Continued
  cardiovascular abnormalities in, 336
  chronic obstructive pulmonary disease, 356–359
  diabetes mellitus, 346–352
  hypertension, 339–346
  hyperthyroidism, 370–373
  hypothyroidism, 368–370
  lupus erythematosus, 373–376
  medical therapy management in, 337
  monitoring in, 338–339
  obesity, 364–366
  preoperative testing in, 335–337
  renal failure, 352–356
  rheumatoid arthritis, 366–368
Systole, 9–10
  ejection phases of, 10
  end systolic volume, 10
  isovolumic phase of, 10
Systolic function, 131
  in aortic regurgitation, 120
  in aortic stenosis, 112
  in cardiomyopathy
    hypertrophic, 204, 205
    ischemic, 194
  in diabetes mellitus, 348
  in hypertension, 340
  in mitral regurgitation, 148–149, 154
  in mitral stenosis, 134

Tachycardia
  atrial
    multifocal, 228
    paroxysmal, 225
  intraoperative, 100
  in mitral stenosis, 141
  in pregnancy, 311
  sinus, 225
    in lupus erythematosus, 375
  supraventricular
    paroxysmal, 225
    in Wolff-Parkinson-White syndrome, 229
  temporary pacing in, 267
  ventricular, 233
    in hypertrophic cardiomyopathy, 206
Tamponade, pericardial, 173–184
  in AIDS, 376
  anesthetic management in, 181–184
  in cancer patients, 174, 182
    example of emergency operation in, 183
  chest films in, 174
  clinical signs of, 174
  echocardiography in, 175
  effects of ventilation in, 177–178
  electrocardiography in, 175
  hemodynamics of fluid status in, 178–179
  monitoring in, 179–180
  pathophysiology of, 175–177
  in pericarditis, 186
  postoperative management in, 184
  preoperative care in, 180–181
  pressure-volume curves in, 179
  release of, in dissection of ascending aorta, 173, 182
Temporal artery cannulation in infants, 401
Tetralogy of Fallot, 452–455
  hypercyanotic state in, 318, 454, 455
  in pregnancy, 318–319
  pulmonary blood flow in, 423
Thallium stress tests, 88, 335
  in pregnancy, affecting fetus, 324
Theophylline, multifocal atrial tachycardia from, 228
Thermodilution curves in children, 410–413
Thiamylal, 28
Thiopental
  cardiovascular effects of, 28–29
  for cerebral protection in aortic arch repair, 252
  dosage in congenital heart disease, 440
Thoracic aortic disorders, 241–260
  anesthetic management in, 249
  in aortic arch repair, 250–253
  in ascending aortic surgery, 249–250
  in descending aortic surgery, 253–259
  in noncardiac surgery, 259–260
  aneurysm, 242–243
    in ascending aorta, 249–250
    in descending aorta, 253–259
  dissection, 243–249
    classification of, 244
    in cystic medial necrosis, 243
    diagnostic techniques in, 246–247
    initial management in, 247–249
    in pregnancy, 244
    signs and symptoms of, 244–246
  traumatic rupture, 243

Thrombocytopenia
  absent radius with, cardiac lesions in, 426
  after cardiac surgery, 291
Thromboembolism
  in mitral stenosis, 131–132
  pulmonary embolism after cardiac surgery, 295–296
Thrombosis from arterial cannulation, 68–69
Thyroid disease, 368–373
  hyperthryoidism, 360–373
  hypothyroidism, 368–370
Timolol in arrhythmias, 222
Tolazoline dosage in congenital heart disease, 440
Torsades de pointes
  from amiodarone, 221
  from quinidine, 218
Torus aorticus, 4
Transfusions, in surgery of descending thoracic aorta, 253
Transposition of great vessels, 455–458
Trauma
  aortic rupture in, 243
  pericardial tamponade in, 174
Tricuspid valve, 6
  atresia of, 458–460
Trimethaphan
  dosage in congenital heart disease, 440
  in pregnancy, placental transfer of, 306
Trisomy 18, cardiac lesions in, 426
Trisomy 21, cardiac lesions in, 426
Tuberous sclerosis, cardiac lesions in, 426
d-Tubocurarine dosage in congenital heart disease, 440
Turner syndrome, cardiac lesions in, 426

Ulcers, gastroduodenal, after cardiac surgery, 292–293
Ulnar artery cannulation in children, 400–401
Ultrasound
  in echocardiography. See Echocardiography
  transcutaneous Doppler for blood pressure measurement, 397
Umbilical artery cannulation, 401
Urinary tract, opioids affecting, 39

Valves of heart, 5–6
  aortic disease, 109–126. See also Aortic valve disease

in lupus erythematosus, 375
mitral disease, 129–165. *See also* Mitral valve disease
in pregnancy, 299, 310–316
in rheumatoid arthritis, 367
tricuspid atresia, 458–460
Vancomycin in endocarditis prophylaxis, 428
Vascular disorders
after cardiac surgery, 288, 295–296
in diabetes mellitus, 347, 348
Vascular resistance
pulmonary
in chronic obstructive pulmonary disease, 358–359
in mitral regurgitation, 149
in mitral stenosis, 134, 140
nitrous oxide affecting, 16, 22
systemic
diazepam affecting, 30, 34
ketamine affecting, 34
midazolam affecting, 33
nitrous oxide affecting, 14, 22
volatile anesthetic agents affecting, 17, 22
systolic, propofol affecting, 37
Vasodilatation after cardiac surgery, 288
Vasodilators
dosage in congenital heart disease, 440
in pregnancy, affecting uterine blood flow, 306
Vasopressors
dosage in congenital heart disease, 440
in pregnancy, affecting fetus, 304–305
Vasospasm in primary pulmonary hypertension, 327
Vater syndrome, cardiac lesions in, 426
Vecuronium
in aortic regurgitation, 126
in aortic stenosis, 119
in cardiomyopathy, ischemic, 197
dosage in congenital heart disease, 440

in ischemic heart disease, 100
in mitral regurgitation, 158
in mitral stenosis, 145
in pericardial tamponade, 183
in pericarditis, 187
Venipuncture sites for central venous pressure monitoring, 70–71
in children, 403–406
Venous system of heart, 6
Ventilation
one-lung, in surgery of descending thoracic aorta, 253–254
positive-pressure, effects in pericardial tamponade, 177–178
Ventricles, 4–5
function abnormalities
after cardiac surgery, 288–290
in diabetes mellitus, 348–349
in ischemic heart disease, 85–86
hypertrophy of. *See* Hypertrophy of heart
left, compliance in hypertrophic cardiomyopathy, 204
outflow tract obstruction
in idiopathic hypertrophic subaortic stenosis, 323
in tetralogy of Fallot, 453
premature contractions, 232–233, 336
in alcoholic heart disease, 363, 364
right, infarction of, 85
Ventricular fibrillation, 233
Ventricular septal defect, 432–433
in pregnancy, 317–318
pulmonary blood flow in, 422
in tetralogy of Fallot, 453, 454
in transposition of great vessels, 455
Ventricular tachycardia, 233
Ventriculography
in diabetes mellitus, 348
in hypertrophic cardiomyopathy, 206
in ischemic heart disease, 88–89
in mitral regurgitation, 149

Ventriculomyectomy in hypertrophic cardiomyopathy, 207
Verapamil
in aortic dissection, 249
in arrhythmias, 222–223
in atrial fibrillation, 226
dosage in congenital heart disease, 440
in hypertrophic cardiomyopathy, 207
in mitral prolapse, 163
in multifocal atrial tachycardia, 228
in pregnancy, affecting fetus, 308
propranolol with, 223
in Wolff-Parkinson-White syndrome, 232
Volatile anesthetic agents, 16–22. *See also* Desflurane; Enflurane; Halothane; Isoflurane; Sevoflurane
in aortic regurgitation, 125
in aortic stenosis, 118
and arrhythmias, 21
bradycardia from, 224
and coronary blood flow, 18–19
and coronary steal, 19–21
hemodynamic effects of, 22
in mitral regurgitation, 157
in mitral stenosis, 144
and myocardial contractility, 16–17
and myocardial oxygen demand, 18
in pericardial tamponade, 182
and peripheral circulation, 17–18

Warfarin in pregnancy, affecting fetus, 307
Wenckebach atrioventricular block, 234
Williams syndrome, 436
Wolf syndrome, cardiac lesions in, 426
Wolff-Chaikoff effect in hyperthyroidism, 373
Wolff-Parkinson-White syndrome, 228–232
in mitral prolapse, 163

RD 87.3 .H43 A49 1993

Anesthesia and the patient with co-existing heart

**NO LONGER THE PROPERTY
OF THE
UNIVERSITY OF R.I. LIBRARY**